Clinical Trials in Neurology

Springer

London
Berlin
Heidelberg
New York
Barcelona
Hong Kong
Milan
Paris
Singapore
Tokyo

Roberto J. Guiloff (Ed)

Clinical Trials in Neurology

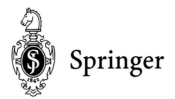

Springer

Roberto J. Guiloff, MD, FRCP
Neuromuscular Unit
West London Neurosciences Centre
Charing Cross Hospital
Fulham Palace Road
London W6 8RF, UK

British Library Cataloguing in Publication Data
Clinical Trials in Neurology
   1. Nervous system – Diseases – Treatment   2. Neurology   3. Clinical trials
   I. Guiloff, Roberto J.
   616.8′06
   ISBN 1852332395

Library of Congress Cataloging-in-Publication Data
Clinical Trials in Neurology / Roberto J. Guiloff (ed).
      p.; cm.
   Includes bibliographical references and index.
   ISBN 1-85233-239-5 (alk. paper)
   1. Neuropharmacology – Methodology.   2. Drugs – Testing.   3. Clinical trials.   I. Guiloff,
Roberto J., 1943–
   [DNLM: 1. Nervous System Diseases.   2. Clinical Trials.   3. Ethics, Medical. WL 140 N4919 2000]
RM315 .N459 2000
616.8′0461 – dc21   00-023917

ISBN 1-85233-239-5 Springer-Verlag London Berlin Heidelberg
a member of BertelsmannSpringer Science+Business Media GmbH
http://www.springer.co.uk

Typeset by Best-set Typesetter Ltd., Hong Kong
Printed and bound at The Cromwell Press, Trowbridge, Wiltshire, England.
28/3830-543210 Printed on acid-free paper SPIN 10532902

Foreword

One of the most important developments in neurology, and medicine generally, has been the advent of the randomised clinical trial. This statement may surprise the casual observer, for modern medicine is enrobed in spectacular and highly visible advances in technology and pharmacology. The clinical trial will seem modest in comparison, yet it remains true that no single technique has had a more beneficial effect in guiding treatment on a broad front. The clinical trial has had a highly meritorious impact, it has provided the definitive measure of quality in assessing the effectiveness of treatment, it has provided evidence of value and, in doing so, the yardstick by which to direct health care resources.

The first-modern randomised trial, the MRC trial of streptomycin in tuberculosis, was reported in 1948 and its findings had an immense impact on health throughout the world. Since then, the extraordinary advance of pharmaceutical science has changed neurology from a diagnostic to a therapeutic specialty. Mant points out in chapter 5 that in 1920, only six drugs made up 60% of British prescribing, and in 1990 there were 3500 compounds listed as available in the UK. I have a figure in my head that 50% of all drugs in the pharmacopoeia were introduced in the past decade. The assessment of the multiplicity of neurological drugs has also required the development of new methods for carrying out clinical trials. Over the 50 years in which modern clinical trials have been conducted, their methodology has grown immensely in sophistication to accommodate ethical, clinical and statistical considerations. Politics and economics however interact with clinical prerogative, and the patchwork of clinical trial practice is the result of an amalgam of different and often competing pressures. Regulatory requirements in different countries vary, and all have become more and more stringent as the expense of now pharmaceuticals increases. Most clinical trial programmes now are conducted in four distinct phases, each with a distinct code of practice. A very important aspect of trials in all phases (with the exception of some phase 1 studies) is randomisation, and in recent years the emphasis placed on randomisation has become profoundly important. It is easy to overlook how much practice has improved in recent times. In 1981, I reviewed all the previously published comparative studies of either carbamazepine and phenytoin, for instance. 155 were found and none were randomised. Furthermore documentation was deficient in most, and basic data was often missing such as the duration of the trial period (missing in 75%), the age range of the patients (missing in 35%), the dose of treatment (missing in 26%) or the drug serum levels (missing in 91%). One recent aspect of clinical trials has been the quest for objective measures of assessment and, in particular, for surrogate rather than direct measures of effectiveness. Issues of sensitivity and specificity, of reliability and standardisation, and of scaling and validity have all become important. Yet at the heart of all clinical trial methodology are the basic issues of ethics and conduct. These issues largely revolve around the conflict between doing what is good for an individual patient – the main duty of any doctor – and what is necessary to advance clinical science. This dilemma is the fundamental reason for the complex nature of most trials.

Clinical trials are thus a compromise – between the requirement for furthering knowledge, the best current interest of the individual patient, the political and legal context, economic and professional forces. All great alterations in human affairs are produced by compromise, and clinical trials are no exception. This is why this book is so valuable. I know of no other major text with such depth and coverage as the current volume. The issues pertaining to this compromise, the issues of ethics, regulation, assessment, statistics and quality control, and analysis are all brilliantly covered in part one. How these are translated to individual neurological diseases form the substance of the second part, and all the major disease areas in neurology are covered. The translation of universal theory into practice varies from disease to disease and this second part is an invaluable guide to the difficulties in such a translation. An impressive team of authors has been assembled, with contributions from neurologists, ethicists, statisticians, members of regulatory authorities, and pharmacologists amongst others. This volume is designed to contribute to improving assessment and evaluation of our future treatments in neurology, and in my opinion the editor has produced what will be a landmark in its field.

Simon Shorvon
London, November 2000

Preface

It was with trepidation but excitement that I accepted the task of editing a book on Clinical Trials in Neurology when approached by Springer-Verlag. The magnitude of the task seemed overwhelming. I was aware of some of the complexities involved in clinical trials and their application in Neurology and agreed with the need for such a book. My previous experience in phase II and III clinical trials in Motor Neuron Disease had shown me the importance of integrating biological and statistical issues in trial design and in data analysis. I had learnt something of the role of the pharmaceutical industry in developing a drug from molecule to clinical trials and then obtaining regulatory approval. As a clinician I was impressed by the differences in outcome variables and designs in clinical trials in various neurological conditions, yet that a broad common ground existed.

Clinical neurologists are expected to analyse clinical trials and, in particular, evidence for the efficacy of a drug. They ultimately prescribe drugs and see for themselves what their effects are. Statisticians are now expected to understand the biological aspects of disease relevant in trial design and data analysis. Regulatory authorities are increasingly facing new assessment methodologies, relevant to outcome measures, that require an understanding of their guiding biological principles and of the statistics subsequently chosen.

This book attempts to bring together the many aspects of clinical trials in neurology that clinical neuroscientists, statisticians and other workers need to understand. It seemed important to have a General Principles section that would cover the traditional topics of ethics, drug development stages, drug regulation, quality control and statistical principles. Assessment measures and clinical scales, a clinician's overview and the Cochrane Collaboration Reviews were included also in the general section as essential general clinical topics. The Disease Applications section deals with the main areas of clinical trials in neurology. An attempt has been made to discuss in each area the specific ethical problems, outcome variables and clinical scales, basic trial designs and sample sizes and experience with large multicentre trials.

A multi-author book of this sort is only possible because of the support and enthusiasm of its authors. I have been fortunate to enrol a most distinguished group of collaborators. I am most grateful to them for their efforts and patience in bringing this project to successful completion.

My thanks are due to Springer-Verlag for their understanding and for facilitating my work as editor, in particular Nick Mowat, Melissa Morton and Roger Dobbing.

Roberto J Guiloff MD, FRCP
London, February 2001

Contents

Contributors

Dr. Sundus H. Alusi
Neurology Specialist Registrar
Morriston Hospital
Swansea SA6 6NL
Wales
UK

Dr. Heather Angus-Leppan
Consultant Neurologist and
Honorary Senior Lecturer
Royal Free Hospital
Pond Street
London NW3 2QG
UK

Dr. Peter G. Bain
Senior Lecturer and Consultant in Clinical
   Neurology
Imperial College School of Medicine
Charing Cross Hospital Campus
Fulham Palace Road
London W6 8RF
UK

Professor H.J.M. Barnett
Professor Emeritus
University of Western Ontario
John P. Robarts Research Institute
100 Perth Drive
London
Ontario N6A 5K8
Canada

D. Belden

Dr. Stavia B. Blunt
Consultant Neurologist
West London Neurosciences Centre
Charing Cross Hospital
Fulham Palace Road
London W6 8RF
UK

Professor Vera Bril
Division of Neurology
EN 11-209
The Toronto Hospital
200 Elizabeth Street
Toronto
Ontario M5G 2C4
Canada

Professor Michael H. Brooke
Chairman
Division of Neurology
2E3 Walter C McKenzie Centre for Health
   Sciences
8440-112 Street
Edmonton
Alberta T6G 2B7
Canada

Professor Benjamin Rix Brooks
Department of Neurology
ALS Clinical Research Center
University of Wisconsin Hospital & Clinics
600 Highland Avenue CSC H6-563
Madison, WI 53792-5132
USA

Dr. Laura Brown
Independent Consultant and Course Director
MSc Clinical Research University of Cardiff
7 Coppice Way
Hedgerley
Buckinghamshire SL2 3YL
UK

Professor Martin M. Brown
University Department of Clinical Neurology
Institute of Neurology
University College London
Queen Square
London WC1N 3BG
UK

Dr. E. Buskens
Epidemiologist
Julius Center for General Practice and Patient
    Oriented Research
University Medical Center Utrecht
PO Box 85500, room D.01.335
3508 GA Utrecht
The Netherlands

Professor Livia Candelise
Istituto Clinica Neurologica
Università degli Studi Milano
Via F. Sforza 35
20122 Milan
Italy

Professor David Chadwick
Department of Neurological Science
Walton Centre for Neurology and Neurosurgery
Lower Lane
Liverpool L9 7LJ
UK

Dr. C.E. Clarke
Reader in Clinical Neurology
City Hospital NHS Trust
Dudley Road
Birmingham B18 7QH
UK

Dr. Jeffrey A. Cohen
Director
Experimental Therapeutics
Mellen Center
9500 Euclid Avenue
Cleveland
Ohio OH 44106
USA

Dr. Alasdair J. Coles
Wellcome Advanced Fellow
University of Cambridge
Neurology Unit, Box 165
Addenbrooke's Hospital
Hills Road
Cambridge CB2 2QQ
UK

Professor D.A.S. Compston
MRC Cambridge Centre for Brain Repair
University Forvie Site
Robinson Way
Cambridge CB2 2PY
UK

Dr. Diane L. Cookfair
Department of Neurology
State University of New York at Buffalo
647 West Delavan Avenue
Buffalo, NY 14222
USA

Dr. Peter James Dyck
Mayo Clinic
200 First Street SW
Rochester
Minnesota, MN 55905
USA

Dr. Michael Eliasziw
Associate Professor
University of Western Ontario
Scientist
John P. Robarts Research Institute
London, Ontario
Canada

Dr. Chris Gennings
Virginia Commonwealth University
Medical College of Virginia
Department of Biostatistics
Richmond, Virginia
USA

Dr. Ajith Goonetilleke
Consultant Neurologist and Honorary
Senior Lecturer
Newcastle General Hospital
Westgate Road
Newcastle upon Tyre NE4 6BE
UK

Dr. Roberto J. Guiloff
Consultant Neurologist
Neuromuscular Unit
1st Floor Pilot Wing
West London Neurosciences Centre
Charing Cross Hospital
Fulham Palace Road
London W6 8RF
UK

Dr. Richard J. Harvey
Director of Research and Alzheimer's
    Society
Senior Research Fellow
Alzheimer's Society
Quality Research in Dementia
Institute of Neurology
Queen Square
London WC1N 3BG
UK

Dr. Jeremy Hobart
Neurological Outcome Measures Unit
Institute of Neurology
Queen Square
London WC1N 3BG
UK

Dr. David Hoberman
Mathematical Statistician
Drug Evaluation and Research
Director of Pharmacological Drug
Products HFD-120
Food and Drug Administration
Woodmount II Building
1451 Rockville Pike
Rockville
Maryland, MD 20852
USA

Dr. Tony Hope
Ethox
Institute of Health Sciences
University of Oxford
Old Road
Headington
Oxford OX3 7LF
UK

Dr. D.B. Jeffreys
Medical Devices Agency
Hannibal House
Elephant & Castle
London SE1 6TE
UK

Professor Gary G. Koch
University of North Carolina
School of Public Health
Department of Biostatistics
Chapel Hill
North Carolina, NC 27599-7400
USA

Dr. J.B.M. Kuks
Department of Neurology
Academisch Ziekenhuis Groningen
Hanzelplein 1
Postbus 30.001
9700 RB Groningen
The Netherlands

Dr. Andrew D. Lawrence
MRC Cognition and Brain Sciences
Unit
15 Chaucer Road
Cambridge CB2 2EF
UK

Dr. Paul Leber
Director Neuro-Pharm Group, LLC
11909 Smoketree Road
Potomac
Maryland 20854
USA

Dr. Roderick J. Little
Department of Biostatistics
University of Michigan
M 4208 SPH II
1420 Washington Heights
Ann Arbor
Michigan, MI 48109-2029
USA

Dr. T.G.K. Mant
Medical Director
Guy's Drug Research Unit
6 Newcomen Street
London SE1 1YR
UK

Dr. Tony Marson
Department of Neurological Science
Walton Centre for Neurology and Neurosurgery
Lower Lane
Liverpool L9 7LJ
UK

Dr. Maureen A. McBride
United Network for Organ Sharing (UNOS)
Richmond
Virginia
USA

Ms. Heather Meldrum
Research Associate
John P. Robarts Research Institute
100 Perth Drive
London, Ontario N6A 5K8
Canada

Dr. Roger Newson
Lecturer in Medical Statistics
Department of Public Health Sciences
Guy's, King's and St Thomas' School of
Medicine
5th Floor, Capital House
Guy's Hospital
42 Weston Street
London 5E1 3QD
UK

Dr. John H. Noseworthy
Mayo Clinic/Mayo Foundation
Department of Neurology
200 First Street SW
Rochester
Minnesota, MN 55905
USA

Dr. Peter O'Brien
Mayo Clinic
200 First Street SW
Rochester
MN 55905
USA

Prof. Dr. H.J.G.H. Oosterhuis
Department of Neurology
Academisch Ziekenhuis Groningen
Hanzelplein 1
Postbus 30.001
9700 RB Groningen
The Netherlands

Dr. Richard W. Orrell
University Department of Clinical
    Neurosciences
Royal Free & UCL Medical School
Rowland Hill Street
London NW3 2PF
UK

Dr. Jackie Palace
Consultant Neurologist and Honorary Senior
    Lecturer
Radcliffe Infirmary
Woodstock Road
Oxford OX2 6HE
UK

Dr. Richard Peatfield
Consultant Neurologist
Charing Cross Hospital
Fulham Palace Road
London W6 8RF
UK

Dr. Anthony C. Pereira
University Department of Clinical Neurology
Institute of Neurology
University College London
Queen Square
London WC1N 3BG
UK

Dr. E.D. Playford
Institute of Neurology
Queen Square
London WC1N 3BG
UK

Professor Martin N. Rossor
Professor of Clinical Neurology
Dementia Research Group
National Hospital for Neurology and
    Neurosurgery
Queen Square
London WC1N 3BG
UK

Dr. Peter M. Rothwell
MRC Senior Clinical Fellow
Department of Clinical Neurology
Radcliffe Infirmary
Woodstock Road
Oxford OX2 6HE
UK

Dr. Barbara J. Sahakian
Department of Psychiatry
Box 189
Addenbroke's Hospital
Hills Road
Cambridge CB2 2QQ
UK

Dr. J.T. Sahlroot
Team Leader
Food and Drug Administration
Woodmount II Building
1451 Rockville Pike
Rockville
Maryland, MD 20852
USA

Professor J.W. Sander
National Hospital for Neurology and
    Neurosurgery
Queen Square
London WC1N 3BG
UK

Mohammel Sanjak
Clinical Associate Professor of Neurology
ALS Clinical Research Centre
University of Wisconsin Hospital and Clinics
600 Highland Avenue CSC 146-563
Madison, WI 53792-5132
USA

Dr. Julian Savulescu
Murdoch Institute
University of Melbourne
Parkville
Melbourne
VIC 3052
Australia

Professor Michael J. Schell
University of North Carolina
School of Public Health
Department of Biostatistics
Chapel Hill
North Carolina, NC 27599-7400
USA

Dr. Kaj Seidelin
Department of Neurology
Bispebjerg Hospital
Bispebjerg Bakke 23
DK-2400 Copenhagen NV
Denmark

Professor Stephen Senn
Department of Statistical Science
University College London
Room 316
1-19 Torrington Place
London WC1E 6BT
UK

Professor S.D. Shorvon
National Hospital for Neurology and
  Neurosurgery
Queen Square
London WC1N 3BG
UK

Dr. T.J. Steiner
Division of Neuroscience and Psychological
  Medicine
Imperial College School of Medicine
St Dunstan's Road
London
UK

Dr. Lesley A. Stewart
Head of Meta-analysis Group
Clinical Trials Unit
222 Euston Road
London NW1 2DA
UK

Dr. Peer Tfelt-Hansen
Department of Neurology
Glostrup Hospital
DK-2600 Glostrup
Denmark

Professor Alan J. Thompson
Neurological Outcome Measures Unit
Institute of Neurology
Queen Square
London WC1N 3BG
UK

J. van Gijn
Professor and Chairman
University Medical Center Utrecht
University Department of Neurology
PO Box 85500, room G.03.228
3508 GA Utrecht
The Netherlands

Dr. Andrew Waclawik
Associate Professor of Neurology
ALS Clinical Research Centre
University of Wisconsin Hospital and Clinics
600 Highland Avenue CSC 146-563
Madison, WI 53792-5132
USA

Dr. M.C. Walker
National Hospital for Neurology and
  Neurosurgery
Queen Square
London WC1N 3BG
UK

Dr. Brian G. Weinshenker
Mayo Clinic/Mayo Foundation
Department of Neurology
200 First Street SW
Rochester
Minnesota, MN 55905
USA

Dr. Bianca Weinstock-Guttman
Experimental Therapeutics
Mellen Center
9500 Euclid Avenue
Cleveland
Ohio, OH 44106
USA

PART I

General

1. Ethical Considerations

T. Hope and J. Savulescu

Introduction

Clinical trials have had enormous impact in several areas of medical practice. Some examples are the trials assessing the value of aspirin and thrombolytic therapy following acute stroke [1–3]. Millions of patients benefit from the knowledge gained from trials. There is, however, a dark side to medical experiments carried out on people.

In 1967 Pappworth [4] published the book *Human Guinea Pigs: Experimentation on Man* that described several hundred allegedly unethical experiments involving people as the subjects of research. A year earlier Beecher [5] had reported 22 examples of what he considered unethical medical research published in prestigious journals. There were two major grounds on which these experiments were considered to be unethical: either they put those participating in the research at an unacceptable level of risk; or they were carried out without adequate consent.

Clinical practice normally has as its aim the benefiting of the individual patient. This aim is the "therapeutic intention". Medical research, including clinical trials, has a different aim: the good of those patients in the future who will benefit from the knowledge gained from the research. This aim is the "research intention". The wishes, and interests, of people who participate in research may conflict with what is best for future patients. It is this potential conflict which gives rise to the special ethical issues raised by medical research carried out with patients.

Therapeutic and Non-therapeutic Research

A doctor might be engaged in either research or clinical practice, or in both at the same time. A neurolo-gist, treating patients within a research trial comparing different therapies, is engaged in both research and clinical practice. A distinction can be made between *therapeutic research* which is carried out with both the research and therapeutic intentions and *non-therapeutic research* in which there is no therapeutic intention. An example of non-therapeutic research is when patients have an investigation done purely to measure a factor for research purposes, and which plays no role in diagnosis or management.

The Regulation of Research on Humans

There are historical reasons why the regulation of research involving people differs from the regulation of normal clinical practice. These historical reasons account for some differences in standards between research and clinical practice.

The appalling experiments carried out by some Nazi doctors led to the first internationally agreed guidelines on research involving people: the Nuremburg Code (1946) [6].

The Nuremburg Code consists of ten principles. These were incorporated into the Declaration of Helsinki first published by the World Medical Association in 1964. The latest version was approved in 1996 [7].

One principle contained in the Declaration of Helsinki is:

> The design and performance of each experimental procedure involving human subjects should be clearly formulated in an experimental protocol which should be transmitted for consideration, comment and guidance to a specially appointed committee independent of the investigator and the sponsor.

Local Research Ethics Committees (LRECs)

The Department of Health [8] has stated that every health district in the UK should have a local research ethics committee to advise National Health Service (NHS) bodies on the ethical acceptability of research proposals involving human subjects. Approval by such a committee should be sought for any research proposal involving:

1. NHS patients;
2. fetal material and in vitro fertilisation involving NHS patients;
3. the recently dead, in NHS premises;
4. access to medical records of past or present NHS patients;
5. access to NHS premises.

Strictly speaking there is no legal requirement for a researcher to submit a proposal to a LREC, neither does approval by a LREC provide a guarantee that the research is lawful. However, most research funding bodies require approval by a LREC, as do most organisations providing indemnity. Furthermore, it is likely that the courts would be more willing to find that a research project has been conducted lawfully if prior approval had been received from the appropriate LREC.

The membership of LRECs include lay people (at least two on each committee, one of whom should be the chairman or vice-chairman), health professionals (including hospital doctors, general practitioners and nursing staff) and researchers. The duties of LRECs are to protect research subjects and maintain proper standards of practice in research, while ensuring that valid and worthwhile research is carried out. The members of the committees themselves are potentially at risk from being sued if they carry out their duties negligently.

Multi-centre Research Ethics Committees (MRECs)

Clinical trials, and some other research projects, may involve patients from many different geographical areas. It can be very tiresome for research workers to submit the same research protocol to a large number of different LRECs. Not only do different LRECs have different forms to complete, but each is autonomous. Researchers may be asked to modify their research proposals in different, and even incompatible ways, by different LRECs. Some LRECs may approve the research, others may not approve it.

To address this problem, multi-centre research ethics committees (MRECs) have been set up by the Department of Health in each Health Region [9]. These examine research protocols which would otherwise need to be seen by five or more LRECs. The relevant LRECs will liaise with the MREC and may make essential, locally applicable changes to the patient information sheet.

Three Approaches to the Ethics of Medical Research Involving People

Well-conducted research has the potential to do a great deal of good as a result of the knowledge gained: if it were not for this good then most research, and especially non-therapeutic research, would not be justified. For this reason there is a moral imperative for the carrying out of valuable research. However, research may be unethical, particularly if the harm or risk of harm to participants is unacceptable, or if there is no valid consent. These three elements – the value of research, harm, and consent – are each highlighted by three different ethical approaches [10].

Rights-Based Approaches

Rights-based approaches emphasise the autonomy of the research participant. The participant needs to give valid consent to take part in the research. If the participant gives such consent then, within broad limits, that research is ethically justified. The main duty on the research worker, therefore, is to ensure that valid consent is given.

Duty-Based Approaches

Duty-based approaches emphasise the duties on the research worker. Precisely what these duties are depends on the specific ethical viewpoint. However, one widely held duty is to ensure that the participant is not exposed to a high risk of harm. A duty-based approach may therefore override patient autonomy and in some instances justify a paternalistic approach.

Rights-based and duty-based approaches lead to similar conclusions over many points. For example both highlight the importance of properly informing the participant about the research – the former because this respects autonomy, the latter because this is a duty of the researcher. However they differ in other respects (see below).

Consequentialist Approaches

Consequentialist approaches (such as utilitarianism) see the outcome – consequences – of our moral choices as of critical importance. An important aspect of a consequentialist approach is that the benefits and harms both to participants and to those in the future are to be considered. Harm to research participants may be justified by the good to people in the future who benefit from the research.

Contrasting These Three Approaches

The differences between these approaches may not be as stark as this outline suggests. Consequentialists, for example, may stress the importance of informed consent on the grounds that giving people control over their lives leads overall to better consequences. In practice elements from all approaches are taken into account in the guidelines and decisions of LRECs and in the Declaration of Helsinki. Most guidelines state that participants should be subjected to minimal risk of harm only (duty-based approach). The importance given to consent and confidentiality reflects a rights-based approach. The Declaration of Helsinki (principle I. 5) states:

> Every biomedical research project involving human subjects should be preceded by careful assessment of predictable risks in comparison with foreseeable benefits to the subject or to others.

This balancing of the value of the research with the risks to the participants reflects a consequentialist approach.

Table 1.1 contrasts these three approaches. We have compared: the libertarian (a rather extreme rights-based position which emphasises informed consent and the right not to be interfered with by others); the paternalist (who has a sense of duty in protecting others from harm); and the utilitarian

who wants the greatest good for the greatest number. The paternalist is particularly concerned about research that exposes participants to significant risk of harm even if the participant is fully aware of these risks and has given valid consent. The libertarian is concerned mainly about the validity of consent. For the libertarian a person should not be prevented from risks that are taken voluntarily and in full knowledge. On the other hand the libertarian insists that valid consent is needed even if there is no significant risk of harm. The utilitarian is concerned with overall good. For him or her, the value of the research to people in the future is of key significance. The utilitarian, like the paternalist, may not be concerned about research that risks little harm to the participants. The utilitarian, however, will be particularly concerned about research which is poor – thus offering little overall benefit. Valuable research which involves little risk and in which participants give valid consent is acceptable to all.

Key Ethical Considerations in Carrying Out Research

One way of seeing these three approaches is as alternatives, one of which must be chosen. Another way is to see each approach as emphasising one or more values, all of which are relevant and need to be taken into account. Table 1.2 summarises the key ethical considerations in carrying out research.

Scientific Validity

The Declaration of Helsinki states:

> The purpose of biomedical research involving human subjects must be to improve diagnostic, therapeutic and prophylactic procedures and the understanding of the aetiology and pathogenesis of disease.

Table 1.1. Three approaches to the ethics of research involving humans

	Research where participants knowingly expose themselves to high risk	Low-risk research where participants are not fully informed	Low-risk research where participants are fully informed	Poor-quality research which is of little value but where participants are fully informed
Libertarian (rights-based)	Yes	No	Yes	Yes
Paternalistic (duty-based)	No	Yes	Yes	?No
Utilitarian (consequentialist)	Yes	Yes	Yes	No

Table 1.2. Key issues in assessing the ethical aspects of a research protocol

Scientific validity
- Are the aims worthwhile?
- Is the method appropriate to the aims?
- Can the research design be improved?
- Is this research unnecessarily repeating work previously carried out?

Safety
- Should any non-human or epidemiological, systematic overview or computer modelling be performed prior to the study to better estimate the risk to participants or obviate the need for the use of human participants?
- What is the degree of risk for participants, and how good is this estimate?
- Could the risks be further reduced?
- Are the benefits of the study worth the risks?
- Are some participants being denied care they should receive?

Consent procedure
Informed
- Is the information clearly written, honest, sufficient, and balanced?

Voluntary (absence of coercion)
- Is it clear to participants that refusal to take part will not affect clinical care?
- Is the relationship between researcher and participant free from potential coercion?
- Is the payment such as to encourage participation "against the person's better judgement"?
- Is the researcher under undue pressure to recruit participants?
- Is there sufficient time after being given information for the person to decide whether to participate?

Competence
- Are the potential participants competent to decide whether or not to take part?
- Is such competence being assessed, when relevant to do so?
- If potential participants are not competent, are they either excluded, or is the recruitment procedure adequate?

Confidentiality
- Have participants given consent for confidential data to be accessed in the research?
- Are there adequate safeguards to prevent those not involved in the research from having access to confidential data?

Dissemination of results
- Will the results be made publicly available in effective ways?

Principle 1 states:

> Biomedical research involving human subjects must conform to generally accepted scientific principles and should be based on adequately performed laboratory and animal experimentation and on a thorough knowledge of the scientific literature.

There are two criteria for scientifically valid research: first, the aims must be worthwhile; second, the methods must be suitable to the aims.

Safety

Neurological trials can involve the possibility of serious harm. For example, thrombolytic therapy for acute ischaemic stroke may cause cerebral bleeding with resulting paralysis, loss of speech or other gross impairments of functioning. Some of the trials of streptokinase in acute stroke raised concerns about safety [11]. The degree of risk of harm to which competent adults may legally expose themselves is uncertain. A potential subject may be fully informed,

and give consent, and yet the risks of taking part may be too great for the research to be lawful. In other words, English law does not take the extreme libertarian view.

The guidance given by The Royal College of Physicians [12] is likely to be considered were the issue of degree of risk of harm to come to court.

> 11.13 Research procedures are more or less substantial in terms of complexity, time and effort involved, but generally they should not involve more than minimal risk either to a patient volunteer or to a healthy volunteer. The term "minimal risk" is used to cover two types of situation. The first is where the level of psychological distress is negligible although there may be a small chance of a reaction which itself is trivial, e.g. a mild headache or feeling of lethargy. The second is where there is a very remote chance of serious injury or death. "We regard this second risk to the healthy volunteer as comparable, for example, to that of flying as passenger in a scheduled aircraft".
>
> 11.14 There are some situations, such as the treatment of serious disease, where it is ethical for

research studies to involve more than minimal risk. These would never involve healthy volunteers.

In the case of clinical trials the issue of safety is unlikely to arise except, perhaps, where a new treatment, which is being compared with a standard treatment, carries high risks – although potentially balanced by expected benefits. Such a situation would probably be covered by the exception stated in paragraph 11.14.

Consent

The involvement of competent adults in medical research is governed mainly by the common law concept of consent. In brief, this means that the potential research subject should be given information about: the nature and purpose of the research procedures; the fact that this is motivated by a research intention; and the pros and cons of taking part in the research. The person could only become a subject for the research if he gave his competent and voluntary consent. In order to be voluntary, it would be important for the subject to know that medical treatment would not be compromised if he refused consent to take part in the research. It would also be important for the subject to be given sufficient time to decide.

It is likely that, in the case of research, the courts would demand a higher level of information concerning risk than they would in the case of ordinary clinical medicine. The researcher must take steps to ensure that the patient understands the information. The provision of information must be sufficiently flexible to take account of the varying needs, and levels of understanding, of different research subjects. Subjects would normally need to understand the design of the research in broad terms; for example whether subjects were randomised to different groups.

It is usual for subjects to be given information both verbally and in written form, and to have an opportunity to ask questions.

The Relationship Between Researcher and Participant

Clearly it is unethical to use force to ensure that someone takes part in a research project. However, the idea of coercion is usually taken to cover much more than the use of force. One consideration is the relationship between the researcher and the participant.

The key question is whether the potential participant is in a special relationship with the researcher so that it might be hard to refuse participation in the study. One example of such a special relationship is that between a patient and doctor. Since, in clinical trials, the patient's own doctor will normally be involved in entering the patient into the trial, particular care needs to be taken with the consent procedure. There is a danger that patients may feel obliged to enter the trial, or they may worry that their doctor will not provide such good care if they do not participate.

Incompetent Adults

Neurological disorders often render patients incompetent to give (or withhold) consent to participate in research. Examples of such conditions are dementia, stroke and encephalitis. The question of research on adults unable to give consent is a difficult area in English law. In the absence of statutory provisions, it is necessary to look to common law. Common law principles have been developed much more extensively in relation to ordinary medical practice than in relation to research. The principles established in clinical practice therefore are likely to apply to research. The key points are these:

1. In English law no one (not even a court) can give consent on behalf of another adult – not even on behalf of an incompetent adult. In the context of medical treatment the clinician should provide the treatment which is in the incompetent patient's best interests.
2. With regard to therapeutic research, the same criteria are likely to be used as with medical treatment.
3. The issue is most problematic with regard to incompetent patients and non-therapeutic research since such research cannot, by definition, be said to be in the patient's best interests.

In the case of a clinical trial, conducted on patients not competent to give consent, the key legal issue is whether entering the trial is "in the best interests" of the patient. If the clinical trial compares two treatments for which there is no good reason to prefer one to the other (see Equipoise below) then it might be said that entering the trial is not against the patient's best interests, although there is no reason to think it is better for the patient to enter the trial than not to enter the trial. It would probably not be illegal to enter an incompetent patient into a trial if it were not against the patient's best interests to do so.

There may be "non-therapeutic" elements to a clinical trial. For example, the trial protocol may involve carrying out investigations on patients which would not be part of normal clinical practice and which are of no benefit to the patient. Various guidelines do countenance non-therapeutic research on incompetent people.

The Royal College of Physicians [13], in its report *Research Involving Patients* recognises that there is value to others in non-therapeutic research carried out on incompetent subjects and suggests that such research should only be carried out in agreement with close relatives or guardians. The Department of Health's guidelines (1991) to local research ethics committees again [8] seem to accept the possibility of non-therapeutic research on incompetent subjects. They state:

> Proposals for research where capacity to consent is impaired will need particularly careful consideration by the LREC, with regard to its acceptability in terms of the balance of benefits, discomforts and risk to the individual patient and the need to advance knowledge so that people with mental disorder may benefit.

The Medical Research Council's guidance (1998) [14] emphasises the benefit from research and suggests that non-therapeutic research on incompetent adults may be permissible if:

1. the knowledge cannot be gained by researching persons able to give consent;
2. the research is approved by the Local Research Ethics Committees;
3. the subject does not object or appear to object in either words or actions;
4. an independent person acceptable to the LREC agrees that the individual's welfare and interests have been properly safeguarded;
5. participation in the research would not place the individual at more than negligible risk of harm and is not against that individual's interests.

The Royal College of Psychiatrists' Guidelines (1988) [15] introduce the idea of "substituted judgement" – i.e. a judgement as to whether the incompetent person would give consent. The guidelines state:

> These people should attempt to form a judgement, based on the patient's known previous opinions about research and on his recent behaviour, as to whether the patient would be likely to consent were he able to do so. Any patient who indicates refusal either in words or in actions should be excluded from the research whatever opinion is voiced by the others who have been consulted.

The Assessment of Competence

The question of competence (or *capacity* to give it the legal term) is a crucial issue in the law relating to medical practice. A competent adult can refuse any medical treatment – even life-saving treatment. An incompetent adult should be treated according to best interests. Competence to give consent to enter a clinical trial (or other research project) is also a key issue in the law relating to medical research, as has been discussed above. It is, therefore, important for clinicians and researchers to be able to assess competence.

Common law has established an approach to the assessment of capacity (competence). First, capacity is specific to the particular issue. Thus, a person may have capacity for one thing, but lack capacity for another. For example, a person may have capacity to make a valid will but lack capacity to refuse specific medical treatment (or vice versa). One implication of this for research is that the specific capacity to give consent to enter a clinical trial needs to be assessed. There are three components to capacity:

1. The person *understands* the relevant information;
2. He *believes* that information;
3. He is able to *weigh up* the information and come to a *decision*.

In the case of a patient being asked for consent to enter a clinical trial, the relevant information would include:

1. the fact that this is a trial;
2. the advantages and disadvantages of entering the trial;
3. the effect of not giving consent (notably that this does not affect normal treatment);
4. the advantages and disadvantages of each of the treatments given within the trial;
5. the method of allocation (e.g. random) of an individual to the various interventions;
6. in broad terms what would be involved in entering the trial – and in not entering the trial.

A person may understand the relevant information but not believe it (for example, because of a delusional belief that he will inevitably die whatever happens). In such a situation, he would not have capacity. People with a degree of cognitive impairment may be able to understand and believe relevant information but not have the capacity to retain and weigh up the information in coming to a decision. In such a situation, the person would not have legal capacity to give consent.

Children

Neurological diseases may, of course, afflict children. Research can be particularly problematic when the disease is serious, and when potential treatments may be dangerous. One example is X-linked adrenoleukodystrophy, for which bone marrow transplantation has been used as a therapeutic intervention. A child may be competent to give valid consent to medical treatment if he has sufficient intelligence to be capable of understanding what is proposed. Competence may be compromised by lack of maturity, pain, drugs or psychiatric condition. The required standard of comprehension is likely to be greater where the child is consenting to participation in a research project than in normal clinical practice, since the child must be capable of understanding that his or her treatment is motivated by a research intention. In relation to non-therapeutic research, where there are no beneficial consequences for the child and there may also be a risk of harm, a high level of comprehension and intelligence is likely to be required by the courts.

If the child is competent, then with regard to therapeutic research the situation is identical to that of normal clinical practice. With regard to non-therapeutic research the situation is in theory similar to that with regard to the competent adult, but courts are likely to impose a high standard of competence. A child not reaching such a high standard would be treated as incompetent. In any case it is probably wise for the research worker to gain consent from the child's parent or guardian. In the case of the competent child who refuses consent, it would probably be unlawful to proceed with the research even if the child's parent or guardian gave consent, unless the procedure was necessary in order to avoid a threat to the child's life or serious threat of permanent physical harm.

When a child is not competent, the parent or guardian may act as proxy for making decisions in relation to the child's medical treatment. The requirements for valid consent (competent, informed, voluntary) apply to the proxy. Consent from a proxy is generally valid only where it accords with the best interests of the child. It will often be difficult to say that research is in the child's best interests. With regard to non-therapeutic research, it will almost always not be in the child's best interests to proceed with the research. The British Paediatric Association's Guidelines (1992) for the ethical conduct of medical research involving children states [16]:

> Parents can consent to research procedures which are intended directly to benefit the child, but that research that does not come into this category can only be validly consented to if the risks are sufficiently small to mean that the research can be reasonably said not to go against the child's interests.

The Value of Clinical Trials

Case Example: Iron Chelation in Friedreich's Ataxia

Both animal and human studies suggest that iron accumulates in the mitochondria of patients with Friedreich's ataxia. One theory proposes that this iron accumulation plays a significant pathogenic role [17,18]. Iron chelation with desferrioxamine has been effective in reducing the problems associated with iron overload in patients with thalassaemia. On the basis of this, the question arises as to whether the effectiveness of desferrioxamine should be studied in a clinical trial. Three arguments against a trial are: first, there is no direct evidence from human studies that iron plays a pathogenic role; second, it is not clear that desferrioxamine would reduce iron levels within mitochondria; third, there are significant side-effects from desferrioxamine, including anaphylaxis and iron depletion. Is it unethical to carry out a randomised controlled trial (RCT) of desferrioxamine? Should patients be given desferrioxamine in the absence of data from an RCT if they request it?

There are two principal reasons for carrying out large randomised trials (RCTs):

1. A large RCT provides very good quality evidence on the effectiveness of a particular intervention compared with an alternative treatment The results from such a trial will therefore provide patients in the future (i.e. after the trial results are known) with good quality evidence on which to base their treatment decisions.
2. The funders of health care, whether these are the state or insurance companies, may reasonably require good-quality evidence for the effectiveness of a health care intervention which they fund.

At root, this is an issue of distributive justice. Suppose, for example, that following the results of early small trials all patients with multiple sclerosis would have chosen to have β-interferon – on the grounds that there is little to lose, and there might be worthwhile gain. Even if all those with the relevant condition would choose the treatment with no further trials, the funding organisations might, reasonably, refuse to fund such treatment until the evidence for effectiveness – and information about the likely degree of benefit – is better characterised. This is because the funds for β-interferon could be used for other types of health care. In deciding how best to use their limited resources, health care funders must take the quality of evidence of health care interventions into account.

The principal reasons against carrying out large clinical trials are:

1. The participants in the trial may not be receiving the best treatment, on the evidence currently available. Thus the quest for very good evidence (which is helpful to patients in the future) may be at the expense of the interests of patients in the trial.
2. Sufficiently good evidence on which to base treatment decisions may be available from trials which are not large RCTs. These other types of trial may better safeguard the interests of the trial participants.

We will consider this second point first.

Are Large RCTs the Only Worthwhile Trials?

There is considerable divergence of opinion with regard to the evidential value of data from different types of study design. There seems general agreement that the strength of evidence can be represented by a hierarchy as illustrated in Table 1.3 [19,20].

Case Example: Lorenzo's Oil and Bone Marrow Transplantation in X-linked Adrenoleukodystrophy (X-ALD)

Adrenoleukodystrophy is characterised by an abnormal accumulation of very long chain fatty acids (VLCFAs) and a pathogenic role has been hypothesised. Lorenzo's oil (a 4:1 mixture of glycerol trioleate:glyceryl trierucate) dramatically reduces VLCFAs.

Table 1.3. A hierarchy of strength of evidence

A systematic review is stronger evidence than unsystematic reviews or single studies

Systematic reviews where all studies yield similar estimates of the effects of the intervention provide better evidence than when studies yield variable estimates

There is a hierarchy of study design in terms of the strength of evidence they provide, as follows:

1. Randomised controlled trials
2. Non-randomised controlled studies
3. Non-controlled studies
4. Anecdotal studies

The dramatic effect of Lorenzo's oil on the plasma levels of VLCFAs led to a series of therapeutic trials that have involved more than 300 patients. For "ethical reasons" these were conducted as non-randomised trials. The consensus view is that when the diet is administered to patients who are already neurologically involved it has little or no effect on the neurological progression [21]. The "ethical reasons" were (H.W. Moser, personal communication):

1. the severity of the illness;
2. the minimal risk of the treatment with Lorenzo's oil;
3. the grounds for believing that Lorenzo's oil might be effective.

Lilford and colleagues [22,23] have argued that although small trials may provide misleading results, they are better than no trial at all. Moreover, small trials are more easily performed, and the results of many small trials can be combined using meta-analyses, especially if randomisation, data collection, analysis and archiving are supervised by a trial centre [22]. These authors emphasise a Bayesian approach to statistical design and inference. In the Bayesian approach, any knowledge or clinical opinion about the treatment effect is summarised, before the trial, as a probability function. This is known as the "prior distribution". The trial results provide data that, combined with the prior distribution, produce the "posterior distribution". This Bayesian approach to clinical trials is in contrast with the more traditional "frequentist" approach. The frequentist approach views the trial as testing the "null hypothesis" that there is no difference between the two treatments which the trial compares [23,24].

Equipoise and Randomised Controlled Trials

Consider a randomised trial which compares two drug treatments, A and B. The term "equipoise" has been coined [25] to describe the state where the evidence to date does not clearly favour one drug over the other. One view is that a RCT is only ethically justified if there is such a state of equipoise. If a state of equipoise does not exist then, by definition, the evidence favours one drug over the other. If this is the case then the better drug should be offered to all patients: it would be unethical to carry out a randomised trial.

This approach is consistent with the Declaration of Helsinki's principle that the interests of participants in the trial are not to be compromised for the sake of future patients. However, the concept of "equipoise" is not as straightforward as it might appear. Who is to decide when "equipoise" exists? How are the different side-effects of the two treatments to be compared and balanced? If equipoise exists at the start of the trial, at what stage during the trial does it cease to exist?

We will outline some different approaches to these issues by considering answers to the question: When should RCTs be stopped? Some of these approaches are relevant also to the question of when such trials should, or should not, be started.

When Should Randomised Controlled Trials Be Stopped?

Once a RCT is under way data are collected, as part of the trial, which may provide evidence that one drug is better than the other. Indeed that is the purpose of the trial. The question then arises: At what point should the trial be stopped?

Four main issues arise:

1. How are the interests of research participants to be balanced against the interests of future patients? In general, future patients benefit from very large trials that provide highly reliable information. However, large trials involve continuing the trial to a time when half of those participating will receive what is almost certainly the inferior treatment.
2. What exactly is "against the best interests" of those participating in the trial given:
   (a) the fact that it is probabilities not certainties with which we are dealing;
   (b) that there are known and unknown short- and long-term side effects, and thus simply focusing on the main, and relatively short-term, outcomes measured as part of the trial is not sufficient;
   (c) different clinicians and patients will be persuaded by different types and amounts of evidence?
3. What are the responsibilities of those running the trial compared with the responsibilities of the clinicians who enter patients into the trial?
4. How should patients be informed and involved?

Seven Potential Criteria for Stopping Randomised Trials

When the Truth Is Known

One approach is to say that the trial should be continued until the right answer is known: until, for example, we know whether intervention A saves more lives than intervention B. However, this criterion is an illusion. The truth can never be known. All we have is greater or lesser degrees of certainty. Strict application of this criterion would lead to infinitely long trials.

Utilitarianism: To Minimise Deaths Overall

One possible rule for stopping a trial would be one that, as a general rule, would lead to the best outcome (fewest deaths) overall – taking both patients in the trial and future patients whose treatment is affected by the trial into account. This criterion gives equal consideration to these two groups of patients.

If minimising deaths overall is the aim, then, in general, the trial should be stopped only when the significance level favouring one drug is very low, much lower than conventional levels (e.g. $p < 0.0001$ rather than $p < 0.05$). In other words the chance of coming to the wrong conclusion should be very small. This is assuming that a large number of patients will be treated with the apparently better drug in the future.

When the Evidence Favours One Drug – The Minimal Evidence Condition

The central criticism for following the "utilitarian" view is that it harms those in the trial for the sake of people in the future. This conflicts with traditional views of research ethics including the principle enshrined in the Declaration of Helsinki: "Concern for the interests of the subject must always prevail over the interests of science and society."

What are the interests of the subject in the situation where there is uncertainty over what is best? Consider two drugs, A and B. For simplicity suppose they have no side effects. The question is simply: do more patients die within 3 months if given A or B? We do not know whether A or B is better. We randomly allocate patients: 10 receive A and 10 receive B. Four of those receiving A die, three of those receiving B die. Do we at this stage have evidence that B is better than A? And if we do, should we stop the trial on the grounds that it is best, on the evidence available, for potential subjects to receive B but not A?

Many people would say that we do not have evidence that one treatment is better than the other. Statistical analyses have been developed to look at this question. It has become traditional to consider a result as not statistically significant if $p > 0.05$.

This level of significance, however, is arbitrary. It is not true to say that there is no evidence that B is better than A when the significance level is high; only that the evidence is not strong. Should a clinician who puts the interests of his patients above all other concerns pull out of the trial at this stage and treat all patients with the "better" drug? In practice if this were to be adopted it would mean few trials would be started because there will almost always be evidence of this minimal degree in favour of one or other already.

Where There Is No Longer "Reasonable Uncertainty" (Equipoise)

The arguments in the subsection above assume no side effects. In practice drugs can have both short- and long-term unwanted effects. Because of this, different clinicians might reasonably differ in their judgement as to when it is in their patients' best interests to have A or B; and justify a clinician in entering a patient into a trial on the grounds that there is reasonable uncertainty as to which is better. This area of reasonable uncertainty is what is termed equipoise (see above). There are, however, limits to this. Surely once we have a significance level of, say, $p < 0.02$ that B is better than A it cannot be right for a clinician, acting in a patient's best interests, to enter that patient into the trial.

Since the larger the trial, the better for future patients, trials should be continued to the limit of the range of equipoise (because trial subjects are not being harmed and future patients will benefit). In general, this range will be roughly until conventional levels of significance are reached in favour of one drug.

What reasons can be given for continuing a trial beyond this point? Four possible reasons are as follows:

1. The good of future patients does have some weight (i.e. to adopt either the utilitarian approach, or a compromise between the "utilitarian" and equipoise approaches).
2. As long as the patients in the trial are fully informed of the current evidence (including the results of the trial so far), are competent and are not coerced, then, if they agree to enter the trial, it is all right for them to do so.
3. The trial may continue as long as there are clinicians willing to enter patients into it. In other words, if a clinician believes that, given the latest information, including that from the trial so far, there is still "equipoise" it is permissible to continue the trial (see Pragmatism below).
4. The best interests of those who take part in the trial are met by continuing the trial. The argument in favour of this is considered below under When Potential Subjects Are Better Off Outside the Trial.

Clinical Autonomy

According to Collins and colleagues [26], the design of RCTs should be governed by "the uncertainty principle" (or "clinician's equipoise"): "patients can only be entered [in a clinical trial] if the responsible clinician is *substantially uncertain* as to which of the trial treatments would be most appropriate for this particular patient"[26].

This position is essentially about responsibility. In a clinical therapeutic trial, it is argued, patients are entered into the trial by the clinicians responsible for their care. These clinicians should act in the best interests of their patients. If the responsible clinician is happy to enter patients then the trial can continue. It is not the role of the trial organisers to tell clinicians whether they are right or wrong – only to provide information.

Pragmatism: What Changes Practice

Doll (1993) gives two justifications for large clinical trials:

1. Large trials provide evidence that is "much more readily accepted by clinicians who have become accustomed, over the past 30 years, to basing their practice on the results of randomised clinical trials".
2. "Involving large numbers of clinicians in the trial predisposes them to accept the results as it is a characteristic of human nature to believe what you have experienced in your own life more readily than what someone else has experienced or told you about. Participation in a large-scale controlled trial constitutes, in practice, one of the best means of continuing medical education."

Large trials are justified because only large trials will, in fact, alter clinical practice. Against this it might be argued that commencement and termination criteria should be chosen according to defensible criteria. It may be true that many clinicians do not change their prescribing habits in the light of reasonable evidence to do so. For such clinicians only the results of excessively large trials would lead to change. But the response to this should not be to continue trials beyond reasonable evidence that one treatment is better than the other. Instead, clinicians' behaviour should be changed by other means, which do not involve giving research participants a known inferior treatment. Examples of such other means are: drug policy regulation, professional practice standards and education.

When Potential Subjects Are Better Off Outside the Trial

We return to the question of what is in the interests of those who take part in the trial. The minimal evidence condition (third strategy) gave these interests paramount importance but was based on the unrealistic assumption that treatments do not have unwanted effects. The fourth strategy (equipoise) was an extension of the third strategy. However this may also lead to trials being stopped too early, even if weight is given only to the best interests of those in the trial. Consider the following hypothetical situation.

An interim analysis of the results during a trial shows that a new treatment, B, is better than the traditional treatment, A (say with p < 0.02). Dr. X is entering people into the trial. Dr. X was treating all patients with A before the trial. On being asked to participate in the trial he considered that there was sufficient uncertainty to randomise patients, but he tends to switch late to new treatments. Suppose that after the interim analysis the trial is stopped, on the grounds that the evidence in favour of B means that it is unethical to continue to give patients A. Suppose further, however, that once the trial has stopped Dr. X will treat all his patients with drug A, as he believes that the possibility of long-term unknown side effects of the new treatment still outweighs giving the treatment. Whether he is right or wrong is not the central point. From the trial leaders' point of view, if the trial is stopped the people who would have been entered by Dr. X into the trial would all receive A. If the trial continues, 50% receive A and 50% receive B. Therefore it is better for the potential subjects of the trial that the trial continue, if, indeed, B is the better treatment.

On this criterion, when the interim analysis shows (with conventional levels of significance) that one treatment is better than the other, the trial leaders should ask the following question to the clinicians involved:

"Given this information, if the trial were stopped now, which treatment would you recommend for your patients?" If the clinician answered A – but was still willing to randomise – then it would be best to continue the trial. If the clinician answered B then it would be best to discontinue the trial even if the clinician were willing to randomise.

Patient Autonomy and Randomised Trials: Are There Double Standards?

The seven strategies, outlined above, for stopping a clinical trial have focused on the perspectives of the trial leaders and clinicians. A central question is how patients should be involved in the decision concerning their entry into the trial.

As has been discussed above, competent patients should be properly informed about the research and given the option as to whether to take part in the trial. This raises the issue as to what is to be "properly informed".

Several researchers [26,28] have argued that different standards of informing are being applied, without good reason, to therapeutic research (such as clinical trials), on the one hand, and to clinical practice, on the other.

Contrast these two situations:

Clinical case: *Dr. A sees patient B in the outpatient department. B is suffering from a condition likely to be helped by a particular class of drugs. There are several slightly different drugs in this class available. Dr. A advises B to take a particular drug (drug X) – the one with which he is most familiar and which is suitable for B. Dr. A informs B about the likely benefits and the side effects of drug X. However, he says nothing about the other drugs in this class which might be prescribed.*

Research case: *A randomised controlled trial is under way to compare two related drugs, X and Y used to treat a particular condition. Although Dr. A tends to prescribe drug X, on reflection he does not think that there is currently good evidence to prefer X to Y. It could be important to establish the relative effectiveness of each. Dr. A therefore agrees to ask suitable patients whether they would be prepared to take part in the trial. Dr. A sees B in the outpatient department. B is suffering from the relevant condition and would be a suitable candidate for the trial. In order to conform to the standards laid down by the LREC Dr. A must obtain valid consent for B to enter the trial. He must inform B about the trial and its purpose. He must also inform B about both drugs X and Y and tell B that a random process will be used to choose which will be prescribed.*

In the case of routine clinical practice it is not normally considered important that the doctor discusses the pros and cons of the various drugs which could reasonably be prescribed. The standard for the provision of information in the case of a trial, however, is normally higher. Some information about a comparison between the drugs would normally be given in the case of a trial.

There are three possible responses to this "double standard":

1. There is no justification for such double standards. Normal clinical practice should raise the

standards, in giving information to patients, to those set by research.

2. The standards set by research are excessively high. Those taking part in clinical trials do not need to be given more information than would currently occur in normal clinical practice.

3. The difference in the standard of information provided between clinical trials and clinical practice is justified because the two situations are different.

This third position might be defended in the following ways.

1. Double masters require double standards. Research trials and clinical practice are critically different. In the case of a trial, a central purpose is to benefit people in the future (the research intention). There is thus a pressure on the doctors and on those running the trial to make decisions which are good for the trial. In the case of ordinary clinical practice the doctor has no double master. His duty is simply to do what is in the best interests of the patient. The requirement for a more careful consent procedure in the case of research arises from this difference and the need to protect those entering the trial.

2. Patients are likely to view the two situations as different. It is likely that if patients were not informed, and subsequently found out, that they had been entered into a trial and that their treatment had been chosen using a random process they would be extremely angry. "How dare you carry out an experiment on me without my consent" might be a typical response. On the other hand, it seems much less likely that patients would be concerned if the doctor, within normal clinical practice, had selected "in good faith" the most appropriate treatment without giving information about similar alternative drugs.

3. If the public were to realise that trials were being conducted without patients' consent then there is likely to be a public reaction against clinical research.

These three reasons can each be criticised. In answer to the first it can be argued that doctors are influenced by many factors when prescribing. One factor is pharmaceutical industry advertising and promotion. This factor is just as likely to distort doctors' assessment of patients' best interests as is the "research intention". In fact, in the case of a RCT there will have been much more careful scrutiny of the objective data regarding efficacy than would be normal in clinical practice.

With regard to reasons 2 and 3, these are both empirical claims which may or may not be true.

The Moral Imperative To Make the Results of Good Research Publicly Accessible

The consequences of failing to publish good research have been well documented and include the fact that patients are subjected to ineffective or dangerous forms of care, or are denied effective forms of care [29]. Failure to make the results of research accessible is a particular problem in neurology, in which research is expensive and under the aegis of large pharmaceutical and biotech companies. Researchers may sign confidentiality agreements and the multi-site nature of modern research means that individual researchers are not privy to all emerging data of the trial. Unfavourable results can be effectively buried, even when patients' care has been adversely affected by participating in the trials, paving the way for approval of trials of related compounds, and the possibility of a lucky strike. Such concerns can only be alleviated when the results of "commercial research", positive or negative, are made publicly accessible. The failure to publish negative results also leads to bias in systematic reviews, which can result in erroneous conclusions. The publication of the results of research is therefore as much an ethical issue as the way in which the research is conducted in the first place.

References

1. Donnan GA, Davis SM, Chambers BR, Gates PC, Hankey GJ, McNeil JJ, et al. Trials of streptokinase in severe acute ischaemic stroke. Lancet 1995;345:578–579.

2. Italy (MAST-I) Group. Multicentre Acute Stroke Trial: randomised controlled trial of streptokinase, aspirin, and combination of both in treatment of acute ischaemic stroke. Lancet 1995;346:1509–1514.

3. Europe Study Group. The Multicentre Acute Stroke Trial. Thrombolytic therapy with streptokinase in acute ischaemic stroke. N Engl J Med 1996;335:145–150.

4. Pappworth MH. Human guinea pigs: experimentation on man. London: Routledge and Kegan Paul, 1967.

5. Beecher HK. Ethics and clinical research. N Engl J Med 1966;274:1354–1360.

6. Annas GJ, Grodin MA, editors. The Nazi doctors and the Nuremberg Code: human rights in human experimentation. Oxford: Oxford University Press, 1992:343–345.

7. World Medical Association. The Declaration of Helsinki. Recommendations guiding physicians in biomedical research involving human subjects. Adopted by the 18th World Medical Assembly Helsinki, 1964 and amended by the 29th World Medical Assembly Tokyo, 1975; 35th World Medical Assembly Venice, 1983; and 41st World Medical Assembly Hong Kong, 1989.

8. Department of Health Circular. Local Research Ethics Committees (HSG(91)5) London: Department of Health, 1991.

9. Department of Health. Health Service Guidelines (HSG (97) 23). Ethics Committee Review of Multi-Centre Research. London: Department of Health, 1997.

10. Botros S. Ethics in medical research: uncovering the conflicting approaches. In: Foster C, editor. Manual for research ethics committees. 4th ed. King's College, London: The Centre of Medical Law and Ethics, 1996.

11. Grotta J. Should thrombolytic therapy be the first-line treatment for acute ischaemic stroke? t-PA: the best current option for most patients. N Engl J Med 1997;337:1310.

12. Royal College of Physicians. Guidelines on the practice of ethics committees in medical research involving human subjects. London: The Royal College of Physicians, 1990.

13. Royal College of Physicians. Research involving patients. Summary and recommendations of a report of the Royal College of Physicians. J R Coll Physicians 1990;24:10–14.

14. Medical Research Council. MRC guidelines for good clinical practice in clinical trials. London: MRC, 1998.

15. Hirsch SR, Harris J, editors. Consent and the incompetent patient. Ethics, law and medicine. London: Royal College of Psychiatrists, 1988.

16. British Paediatric Association. Guidelines for the ethical conduct of medical research involving children. V.27.1. London: British Paediatric Association, 1992.

17. Babcock M, de Silva D, Oaks R, Davis-Kaplan S, Jiralerspong S, Montermini L, et al. Regulation of mitochondrial iron accumulation by Yfh1p, a putative homolog of frataxin. Science 1997;276:1709–1712.

18. Koenig M, Mandel J-L. Deciphering the cause of Friedreich's Ataxia. Curr Opin Neurol 1997;7:689–694.

19. Chalmers I. Evaluating the effects of care during pregnancy and childbirth. In: Chalmers I, Enkin M, Keirse M, editors. Effective care in pregnancy and childbirth. 1989:3–38

20. Hope T. Evidence-based patient choice. London: The King's Fund, 1996.

21. Moser HW. Adrenoleukodystrophy: phenotype, genetic, pathogenesis and therapy. Brain 1997;120:1485–1508.

22. Edwards SJL, Lilford RJ, Braunholtz D, Jackson J. Why "underpowered" trials are not necessarily unethical. Lancet 1997; 350: 804–807.

23. Lilford RJ, Thornton JG, Braunholtz D. Clinical trials and rare diseases: a way out of a conundrum. BMJ 1995;311:1621–1625.

24. Piantadosi S. Clinical trials: a methodologic perspective. New York: Wiley, 1997.

25. Freedman B. Equipoise and the ethics of clinical research. N Engl J Med 1987;317:141–145.

26. Collins R, Doll R, Peto R. Ethics of clinical trials. In: Williams CJ, editor. Introducing new treatments for cancer: practical, ethical and legal problems. Wiley, 1992:50.

27. Doll R. Summation of the conference. In: Warren KS, Mosteller F, editors. Doing more good than harm: the evaluation of health care interventions. Ann N Y Acad Sci. 1993;703:310–313.

28. Chalmers I, Silverman WA. Professional and public double standards on clinical experimentation [commentary]. Control Clin Trials 1987;8:388–391.

29. Savulescu J, Chalmers I, Blunt J. Are research ethics committees behaving unethically? Some suggestions for improving performance and accountability. BMJ 1996;313:1390–1393.

2. Assessment Measures and Clinical Scales

J.C. Hobart and A.J. Thompson

Introduction

Increasingly, clinical trials in neurology are using standardised scales and assessment measures to determine the effectiveness of therapeutic interventions. To justify this important role in research these measurement methods must demonstrate that they are reliable and valid indicators of abstract and unobservable variables such as disability, mood and health-related quality of life. In this chapter we begin by defining measurement and outlining the advantages of using standardised measurement methods. Then, we explain why it is important to measure variables such as disability and how they can be measured rigorously using Likert scales.

Next, rather than recommend a list of good instruments we offer a framework for assessing intelligently the available measures. We have taken this approach for two reasons. First, the clinical trialist in neurology is often faced with a choice: "Which of the many measures available do I select for my study?" Second, no instrument has universal usefulness so each measure must be assessed in the light of the study design for which it is being considered.

Finally, we outline the process of instrument development. This is not to encourage trialists to develop new measures (it is more likely to have the opposite effect) but to demonstrate that the process requires considerable expertise and also to enable trialists to determine whether available instruments have been developed in accordance with standard principles.

Measurement

Measurement is an essential component of scientific research and is approached through the development of appropriate instrumentation. Some authors go as far as saying that all science is measurement [1]. This highlights the underlying philosophy that variables must be adequately measured before relations between them can be studied in detail and results can be interpreted with confidence.

A widely used definition of measurement is "rules for assigning numbers to objects in such a way as to represent quantities of attributes" [2]. The term "rules" indicates that the procedures for assigning numbers must be explicitly formulated. Rules for measuring variables such as length, height and weight are very obvious; however, rules for measuring abstract clinical variables such as health status are not intuitively obvious. The term "attributes" indicates that measurement always concerns some particular feature of objects, that is, one does not measure objects, one measures their attributes.

Advantages of Standardised Measures

Without standardised measures we would be left with subjective appraisals and personal judgements: for example, the neurologist on a ward round trying to decide whether a patient is more or less disabled since a treatment was started. In contrast to these intuitive processes, standardised measures offer objectivity, quantification, communication and economy [2]. They take the guess-work out of scientific observation and allow unambiguous procedures for documenting empirical events. Scientific results are inevitably reported in terms of functional relations between measured variables. Consequently, the science of medicine can only progress when important variables can be measured rigorously.

Numerical results provided by standardised measures have two advantages. First, numerical indices allow more detailed reporting than would be possible with personal judgements. Second, quantification permits the use of powerful methods of mathematical analysis which are necessary to assess the results of research. Communication is greatly facilitated when standardised measures are available. The rate of scientific progress in a particular area is limited by the efficiency with which scientists can communicate their results to one another.

Although a great deal of work is often required to develop standardised measures, once developed they are usually more economical of time and money than subjective evaluations. In addition, standardised measures often free highly trained professionals for more important work.

Why Measure Clinical Variables?

Traditionally, medicine has assessed the effectiveness of therapeutic interventions using measurements made by machines or by documenting simple clinical end points. For example, studies of interferons in multiple scleroris have measured MRI appearances and relapse rate; studies of interventions in stroke have measured mortality rates, stroke recurrence rates and incidence of cerebral haemorrhage as a complication of treatments; studies of epilepsy have measured seizure frequency; and studies of cancer chemotherapy have measured mortality rates, duration of survival and 5-year survival rates.

Recently the inadequacy of traditional outcomes has been highlighted as, despite their undoubted importance, these measures provide little information about the diverse consequences of disease and fail to incorporate the patient perspective. Consequently, there is a need to measure more pertinent but abstract health status concepts such as disability, handicap and health-related quality of life. As neurology is a specialty with few cures and a large proportion of chronic disorders this change in focus from measuring quantity of life towards assessing aspects of the quality of life is particularly appropriate.

Many clinicians hold the point of view that aspects of health status and health-related quality of life cannot be measured rigorously because they are abstract and subjective concepts [3]. Others consider that the patient's perspective can only provide meaningful data after interpretation through the physician's objective filter [4]. Some feel that the psychosocial consequences of disease do not assume the same scientific importance as basic concepts [5]. However, there is ample evidence that abstract concepts can be measured rigorously. Psychologists have been wrestling with similar issues since the turn of the century and out of their need to measure attitudes, personalities and emotional states, methodologies have developed enabling their reliable and

valid measurement to be guaranteed [6,7]. Unfortunately, the knowledge required to ensure that these complex entities are being measured with the necessary scientific rigour has yet to transfer fully from the social sciences and is generally unavailable to most clinicians.

Measuring "Latent Variables"

Unlike height, weight and blood pressure, many aspects of health status are impossible to measure explicitly because they are unobservable [8]. They are often known as theoretical constructs or latent variables and cannot be measured until reliable and valid indicators are available. Empirical indicators of theoretical constructs can be referred to as scales [9]. (A construct is a variable that is relatively abstract as opposed to concrete, and is defined or operationalised in terms of observed indicators [10].)

Latent variables can be measured indirectly by asking questions intended to capture empirically the essential meaning of the construct. The simplest way to do this is to ask a single straightforward question (item). For example, rate patient X's degree of disability on a scale of 1 (no disability) to 5 (extremely disabled). The Ashworth scale (Table 2.1), which grades spasticity from 0 (no increase in tone) to 4 (limb rigid in flexion or extension), is an example of a single-item measure [11,12].

Although single-item measures are simple, userfriendly and appropriate for measuring some individual properties, they have a number of scientific limitations when measuring complex clinical variables. Single items are unlikely to represent well the broad scope of a complex theoretical construct and are likely to interpreted in many different ways by respondents. In addition, single items are imprecise as they cannot discriminate the fine degree of an attribute (the Ashworth scale categorises patients into five levels only), and are notoriously unreliable

Table 2.1.   Ashworth scale of spasticity

0	No increase in tone
1	Slight increase in tone giving a "catch" when the limb is moved in flexion or extension
[1+ᵃ	Slight increase in tone, manifested by a catch, followed by minimal resistance throughout the remainder (less than half) of the range of movement]
2	More marked increase in tone but the limb easily flexed
3	Considerable increase in tone, passive movement difficult
4	Limb rigid in flexion or extension

ᵃ The modified Ashworth scale includes the 1+ rating.

(prone to random error) as they do not produce consistent answers over time [13]. Finally, it is difficult to estimate the measurement properties of single-item measures [9].

Visual analogue scales are special versions of single-item measures where respondents are required to indicate the extent of the problem on a line usually 100 mm long. They have been used extensively in health measurement. Although visual analogue scales enable better precision than a fixed number of response categories, they still suffer from problems of limited scope, variable interpretation and unreliability [14].

Multi-item instruments, where each item addresses a different aspect of the same underlying construct, are able to overcome the scientific limitations of single items and are superior measures of latent variables. More items increase the scope of the measure, are less open to variable interpretation, enable better precision, and improve reliability by allowing random errors of measurement to average out [13]. The Barthel Index [15] is an example of a multi-item measure covering 10 items feeding, grooming, dressing, bathing, walking, transfers, stairs, toilet use, bladder and bowels.

There are many methods, termed scaling models, for combining multiple items into scales depending on the purpose the resulting scale is to serve [16–20]. The most widely used scaling model in health measurement is the method of summated rating proposed by Likert in 1932 [21,22].

Likert Scaling

Four characteristics constitute a summated rating scale. First, there are multiple items whose scores are summed, without weighting, to generate a total score. Second, each item measures a property that can vary quantitatively (e.g. difficulty walking ranges from none to unable to walk). Third, each item has no right answer. Fourth, each item in the scale can be rated independently. Examples of Likert scales in health measurement are: the Barthel Index (BI) [15], Functional Independence Measure (FIM) [23], Medical Outcomes Study 36-item Short Form Health Survey (SF-36) [24,25], EuroQol [26], General Health Questionnaire (GHQ) [27], Hospital Anxiety and Depression Scale (HADS) [28] and the Parkinson's Disease Questionnaire (PDQ-39) [3].

Likert scales are popular because they are simple, easy to administer, user-friendly, cheap, and relatively straightforward to develop. More importantly, it is possible to develop Likert scales that are reliable and valid indicators of latent variables, that is, instruments with good measurement (psychometric) properties [13]. The limitations of Likert scales are that they require a degree of literacy to complete, and a level of expertise and statistical sophistication to develop [29].

The items in a Likert scale usually have the same type and number of response options, although this is not essential. The four most commonly used response categories are agreement, intensity, evaluation and frequency. Agreement response categories ask respondents to indicate the extent they agree with items. For example: "My health is excellent". (agree strongly, agree, neither agree nor disagree, disagree, disagree strongly). Intensity asks respondents to indicate the extent of a problem. For example: "How severe has your pain been?". (none, very mild, mild, moderate, severe). Evaluation response categories ask for an evaluative rating of each item. For example: "In general would you say your health is". (poor, fair, good, very good, excellent). Frequency response categories ask for a judgement of how often each item occurs. For example: "I have difficulty getting dressed". (all the time, most of the time, some of the time, a little of the time, never). The number of response options usually ranges from four to seven.

There is a misconception in the medical literature about the statistics that can be applied to data generated by Likert scales. Two schools of thought exist. One school argues that only non-parametric tests can be applied to the data as the measurements are ordinal in nature [30–32]. The other school argues that it is entirely appropriate to apply parametric statistical tests as the data, though theoretically ordinal, behave in an interval manner [13,33]. The latter school of thought is supported by theoretical [34] and extensive empirical evidence [35–40]. In addition, there is considerable evidence that assumptions of interval level measurement and normally distributed data can be violated with little effect on t-tests [41,42], analysis of variance [43,44], and Pearson's product-moment correlation coefficients [45].

Types of Clinical Scales

There is no widely accepted classification of health measures. However, two important methods for classifying scales are considered below.

Generic and Disease-Specific Scales

Clinical scales can either be generic or disease-specific [46]. Generic measures can be used in any disease group provided they are appropriate (see later). They enable comparisons between different disease groups. For example, the SF-36 is a generic measure of health status. Freeman et al. [47] demonstrated the profound impact of multiple sclerosis on health status compared with other disease groups. In contrast, disease-specific measures such as the PDQ-39 are designed for use in a specific disease and have the theoretical advantage of being more relevant and more responsive than generic measures. It is recommended that generic and disease-specific measures are used in parallel [46].

Purpose of Measurement

Health measurement instruments can have one (or more) of three purposes [48]. Discriminative instruments distinguish between groups or individuals on an underlying dimension. Predictive measures attempt to classify individuals into predefined measurement categories. Evaluative instruments are used to measure the magnitude of longitudinal change in an individual or group on the dimension of interest [49]. There are two reasons for highlighting different measurement purposes. First, measures for one purpose cannot be assumed to be measures of another; this must be formally proven. This is not the same for laboratory measures, where the process of development, and the requirements for successful application, may be identical for discrimination, prediction and evaluation [48]. For example, MRI can be used to discriminate between people who do and do not have multiple sclerosis, predict people presenting with isolated neurological syndromes who may develop multiple sclerosis, and to evaluate whether there has been progression of disease over time. This is not true for health measures.

The second reason for highlighting the purpose of health measures is that different methods are required to develop measures for different purposes [49]. For example, when developing an evaluative measure it is appropriate to select from the item pool (see later) those items that demonstrate change over time (i.e. empirically responsive items). In contrast, when developing a discriminative measure it is appropriate to select those items that discriminate between individuals at one point in time (i.e. items with good distributions among the different response categories).

How To Choose a Clinical Scale

Clinical trialists often have to choose one scale from among many potential candidates. There are now a number of texts listing health measures [50–55] and journals continually report newly developed measures. However, not all published measures are good and many have been published with inadequate

research and evaluation. Different scales have different virtues, there is no one scale which is the best for all purposes, and instruments that are useful for one clinical trialist may not be useful for others. No one scale exhibits all desirable qualities and although new scales tend to improve some characteristics at the expense of others there is always some trade-off between properties. Therefore, scales must be selected for the particular purpose for which they are to be used and the scale user must be able to choose measures intelligently based on his or her needs.

For success in clinical trials instruments must be clinically useful and scientifically sound. Clinical usefulness refers to the successful incorporation of an instrument into clinical practice and its appropriateness to the study sample. Scientific soundness refers to the demonstration of reliable, valid and responsive measurement of the outcome of interest. It is important to note that clinical usefulness does not guarantee scientific soundness nor vice versa.

Clinical Usefulness

Factors that determine whether an instrument can be successfully incorporated into clinical practice are method of administration and user acceptability. Factors that determine appropriateness to the study sample are content and score distributions.

Method of Administration and User Acceptability

There are many methods by which an instrument can be administered, each of which has advantages and disadvantages. The most widely used methods are: patient-completion, e.g. SF-36, and PDQ-39; interviewer rated, e.g. neuropsychological testing; rating by observation of behaviour, e.g. Barthel Index; rating from examination, e.g. Ashworth scale and Kurtzke's Expanded Disability Status Scale [56]; and team consensus rating from observation of behaviour by trained observers, e.g. FIM.

The method of administration of an instrument should not be changed from that recommended by the instrument developers in order to suit the needs of a study. This is because altering the method of administration may affect the scientific properties (reliability and validity) of a measure. If an alternative method of administration is considered necessary the validity of this method needs to be evaluated before the instrument is used. This can be achieved by correlating scores for patients obtained by the two methods; the higher the correlation the greater the validity of the alternative method of administration.

The method of administration of an instrument has important implications for study design and cost. For example, the use of self-report questionnaires allows data to be collected from large samples in geographically disparate areas and reduces patient inconvenience. These studies can usually be co-ordinated by a single investigators who rely only on patients returning completed questionnaires. In contrast, rating by trained observer requires training, proof of success of training, and usually multiple raters in multiple centres to attain large sample sizes. If an instrument with limited responsiveness is being used, a large sample may be essential to have any hope of demonstrating significant results.

Although physicians have tended to favour clinician-report measurement the current trend in health measurement is towards patient-report questionnaires. There are many reasons for this, the most compelling being the library of information indicating that patients and clinicians often have widely differing perceptions as to the impact of disease [57–60].

User acceptability is important in obtaining the cooperation of persons in the study. Patients in clinical trials are ill and their tolerance for completing long and complex questionnaires may be limited. Seemingly irrelevant items arouse criticism. Busy clinicians with no ownership of a study have little personal gain from the results. These factors influence the interest of patients and clinicians in participating in clinical trials, the reliability and validity of scores, and also the relationships between the investigators, clinicians and patients.

Content and Score Distributions

The content of the instrument must be relevant to the study, the items must reflect problems encountered by the study group, and must also measure aspects of health that the intervention is expected to change. This is logical but the current vogue for measuring "quality of life" in treatment trials could result in the blind use of inappropriate instruments.

If an instrument is to be a useful measure of an attribute (e.g. disability) in a clinical trial it must adequately represent the true distribution of that attribute in the study sample [61]. In addition, it must also be able to discriminate between individuals in the study sample, and have the capacity to detect change in the attribute being measured. Important information concerning these issues can be provided by simply examining the score distributions in the sample of interest. That is, the range of scores, mean score, standard deviation, floor and ceiling effects, and extent of skewness.

Range of scores indicates the actual range of the attribute in the sample. The nearer the actual range approximates to the possible range of a scale the more likely it is that an instrument is able to dis-

criminate between individuals on the attribute being measured. The mean score indicates the central tendency of the sample. Mean scores near the mid-point of the possible scale range suggest that scores on an instrument may have a near-normal distribution and that there is good potential for change to be detected. Standard deviations indicate the spread of the sample. As the aim of many studies is to detect change and discriminate between individuals, scales should demonstrate variability in the attribute being measured. Small standards deviation indicate limited variability.

Floor and ceiling effects are calculated as the percentage of subjects scoring the minimum and maximum possible scores respectively. They indicate the extent to which the measured range of an attribute is restricted [62]. It is recommended that floor and ceiling effects should not exceed 15% as they compromise the capacity of an instrument to detect change in the attribute being measured [63]. Floor effects, although indicating patients with the maximum potential for change, also indicate a group which may change clinically but still not improve in scale terms [64,65]. Ceiling effects indicate patients whose scores cannot increase, and therefore can not register improvement on the scale even if clinical improvement occurs.

Skewness summarises the extent to which score distributions are non-normal and indicates the extent to which distributions are bunched at one end. A positive value indicates that scores cluster to the left of the mean, and a negative value indicates that scores cluster to the right of the mean [10]. Ideally, skewness statistics should be in the range −1 to +1 [62]. Scores need not be normally distributed; in fact a rectangular distribution of scores gives the best discrimination between subjects [33]. If score distributions are not available for the sample of interest, those from related samples give at least some useful information.

Table 2.2 presents results from an unpublished study and illustrates the importance of examining score distributions. Score distributions for 64 multiple sclerosis patients undergoing in-patient neuro-rehabilitation are presented for three disability measures: the Kutzke Expanded Disability Status Scale (EDSS), Barthel Index (BI), and Functional Independence Measure (FIM). No scale has notable floor or ceiling effects. These results indicate that the range of disability in the sample is adequately covered by all three instruments. However, the sample spans the whole range of the BI and FIM but only 50% of the EDSS scale range. These results indicate that the EDSS covers a greater range of disability than the BI and FIM. More importantly these findings indicate that the EDSS does not discriminate

Table 2.2. Score ranges, means, standard deviations, floor and ceiling effects for EDSS, Barthel Index, and FIM ($n = 197$)

Instrument	Admission score			Floor effect n (%)	Ceiling effect n (%)
	Range		Mean (SD)		
	Scale	Sample			
EDSS	0–10	5.0–9.0	7.1 (0.9)	0	0
Barthel Index	0–20	0–20	12.02 (5.7)	5 (2.5)	10 (5.4)
FIM	18–126	24–122	89.42 (23.6)	0	0

EDSS, Kurtzke Expanded Disability Status Scale; FIM, Functional Independence Measure.

as well as the BI and FIM between different levels of disability.

It is important to note that score distributions, like all measurement properties, are sample dependent. More and less disabled samples may have significant floor and ceiling effects on the BI but not the EDSS, suggesting that the latter instrument may be the better choice.

Scientific Soundness

Scientific soundness is the demonstration that an instrument measures in a reliable and valid manner. In addition, instruments whose role is to evaluate the effectiveness of interventions must also demonstrate responsiveness, i.e. the ability to detect change in the attribute being measured.

Reliability

Reliability concerns the extent to which random (measurement) error is associated with a measurement instrument (high reliability = low error). The lower an instrument's reliability the greater the influence of measurement error on scale scores, and the less "true" information is provided. Random error refers to all chance factors that cause variations in repeated measurement producing results that are inaccurate, inconsistent, unstable over time and not reproducible. Poor reliability can have serious effects on all types of scientific inquiry by reducing the overall power of randomized studies [66], attenuating the level of associations in observational studies [67], and biasing conclusions in an unpredictable manner when confounding variables are present [68–70]. Most importantly no measure can have validity unless it measures accurately [2]. Demonstration of reliability is therefore a prerequisite for validity [71] and the first property that needs to be assessed.

Measurement error is common in health measurement as there are many sources of error associated with a person's behaviour. For example, consider the random errors at play when a patient's disability is measured using a self-report scale. The scale consists of a finite number of items representing an individual's ability to undertake tasks. These items are only a sample of all possible disability items and therefore the scale will give an erroneous score if the items represent a combination of tasks that are easy (or difficult) for the patient to perform. In addition, a patient's score represents a sample of their disability at one point in time. We assume that the situation would be similar if the patient's disability were measured at another point in time. The score will not be representative if the patient is measured on an off-day, lacked interest and guessed answers, or misread the questionnaire. Random error is equally at play for other methods of administration.

When evaluating reliability data available for instruments, investigators should try to answer three questions: first, have the appropriate types of reliability been examined; second, were the reliability studies conducted in appropriate samples (type and size); and third, do the results achieve recommended minimum requirements for the type of study being conducted.

Have the Appropriate Types of Reliability Been Assessed? The reliability of a measure is expressed as a reliability coefficient. However, reliability is a generic term, and multiple types (and therefore many coefficients) exist for each instrument. Each type of reliability addresses a different source (or sources) of random error. It is a common misconception that providing evidence for one type of reliability is sufficient. Ideally, all relevant types of reliability should be quantified. If a comprehensive evaluation does not exist, investigators must satisfy themselves that the major sources of random error appropriate to an instrument and the purpose to which it is being used have been determined.

For health measures the most important (but not the only) types of reliability are internal consistency and reproducibility (test–retest, inter-rater and intra-rater). Other types of reliability are beyond the scope of this chapter but are detailed in standard texts [72–74]. Internal consistency is the extent to which items within a scale are reliable measures of the same construct. This type of reliability only applies to multi-item measures such as the SF-36 and Barthel Index and is determined using Cronbach's alpha coefficient [75]. Reproducibility is the agreement between two or more ratings on the same person. Test–retest reliability is the agreement between two or more self-report ratings for the same patient. Intra-rater reproducibility is the agreement between two or more ratings for the same patient made by the same observer. Inter-rater reproducibility is the agreement between two or more ratings for the same patient made by the different observers. Reproducibility should be reported as an intraclass correlation coefficient for continuous data [76], and Kappa coefficients for dichotomous data [77].

Comprehensive reliability assessment for single item measures consists of determining intra-rater and inter-rater reproducibility, and for multi-item measures consists of determining internal consistency, intra-rater and inter-rater reproducibility. However, it is unusual to find instruments where the assessment of reliability is comprehensive. For multi-item measures the most useful index of reliability is the internal consistency. This is because the major source of error is item sampling. A full explanation of this can be found in Nunnally [13]. Second, there is good evidence that estimates of internal consistency and reproducibility are similar [61,78]. Third, high test–retest reliability with low internal consistency is much more likely than low internal consistency with high test–retest reliability. Finally, Cronbach's alpha tends to provide a conservative reliability estimate [79].

Were the Reliability Studies Conducted in Appropriate Samples? All psychometric properties are dependent upon the samples from which they were determined. Therefore, results can only be generalised from one sample to another if the reliability in the two samples is expected to be similar. For example, demonstration of high reliability for a self-report health measure in persons with cervical myelopathy cannot be assumed to indicate high reliability in persons with dementia. However, evidence of reliability from multiple studies in different groups suggests reliability is a stable property for the instrument. There are no clear guidelines as to the sizes of samples for reliability studies though it is generally recommended that they should exceed 50 patients.

Has Adequate Reliability Been Demonstrated? Widely recommended minimum requirements are reliability coefficients >0.70 (ideally 0.85 [13]) for group comparison studies, and >0.90 (ideally >0.95) for individual comparison studies [13,80]. The need for high reliability in individual comparison studies is clear when confidence intervals around individual scores are calculated. Confidence intervals are calculated from the standard error of measurement (SEM). This estimates the standard deviation of scores obtained if an instrument were administered repeatedly to the same individual [13]. Therefore, the SEM is a direct indicator of the probable extent of random error associated with scores [33] and can be used to calculate confidence intervals around individual patient scores. Standard errors of measurement are calculated using the formula: $SEM = SD \times \sqrt{(1 - reliability)}$; 95% confidence intervals (± 1.96 SEM). Confidence intervals reflect the accuracy for individual-patient assessment and clinical decision-making [81]. Table 2.3 illustrates the effect of decreasing reliability on the confidence intervals of Barthel Index (BI) scores. For example, even with a reliability coefficient of 0.90 the 95% confidence interval around an individual BI score of 10 ranges from 6.3 to 13.7, indicating why scores for individual patients should be interpreted with extreme caution [74].

Validity

The validity of a health measure is defined as the extent to which it measures what it purports to measure [13]. Determining the validity of a health measure is the most difficult of the psychometric properties. This is for the following reasons. First, validity cannot be proven it can only be supported or refuted by evidence. Second, unlike reliability there is no consensus as to the minimum requirement of evidence to satisfy validity. Third, support for validity in one context does not guarantee validity for another.

Table 2.3. Effect of different levels of reliability on the confidence intervals around individual patient scores for the Barthel Index

Reliability	95% confidence interval
0.95	±2.6
0.90	±3.7
0.80	±5.2
0.70	±6.3
0.60	±7.3
0.50	±8.2

Barthel Index scores: $n = 149$; mean score = 11.5; SD = 5.9; sample range 0–20; floor effect = 2.5%; ceiling effect = 5.4%.

To determine whether an instrument is valid for a specific purpose, clinical trialists must assess the strength of empirical evidence available. This is done by reviewing three types of evidence gathered from multiple studies: content validity, criterion-related validity and construct validity.

Content validity concerns the extent to which the content of the instrument reflects the domain of content (all possible items) of the attribute being measured. For example, the BI is purported to be a measure of personal activities of daily living (PADL). As the 10 items of the BI are a sample of all possible PADL tasks, evidence is required to support the extent to which these items reflect the entire domain of content of PADL. Simply reading the items tells us that they are intuitively sound, thus providing evidence for face validity, a weak form of content validity. Strong evidence for content validity is provided by examining the methodology of instrument construction. If the method of construction of the BI were by the generation of a large pool of PADL items from literature review, expert opinion, and semi-structured patient interviews followed by item reduction from item analysis techniques strong evidence for the content validity would be provided. However, the 10 items of the BI were chosen by clinicians who perceived them to be important and no statistical evidence of item analysis was presented [15]. Consequently, the evidence for content validity of the BI is limited.

Criterion-related validity is defined as the extent to which the instrument under study correlates with a gold standard (the criterion) [13]. Examination of criterion-related validity is unlikely to be possible for health measures as gold standard instruments rarely exist [10]. Under these circumstances a different type of evidence, construct validity, is required to support the supposition that a measure is valid for a particular purpose [82].

Construct validity is defined as the extent to which the scores generated from an instrument conform with those predicted from hypotheses based on theoretical knowledge of the construct under study [82]. Simply, we make predictions as to how an instrument should behave if it were a valid measure of the construct. The validity of the instrument is the extent to which empirical data conform to these theoretical predictions. As such data can come from many sources it is useful to consider evidence of construct validity as being of two complementary types: internal and external construct validity [1].

Internal construct validity involves statistical analyses of scale scores to determine whether hypotheses concerning the theoretical structure of the instrument are supported. In contrast, external construct validity examines the relationships between scores on the instrument of interest and external variables to determine whether hypotheses concerning the interpretation of scores are supported by empirical data. Ideally both types of evidence are required as each has its limitations.

Evidence for internal construct validity is provided by analyses of internal consistency, intercorrelations between the different subscales of an instrument for multi-dimensional measures, and analyses of group differences validity. The interpretation of internal consistency as evidence for reliability and validity is a source of confusion. However, the higher the internal consistency the higher the relationships between the items and the greater the evidence that they measure a single construct. For data to be interpreted accurately an instrument should measure a single construct.

If an instrument measures multiple dimensions of health (e.g. SF-36 or PDQ-39) these dimensions must be shown to be empirically distinct constructs. Intercorrelating the scores of the different subscales indicates the extent to which they measure related subconstructs. Ideally correlations should be moderate (say 0.30–0.70) indicating that the different subscales measure related but different subconstructs. High correlations between subscales indicate that they measure closely related constructs and thus questions whether they are conceptually separate.

Group differences validity is supported by demonstrating that groups known to differ in the construct being measured generate predictably different scores on the instrument under study. For example, quadriplegic patients should demonstrate greater physical disability than paraplegic patients.

Whilst studies providing evidence of internal construct validity support the validity of an instrument they are limited as they provide no specific evidence of the construct being measured. For example, demonstration that the FIM scales are internally consistent, that the total, motor and cognitive scales measure related but different constructs, and that quadriplegic patients have statistically lower mean FIM motor scores than paraplegic patients (indicating greater motor disability), does not provide evidence that the FIM measures disability.

Studies of external construct validity examine the relationships (in the form of correlations) between the instrument under study and other measures of related and unrelated constructs. To the extent that correlations conform with the direction, pattern and magnitude of predictions, validity is supported. The statistical significance of these correlations is of limited importance. For example, Table 2.4 presents correlations between the FIM and a selection of other scales in 64 multiple sclerosis patients undergoing in-patient rehabilitation. If the FIM measures dis-

Table 2.4. Product-moment correlations between the FIM, other measures of disability, and measures of handicap, psychological well-being, health status and age

	Barthel Index	EDSS	LHS	GHQ	Age
FIM	0.94	0.87	0.42	0.13	−0.05

EDSS, Kurtzke Expanded Disability Status Scale; LHS, London Handicap Scale; GHQ, General Health Questionnaire; SF-36 PCS, Medical Outcomes Study 36-item Short Form Health Survey Physical Component Summary Score; SF-36 MCS, Medical Outcomes Study 36-item Short Form Health Survey Mental Component Summary Score; FIM, Functional Independence Measure.

ability we would predict: high correlations with other measures of physical disability (BI, EDSS); higher correlation with measures of disability than with measures of handicap (LHS), and psychological well-being (GHQ); and low correlations with age. The data in Table 2.4 conform with these predictions and therefore provide strong evidence for the validity of the FIM as a measure of disability in multiple sclerosis patients.

Studies of external construct validity are limited as the validating instruments themselves have often not been comprehensively validated. Consequently, it is important to have results from multiple studies of both internal and external construct validity.

Responsiveness

Responsiveness is defined as the ability of an instrument to detect clinically significant change in the attribute measured [83]. There is debate (largely academic) as to whether responsiveness should be considered an aspect of construct validity [84] or a separate psychometric property [85]. The value of considering responsiveness as a separate psychometric property is that it highlights the importance of the ability of instruments to detect change over time. As clinical trials usually evaluate the effectiveness of interventions to induce change this seems sensible.

Responsiveness methodology is less well advanced than that for reliability and validity. This is partly because the measurement of change is less pertinent to psychological than to health measurement. As the intention of therapeutic interventions is largely to evoke change, health measurement instruments must be able to detect those changes. Consequently, responsiveness has become a key methodological issue in the last few years.

Several methods have been proposed for determining the responsiveness of health measures and there is no clear consensus as to which is the optimal one [86]. Most methods examine scores at two points in time, usually before and after an intervention

thought to alter the attribute being measured. Responsiveness is reflected by the magnitude of the standardised change score.

Reporting raw change scores as indices of responsiveness is limited for two reasons. First, they do not take into account the sample studied. Second, they do not allow comparison between different instruments. The latter is important as investigators are often faced with a choice between different instruments. Reporting the statistical significance of change scores as an index of instrument responsiveness is also limited for two reasons. First, statistical significance is dependent upon the sample size. Second, statistical significant change does not guarantee clinically significant change [87,88].

For these reasons it is recommended that responsiveness is reported in the form of an effect size (standardised change score). The formula for the most commonly reported effect size is: mean change score divided by the standard deviation of the baseline scores [89]. This effect size therefore standardises the change score to standard deviation units. A value of 1.0 indicates that the mean change is equivalent to the standard deviation of the baseline sample. The larger the effect size the greater the responsiveness of an instrument.

To aid the clinical interpretation of effect size values it has been recommended that Cohen's arbitrary criteria are applied: 0.20 = small; 0.50 = medium; 0.80 = large [89,90]. However, when comparing instruments the strongest evidence for the superior responsiveness of an instrument comes form head-to-head comparisons of instruments.

Developing Scales

Developing clinical scales is a labour-intensive process requiring considerable expertise in health measurement [29]. Therefore, clinical trialists are advised to carefully evaluate available measures before abandoning them. The psychometric properties of available measures can be determined more quickly. A detailed account of instrument development is beyond the scope of this chapter. However, a thumb-nail sketch is presented to highlight important areas.

Development of a measurement instrument in accordance with psychometric theory involves four stages: first, defining a conceptual model; second, generation of an item pool; third, reduction of the item pool to form an instrument; fourth, testing the reliability, validity and responsiveness of the final instrument.

A conceptual model is the rationale for, and description of the concept(s) that the measure is intended to assess [80]. The importance of a conceptual basis for the measurement of latent variables cannot be overemphasised [91,92]. However, this is often absent or poorly defined for health measurement instruments [53]. For example, a clinical trialist may wish to develop a measure of disability for multiple sclerosis. The trialist must firstly define disability in multiple sclerosis and decide which aspects to measure. Only when this has been done can a comprehensive approach to item generation be undertaken.

There are four sources from which candidate items can be generated: semi-structured interviews of patients with the disorder under study, consensus opinion of experts in the field, literature review and examination of available measures. Patient interviews are very valuable as they help to identify areas that are important to them – a process that maximises the validity of an instrument.

From these four sources items are devised aiming to address the appropriate range and depth of concept/s to be measured. These items are then pretested on a small sample to assess how easily they can be understood and completed. Appropriate alterations are made and this version is used in the preliminary field test.

The purpose of the preliminary field test phase is to reduce the number of items and to develop a scale. The instrument is administered to a large sample of patients and the results are analysed using standard psychometric techniques for item analysis [14,72]. The aim of item reduction is to select, on an empirical basis, the items that measure the construct of interest, that is items that discriminate between individuals, are stable over time and measure the same underlying construct. The importance of selecting items on an empirical basis is that approaches to measurement on an intuitive basis often fail to produce the desired empirical results [2].

After items have been reduced they may need to be grouped into scales if it is anticipated that the instrument may measure more than one related but different construct. Items can be grouped in two ways: first, on a theoretical basis, and second, on an empirical basis using item-level exploratory factor analysis. Item groupings, both hypothesised and empirically defined, are then tested using multitrait scaling techniques to define which method of grouping items produces the best empirical measurement instrument [93].

When items have been reduced and scales formed the final instrument must be tested on an independent sample for its clinical usefulness and scientific soundness (reliability, validity and responsiveness) using the techniques outlined above.

Conclusions

Latent variables can be measured rigorously using Likert scales and should be used as outcomes in the evaluation of therapeutic interventions in neurology. When assessing available instruments clinical trialists must evaluate their clinical usefulness and scientific soundness with respect to a particular study. First, find instruments that can be incorporated into the study design, whose items look like they measure the required constructs for the study (do not be misled by instrument names) and are appropriate to the study sample.

Next, examine the empirical evidence that these measures are reliable, valid and responsive in the study sample. Start with evidence for reliability as this is a prerequisite for (but not sufficient for) validity and responsiveness. Have the important types of reliability been determined in appropriate samples, and have minimum criteria for the type of study (group or individual comparisons) been satisfied? Next, examine the empirical evidence that the instrument measures what it purports to measure. What type of evidence supports the instrument's validity and how strong is this evidence? Finally, what evidence is there that the instrument has the ability to detect change over time?

The trialist is commonly left with no instrument fulfilling all the above criteria. Can further evaluative studies be undertaken on available instruments, or does the study design need to be re-considered? If no instrument exists and no compromise is acceptable a new instrument may need to be developed. Be sure to collaborate with a health measurement expert, but also be sure that they have one foot in clinical reality [94].

References

1. Bohrnstedt GW. Measurement. In: Rossi PH, Wright JD, Anderson AB, editors. Handbook of survey research. New York: Academic Press, 1983:69–121.
2. Nunnally JC Jr. Introduction to psychological measurement. New York: McGraw-Hill, 1970.
3. Peto V, Jenkinson C, Fitzpatrick R, Greenhall R. The development and validation of a short measure of functioning and well-being for individuals with Parkinson's diseases. Qual Life Res 1995;4:241–248.
4. Devinsky O. Outcomes research in neurology: incorporating health-related quality of life. Ann Neurol 1995;37:141–142.
5. Deyo R, Patrick D. Barriers to the use of health status measures in clinical investigation, patient care and policy research. Med Care 1989;27(3 Suppl):S254–S268.
6. Du Bois PH. A history of psychological testing. Boston: Allyn and Bacon, 1970.
7. Rogers T. The psychological testing enterprise: an introduction. Pacific Grove, CA: Brooks Cole, 1995.

8. Bland J, Altman D. Cronbach's alpha. BMJ 1997;314:572.
9. McIver JP, Carmines EG. Unidimensional scaling. Sage university paper series on quantitative applications in the social sciences, 07-024. Newbury Park, CA: Sage, 1981.
10. Stewart AL, Ware JE Jr, editors. Measuring functioning and well-being: the Medical Outcomes Study approach. Durham, NC: Duke University Press, 1992.
11. Ashworth B. Preliminary trial of carisoprodol in multiple sclerosis. Practitioner 1964;192:540–542.
12. Bohannon RW, Smith MB. Inter-rater reliability of a modified Ashworth scale of spasticity. Phys Ther 1987;67:206–207.
13. Nunnally JC. Psychometric theory, 2nd ed. New York: McGraw-Hill, 1978.
14. Streiner DL, Norman GR. Health measurement scales: a practical guide to their development and use, 2nd ed. Oxford: Oxford University Press, 1995.
15. Mahoney FI, Barthel DW. Functional evaluation: the Barthel Index. Maryland State Med J 1965;14:61–65.
16. Thurstone LL. A law of comparative judgement. Psychol Rev 1927;34:273–286.
17. Guttman L. A basis for scaling qualitative data. Am Sociol Rev 1944;9:139–150.
18. Gulliksen H. Theory of mental tests. New York: Wiley, 1950.
19. Edwards AL. Techniques of attitude scale construction. New York: Appleton-Century-Crofts, 1957.
20. Torgerson WS. Theory and methods of scaling. New York: Wiley, 1958.
21. Likert RA. A technique for the development of attitudes. Arch Psychol 1932;140:5–55.
22. Likert RA, Roslow S, Murphy G. A simple and reliable method of scoring the Thurstone attitude scales. J Soc Psychol 1934;5:228–238.
23. Granger CV, Hamilton BB, Keith RA, Zielezny M, Sherwin FS. Advances in functional assessment for medical rehabilitation. Topics in Geriatric Rehabilitation. Aspen, MD: Rockville, 1986:59–79.
24. Ware JE Jr. SF-36 Health Survey manual and interpretation guide. Boston, MA: Nimrod Press, 1993.
25. Ware JE Jr, Kosinski MA, Keller SD. SF-36 physical and mental health summary scales: a user's manual. Boston: The Health Institute, New England Medical Centre, 1994.
26. EuroQol Group. EuroQol: a new facility for the measurement of health-related quality of life. Health Policy 1990;16:199–208.
27. Goldberg D. Manual of the General Health Questionnaire. Windsor: NFER-Nelson, 1978.
28. Zigmond AS, Snaith RP. The Hospital Anxiety and Depression Scale. Acta Psychiatr Scand 1983;67:361–370.
29. Spector PE. Summated rating scale construction: an introduction. Quantitative applications in the social sciences, 07-082. Newbury Park, CA: Sage, 1992.
30. Stevens SS. On the theory of scales of measurement. Science 1946;103:677–680.
31. Merbitz C, Morris J, Grip J. Ordinal scales and foundations of misinference. Arch Phys Med Rehabil 1989;70:308–312.
32. Wright BD, Linacre JM. Observations are always ordinal: measurements, however, must be interval. Arch Phys Med Rehabil 1989;70:857–860.
33. Guilford JP. Psychometric methods, 2nd ed. New York: McGraw-Hill, 1954.
34. Lord FM. On the statistical treatment of football numbers. Am Psychol 1953;8:750–751.
35. Burke CJ. Additive scales and statistics. Psychol Rev 1953;60:73–75.
36. Gaito J. Non-parametric methods in psychological research. Psychol Rep 1959;5:115–125.
37. Gaito J. Scale classification and statistics. Psychol Bull 1960;67:277–278.
38. Baker B, Hardyck C, Petronovich L. Weak measurement vs. strong statistics: an empirical critique of S.S. Stevens proscritions on statistics. Educ Psychol Meas 1966;26:291–309.
39. Gaito J. Measurement scales and statistics: resurgence of an old misconception. Psychol Bull 1980;87:564–567.
40. Gaito J, Yokubynas R. An empirical basis for the statement that measurement scale properties (an meaning) are irrelevant in statistical analyses. Bull Psychon Soc 1986;24:449–450.
41. Boneau CA. The effects of violations of assumptions underlying the t-test. Psychol Bull 1960;57:49–64.
42. Havlicek L, Peterson N. Robustness of the t-test: a guide for researchers on effect of violations of assumptions. Psychol Rep 1974;34:1095–1114.
43. Kenny D, Judd C. Consequences of violating the independence assumptions in analysis of variance. Psychol Bull 1986;99:422–431.
44. Cochran W. Some consequences when the assumptions for the analysis of variance are not satisfied. Biomterics 1947;3:22–38.
45. Havlicek LL, Peterson NL. Effect of the violation of assumptions upon significance levels of the Pearson r. Psychol Bull 1977;84:373–377.
46. Patrick D, Deyo R. Generic and disease-specific measures in assessing health status and quality of life. Med Care 1989;27(Suppl):S217–S232.
47. Freeman JA, Langdon DW, Hobart JC, Thompson AJ. Health-related quality of life in people with multiple sclerosis undergoing inpatient rehabilitation. J Neurol Rehabil 1996;10:185–194.
48. Kirshner B, Guyatt G. A methodological framework for assessing health indices. J Chron Dis 1985;38:27–36.
49. Guyatt GH, Krishner B, Jaeschke R. Measuring health status: what are the necessary measurement properties. J Clin Epidemiol 1992;45:1341–1345.
50. Bowling A. Measuring health: a review of quality of life measurement scales. Buckingham, UK: Open University Press, 1991.
51. Bowling A. Measuring disease: a review of disease-specific quality of life measurement scales. Buckingham, UK: Open University Press, 1995.
52. Herndon RM, editor. Handbook of neurological rating scales. New York: Demos, 1997.
53. McDowell I, Newell C. Measuring health: a guide to rating scales and questionnaires, 2nd ed. Oxford: Oxford University Press, 1996.
54. Wilkin D, Hallam L, Doggett M-A. Measures of need and outcome for primary health care. Oxford: Oxford University Press, 1992.
55. Wade DT. Measurement in neurological rehabilitation. Oxford: Oxford University Press, 1992.
56. Kurtzke JF. Rating neurological impairment in multiple sclerosis: an expanded disability status scale (EDSS). Neurology 1983;33:1444–1452.
57. Sprangers MAG, Aaronson NK. The role of health care providers and significant others in evaluating the quality of life of patients with chronic disease: a review. J Clin Epidemiol 1992;45:743–760.
58. Reiser SJ. The era of the patient. JAMA 1993;269:1012–1017.
59. Hobart JC, Freeman JA, Lamping DL. Physician and patient oriented outcomes in chronic and progressive neurological disease: which to measure? Curr Opin Neurol 1996;9:6.
60. Rothwell PM, McDowell Z, Wong CK, Dorman PJ. Doctors and patients don't agree: cross sectional study of patients' and doctors' perceptions and assessments of disability in multiple sclerosis. BMJ 1997;314:1580–1583.
61. Ware JE Jr, Davies-Avery A, Donald C. Conceptualization and measurement of health for adults in the health insurance study, vol V, General health perceptions. Santa Monica, CA: Rand Corporation, 1978.

62. Holmes WC, Bix B, Shea JA. SF-20 score and item distributions in a human immunodeficiency virus seropositive sample. Med Care 1996;34:562–569.

63. McHorney CA, Tarlov AR. Individual-patient monitoring in clinical practice: are available health status surveys adequate? Qual Life Res 1995;4:293–307.

64. Bindman AB, Keane D, Lurie N. Measuring health changes among severely ill patients: the floor phenomenon. Med Care 1990;28:1142–1152.

65. Baker D, Hays R, Brook R. Understanding changes in health status: is the floor phenomenon merely the last step of the staircase. Med Care 1997;35:1–15.

66. Fleiss JL. The design and analysis of clinical experiments. New York: Wiley, 1986.

67. Allen MJ, Yen WM. Introduction to measurement theory. Monterey, CA: Brooks Cole, 1979.

68. Lui K. Measurement error and its impact on partial correlation and multiple linear regression analysis. Am J Epidemiol 1988;127:864–874.

69. Kupper LL. Effects of the use of unreliable surrogate variables on the validity of epidemiological research. Am J Epidemiol 1984;120:643–648.

70. Greenland S. The effect of misclassification in the presence of covariates. Am J Epidemiol 1980;112:564–569.

71. Lord FM, Novick MR. Statistical theories of mental test scores. In: Mosteller F, editor. Behavioural science: quantitative methods. Reading, MA: Addison-Wesley, 1968.

72. Nunnally JC, Bernstein IH. Psychometric theory, 3rd ed. New York: McGraw-Hill, 1994.

73. Cronbach LJ. Essentials of psychological testing, 5th ed. New York: Harper Collins, 1990.

74. Anastasi A, Urbina S. Psychological testing, 7th ed. Upper Saddle River, NJ: Prentice-Hall, 1997.

75. Cronbach LJ. Coefficient alpha and the internal structure of tests. Psychometrika 1951;16:297–334.

76. Shrout PE, Fleiss JL. Intraclass correlations: uses in assessing rater reliability. Psychol Bull 1979;86:420–428.

77. Cohen J. A coefficient of agreement for nominal scales. Educ Psychol Meas 1960;20:37–46.

78. Ware JE Jr, Johnson S, Davies-Avery A, Brook R. Conceptualization and measurement of health for adults in the health insurance study, vol III, Mental health. Santa Monica, CA, Rand Corporation, 1979.

79. Bravo G, Potvin L. Estimating the reliability of continuous measures with Cronbach's alpha or the intraclass correlation coefficient: toward the integration of two traditions. J Clin Epidemiol 1991;44:381–390.

80. Scientific Advisory Committee of the Medical Outcomes Trust. Instrument review criteria. Med Outcomes Trust Bulletin 1995;3:I–IV.

81. Williams JI, Naylor CD. How should health status instruments be assessed? Cautionary notes on procrustean frameworks. J Clin Epidemiol 1992;45:1347–1351.

82. Cronbach LJ, Meehl PE. Construct validity in psychological tests. Psychol Bull 1955;52:281–302.

83. Guyatt GH, Walter S, Norman G. Measuring change over time: assessing the usefulness of evaluative instruments. J Chron Dis 1987;40:171–178.

84. Hays R, Hadorn D. Responsiveness to change: an aspect of validity, not a separate dimension. Qual Life Res 1992;1:73–73.

85. Guyatt GH, Deyo RA, Charlson M, Levine MN, Mitchell A. Responsiveness and validity in health status measurement: a clarification. J Clin Epidemiol 1989;42:403–408.

86. Liang MH. Evaluating instrument responsiveness. J Rheumatol 1995;22:1191–1192.

87. Cohen J. The earth is round ($p < 0.05$). Am Psychol 1994;49:997–1003.

88. Cortina JM, Dunlap WP. On the logic and purpose of significance testing. Psychol Methods 1997;2:161–172.

89. Kazis LE, Anderson JJ, Meenan RF. Effect sizes for interpreting changes in health status. Med Care 1989;27(3 Suppl):S178–S189.

90. Cohen J. Statistical power analysis for the behavioural sciences. Hillsdale, NJ: Lawrence Erlbaum, 1988.

91. DeVellis RF. Scale development: theory and applications. London: Sage, 1991.

92. Kopec JA, Esdaile JM, Abrahamowicz M, et al. The Quebec Back Pain Disability Scale: measurement properties. Spine 1995;20:341–352.

93. Ware JE Jr, Harris WJ, Gandek B, Rogers BW, Reese PR. MAP-R for Windows: multitrait / multi-item analysis program: – revised user's guide. Boston, MA: Health Assessment Lab, 1997.

94. Aaronson NK. Quantitative issues in health-related quality of life assessment. Health Policy 1988;10:217–230.

3. Ethics, Outcome Variables and Clinical Scales: The Clinician's Point of View

E. Buskens and J. van Gijn

Ethics

"Ethics" in the context of medical research refers to a code of moral obligations towards not only patients but also colleagues and the (scientific) community. Some important rules for conduct of scientific research, e.g. clinical trials, arise from these obligations. Occasionally there may be a conflict between the different kinds of loyalty that medical scientists are supposed to cultivate. Obviously the obligations towards individual patients should predominate in such instances. In terms of the Declaration of Helsinki: "Concern for the interest of the subject must always prevail over the interests of science and society" [1,2]. The ethical aspects of research in neurology in no way differ from those in most other branches of medicine.

The Uncertainty Principle

The prime interest of physician-scientists must lie with their patients' health and well-being. Accordingly, the motive for starting a therapeutic trial should be genuine uncertainty: sincere doubt whether treatment regimen X is better or worse than no treatment (if there is no treatment of proven efficacy), or better than regimen Y (if some treatment is of proven value but less than ideal). Such doubts should have their origin not only in intuitive scepticism, but should preferably be backed up by a formal meta-analysis of the existing evidence. It follows from this principle of uncertainty that physicians with strong beliefs (founded or unfounded) are excluded from participating in clinical trials in which a favourite belief is at stake. Nevertheless, having strong but unfounded beliefs in medicine may be considered unethical in itself. To illustrate the limitations of medical reasoning it is not neces-

sary to go back to enemas and leeches. Within our lifetime, patients have been infected with malaria to cure neurosyphilis, have been treated with X-rays for sciatica, and have had their internal mammary artery ligated to improve blood flow to the heart and alleviate the symptoms of angina; up to the present day patients with severe head injury are subjected to profound hyperventilation in intensive care units to bring the intracerebral pressure down at the expense of what little perfusion of the brain is left. Theories are there to be put to the test, but dogmatists cling to their deductive theories and act on them; only when a theory has been proved ostentatiously wrong (by others, necessarily) do they desert it. Some will have learned from the experience and be converted to doubt and empiricism, others will immediately embrace the next theory. No one has said it better than William Cowper (1731–1800):

> Knowledge and wisdom, far from being one,
> Have oft-times no connexion. Knowledge dwells
> In heads replete with thoughts of other men;
> Wisdom in minds attentive of their own.
> Knowledge is proud that he has learned so much;
> Wisdom is humble that he knows no more.

"Wisdom" or uncertainty does not always come naturally to physicians; in many cases the seed of doubt has to be sown across a continent before a trial gets off the ground – as C.P. Warlow did for trials of carotid endarterectomy [3].

In clinical reality the uncertainty relates to a defined type of patient with a particular health problem. The next step is meticulously working out the design of the study. In fact an improper design generating flawed results can also be considered unethical, as useless information is produced and resources, time, effort and possibly patient benefit is wasted.

Informed Consent

Before being invited to participate in a study the potential subjects need to be extensively informed about the fundamental question they are about to be asked. In order to be able to decide whether the procedure or medication under trial would merit being tested on themselves subjects must be able to weigh potential drawbacks and benefits. Initially an oral explanation by the trial physician should be provided. In addition the subjects should at least be provided with written explanation of the research question and the potential discomfort, risks and gain. Also, the entirely voluntary nature of participation must be stressed, as well as the fact that subjects will receive the currently accepted alternative treatment if they decided not to participate or later to drop out of the trial for whatever reason. This in fact is conveyed in the Helsinki Declaration, which specifies that patients "must be adequately informed of the aims, methods, anticipated benefits, and potential hazards of the study and the discomfort it may entail" [4].

Physician-investigators may feel uncomfortable with this obligation. In a survey covering eight Western countries 22% of physicians indicated that they never asked for informed consent when entering patients in a clinical study, and many also doubt whether patients really want to be fully informed about their disease, treatment and study procedures, and whether patients sufficiently understand the information [5]. Indeed, fears that patients have difficulty with the information provided in consent procedures have repeatedly been shown to be justified. In one example, in which 81 patients were interviewed some 18 months, on average, after having consented to participate in a trial comparing two doses of aspirin in the secondary prevention of stroke, 12% did not know they were in a study, 8% thought participation was compulsory, and 27% were uncertain whether they could withdraw from the study [6]. On the other hand, the public attitude towards clinical trials and participation in such studies is very positive [7], the patients' altruistic motives are high, and well-informed patients often feel that the additional medical monitoring, the opportunity for a second opinion, and reassurance are more important benefits than the actual improvement in health [8]. It is the task of the investigators to optimise the procedures for informing patients, including the provision of written information. The text should consist of short sentences, short words, and concepts that average readers will understand [9]. Testing of written information in a sample of lay-persons before actual application in clinical research is advisable. Also, once patients have been enrolled, the investigators should check whether potential subjects have understood the information provided. If necessary, additional explanation and reworded repetition of information should be provided. Then and only then can actual informed consent be obtained and confirmed by a written agreement.

In this regard a potential problem in some neurological disorders may be that eligible candidates are unable to give informed consent as a result of the condition the trial addresses. For instance, patients having suffered a stroke or subarachnoid haemorrhage may in the acute phase be unconscious. In addition, or in a later phase, they may be cognitively impaired or aphasic. This problem is not specific for patients with neurological disorders. A great number of diseases may involve loss of consciousness or involve patients that can not be considered responsible for their actions or decisions. For instance, in paediatrics or psychiatry comparable problems of competence occur. Roth et al. [10] assessed the ability of depressed patients to decide on application of ECT and found that approximately 1 in 4 may be considered incompetent. Surrogate or proxy consent by relatives, knowledgeable colleagues or expert committees may solve part of the problem but raises ethical issues about autonomy and confidentiality. Also, obtaining surrogate consent may cause a delay in treatment and thereby induce more extensive harm. Regrettably, no simple solution is available [11]. Still, depending on the disorder of interest, the type of intervention under investigation, and local or national ethical and legal standards, a solution has to be found for subjects eligible but possibly incompetent.

Control Treatment

A problem of an entirely different order yet with ethical implications is the control treatment applied. It is a fallacious notion that all controlled trials need to be placebo-controlled. The experimental treatment should be compared with standard treatment, according to the current state-of-the art treatment. No one would dare to propose a trial of a new antibiotic against placebo, instead of against the currently established drug. For the same reason it is unethical to test drugs for the secondary prevention of stroke against placebo in the 1990s, given the proven efficacy of aspirin [12]. By the same token, it is irrational for those who were among the first to prove this to castigate later trialists that their studies were not placebo-controlled! The misunderstanding about the need for placebo has to do with the difference between pragmatic and explanatory trials [13]. The aim of an explanatory trial is to study a biological effect in its own right, which implies placebo treatment in the control group (also there are other consequences such as exclusion of incompletely treated subjects). But explanatory trials are not always relevant to clinical practice. For clinical practice the study setting should be that of the "real world", in which some drugs for the disease in question may already exist (and in which diagnosis and drug administration may be imperfect).

Responsibility for Trial Conduct

The actual daily conduct of a trial also has ethical implications. Though sponsors derive certain rights from their investments this does not include the right to exclude clinicians from core activities that should guarantee the quality and credibility of the trial. Not only drawing up the protocol but also storage of the data, planning of interim analyses, and prior definition of subgroups are grave responsibilities that should be shared between sponsor and participants. This shared responsibility should be reflected in the creation of a single steering committee as the highest authority of the study, a body in which all parties are represented. The selection of clinicians in the steering committee should be made by the participants, and not by the sponsoring company.

In this day and age it is unacceptable for responsible clinicians to be confronted by changes in the protocol or interim analyses which have been initiated almost entirely by the company in question, without involvement of an independent steering committee in which the participating physicians are represented. It is not sufficient for the company to appoint one or two clinicians only to keep up appearances while the operation of the trial remains hidden from the participants to such an extent that great damage is done to the reputation of the trial as well as of the physicians at the masthead. At medical conferences one may still be embarrassed by a colleague presenting an ostensibly poor trial where scientific independence has been sacrificed to other interests.

Similarly, trial forms should be sent for checking and inclusion in the data base not to the sponsoring company, but to an independent office, run under the direction of one of the clinical participants or of an epidemiologist – provided the people involved have a good track record in independent research. It has been rightly argued that the group responsible for data collection and analysis should be financially independent from the results of the trial [14].

Interim Analyses and Stopping Rules

One specific problem under the responsibility of the steering committee is dealing with evidence becoming available before the anticipated number of subjects has been included. Obviously, continuation of a trial can not be considered ethical in the case where a clear and highly significant result has emerged. Premature termination of a trial is a topical subject, given the recent fate of several trials of thrombolytic agents after acute stroke [15]. Serving the patients' best interest requires that a treatment is no longer continued after it has been proven definitely harmful or, conversely, definitely beneficial. Interim analyses are therefore clearly required, but the problem is the definition of "definite". In this way ethical principles are converted into statistical problems: the patients' best interests also require that random variations or inappropriate subgroup analyses (such as myocardial infarction only or stroke only or other non-fatal events only) lead to premature conclusions. In general, the thresholds at which differences are regarded as sufficiently large to stop a trial should be asymmetrical, that is, lower for adverse effects (safety aspects) than for beneficial effects (efficacy); for efficacy the thresholds for statistical significance are set higher in interim analyses than at the predetermined end of a study, and again higher at each subsequent analysis. Usually interim analyses are performed at fixed intervals that have been defined in advance, but techniques exist also for sequential analysis [16]. Although performed under the responsibility of the steering committee, interim analyses should preferably be executed and, in case of conclusive results, co-reported by an independent body to ascertain unbiased decisions.

Reporting of Results

As is the case in unexpected results detected at interim analysis, unexpected or unwelcome end results should nevertheless be reported. If the result of a trial is disappointing, investigators and especially sponsoring companies may be tempted to bury the entire project in a drawer and try to forget about it, so that at least other physicians' hopes are kept alive. It hardly needs to be emphasised that ethical obligations towards the patients who took part in the negative trial as well as towards society in general make it mandatory to report the results or at least to make them available to all interested parties, especially to meta-analysts.

Also, trial reports should honestly include every relevant error, however embarrassing. Mistakes are likely to occur in studies with large numbers of patients, especially if many different centres are involved: erroneous diagnoses (most trials of patients with presumed transient ischaemic attacks (TIAs) have inadvertently included subjects with brain tumour, multiple sclerosis, myasthenia gravis, etc.), or silly mistakes (in the Dutch TIA trial the compound calcium carbasalate was supposed to be equivalent to 300 mg of acetylsalicylic acid, but the precise quantity turned out to be 283 mg) [17], or a few patients in a placebo group getting the active drug because the nursing staff administered not the trial medication but proprietary drugs from the hospital pharmacy [18].

A further point of concern in reporting may be that trials are usually undertaken because the organisers strongly believe the treatment under study might represent an important therapeutic advance. This may lead investigators to put a greater emphasis on positive findings than is actually justified. If the primary analysis outlined in the study protocol fails to show a statistically significant advantage for the experimental treatment, investigators may be tempted to deviate from the path chosen before the results are known and to try alternative routes, in a desperate search to confirm the original hypothesis. The most serious flaw is to limit the analysis to certain subgroups in terms of baseline characteristics that differ from those in the original hypothesis [19]. Another method of "data dredging" is to limit the analysis to certain outcome events, with exclusion of other events that were specified in the original protocol. In the Dutch TIA trial, we could have claimed a statistically significant advantage for 30 mg of aspirin over 283 mg in the secondary prevention of stroke (in terms of hazard ratio, adjusted for baseline imbalances) if the primary outcome event had been stroke alone (fatal or non-fatal) [17]. Such findings are hypothesis-generating only and should not be confused with conclusive research evidence. Also with respect to secondary analyses data-ownership merits further attention. Even if the expenses of a trial have been funded by a pharmaceutical company, the steering committee should insist that the definitive trial data are eventually retained by the investigators – for preliminary testing of new questions that come up, or for inclusion in formal meta-analyses as carried out by the Cochrane Collaboration [20]. Institutions such as the Medical Research Council or the Dutch Heart Fund have never claimed exclusive ownership of trials financed by their grants. Although the interests of drug firms are clearly different it should be considered unethical if clinicians agree to contracts by which trial data are kept locked away, outside the domain of the scientific community.

Quality Control

One may wonder briefly what validity and the instrument of quality control to assess validity has to do with ethics in trials in progress. We feel impelled, however, to note the naivety if not gullibility of many practising clinicians (the "consumers" of trials) to have instinctive confidence in the integrity of the trial organisers and participants. Regrettably human nature is not always impervious to the great financial interests that may be at stake. In the US, the Food and Drug Administration (FDA) performs routine checks on clinical investigators of new drugs. In the course of these regulatory activities some appalling examples of scientific misconduct have been uncovered. An obstetrician gave false information about having used a particular analgesic during delivery, a psychiatrist with a good reputation for his prompt reporting of the results of antidepressants was found in a completely empty office, a rheumatologist supplied faked laboratory results, a neurologist was found to have submitted identical reports about patients with Parkinson's disease in two different studies, with two different sponsors, and a cardiologist involved in a study of a drug for congestive heart failure changed the radiologist's report about chest radiographs so that the drug would seem more effective [21]. This list of forgeries is far from exhaustive, and can be extended with many examples in another category, where investigators were not outright dishonest but definitely careless.

It is a disturbing thought that in Europe many national licensing bodies take a rather cavalier attitude towards the conduct of clinical investigations. While critique is sometimes levelled at the interpretation of trial results, the results themselves are often accepted on trust, even if the potential market for the new drug in question is vast and huge profits are at stake. Things may be on the mend by directives from Brussels, but it will be a long time before all European countries have reached the required level of quality control. It is honourable but slightly naive to have so much faith in people's morals when the enticements are so great. At any rate quality control helps clinicians to remain ethical.

Financial Reimbursement

If a trial is sponsored by a pharmaceutical company, it may be in order for clinicians to be reimbursed for the time they invest and the expenses they incur in entering patients in the trial. An ethical problem arises, however. Entering patients into a sponsored trial is much more profitable per unit of time than seeing patients, teaching – or entering patients into a non-commercial trial! Current medical practice is still replete with treatment regimens inherited from the pre-trial era, and present generations have to work their way through a backlog of trials that would have been done decades ago had the appropriate methodology and insight been available. Recent examples of such "catching-up trials" where financial incentives are either lacking or limited to insurers are the benefits of carotid endarterectomy [22], or of anticoagulant treatment in patients with atrial fibrillation and a TIA or non-disabling ischaemic stroke [23]. Things are hardly made easier if the money does not go to the doctor's own pocket but to the departmental research fund, as is often the case. The success of a clinical department, particularly in a university hospital, is intricately linked with tangible and intangible gains of the persons involved: tenure, promotion, and the esteem of one's colleagues. In those cases an impartial outsider might wonder whether the attempt to obtain the patient's consent is really as dispassionate and harmless as it should be.

The choice of clinicians about which clinical trials they wish to join should be motivated not by worries about where to find next year's salaries for their data managers or trusted colleagues, or how to fund the type of research they really want to do [24]. Rather, such decisions should have to do with how burning the issue under investigation is, from the perspective of health care, science, or both. Over-payment may therefore be unethical.

Outcome Variables and Scales

However well designed and ethically well thought out, any result obtained in (clinical) research needs to be considered from the perspective of future patients. Accordingly, the effect of the proposed intervention should be relevant to patients. How then should effect be measured? What outcome is relevant and from which or whose perspective?

Assessing how individual patients are doing is not at all unusual for the neurologist, because this is the basis of day-to-day management: the patient with a ruptured aneurysm who becomes drowsy and hemiplegic probably suffers from delayed ischaemia and is a candidate for hypervolaemic treatment; the myasthenic patient who cannot chew or articulate properly may again improve after an increase in the dose of cholinesterase inhibitors; the patient with Parkinson's disease who starts needing help with dressing and bathing may require more levodopa or the addition of another drug; the patient with multiple sclerosis who has difficulty getting on buses might be advised to apply for a private parking space; and the octogenarian with a large hemispheric infarct who has been refusing food for several days deserves reconsideration of his antibiotic drug regimen.

Despite the familiarity of such assessments, many neurologists are not aware that the examples given

Table 3.1. Levels of assessment of outcome

I	The disease process (occurrence of biological events)
II	Impairments (performance at the level of the organ)
III	Disability (performance at the level of the person)
IV	Handicap (performance at individual and social level)
V	Quality of life (subjective well being)

above represent different levels of measurement (Table 1) [25,26], the *disease process* (ischaemia after subarachnoid haemorrhage), specific *impairments* from the clinical manifestations of disease (difficulty with chewing in myasthenia gravis), the patient's *disability* in daily living (the patient with Parkinson's disease who cannot bathe or dress without the help of others), *handicap* if the disease interferes with the patient's social roles (the patient with multiple sclerosis who no longer manages the use of public transport), and finally *quality of life* (the aged and unhappy stroke victim).

The boundaries between these five levels of measurement are not always sharp; together they represent a continuum in which the disease can be viewed in a wider or narrower perspective, as though through an imaginary bird's eye. At first the observer's position is quite nearby, with a view of the disease process but not of the patient, then at slightly greater distance, which allows assessment of the effects of the disease at the level of the organ, with disturbance of one or more specific functions (impairments), then from still greater distance at the level of the person (disability), then, as though seated on a tree nearby, that of the patient in the context of his environment (handicap), and finally, the most distant or intangible view, where facts no longer count but only the patient's feelings (quality of life).

Below we shall elaborate on these five levels of measurement and some specific instruments in detail. Particularly when groups of patients are studied, in clinical trials of treatment but also in analyses of prognostic factors, it is essential that the level chosen for the measurement of outcome does not have too narrow a view for the purpose of the study; otherwise the results may well be difficult to apply to real life.

The Disease Process: Choosing Outcome Events

Some clinical trials of stroke prevention (a field from which many of our examples come) have included transient ischaemic attacks (TIAs) as an outcome event [27], because this would indicate that the disease process is still unstable. A practical difficulty with TIAs is that these are difficult to define, but a much more fundamental problem is that TIAs do not affect patient's lives other than by causing some additional worry. For that reason, events such as TIAs are appropriate measures of outcome only in the early phases of pharmacological research, where the influence of the drug on the disease process is the actual purpose of the study. But TIAs are irrelevant as measures of outcome in studies addressing the question whether some mode of treatment should be applied in clinical practice.

Another fundamental problem with counting events is that there is usually more to a disease process than whether or not a specific event occurs. Imagine that one is embarking on a trial of a new pharmacological agent to prevent rebleeding after subarachnoid haemorrhage. The obvious measure of outcome in a clinical trial of this drug would be the incidence of rebleeding. But on reflection there are several problems with this approach. The first problem is that patients may suffer more than one rebleed, and that three rebleeds in one patient is not the same thing as one rebleed in three patients. Second, a disease process may be complicated by different kinds of events; after subarachnoid haemorrhage, for instance, not only rebleeds may occur but also ischaemia or hydrocephalus. In fact, one previous trial with antifibrinolytic drugs would have shown a spectacular result if the analysis had been restricted to rebleeding, but these benefits were completely offset by an increase in the incidence of ischaemic complications [18].

Finally, the patient may die from events other than the one under consideration. The intercurrent disease may not be directly related to the primary question, but on the other hand one can hardly dismiss a death as irrelevant. The Canadian trial of aspirin (and sulphinpyrazone) in the prevention of threatened stroke evoked much discussion at the time (1978) because it included not only stroke but also death as a primary outcome event [28]. Meanwhile it has become generally accepted that most deaths in patients with TIAs are caused by ischaemic heart disease, and also that neurologists treat patients rather than brains.

It is particularly in trials of cardiovascular disease that combinations of the most relevant events are chosen as the primary measure of outcome. In stroke prevention trials, for instance, increasing use is made of the composite endpoint "vascular death, stroke or myocardial infarction" [12,29]. Other deaths, however, always have to be specified; after all, the treatment under study may have unexpected side effects.

There are two points of view that argue in favour of always including death, or at least vascular death, in a composite measure with non-fatal events. The first and most important is that of the patient, for whom it counts not only to avoid having a stroke, but also to stay alive. Otherwise a therapy that kills patients before they have had a chance to have a stroke could appear to be beneficial [30]. The second point of view is that of pathophysiology: ischaemic heart disease is undoubtedly the leading cause of death in patients with transient or non-disabling cerebral ischaemia [31], and trial drugs aimed at the prevention of stroke may affect fatal atherothrombosis in the coronary vessels differently from non-fatal embolisation in the cerebral vasculature. In addition these drugs might cause not only haemorrhages but also unexpected complications in other organ systems. Nowadays there is no justification for looking at non-fatal events in isolation.

Although the fact of death is more important than its cause [30], it often remains desirable to classify death, in order to understand the effect of the treatment that is being tested. One way of doing this is to distinguish cerebral deaths and cardiac deaths (and other deaths); non-fatal events can be added for the comparison of all cerebral events or all cardiac events between the treatment groups. Another possibility is to analyse vascular death rather than death from all causes. One should of course first make sure that the rate of non-vascular death is similar across the treatment groups, in order not to overlook iatrogenic adverse effects, teratogenic or other. If this condition is fulfilled, or if one is certain that any difference is the result of chance, the removal of this "noise" from the analysis of deaths makes the comparison more sensitive. For instance, if there are 1000 patients in each of two treatment groups a difference between 35 deaths in the experimental group and 50 in the control group is not statistically significant (relative risk 0.70, 95% confidence interval 0.46–1.07), whereas subtraction of 20 non-vascular deaths from both groups leaves 15 vascular deaths in the experimental group and 30 in the control group, and this difference does reach statistical significance (relative risk 0.50, 95% confidence interval 0.27–0.92). Note, however, that in view of the danger of random hits from multiple analyses the choice between the primary and secondary methods of analysis should be made in advance.

Assigning specific causes to deaths may turn out to be more difficult than one might anticipate. If a patient suffers a stroke, remains bedridden and dies 3 weeks later from an infection, most trialists would regard this as death caused by stroke, despite the terminal disease being an infectious complication. But what if the interval is not 3 weeks but 9 months, while the patient has also been completely dependent in the mean time? An arbitrary time limit is a possible but probably not the best solution to this problem. The most sensible view to be adopted by members of the auditing committee is to consider whether such an event of death would be likely to have occurred if there had been no previous stroke. A second problem is what to include under the heading of vascular death. Congestive heart failure and massive haemorrhage from a ruptured aneurysm of the abdominal aorta can reasonably be regarded as such, but some would feel differently about fatal pulmonary embolism or about fatal gastrointestinal haemorrhage. In those cases it might be argued that it is arterial disease rather than vascular disease in general that is most naturally related with stroke and stroke prevention.

"Sudden death", with the implication of ischaemic heart disease and subsequent dysrhythmia, is included as one of the categories of vascular death. By convention it is regarded certain when natural death occurred within 1 hour of the onset of symptoms, and probable when the victim has been seen to be well within the preceding 24 hours [32]. Nevertheless, death from stroke may occur in a matter of hours [33], and if a patient is found dead several days after having last been seen in his or her normal state there are, of course, many other explanations. Some degree of misclassification has to be accepted, but all available evidence should be collected before submission to the members of the auditing committee of the trial.

A problem of yet another category are patients who have suffered more than one event. A feasible solution would be to include either the first or the worst event; in time-dependent analyses (survival curves) the first event is most often chosen. Even with a meticulous account of all deaths and relevant events in a clinical trial, it is desirable to supplement these results with a global measure of the patient's condition [17].

The Disease Process: Distinguishing Outcome Events

Most clinical features of disease can be measured and quantified, though a particular measure should not be recommended unless validity and reliability have been scrutinised. Stroke, for instance, may seem a simple diagnosis but can still yield considerable difficulty if further specification is required. In the mind of steering committees who write trial protocols it is easy to draw a picture of an ideal world, in which every patient in the trial pays regular visits to the neurologist and in case of symptoms immediately presents to hospital for a full investigation, including a computed tomography (CT) scan. But real life can

be quite different. One example is that of an eldely woman who enters a drug trial with a non-disabling right hemiparesis from a small capsular infarct, agrees to participate in the trial but subsequently declines further visits to hospital. She receives the trial drugs from her general physician, and on one of the follow-up visits, about a year later, she complains that the right leg has been weaker for a week or so, and that this limits her walking; her doctor confirms that she seems to drag the leg more than she used to, and reports this on the form sent to him from the trial office. Should this be judged a stroke? Another difficult decision is the terminal illness of an old man who was randomised into a medical trial after a left-sided hemiparesis of about 2 hours' duration; he was already handicapped by osteoarthritis of the hip joints and when his wife suddenly died he could no longer live on his own and was transferred to a nursing home. There he also seemed depressed and he hardly moved from his chair during the daytime. One day he felt unable to get up because of a headache and difficulty in breathing; he vomited once. In the course of that day he became more and more drowsy and also dyspnoeic; one of the nurses thought he moved his left arm less than the right one. The next morning he was found dead.

Fortunately such mysterious events are exceptional, but they do occur. As decisions based on a limited amount of information are bound to be arbitrary it is best to invoke the wisdom of more than one person, in that at least three members of the "auditing committee" give their independent opinion in writing. Before this procedure is started, it is important to collect every scrap of evidence available; diagnoses of general practitioners on death certificates should not be taken for more than an educated guess, nursing reports are much more helpful, and an eyewitness account from a relative is invaluable. In order to obtain this kind of information and also to keep track of patients in general it is very helpful to include an entry in the notification form about the address and telephone number of a relative who can be expected to follow the patient's whereabouts (but does not live in the same house, otherwise in case of the patient moving house the informant disappears at the same time). The final decision about difficult outcome events is often based on a majority vote, on review of the different opinions by the "executive committee" responsible for the day-to-day running of the trial (provided they are still blinded to the treatment allocation).

The pathology of the disease under study may also be important. From the patient's perspective – which should be adopted first in any trial aimed at finding the optimal treatment in clinical practice – a stroke is an unqualified disaster, and it does not then matter a great deal whether a stroke is haemorrhagic or ischaemic and in what part of the brain the lesion is. From the clinical scientist's perspective, however, these distinctions can be useful because the treatment under study may affect the risk of stroke in different ways, dependent on the type of stroke. Antithrombotic treatment but also carotid endarterectomy or extracranial–intracranial bypass surgery are examples of treatments that may prevent ischaemic stroke at the expense of an increased number of intracranial haemorrhages, and for a proper assessment of the balance of risks these two types of stroke need to be distinguished. Moreover, different subtypes of ischaemic stroke may or may not be prevented by the treatment under study. For instance, it is implausible that carotid endarterectomy would alter the risk of infarction in the contralateral hemisphere, in the occipital lobes or the posterior fossa, or even the risk of lacunar infarction in the deep regions of the hemisphere in question. And medical treatment should not too readily be expected to affect the risk of lacunar infarction and cortical infarction in exactly the same fashion, as the process of atherosclerosis and subsequent thrombosis or embolism may evolve differently in small perforating vessels and in large extracranial arteries.

Ideally, the results of stroke trials should provide both practical guidelines, which can be applied directly in clinical practice, and an improvement in our understanding of the pathophysiology of stroke, which can be incorporated into the design of new trials, years later. These two perspectives have been termed "pragmatic" and "explanatory" by Schwartz and Lellouch [13], and it should be emphasised that this distinction affects many aspects of trial design other than the assessment of outcome. In case of a conflict of interest, the primary and secondary aims of a study should be clearly distinguished, also in the choice of measures of outcome: a "pragmatic" trial without CT scanning is better than no trial at all. Conversely, if the crucial question is "explanatory", that is, whether the treatment under study has any biological effect at all, one may choose to select a specific subtype of stroke and even to ignore whether or not the individual patient benefits, as long as the temptation is resisted to extrapolate the results of such a study to the consulting room.

Impairments

The next step in the spectrum of outcome measures is the effect the condition has on patients. By convention, any neurological deficit of focal nature and sudden onset that lasts longer than 24 hours is classified as a stroke, but this term encompasses a vast

spectrum of severity, ranging from, for instance, a clumsy hand and wry mouth recovering within 2 weeks at one end and a bedridden existence with a dense hemiplegia, global aphasia and loss of initiative on the other. A treatment that would change future (or present) strokes from big to small ones would still be worthwhile, and from the very beginning of stroke research the need has been felt to quantify the severity of strokes. The clinical impact of a stroke is, not surprisingly, related to the amount of brain tissue lost [34], but quite apart from practical problems with CT scanning the complex balance between functional differentiation and the capacities for compensation within the brain make it mandatory to assess primarily the patient and not the CT scan after a stroke. A similar need to measure the severity of stroke by clinical means exists in the case of trials of treatment immediately after the stroke has occurred, whether the measurement is performed in the first few days or in the stage of rehabilitation.

Scales have been designed for measuring tremor, aphasia, muscle power, intellectual performance, and many other specific functions that can be disturbed by disease. Doctors are often attracted to this kind of measurement, because the grades of these scales seem to lend some kind of objectivity to clinical impressions. In an attempt to overcome the limitations of measuring only a single function, many groups of researchers have developed composite scales, in which many different impairments have been incorporated. Such composite scales exist for Parkinson's disease, motor neurone disease, multiple sclerosis, brain infarction, and many other diseases – up to cerebral vein thrombosis! The neurologists who have designed or used these scales assume that the sum of all the separate elements in the scale will add up to a meaningful picture of the patient as a whole. Regrettably, this assumption is incorrect.

The first problem with disease-specific scales is the choice of the separate elements. Many scales ignore important aspects. For instance, no scale for Parkinson's disease includes the factor pain, because "officially" this is purely a disorder of the motor system; yet pain can be very troublesome in Parkinson's disease. On the other hand, disease scales often include some elements of the neurological examination that are quite useful for localising a lesion in the nervous system but that are completely irrelevant from the patient's point of view, such as Babinski signs, muscle rigidity or fasciculations.

The most serious deficiency of composite scales for specific diseases is that the scores for separate functions can never add up to something meaningful [35]. Weighting of different items is a futile attempt to solve this problem, because overall performance results from a complex interaction between different "functions". Not the least of this is intellectual function, which is grossly neglected in many scales of neurological disease, whereas motor aspects are overrated. Everyday life consists of a multitude of tasks that are integrated and difficult to separate. This applies to something as seemingly trivial as putting the waste bags on the pavement to be collected, which requires an adequate memory to do it on the right day of the week, the dexterity and visuospatial ability to tie the tops with small pieces of wire, and the power and balance to carry the sacks outside. It would require extensive neurological and neuropsychological testing to assess all the separate aspects of brain function involved in this simple act.

Again, as with assessing outcome on the basis of specific events, quantification of separate functions can be useful in the early stages of research, when the question is whether a particular mode of treatment has any biological effect at all [13]. For instance, if some imaginary new drug might favourably influence the muscle defect in Duchenne muscular dystrophy, it is reasonable to start by studying the effects on the power of one particular muscle. But when the question is whether the drug should be given to all patients with the disease the measure of outcome should at least include disability, and preferably handicap. In short, the patient is more than the sum of his or her signs [35]. A higher, more integrated level of measurement is needed, that is, scales should measure function not at the level of the organ (impairments) but at the level of the person (disability scales), or even at the level of social interaction (handicap scales) [36]. What really counts for patients is what they can do in life, compared with what they want to do, or were once able to do.

Many pharmaceutical companies are fond of outcome measures at a low level of integration; though these are of little relevance to the patient, they are objective, they can be quantified and even with small trials they lend themselves to statistical massage from which some significant advantage can be made to emerge. Not all licensing bodies are equally quick in perceiving how completely meaningless these calculations are. In many Western countries drugs have been licensed merely on the basis of effects on specific functions, or with even less reliable evidence, of effects on MRI scans (beta interferon in multiple sclerosis!), laboratory animals, or cell cultures. The FDA has now firmly and sensibly taken the position that new drugs for neurological diseases are allowed only if an effect on disability has been demonstrated.

Disability

Disability, according to the international classification of the World Health Organization [26], represents function at the level of the person; it is "the restriction or lack (resulting from an impairment) of the ability to perform tasks, within the physical and social environment". A great advantage of disability scales is that these integrate not only different impairments but also different diseases; it is often thought that this generalisability is at the cost of sensitivity, but with a sufficient number of patients a simple scale with a few meaningful categories may suffice.

Most disability scales measure essential tasks in activities of daily living (ADL), such as toilet use, walking, dressing and managing stairs. The large number of existing ADL scales indicates that this level of measurement has its own difficulties, but the Barthel index is the most widely used, and it has proved reliable on repeated testing [37,38]. The scale is hierarchical, in the sense that an ascending order of difficulty can be attributed to the activities listed, from bowel continence to taking a bath [39]. Cultural differences may interfere with this fixed order. For instance, bathing is relatively easy in the United States, because this means taking a shower rather than immersing oneself in a tub from the neck down. In Japan feeding oneself is the easiest activity instead of being moderately difficult, because this involves picking up pieces of meat without the necessity of cutting it [40].

Yet there is more to life than getting into the bath on one's own. A further disadvantage of ADL scales is that these measure only what patients can do, and not what they actually do do when left to care for themselves. The true degree of independence is more accurately reflected by scales that do not specify separate tasks, such as the Rankin scale, the Glasgow Outcome Scale and the Karnofsky Index. Some have called this type of scales performance scales, as opposed to capacity scales [41]. The Karnofsky Index proved disappointing in a study of interobserver variability [42], whereas the Rankin scale stood up rather well to such a test [43]. In its original form the Rankin scale contained the term "walking" and was therefore something of a hybrid with ADL scales, but this has been remedied in a recent modification named the Oxford Handicap Scale (Table 2) [44].

Although some of the elements of this scale indeed refer to social roles ("lifestyle") or even to quality of life (symptoms without impairment or disability), the emphasis is on (in)dependence and it should perhaps more appropriately be classified among the disability scales. Some other performance scales

Table 3.2. Oxford Handicap Scale [44]

Grade	Description (abridged)
0	No symptoms
1	Only symptoms
2	Some restriction of lifestyle, but independent
3	Partly dependent
4	Dependent, but no constant attention required
5	Fully dependent

also overlap with the measurement of handicap because they refer to work (Karnofsky Index) or to other social interactions (Frenchay Activities Index and Nottingham extended ADL Index). The Glasgow Outcome Scale is more exclusively concerned with (in)dependence [45], and is reasonably reliable [46]. A great advantage of performance scales in multi-centre trials is that these can be applied without the patient being examined or even seen; interviews by telephone proved satisfactory in one study [47], and probably even postal questionnaires can be used.

Handicap and "Quality of Life"

Impairment, although often less relevant from the patient's point of view, can be assessed more or less objectively. Measuring handicap, however, entails considerable difficulties. Handicap represents the social consequences of impairment and disability, in the domains of, for instance, family relationships, sexual relations, occupation and economic independence, social contacts outside the family circle, and leisure activities. Obviously all these dimensions are very relevant to the patient. Yet, interpreting and measuring them is rather subjective, depending on personal and socio-cultural standards. Many of the dimensions of handicap have been listed in the classification of the World Health Organization [26]. An instrument which incorporates many of these domains may be the Level of Rehabilitation Scale (LORS) [48]. Subscales for five domains – ADL, cognition, home activities, outside activities and social interaction – are included. A new version has subsequently been developed (LORS-II) [49]. On the whole, the measurement of handicap has been less well conceptualised and tested than that of impairments or disabilities. The most comprehensive and at the same time most subjective measure of outcome is quality of life. It refers to a person's sense of well-being and life satisfaction, and includes all physical, social and emotional domains of life. At this level of measurement it is the patient and no longer the doctor who determines to what extent the disease

interferes with the desired lifestyle. Oncologists have been leading this field of research, because they are continuously confronted by the question at what cost prolongation of life should be obtained [50]. Quality of life depends on many more factors than those determining disability or handicap, for instance the coping behaviour of the patient. This explains why a careful study about the quality of life of patients in a wheelchair failed to detect marked differences with ambulant controls [51]. Measuring quality of life as the ultimate index of medical interventions is obviously even more difficult than measuring handicap. Several instruments have, however, been developed. Quality of life has been measured by means of extensive questionnaires such as the Sickness Impact Profile or the Nottingham Health Profile [52,53], or something as simple as a visual analogue scale [54].

If quality of life is measured separately for different domains of life [55], the difficulty of weighting these components looms again. Some attempts have been made though, yielding one overall dimensionless measure of quality of life – a so-called utility. Initially, specific interview techniques have been developed. For instance, standard gamble, allowing subjects to choose between a certain sub-optimal outcome and a two-way chance outcome of either perfect health or death supposedly yields the utility of the sub-optimal outcome at the point (or chance) where subjects are indifferent between the two options. [56,57]. Time trade-off is a comparable technique allowing subjects to choose between life in a certain period of time in a particular sub-optimal state of health and life in a shorter period of time in optimal health. Again at the point of indifference the ratio of the two periods (short – "optimal"/long – "sub-optimal") yields the utility of life in the sub-optimal state of health [58]. In addition written questionnaires are currently available to assess the utility of outcome. The Health Utility Index and the EuroQol questionnaire are examples of instruments designed to provide a single numerical index of outcome [57,59]. Usually a fraction between 0, as the worst possible state (death), and 1, as optimal state, is generated by means of a specific algorithm. This fraction may be perceived as a general weight of the time alive in a certain state of health, thus yielding quality adjusted survival time – so-called Quality Adjusted Life Years (QALY). However, some outcomes may be perceived as worse than death. This would yield a negative utility. As one might anticipate, there are many other pitfalls [60].

So far quality of life has not been extensively studied in patients with stroke or other diseases of the brain. A specific problem in these patients is that to obtain a subjective judgement about the predicament of disease may be difficult or even impossible because of aphasia or dementia, and even in the remaining patients the perception of their own condition may differ from what they would have thought of it with an intact brain.

General Comments

The Choice of the Measure of Outcome

No single instrument or scale is perfect. Varying perspectives – recall the bird's eye – imply that often a compromise will have to be made between objectivity and relevance; availability of a validated version in the national language and applicability in the patients and/or disease under study are important factors determining the choice.

In general the solution lies in combining several instruments or questionnaires to assess outcome in all relevant domains. Well-known clinical measures of the disease process do not require an additional explanation. However, to measure the disability caused by the disease process a specific instrument has to be used. Similarly, handicap and quality of life can be assessed by means of specific instruments. Particular disease-specific instruments will accurately indicate the impact of disease on relevant (sub)domains, whereas generic instruments yield less detailed information about several domains. In that sense the instruments generating utility as outcome are also generic instruments. In principle, such generic measures allow comparison of the impact of disease across various disorders because a dimensionless utility is generated.

In conclusion, measuring health-related quality of life usually implies applying a generic instrument to assess the integrated impact of disease in all domains, applying a disease-specific instrument to assess the impact of disease in more detail, and finally an additional generic instrument with utility as outcome.

Statistics with Scales

If the main measure of outcome in a study is some kind of scale, it invariably involves an assortment of categories or subcategories, which are designated by numbers. This use of numbers rather than letters or other hierarchical symbols reflects the desire of doctors to convert the complexities of disease into a limited number of grades in an ordered system. But the dangerous pitfall to be avoided with these numbers is to treat them statistically as though they represented true values. That assumption is valid only for so-called interval scales, on which each cat-

egory differs as much from the previous as from the following step. A good example is a tape measure, on which, for instance, 10 cm truly represents twice as much length as 5 cm. In contrast, categories in the hierarchical rating systems used in medicine form so-called ordinal scales, in which the numbers indicate classes, with distances of unequal magnitude between the different steps. Examples of ordinal scales are the Beaufort scale for wind force, in which grade 10 (gale) is many times more powerful in a physical sense than a fresh breeze of wind force 5 [61], and the Glasgow Coma Scale (GCS) [62], in which a patient who swears, localises and opens his eyes to painful stimulation (GCS of 10) cannot be said to be twice as awake as someone with a GCS of 5, who does not open his eyes, does not make a sound and only flexes the arm to pain.

Yet, many doctors are so eager to exchange the disorderly characteristics of neurological illness for neat figures and are at the same time so poorly trained in even elementary statistics that numbers derived from ordinal scales are entered into unprotesting pocket calculators to produce means, standard deviations, or parametric testing of differences with other groups of patients. Perhaps the most surprising aspect is that papers with those kinds of calculations are still being accepted by respectable journals. Such errors are unnecessary, as suitable (non-parametric) methods for the analysis of ranked data can be found in every handbook of statistics.

Conclusions

(1) For some clinical trials, the principal measure of outcome will be a combination of specific events. These should always include death; if only specific deaths are included in the primary analysis, deaths from other causes still have to be accounted for. In case of multiple events per patient, only one is counted.

(2) Scales for measuring not the disease process but a patient's overall condition can be classified into (a) *impairment scales*, which are disease-specific and assess a combination of separate functions, such as limb strength or language in brain disease; (b) *disability scales*, which operate at the level of the person and measure either the capacity to perform defined tasks (Activities of Daily Living scales) or the actual degree of (in)dependence in the patient's own environment (performance scales); (c) *handicap scales*, which address the disadvantage for the individual in the fulfilment of roles in the family and in society; and (d) *scales for quality of life*, which aim at reflecting the individual's sense of well-being and life sat-

isfaction. **Across the spectrum from impairment to quality of life the measures become applicable to more than one disease but less sensitive, and less objective but more relevant.**

(3) Impairment scales have many more disadvantages than advantages, the main problem being that sum scores of clinical features are meaningless, whether or not some sort of weighting has been attempted. Although some of these scales have been hallowed by tradition, they should be ruthlessly abandoned.

(4) For many clinical trials performance scales (the modified Rankin scale or the Glasgow Outcome Scale) are the most suitable primary measure of outcome. Disability from all causes contributes to the level of performance, and specific events may be used as a secondary measure of outcome.

(5) Clinical scales often contain numbers but these represent classes, not mathematical values. The statistical methods should be appropriate for ranked data (median, interquartile range, etc.), and calculations such as means and standard deviations are meaningless.

References

1. Vinuela FV, Debrun GM, Fox AJ, Girvin JP, Peerless SJ. Dominant-hemisphere arteriovenous malformations: therapeutic embolization with isobutyl-2-cyanoacrylate. AJNR 1983;4:959–966.
2. Kayembe KN, Sasahara M, Hazama F. Cerebral aneurysms and variations in the circle of Willis. Stroke 1984;15:846–850.
3. Warlow C. Carotid endarterectomy: does it work? Stroke 1984;15:1068–1076.
4. World Medical Association. Human experimentation. Code of ethics of the world medical association – Declaration of Helsinki. BMJ 1964;ii:1977–1979.
5. Taylor KM, Kelner M. Informed consent: the physician's perspective. Soc Sci Med 1987;24:135–143.
6. Oddens BJ, Algra A, Van Gijn J. [How much information is retained by participants in clinical trials?] Hoe goed zijn deelnemers aan een klinisch onderzoek geinformeerd? Ned Tijdschr Geneeskd 1992;136:2272–2276.
7. Cassileth BR, Lusk EJ, Miller DS, Hurwitz S. Attitudes towards clinical trials among patients and the public. JAMA 1982;248:968–970.
8. Mattson ME, Curb JD, McArdle R, the AMIS and BHAT research groups. Participation in a clinical trial: the patients' point of view. Control Clin Trials 1985;6:156–167.
9. Albert T, Chadwick S. How readable are practice leaflets? BMJ 1992;305:1266–1268.
10. Roth LH, Lidz CW, Meisel A, et al. Competency to decide about treatment or research – an overview of some empirical data. Int J Law Psychiatry 1982;5:29–50.
11. Taylor PJ. Consent, competency and ECT: a psychiatrist's view. J Med Ethics 1983;9:146–151.
12. Antiplatelet Trialists' Collaboration. Collaborative overview of randomised trials of antiplatelet therapy. I. Prevention of death, myocardial infarction, and stroke by prolonged antiplatelet therapy in various categories of patients. BMJ 1994;308:81–106.
13. Schwartz D, Lellouch J. Explanatory and pragmatic attitudes in therapeutical trials. J Chronic Dis 1967;20:637–648.
14. Bogousslavsky J. Acute stroke trials: from Morass to Nirvana? Cerebrovasc Dis 1995;5:3–6.
15. Van Gijn J. Thrombolysis in ischemic stroke: Double or quits? Circulation 1996;93:1616–1617.
16. Emerson SS. Stopping a clinical trial very early based on unplanned interim analyses: A group sequential approach. Biometrics 1995;51:1152–1162.
17. The Dutch TIA Trial Study Group. A comparison of two doses of aspirin (30 mg vs 283 mg a day) in patients after a transient ischemic attack or minor ischemic stroke. N Engl J Med 1991;325:1261–1266.
18. Vermeulen M, Lindsay KW, Murray GD, et al. Antifibrinolytic treatment in subarachnoid hemorrhage. N Engl J Med 1984;311:432–437.
19. Van Gijn J, Algra A. Ticlopidine, trials, and torture [editorial comment]. Stroke 1994;25:1097–1098.
20. Counsell C, Warlow C, Sandercock P, Fraser H, Van Gijn J. The Cochrane Collaboration Stroke Review Group. Meeting the need for systematic reviews in stroke care. Stroke 1995;26:498–502.
21. Kohn A. False prophets – fraud and error in science and medicine. Oxford: Basil Blackwell, 1986.
22. European Carotid Surgery Trialists' Collaborative Group. MRC European Carotid Surgery Trial: interim results for symptomatic patients with severe (70–99%) or with mild (0–29%) carotid stenosis. Lancet 1991;337:1235–1243.
23. EAFT (European Atrial Fibrillation Trial) Study Group. Secondary prevention in non-rheumatic atrial fibrillation after transient ischaemic attack or minor stroke. Lancet 1993;342:1255–1262.
24. Fergus M, Stephens R. Marketing clinical trials. Lancet 1996;348:111–112.
25. Stein RE, Gortmaker SL, Perrin EC, et al. Severity of illness: concepts and measurements. Lancet 1987;II:1506–1509.
26. World Health Organization. International classification of impairments, disabilities, and handicaps. Geneva: WHO, 1980.
27. Hankey GJ, Warlow CP, Sellar RJ. Cerebral angiographic risk in mild cerebrovascular disease. Stroke 1990;21:209–222.
28. The Canadian Cooperative Study Group. A randomised trial of aspirin and sulfinpyrazone in threatened stroke. N Engl J Med 1978;299:53–59.
29. Antiplatelet Trialists' Collaboration. Secondary prevention of vascular disease by prolonged antiplatelet treatment. BMJ 1988;296:320–331.
30. Sackett DL, Gent M. Controversy in counting and attributing events in clinical trials. N Engl J Med 1979;301:1410–1412.
31. Heyman A, Wilkinson WE, Hurwitz BJ, et al. Risk of ischemic heart disease in patients with TIA. Neurology 1984;34:626–630.
32. Myerburg RJ, Castellanos A. Cardiac arrest and sudden cardiac death. In: Braunwald E, editor. Heart disease: a textbook of cardiovascular medicine. Philadelphia: Saunders, 1986;742–777.
33. Phillips LH, Whisnant JP, Reagan TJ. Sudden death from stroke. Stroke 1977;8:392–395.
34. Miller LS, Miyamoto AT. Computed tomography: its potential as a predictor of functional recovery following stroke. Arch Phys Med Rehabil 1979;60:108–109.
35. Van Gijn J, Warlow CP. Down with stroke scales! Cerebrovasc Dis 1992;2:244–246.
36. Wood PNH, Badley EM. People with disabilities: toward acquiring information which reflects more sensitively their problems and needs. New York: World Rehabilitation Fund, 1980.

37. Granger CV, Dewis LS, Peters NC, Sherwood CC, Barrett JE. Stroke rehabilitation: analysis of repeated Barthel index measures. Arch Phys Med Rehabil 1979;60:14–17.

38. Collin C, Wade DT, Davies S, Horne V. The Barthel ADL Index: a reliability study. Int Disabil Stud 1988;10:61–63.

39. Wade DT, Langton Hewer R. Functional abilities after stroke: measurement, natural history and prognosis. J Neurol Neurosurg Psychiatry 1987;50:177–182.

40. Chino N. Efficacy of Barthel index in evaluating activities of daily living in Japan, the United States, and United Kingdom. Stroke 1990;21:II64–5.

41. Task force on stroke impairment, task force on stroke disability, and task force on stroke handicap. Symposium recommendations for methodology in stroke outcome research. Stroke 1990;21(Suppl 2):68–73.

42. Hutchinson TA, Boyd NF, Feinstein AR, Gonda A, Hollomby D, Rowat B. Scientific problems in clinical scales, as demonstrated in the Karnofsky index of performance status. J Chronic Dis 1979;32:661–666.

43. van Swieten JC, Koudstaal PJ, Visser MC, Schouten HJ, Van Gijn J. Interobserver agreement for the assessment of handicap in stroke patients. Stroke 1988;19:604–607.

44. Bamford JM, Sandercock PA, Warlow CP, Slattery J. Interobserver agreement for the assessment of handicap in stroke patients [letter]. Stroke 1989;20:828.

45. Jennett B, Bond M. Assessment of outcome after severe brain damage: a practical scale. Lancet 1975;I:480–484.

46. Maas AI, Braakman R, Schouten HJ, Minderhoud JM, van Zomeren AH. Agreement between physicians on assessment of outcome following severe head injury. J Neurosurg 1983;58: 321–325.

47. Italian Acute Stroke Study Group. Haemodilution in acute stroke: results of the Italian haemodilution trial. Lancet 1988;I: 318–321.

48. Carey RG, Posavac EJ. Program evaluation of a physical medicine and rehabilitation unit: a new approach. Arch Phys Med Rehabil 1978;59:330–337.

49. Carey RG, Posavac EJ. Rehabilitation program evaluation using a revised level of rehabilitation scale (LORS-II). Arch Phys Med Rehabil 1982;63:367–370.

50. Spitzer WO. State of science 1986: quality of life and functional status as target variables for research. J Chronic Dis 1987;40: 465–471.

51. Stensman R. Severely mobility-disabled people assess the quality of their lives. Scand J Rehabil Med 1985;17:87–99.

52. Bergner M, Bobbitt RA, Carter WB, Gilson BS. The Sickness Impact Profile: development and final revision of a health status measure. Med Care 1981;19:787–805.

53. Hunt SM, McKenna SP, McEwen J, Backett EM, Williams J, Papp E. A quantitative approach to perceived health status: a validation study. J Epidemiol Community Health 1980;34: 281–286.

54. Ahlsiö B, Britton M, Murray V, Theorell T. Disablement and quality of life after stroke. Stroke 1984;15:886–890.

55. Niemi ML, Laaksonen R, Kotila M, Waltimo O. Quality of life 4 years after stroke. Stroke 1988;19:1101–1107.

56. von Neumann J, Morgenstern O. Theory of games and economic behaviour. Princeton, NJ: Princeton University Press, 1944.

57. Torrance GW. The measurement of health state utilities for economic appraisal. J Health Econ 1986;5:1–30.

58. Sackett DL, Torrance GW. The utility of different health states as perceived by the general public. J Chronic Dis 1978;31:697–704.

59. EuroQuol Group. Euroquol – a new facility for the measurement of health-related quality of life. Health Policy 1990;16: 199–208.

60. Fletcher AE, Hunt BM, Bulpitt CJ. Evaluation of quality of life in clinical trials of cardiovascular disease. J Chronic Dis 1987;40:557–569.

61. Wulff HR. Rational diagnosis and treatment – an introduction to clinical decision-making. Oxford: Blackwell, 1981.

62. Teasdale G, Jennett B. Assessment of coma and impaired consciousness – a practical scale. Lancet 1974;ii:81–84.

4. The Cochrane Collaboration Reviews in Neurology

L. Candelise

Introduction

Evidence-based medicine is the process of systematically finding, evaluating and utilising updated and good-quality research as the basis for clinical decision making [1].

Most clinicians seem to support this concept, receiving continuous pressure from both patients and government to practise it. Although we clearly need this new evidence daily, very often we fail to get it [2]. Textbooks are usually out of date by the time they are published and are subject to considerable bias.

On the other hand there is an explosion of bio medical literature which makes it difficult in practice for clinicians to keep up to date. A MEDLINE search may locate many randomised controlled trials, but most search strategies will miss a large proportion of studies which have not been appropriately coded. Yet, unfortunately, only 1% of articles published in medical journals are judged to be scientifically sound [3]. Basing an appraisal of the literature on this type of search is therefore prone to considerable inaccuracy and bias. Neurology is not immune from these problems; in fact it is rapidly evolving from a descriptive discipline to one of increasing epidemiological research mostly related to diagnosis and therapy. New types of evidence have been generated and might create significant changes in the way we care for our neurological patients.

Due to the above-described difficulties neurologists make suboptimal use of the available evidence. A clear demonstration of this is the large variation in neurological practice not only between different countries but also between clinicians working in the same institution. Until recently the treatment of a large number of neurological diseases was disappointing, and therapeutic nihilism dominated neurological practice. Due to a better knowledge of disease processes new treatments have been proposed recently. Unfortunately many of the new experimental interventions have a marginal efficacy, requiring large randomised multicentre studies rather than single personal experience to reach a reliable conclusion regarding treatment benefit.

At present randomised clinical trials (RCTs) are considered the "gold standard" for therapeutic decision-making. All neurologists should be familiar with the major RCTs related to their clinical practice [4]. The number of neurological RCTs is in fact, very large. The Cochrane Controlled Trials Register (CCTR) of the Cochrane Library (Issue 1, 2000) includes many neurological references (Table 4.1). The number of the articles increased for many diseases from 1990 to 2000. There were 825 studies on epilepsy, 641 on dementia and 1365 on multiple sclerosis, to mention just some of the major neurological diseases. These figures give an idea of the amount of work that needs to be done by neurologists involved in clinical practice to evaluate the research on treatment of neurological patients. The identification and selection of more relevant articles is a time-consuming process. To obtain rapid, up-to-date information on the best literature evidence neurologists make diffuse use of reviews of RCTs performed by leading researchers in the field, either published in journals or presented at medical meetings. Teaching courses in the United States (American Academy of Neurology) and Europe (European Neurological Society and European Federation of Neurological Societies) are attended by an increasing number of neurologists. They appreciate this type of review because it seems to combine the literature data with the personal opinion of an expert in the area. However, reviews by opinion leaders may in many instances be misleading [5]. The identification and selection of clinical trials are frequently incomplete and biased, rarely is there a quality assessment of included trials, and frequently a quantitative summary of treatment effect is lacking.

Table 4.1.   References to neurological RCTs on the Cochrane Library

Keywords	1990	1998	2000
Epilepsy	263	360	825
Dementia	237	247	641
Movement disorders	138	57	227
Back pain	200	381	730
Multiple sclerosis	198	252	1365
Cerebrovascular diseases	96	145	130

There is a valid alternative to a traditional review. A new methodology, the systematic review or meta-analysis, is starting to be used more frequently. Such systematic reviews should give explicit criteria for the inclusion of every single study, use extensive search strategies to identify all the potentially eligible studies and, when possible, use appropriate statistical methods to pool the data, to derive a best estimatation of treatment effect. There are some examples of systematic reviews in various neurological areas. In 1994 Counsell et al. [6], using a MEDLINE search and personal knowledge, identified only 35 systematic reviews relevant to neurology and neurosurgery. They stress that there is a need for systematic reviews in many other areas. In fact many reviews are published in very important journals but few of them are systematic.

At our Institute we have organised a comprehensive database of all systematic and non-systematic reviews in neurology. The aim was to assess the number and quality of published reviews for all types of neurological interventions including medical, surgical, palliative and service organisations. We identified the articles by means of a systematic search of MEDLINE, EMBASE and the Cochrane Library database from January 1996 to April 1997. The reviews were accepted if at least two clinical trials were evaluated. Reviews on experimental animals, and with a prominent pharmacological approach, were excluded as were articles in languages other than English, German, French, Italian and Spanish. The papers were classified according to disease groups: cerebrovascular disease, subarachnoid haemorrhage, epilepsy, migraine and headache, brain and spinal cord tumour, CNS infection, dementia, movement disorders, neurosurgery, multiple sclerosis, motor neurone disease, back pain, peripheral neuropathy, neurological pain, neuromuscular disease, head and spinal injury, rare and hereditary disease, symptomatic treatment, intensive care, and neurological services. We defined as "good-quality reviews" those either performed by the Cochrane Collaboration or included in the Database of Abstracts of Reviews and Effectivness in the Cochrane Library. Thus probably a minority of reviews that may be identified by

means of an electronic search are of good quality. Therefore, we must recognise that the identification and selection of good-quality clinical trials and reviews is a difficult and time-consuming job. Neurologists will hardly be able to perform this task by themselves, particularly at a time when they are being asked to see new patients and take on more management responsibilities. There is a need for reliable people and an organisation that can synthesise systematically the best research data in neurology and keep it up to date.

The Cochrane Collaboration

These problems were recognised many years ago by a respiratory epidemiologist, Archie Cochrane: "It is surely a great lack of our profession that we have not organised a critical summary, by speciality or subspecialty, adapted periodically, of all relevant randomised trials" [7]. In October 1993, a group of committed individuals met in Oxford and created an international network to perform, maintain and disseminate systematic reviews of all health care interventions, thereby founding the Cochrane Collaboration [8]. The Cochrane Collaboration is an international organisation that aims to help people make well-informed decisions about health care by preparing, maintaining and promoting the accessibility of systematic reviews of the effects of health care intervention. The Cochrane Collaboration's work is based on eight key principles: collaboration, building on the enthusiasm of individuals, avoiding duplication, minimising bias, keeping up to date, striving for relevance, promoting access and ensuring quality.

The Collaboration has increased rapidly. Fifteen Cochrane centres are already active in different countries. There are 51 Collaborative Review Groups and numerous people working within the Collaboration helping in different and important ways such as hand-searching medical journals for RCTs. Progress is being made in producing a mega-database of trials called CENTRAL that includes 268 827 trials up to January 2000. Many people will use the Cochrane Library reviews, often to make decisions which could dramatically affect their life or the lives of others. Nowadays the Cochrane Collaboration includes a number of structures and activities that exist to support and encourage individual workers in the preparation and maintenance of systematic reviews.

Cochrane Centres

The Centres encourage the formation of the various groups within the Collaboration and help to support their activities. At present there are 15 Cochrane

Centres in Australia, Brazil, Canada, Denmark, France, Germany, Italy, The Netherlands, UK, USA (four), South Africa and Spain. The address of the Oxford Centre is given in the Appendix.

Collaborative Review Group

The Collaborative Review Group (CRG) prepares and maintains systematic reviews in a specific disease area. The prototype CRG was the Pregnancy and Childbirth Group, followed by the Subfertility, Schizophrenia, Stroke and Parasitic Disease CRGs. Each Group is comprised of individuals who have sufficient enthusiasm to convene an exploratory meeting under the supervision of a local Cochrane Centre. When the Group has sufficient support, it prepares an application for registration with the Cochrane Collaboration. This must be formally approved by the Steering Group of the Cochrane Collaboration before the Group can commence its review work. The three to six Editors in a Group are volunteers drawn from various parts of the world and various disciplines. The Editorial Base is constructed and coordinated by one of the Editors. The base is responsible for computer searches for the Group, coordinating hand searches of relevant journals for RCTs, housing a computerised register of relevant RCTs, providing individual reviewers with papers, newsletters and statistical support and liaison with their local and other Cochrane Groups. The Editor of the Editorial Base is reliant on a full-time Administrator, usually with part-time support from research workers, a statistician and a computer scientist. In order to set up and run the Editorial Base, the Group must first find sufficient financial support.

Review Process

The review process commences with an individual Reviewer registering the title of his or her review with the Group. This prevents unnecessary repetition by others. A protocol for the review is then constructed which details the search strategy, inclusion and exclusion criteria for RCTs and the method of statistical overview, if appropriate. The protocol must be approved by the Editors. It is at this stage that some Groups have chosen to submit work to an advisory panel of health care professionals and even patient groups to provide consumer input. With the protocol approved, the review can be performed. The data from individual RCTs is entered into specifically designed software called Review Manager. This presents the review and its meta-analysis in a standard format which can be entered in the Cochrane Database of Systematic Reviews (CDSR) after approval by the Editors. Training in the writing of protocols, performance of reviews and the use of the software is provided by the Cochrane Centres. Reviewers must update their reviews when new RCTs become available.

Cochrane Library

The reviews are disseminated in the CDSR, which is part of the Cochrane Library. The latter is a package of databases concerned with evidence-based medicine. In addition to the CDSR, it has the Database of Abstracts of Reviews of Effectiveness (DARE), the Cochrane Review Methodology Database (CRMD) and the Cochrane Controlled Trials Register (CENTRAL). This register is a fundamental part of the work of the Cochrane Collaboration. The records for CCTR have primarily been identified through hand-searching of journals within the Cochrane Collaboration. They include records from the specialised registers of trials that are maintained by the CRGs, records supplied from elsewhere, both inside and outside the Collaboration, and references to clinical trials identified on MEDLINE and EMBASE.

The Cochrane Library is published quarterly on CD-ROM and is now available on the Internet. To allow the widespread dissemination of the results of Cochrane systematic reviews, publication of reviews in paper format is encouraged. Arrangements have been reached with some journals for simultaneous publication of important reviews.

Cochrane Neurological Review Groups

The Cochrane Collaboration is evolving at a tremendous pace in general, but neurology is advanced in comparison with many other specialities. Nine neurological CRGs (Stroke; Dementia and cognitive impairment; Back; Movement disorders; Epilepsy; Injuries; Neuromuscular disease; Multiple sclerosis; Pain, palliative and supportive care) are already registered with the Cochrane Collaboration (Table 4.2). Table 4.2 gives information about the neurological groups and the number of reviews and protocols. The nine CRGs that are mainly working on topics of neurological interest represent a heterogeneous group and some of them include, among their purposes, non-neurological topics also. Only four of them have a neurological editorial basis: Stroke, Epilepsy, Multiple sclerosis and Neuromuscular disease. The other groups are run by epidemiologists (Injuries) pharmacologists (Movement) or professionals from other medical areas (Pain, Spinal disorders, Dementia). Though having different starting points all these groups analyse, using common Cochrane methodology, the effect of interventions

Table 4.2. Neurological Collaborative Cochrane Review Groups

	Cochrane Stroke Group	Cochrane Back Review Group for Spinal Disorders	Cochrane Dementia and Cognitive Impairment Group	Cochrane Movement Disorders Group
Date of registration:	August 1993	November 1993	August 1995	June 1996
Editorial base address:	Department of Clinical Neurosciences, Western General Hospital, Crewe Road, Edinburgh EH4 2XU, UK	Research Department, Institute for Work and Health, 250 Bloor Street East, Suite 702, Toronto M4W 1E6, Canada	Department of Clinical Gerontology, Radcliffe Infirmary, Woodstock Road, Oxford OX2 6HE, UK	Faculty of Medicine, Institute of Pharmacology & Therapeutics, Hospital de Santa Maria, 1600 Lisbon, Portugal
Review Group Coordinator	Mrs Hazel Fraser	Mrs Andrea Furlan	Mr Peter Smith	Dr Joaquim Ferreira
Telephone:	+44 (0)131 5372273	+1 416 927 2027 ext. 2171	+44 (0)1865 224863	+351 1 7973453
Fax:	+44 (0)131 332 5150	+1 416 927 4167	+44 (0)1865 224108	+351 1 7930629
e-mail:	hf@skull.dcn.ed.ac.uk	afurlan@iwh.on.ca	cdcig@geratology.ox.ac.uk	movementdisord@mail.telepac.pt
Reviews on Library:	41	8	20	6
Protocols on Library:	22	14	7	10

specific for the group as well as problems that are common to all types of neurological patients such as the evaluation of care services, the management of the acute phase, specific symptomatic therapies, and rehabilitation. Detailed information on the neurological CRGs as presented in the latest issue of the Cochrane Library (2000, Issue 1) follows and is also presented in Table 4.2.

Cochrane Stroke Group

The Cochrane Stroke Group covers care interventions for prevention and acute treatment of stroke and subarachnoid haemorrhages [9]. As part of Cochrane Collaboration the Cochrane Stroke Group seeks to facilitate the production of high-quality systematic reviews based on the best available evidence and, if possible, on RCTs. The group has completed 41 reviews. These cover many aspects of secondary prevention and acute phase treatment. Five very recent reviews are: Calcium antagonists for acute ischaemic stroke, Carotid endarterectomy for asymptomatic carotid stenosis, Oral anticoagulants, Antiplatelet therapy, and Thienopyridine for prevention of stroke.

Cochrane Dementia and Cognitive Impairment Group

The principal aim of the Dementia and Cognitive Impairment Group is to contribute to the improvement of health care by producing high-quality systematic reviews of the available evidence in response to relevant health care questions for both age-associated cognitive decline and dementia. Twenty reviews, 7 protocols and 17 titles are published and registered in the latest issue of the Cochrane Library (Issue 1, 2000): drug treatments for dementia and Alzheimer's disease, reality orientation, reminiscence therapy, validation therapy, music therapy, and support for carers and others. Three revised protocols on treatment for agitation, vitamin E and NSAIDs for dementia are near completion and should be ready for the next Issue.

Cochrane Movement Disorders Group

The overall plan of the Movement Disorders Group includes Parkinson's disease, spasticity, Huntington's disease, tardive dyskinesia, dystonia, and other movement disorders. The aim of the group is to perform systematic reviews of all health care interventions in prevention, treatment and rehabilitation of movement disorders, by using randomised trials. Where RCTs may not exist, as for neurosurgical interventions, it was agreed to explore the posssibility of using observational data as the basis for systematic reviews [10]. In Issue 1 2000 of the Cochrane Library there is one new review: Botulinum toxin type A in the treatment of lower limb spasticity in cerebral palsy.

Cochrane Epilepsy Group

After the exploratory meeting of the Cochrane Epilepsy Group the members decided that the scope

Table 4.2. (Continued)

Cochrane Epilepsy Group	Cochrane Injury Group	Cochrane Multiple Sclerosis Group	Cochrane Pain, Palliative and Supportive Care Group	Cochrane Neuromuscular Disease Group
September 1996	February 1997	December 1997	January 1998	March 1998
Department of Neurological Sciences, Walton Centre of Neurology and Neurosurgery, Rice Lane, Liverpool L9 1AE, UK	Insistute of Child Health, Epidemiology, 30 Guilford Street, London WC1N 1EH, UK	Epidemiology Laboratory, Istituto Nazionale Neurologico C. Besta, via Celoria 11, Milan 20133, Italy	Pain Research Unit, Churchill Hospital, Old Road, Headington, Oxford OX3 7LJ, UK	Department of Neurology, UMDS – Guy's Hospital, St Thomas Street, London SE1 9RT, UK
Mrs Vicki Quinn	Mrs Frances Bunn	Mrs Liliana Coco	Mrs Frances Fairman	Prof. Richard Hughes
+44 (0)151 5295462	+44 (0)171 9052655	+39 02 239 4381	+44 (0)1865 225762	++44 (0)171 955 4398
+44 (0)151 5295465	+44 (0)171 2422723	+39 02 706 38 217	+44 (0)1865 225775	++44 (0)171 378 1221
VickiQuinn@compuserve.com	f.bunn@inch.ucl.ac.uk	neuroepidemiology@interbusiness.it	phil.wiffen@pru.ox.ac.uk	r.hughes@umds.ac.uk
3	15	0	6	3
20	17	5	6	9

of the group should be to "investigate the outcomes of interventions designed to prevent and manage childhood and adult seizures and epilepsy" [11]. Preliminary work was done to organise a database of RCTs in epilepsy and 360 RCTs were identified; the majority of these trials investigated anti-epileptic drugs. The aim of the Group is to conduct systematic reviews of both RCTs and controlled clinical trials assessing the outcomes (including harm) of interventions designed to prevent and manage childhood and adulthood seizures and epilepsy. The Group registered within the Collaboration in 1996. In Issue 1 2000 the Group had three reviews published: Yoga for epilepsy, Topiramate in drug-resistant partial epilepsy, and Gabapentin for drug resistant partial epilepsy. It also had 8 protocols published, 6 ongoing reviews and 12 ongoing protocols.

Cochrane Injuries Group

The aim of the Cochrane Injuries Group is to produce systematic reviews on interventions in the prevention, treatment and rehabilitation of traumatic injury, including the emergency resuscitation of seriously injured and burned patients. The group produces reviews for neurologists and neurosurgeons as well as for others professional categories. It registered within the Cochrane Collaboration in 1997. In Issue 4 1999 of the Cochrane Library there are 15 reviews and eight protocols. Of the 15 reviews published so far the following are of neurological interest: four reviews about acute brain injury, and one for spinal cord injury; there is also a review on

prophylactic anti-epileptic agents following acute traumatic brain injury, and one on fluid infusion in resuscitation of critically ill patients. Among current protocols there is one related to pharmacological treatment of spasticity.

Cochrane Neuromuscular Disease Group

The aim of the Cochrane Neuromuscular Disease Group is the management of the whole range of neuromuscular diseases including disorders of muscle, the neuromuscular junction, peripheral nervous system and motor neurones. It registered with the Collaboration on 27 March 1998. The primary target for reviews is currently RCTs. For diseases without RCTs the group will consider systematic review of other forms of evidence. In Issue 1 2000 of the Cochrane Library there are three reviews: Corticosteroid treatment for Guillain–Barré syndrome, Nocturnal mechanical ventilation for chronic hypoventilation in patients with neuromuscular and chest wall disorders, and Riluzole for amyotrophic lateral sclerosis (ALS)/motor neuron disease (MND).

Cochrane Multiple Sclerosis Group

The aim of the Cochrane Multiple Sclerosis Group is to produce and publish critical and systematic reviews for multiple sclerosis (MS) and other demyelinating and inflammatory diseases of the central nervous system. The Group covers treatments designed to: (i) improve recovery from acute exacerbations; (ii) decrease the number or the severity of exacerbations; (iii) prevent or delay the onset of the progressive phase; (iv) prevent further progression in patients with primary progressive MS. The organisation of the reviews concern all aspects of the disease process, i.e. secondary prevention, acute treatment of exacerbations, chronic treatment, rehabilitation, curative and symptomatic and palliative treatments. The Group has five new protocols in Issue 1 2000 of the Cochrane Library: two on symptomatic treatment and two on pathogenesis.

Cochrane Pain, Palliative and Supportive Care Group

The scope of the Cochrane Pain, Palliative and Supportive Care Group is to review randomised controlled trials concerning pain and palliative care, including: (i) the prevention and treatment of acute and chronic pain; (ii) the control of symptoms resulting both from the disease process as well as from interventions used in the management of the disease; (iii) the support of patients and carers through the disease process. The first review of the group is on the use of anticonvulsant drugs for the management of acute and chronic pain. Several topics could be of neurological interest, in particular headache treatment.

Cochrane Back Review Group for Spinal Disorders

The aim of the Cochrane Back Review Group for Spinal Disorders is to conduct reviews on pharmacological, physical, surgical, behavioural and educational interventions for neck pain, back pain and other spinal disorders excluding inflammatory disease and fractures. Eight reviews are available and 14 protocols; two reviews are concerned with the conservative management of neck disorders (patient education and physical treatment) and one with the effectiveness of TENS and ALTENS (acupuncture-like transcutaneous electrical nerve stimulation) in chronic low back pain.

Other Neurological Activities Within the Cochrane Collaboration

The Cochrane Library includes, in addition to the reviews (that are the main product of the Cochrane Collaboration), other important information that may be of interest to neurological professionals. Other Collaborative Review Groups have produced or are producing reviews useful for neurological patients. An example of this is the review on the treatment of diabetic neuropathy edited by the Cochrane Diabetes Group. A complete list of titles of the reviews on neurological subjects are available on the Cochrane Library (2000, Issue 1) and is presented in Table 4.3.

The Database of Abstracts of Reviews of Effectiveness (DARE) is also published in the Library. Issue 1 2000 includes more than 100 systematic neurological reviews conducted outside the Cochrane Collaboration. A structured abstract of the reviews gives useful information on the content and methodological quality of the original papers.

Conclusion

The adoption of the principles and practices of evidence-based medicine is clearly a timely and worthwhile venture for the discipline of neurology although some notes of caution should be sounded. It is hoped that over the next decade the Cochrane Collaboration will be developed in all areas of neurology, where preventive measures, treatments and rehabilitation will be available. Neurologists and neurological professional operators should also define better the areas of neurological interest independently of what is defined in text-books or found in electronic data banks of clinical trials. In fact, many aspects of clinical practice are usually not considered by current clinical research or by people running new clinical trials or performing systematic reviews.

In a recent editorial Demaerschalk and Hachinsky [12] argued that a strong methodological process is not a complete substitute for clinical practice. Neurologists have been amongst the last to embrace evidence-based medicine, perhaps because of a tendency towards conservatism and resistance to change. This cautious approach has the advantage of resisting a blind adoption of unproved principles. Applying critical appraisal guidelines to external clinical evidence can inform a neurologist's individual clinical expertise. This expertise may help the clinician to decide whether the evidence applies to a patient, how it might be best integrated into a clinical decision, match a patient's clinical state, predicament, and preferences, and therefore whether it should ultimately be applied. This process could also provide feedback to the researchers who dedicate time to performing new reviews. New types of needs could be generated which could create significant changes in the types of evidence sought by clinical research. For these reasons it is hoped that the widespread dissemination and use in clinical practice of

Table 4.3. Reviews of neurological interest available on the Cochrane Library (1999, Issue 4)

A. Cerebrovascular disease: Prevention

A1. Hypertension
1. Pharmacotherapy for hypertension in the elderly. CDSR 02-1999, CL 4 99.

A2. Atrial fibrillation
1. Antiplatelet therapy for preventing stroke in patients with nonrheumatic atrial fibrillation and a history of stroke or transient ischemic attack. CDSR 03-1999; CL 4 99.
2. Anticoagulants for preventing stroke in patients with nonrheumatic atrial fibrillation and a history of stroke or transient ischemic attack. CDSR 03-1999; CL 4 99.
3. Anticoagulants versus antiplatelet therapy for preventing stroke in patients with nonrheumatic atrial fibrillation and a history of stroke or transient ischemic attack. CDSR 03-1999; CL 4 99.

A3. Antithrombotic
1. Anticoagulants for preventing recurrence following ischaemic stroke or transient ischaemic attack. CDSR 02-1999; CL 4 99.

A4. Surgical/radiological intervention
1. Patch angioplasty vs primary closure for carotid endarterectomy. CDSR 02-1999; CL 4 99.
2. Patches of different types for carotid patch angioplasty. CDSR 02-1999; CL 4 99.
3. Percutaneous transluminal angioplasty and stenting for carotid artery stenosis. CDSR 02-1999; CL 4 99.
4. Percutaneous transluminal angioplasty and stenting for vertebral artery stenosis. CDSR 02-1999; CL 4 99.
5. Local vs general anaesthesia for carotid endarterectomy. CDSR 03-1999; CL 4 99.
6. Carotid endarterectomy for symptomatic carotid stenosis. CDSR 05-1999; CL 4 99.

B. Cerebrovascular disease: Acute treatment

B1. Intracerebral haemorrhage
1. Intraventricular streptokinase after intraventricular hemorrhage in newborn infants. CDSR 11-1998; CL 4 99.

B2. Drugs
1. Piracetam for acute ischaemic stroke. CDSR 02-1999; CL 4 99.
2. Nitric oxide donors (nitrates), L-arginine, or nitric oxide synthase inhibitors for acute ischaemic stroke. CDSR 02-1999; CL 4 99.
3. Glycerol for acute ischaemic stroke. CDSR 02-1999; CL 4 99.
4. Low-molecular-weight heparins or heparinoids vs standard unfractionated heparin for acute ischaemic stroke. CDSR 02-1999; CL 4 99.
5. Haemodilution for acute ischaemic stroke. CDSR 03-1999; CL 4 99.
6. Antiplatelet therapy for acute ischaemic stroke. CDSR 03-1999; CL 4 99.
7. Fibrinogen depleting agents for acute ischaemic stroke. CDSR 03-1999; CL 4 99.
8. Vinpocetine for acute ischaemic stroke. CDSR 03-1999; CL 4 99.
9. Pentoxifylline, propentofylline and pentifylline in acute ischaemic stroke. CDSR 03-1999; CL 4 99.
10. Corticosteroids for acute ischaemic stroke. CDSR 04-1999; CL 4 99.
11. Theophylline, aminophylline, caffeine and analogues, for acute ischaemic stroke. CDSR 05-1999; CL 4 99.
12. Gangliosides for acute ischaemic stroke. CDSR 05-1999; CL 4 99.
13. Anticoagulants for acute ischaemic stroke. CDSR 05-1999; CL 4 99.
14. Thrombolysis for acute ischaemic stroke. CDSR 07-1999; CL 4 99.
15. Prostacyclin and analogues for acute ischaemic stroke. CDSR 07-1999; CL 4 99.

B3. Others and general
1. Interventions for deliberately altering blood pressure in acute stroke. CDSR 02-1997; CL 4 99.
2. Services for reducing duration of hospital care for acute stroke patients. CDSR 05-1999; CL 4 99.
3. Services for helping acute stroke patients avoid hospital admission. CDSR 05-1999; CL 4 99.

C. Cerebrovascular disease: Rehabilitation

C1. Rehabilitation
1. Bladder training for urinary incontinence. CDSR 05-1999; CL 4 99.
2. Speech and language therapy for aphasia following stroke. CDSR 07-1999; CL 4 99.

D. Subarachnoid haemorrhage
1. Calcium antagonists for aneurysmal subarachnoid haemorrhage. CDSR 07-1999; CL 4 99.
2. Antifibrinolytic therapy for aneurysmal subarachnoid haemorrhage. CDSR 07-1999; CL 4 99.

E. Epilepsy
1. Yoga for epilepsy. CDSR 05-1999; CL 4 99.
2. Topiramate in drug resistant partial epilepsy. CDSR 07-1999; CL 4 99.
3. Gabapentin for drug resistant partial epilepsy. CDSR 07-1999; CL 4 99.

F. CNS infection
1. Vaccines for preventing tick-borne encephalitis. CDSR 02-1999; CL 4 99.
2. Drugs for preventing tuberculosis in HIV infected persons. CDSR 05-1999; CL 4 99.
3. Steroids for treating cerebral malaria. CDSR 05-1999; CL 4 99.
4. Drug for treating neurocysticercosis (tapeworm infection of the brain). CDSR 07-1999; CL 4 99.

Table 4.3. (*Continued*)

G. Dementia

1. CDP-choline for cognitive and behavioural disturbances associated with chronic cerebral disorders in the elderly. CDSR 02-1999; CL 4 99.
2. Reminiscence therapy for dementia. CDSR 02-1999; CL 4 99.
3. Validation therapy for dementia. CDSR 02-1999; CL 4 99.
4. Thioridazine for dementia. CDSR 02-1999; CL 4 99.
5. Aspirin for vascular dementia. CDSR 02-1999; CL 4 99.
6. Multidisciplinary team interventions for delirium in patients with chronic cognitive impairment. CDSR 05-1999; CL 4 99.
7. Music therapy for dementia symptoms. CDSR 05-1999; CL 4 99.
8. Rivastigmine for Alzheimer's disease. CDSR 05-1999; CL 4 99.
9. Nicotine for Alzheimer's disease. CDSR 05-1999; CL 4 99.
10. Reality orientation for dementia. CDSR 07-1999; CL 4 99.
11. Nimodipine for primary degenerative, mixed and vascular dementia. CDSR 07-1999; CL 4 99.
12. Dehydroepiandrosterone supplementation (DHEA) for cognition and well-being. CDSR 07-1999; CL 4 99.
13. Hydergine for dementia. CDSR 07-1999; CL 4 99.
14. Selegiline for Alzheimer's disease. CDSR 07-1999; CL 4 99.
15. Antioxidant vitamin and mineral supplements on the progression of age-related macular degeneration. CDSR 07-1999; CL 4 99.
16. Piracetam for dementia or cognitive impairment. CDSR 07-1999; CL 4 99.
17. Lecithin for dementia and cognitive impairment. CDSR 07-1999; CL 4 99.
18. Tacrine for Alzheimer's disease. CDSR 07-1999; CL 4 99.
19. Donepezil for mild and moderate Alzheimer's disease. CDSR 07-1999; CL 4 99.
20. Thiamine for Alzheimer's disease. CDSR 07-1999; CL 4 99.

H. Movement disorders

1. Lisuride for levodopa-induced complications in Parkinson's disease. CDSR 12-1998; CL 4 99.
2. Pergolide vs bromocriptine for levodopa-induced motor complications in Parkinson's disease. CDSR 12-1998; CL 4 99.
3. Lisuride versus bromocriptine for levodopa-induced complications in Parkinson's disease. CDSR 12-1998; CL 4 99.
4. Neuroleptic reduction and/or cessation and neuroleptics as specific treatment for tardive dyskinesia. CDSR 02-1999; CL 4 99.
5. Pergolide for levodopa-induced complications in Parkinson's disease. CDSR 01-1999; CL 4 99.
6. Cholinergic medication for neuroleptic-induced tardive dyskinesia. CDSR 02-1999; CL 4 99.
7. Vitamin E for neuroleptic-induced tardive dyskinesia. CDSR 02-1999; CL 4 99.
8. Diltiazem, nifedipine, nimodipine or verapamil for neuroleptic-induced tardive dyskinesia. CDSR 02-1999; CL 4 99.
9. Miscellaneous treatments for neuroleptic-induced tardive dyskinesia. CDSR 02-1999; CL 4 99.
10. GABA agonist medication for those with neuroleptic-induced tardive dyskinesia. CDSR 02-1999; CL 4 99.
11. Benzodiazepines for neuroleptic-induced tardive dyskinesia. CDSR 02-1999; CL 4 99.
12. Anticholinergic medication for neuroleptic-induced tardive dyskinesia. CDSR 07-1999; CL 4 99.
13. Bromocriptine for levodopa-induced motor complications in Parkinson's disease. CDSR 07-1999; CL 4 99.

I. Peripheral neuropathy

1. The efficacy of aldose reductase inhibitors in the treatment of diabetic peripheral neuropathy. CDSR 01-1997; CL 4 99.
2. Corticosteroid treatment for Guillain–Barré syndrome. CDSR 07-1999; CL 4 99.

L. Neurological pain

1. Anticonvulsant drugs for acute and chronic pain. CDSR 07-1999; CL 4 99.

M. Back pain

1. Transcutaneous electrical nerve stimulation (TENS) and acupuncture-like transcutaneous electrical nerve stimulation (ALTENS) for chronic low back pain. CDSR 02-1999; CL 4 99.
2. Surgery for lumbar disc prolapse. CDSR 02-1999; CL 4 99.
3. Physical medicine modalities for mechanical neck disorders. CDSR 02-1999; CL 4 99.
4. Injection therapy for subacute and chronic benign low back pain. CDSR 07-1999; CL 4 99.

N. Head and spinal injury

1. Calcium channel blockers for acute brain injury. CDSR 02-1999; CL 4 99.
2. Anti-epileptic drugs for preventing seizures following acute traumatic brain injury. CDSR 02-1999; CL 4 99.
3. Hyperventilation therapy for acute traumatic brain injury. CDSR 05-1999; CL 4 99.
4. Barbiturates for acute traumatic brain injury. CDSR 05-1999; CL 4 99.
5. Pharmacological interventions for acute spinal cord injury. CDSR 05-1999; CL 4 99.
6. Interventions for preventing injuries in problem drinkers. CDSR 07-1999; CL 4 99.
7. Corticosteroids for acute traumatic brain injury. CDSR 07-1999; CL 4 99.

high-quality clinical trials and reviews will lead to a better standard of care for patients in the near future, but will also increase the quality and insight of neurological clinical research.

Appendix: Useful Addresses

The Cochrane Library
Update Software Ltd
Summertown Pavilion
Middle Way, Summertown
Oxford OX2 7LG, UK
Tel: +44 (0)1865 513902
Fax: +44 (0)1865 516918
e-mail: info@update.co.uk
http://www.cochrane.co.uk

UK Cochrane Centre
Summertown Pavilion
Middle Way
Oxford OX2 7LG, UK
Tel: +44 (0)1865 516 300
Fax: +44 (0)1865 516 311
e-mail: crouse@cochrane.co.uk

Cochrane Handbook and the latest information on the Cochrane Collaboration
Including links to web sites maintained by the Collaborative Review Groups can be found at:
http://www.cochrane.org

References

1. Sackett DL, Rosenberg WMG, Gray JAM, et al. Evidence based medicine: what it is and what it isn't. BMJ 1996;312:71–72.
2. Covell DG, Uman GG, Menning PR. Information needs in office practice: are they being met? Ann Intern Med 1985;103:596–599.
3. Smith R. Were is the wisdom? The poverty of medical evidence. BMJ 1991;303:798–799.
4. Demaerschalk BM, Wiebe S. Evaluating the relevance of evidence based medicine in a neurology residency program. Can J Neurol Sci 1998;25:S79–80.
5. Altman EM, Lau J, Kupelnick B, Mosteller F, Chalmers TC. A comparison of results of meta-analyses of randomised trials and recommendations of clinical experts: treatment of myocardial infarction. JAMA 1992;268:240–248.
6. Counsell CE, Fraser H, Sandercock PA. Archie Cochrane's challenge: can periodically updated reviews of all randomised controlled trials relevant to neurology and neurosurgery be produced? J Neurol Neurosurg Psychiatry 1994;57:529–533.
7. Cochrane AL. 1931–1971: a critical review with particular reference to the medical profession. In: Medicine for the year 2000. London: Office of Health Economics, 1979:1–11.
8. Bero L, Drummond R. The Cochrane Collaboration: preparing, maintaining, and disseminating systematic reviews of the effects of health care. JAMA 1995;274:1935–1964.
9. Counsell C, Warlow C, Sandercock P, Fraser H, van Gijn J. The Cochrane Collaboration Stroke Review Group: meeting the need for systematic reviews in stroke care. Stroke 1995;26:498–502.
10. Clarke CE, Sampaio C. Movement Disorders Cochrane Collaborative Group. Mov Disord 1997;12:477–482.
11. Marson A, Beghi E, Berg A, Chadwick D, Tonini C. The Cochrane Collaboration: systematic reviews and their relevance to epilepsy. Epilepsia 1996;37:917–921.
12. Demaerschalk BM, Hachinski V. Evidence Based Neurology (EBN): the foundations of progress. Cochrane Neurol Newsletter 1998;2:6–8.

5. Drug Development Stages

T.G.K. Mant

Background

Prehistoric man recognised the medicinal value of various plant extracts containing active drugs such as opium, cocaine and digitalis thousands of years ago [1]. Effective drugs were, however, sparse until this century despite the advances of civilisation and science. Many ineffective remedies survived, the early physicians and patients being deluded by the self-limiting nature of many diseases and the "placebo effect". Progress was often precipitated by the desperation and deprivation of war. The first true chemotherapeutic agent, Salvarsan, for use against syphilis, was synthesised by Ehrlich as recently as 1909. In the 1920s only six drugs, either singly or in combination, made up 60% of all British prescriptions [2].

The recent extraordinary multiplication of new pharmacological agents and the inception of the modern pharmaceutical industry began with the introduction of the sulphonamide antibacterial drugs in the 1930s. Infectious diseases were a major cause of morbidity and mortality and the discovery of penicillin in 1939 (which had probably been present in some mould poultices more than a thousand years before) was a further breakthrough. The introduction of chlorpromazine in the 1950s revolutionised the treatment of schizophrenia and marked the beginning of the end of the enormous mental asylums so prominent in Victorian literature. New drugs for numerous indications flowed from the remarkably successful and innovative pharmaceutical industry. Whereas 213 products, of which only 36 were synthetic drugs, were listed in the 1932 *British Pharmacopoeia*, approximately 3500 licensed products were available in the UK in 1990[2]. The dramatic advances in drug therapy with their major impact on clinical practice appeared limitless. The opposite side of the coin, namely the appalling potential of drug-induced disease, was not widely recognised until the thalidomide catastrophe in the 1960s. This shocked the medical profession, pharmaceutical industry and the public, and led to the Medicines Act (1968) which provides for the licensing of medicinal products in the UK. Until this Act was passed, no statute in the UK required pre-marketing approval of medicines on the grounds of their safety. The UK is also subject to the European Union Pharmaceutical Directives and, at present, the International Congress for Harmonisation (ICH) is attempting to achieve worldwide standards for drug development.

The process of drug development has evolved since the trial and error approach of primitive man to a regulated system, which it is hoped encourages innovative and ethical drug development whilst minimising risk to patients. The concept of clinical trials was first utilised in the identification of the value of limes proposed by Lind to prevent scurvy in English sailors in the eighteenth century (hence the US term "limeys"). Although much of clinical practice and drug research is still based upon empirical evidence, the availability of different more effective therapies, and the recognition that patients may improve spontaneously and not due to drug therapy, emphasised the need for the structured approach of controlled, randomised clinical trials[3] in drug evaluations by the medical profession, pharmaceutical industry and government regulatory authorities. Controlled randomised clinical trials are now the cornerstone of drug development.

Before a new chemical entity (NCE) becomes a licensed medicine, it undergoes in vitro/ex vivo testing to determine its potential clinical utility followed by rigorous pre-clinical studies in animals and clinical studies in humans.

The Tufts Center for the Study of Drug Evaluation has estimated that the time taken from drug synthesis to drug approval in the USA for company-originated new chemical entities averaged 8–12 years in the early 1990s [4].

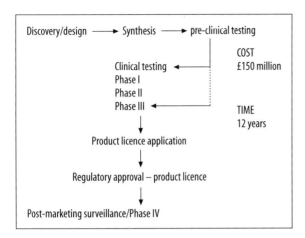

Fig. 5.1.   The process of drug development.

Table 5.1.   Some biotechnology products currently in use or development

Calcitonin gene-related peptide
Luteinising hormone-releasing factor
Granulocyte colony-stimulating factor
Interferons
Interleukins
Human insulin
Growth hormone
Hirudin
Haemoglobin
Factors VIII and IX
Epoetin
Anti-thrombin III

In the USA, it takes on average £86 million and just over 9 years to go from the first human tests to final regulatory approval. For every five compounds entering human studies, usually only one is subsequently marketed [5]. The international patent life is 20 years; hence there are constant pressures not only clinical (to benefit patients) but also financial (to reduce the cost of medical care whilst repaying the investors in pharmaceutical research) to expedite the process without compromising safety. With this objective and also in response to new technologies resulting from the molecular biology "revolution", the development process is continually being refined but can still be conveniently summarised by the stages indicated in Fig. 5.1 and described below.

Discovery/Design

The discovery of most new drugs originates in the major research-based pharmaceutical companies. Whereas up until the last quarter of the twentieth century the majority of new drugs evolved from random screening, serendipity and essentially empirical drug design, advances in analytical techniques, computer-aided graphics and more recently the revolution in biotechnology have resulted in much more focused and specific drug design. This has been assisted by the parallel advances in the understanding of pathophysiology and receptor pharmacology. Complex organic chemicals can be identified and characterised. Naturally occurring enzymes, newly identified receptors, agonists and antagonists can be studied, the drugs synthesised and potential clinical usage investigated more precisely. The ability to splice human genes into bacterial, yeast and non-human mammalian chromosomes

to produce bulk quantities of natural human and other proteins has extraordinary potential. Some biotechnology products currently in use or development are listed in Table 5.1.

Synthesis

Once the new chemical entity has been characterised, the process for its synthesis must be developed. The synthesis of chemical and biotechnological drugs by the pharmaceutical industry is under the stringent regulation of good manufacturing practice (GPMP) to ensure consistent, reliable and accurate chemical composition. Pharmaceutical scientists will be involved in the initial formulation of the drugs. Whatever the route of administration, this is a complex process of many stages [6]. Most new chemical entities are either weak acids or bases or salts. Chemical stability and physical/chemical properties including chiral properties must be established. A new chemical entity needs to be formulated in a manner appropriate to its route of administration which, at an early stage, may not be known. Stability, compatibility in solution and exipient mixtures must be studied. The single commonest formulation marketed in the UK is a tablet. Even simple tablets may contain a myriad of additional chemicals. Initially, the drug is often produced as a powder and placed in a gelatin capsule for oral studies.

Pre-clinical Testing

Animal studies are performed to investigate the pharmacology, toxicology and pharmacokinetics of new chemical entities. The types of pre-clinical studies are summarised in Table 5.2. The ICH guidelines for repeated-dose toxicity studies to support

Table 5.2. Pre-clinical studies

Pharmacology
Acute toxicity
Chronic toxicity
Mutagenicity
Carcinogenicity
Reproductive testing

Table 5.3. Duration of repeated-dose toxicity studies to support phase I and II trials in the European Union

Duration of clinical trials	Minimum duration of repeated-dose toxicity studies	
	Rodents	Non-rodents
Single dose	2–4 weeks	2 weeks
Up to 2 weeks	2–4 weeks	2 weeks
Up to 1 month	1 month	1 month
Up to 3 months	3 months	3 months
Up to 6 months	6 months	6 months
>6 months	6 months	Chronic

phase I and II trials in the EU are indicated in Table 5.3. The timing and duration of toxicity testing in animals varies between nations. The toxicity programme in the UK is usually dependent on the number of doses/duration of treatment to be investigated in humans and the longer-term studies are not considered necessary before administering the drug in restricted doses and for restricted duration in humans. The timing of toxicological studies to support clinical trials has been well covered in the Centre for Medicines Research publication [7] and is described in ICH4 [8].

Although the rationale and value of much animal testing is controversial in view of the remarkable safety record of human clinical trials, it is unlikely there will be dramatic changes in the requirements other than harmonisation in the near future. The investigator conducting early-phase human studies must be cognisant of the pre-clinical data and, in particular, of the "target organ" in the toxicology studies. Appropriate species selection (e.g. primates for immunomodulatory agents) and testing of drugs on cell cultures may help reduce the number of animals sacrificed during drug development. The timing of the toxicity testing may be altered. For example, if there are equivocal results in mutagenicity testing then long-term carcinogenicity tests may be required before the drug is administered to humans.

Clinical Drug Development

Human clinical trials proceed through four distinct phases.

Phase I

Phase I encompasses the initial study of drugs in human volunteers. The principal objective is human tolerability. With the vast majority of drugs, healthy "non-patient" subjects will participate in these studies. The reasons for this are summarised in Table 5.4. In such "non-therapeutic" research to be ethical the risk to the research subject should be "minimal" and consistent with normal activities and occupations such as driving in a private car or travelling on public transport [9]. Subjects are usually paid for their participation in such studies. The payment and any advertising used to recruit subjects must be reviewed by the Research Ethics Committee. The payment should be related to time and discomfort and never risk [9]. It is the responsibility of the investigator, Research Ethics Committee and the sponsor of the research (e.g. pharmaceutical company, MRC, NIH) to ensure such research is ethical and is consistent with the Declaration of Helsinki and subsequent amendments. Written informed consent should be obtained. In the UK there is no specific law covering phase I studies in healthy volunteers, although this is likely to be addressed by the Medicines Control Agency under EU directives in line with ICH guidelines. Certain drugs, including most chemotherapeutic agents for malignant disease, have predictable toxicity at therapeutic doses so their use in healthy subjects would be unacceptable. For such drugs, patients whose disease may benefit from such a drug are chosen for these phase I studies. These studies do fall within the Medicines Act (1968) and regulatory approval is required before commencement. Such studies, where adjustment of dose regimes during a study to maximise therapeutic benefit and minimise toxicity are the rule rather than the exception, require a different strategy in study design compared with phase I studies on healthy subjects. The critical role of phase I studies in oncology is covered in an article by the American Society of Clinical Oncology [10].

Healthy volunteer studies are usually performed in two stages: single rising dose and repeated administration [11]. Parallel or an incremental dose crossover design are commonly employed. Both should be double-blind and placebo-controlled to minimise the risk of non-drug effects confusing the interpretation of results. If it is an oral formulation, then it is common practice to conduct a food inter-

Table 5.4. Young healthy volunteers in phase I studies

Advantages	Disadvantages
1. Avoids the ethical problem associated with the administration of unproven therapy in disease states that require treatment 2. More homogeneous 3. More able to withstand potentially harmful drug effects 4. More able to comply with time consuming and complicated studies and procedures 5. Often impractical to find adequate numbers of patient volunteers 6. No concomitant disease, no concomitant medication, therefore fewer factors to complicate interpretation of results	1. No therapeutic benefit 2. Not "target population" 3. Patients are not homogeneous, so care is needed in extrapolating data

action study before commencing the multiple dose studies. The first dose is usually a fraction, (e.g. 1/50th to 1/100th) of the dose that produced an effect in the most sensitive animal species studied. The dose is increased, with the safety of each dose level being assessed before a dose increment occurs. Dose increments cease at a pre-determined dose level or when a particular plasma concentration or pharmacodynamic effect is achieved or when the maximum tolerable dose is realised.

The doses and dose interval for the repeated-administration phase I studies will be determined by the tolerance, effects and pharmacokinetic results from the single-dose data. It is important that steady-state plasma concentrations are shown to be attained. If non-linear pharmacokinetics are observed at possible therapeutic doses, it is a major disadvantage. Repeated-administration studies usually provide more opportunity to measure surrogate markers of efficacy such as effects on cognitive function, cardiac output, sleep electroencephalogram and positron emission tomography studies to identify receptor occupancy. Challenge studies are usually conducted after the tolerance of single- and repeated-administration studies has been assessed.

Both single- and repeated-administration studies are usually conducted on subjects as "inpatients" to maximise safety and help ensure compliance.

Phase II

Phase II describes the early therapeutic trials, usually in a small number of closely monitored patients, to explore efficacy, safety, and their relationship with dose [9]. Phase II studies may be conducted in more than one indication with the same drug. In these studies, the number of patients tends to be small. The

studies are very closely monitored, often at a single hospital site under an investigator who has particular expertise in that indication. Occasionally, these studies are impractical or unethical to conduct in double-blind fashion with a reference treatment for comparison but, whenever possible, a double-blind design should be used.

The selection of doses and dose frequency will depend on the results of the phase I data. Initial "dose-ranging" phase II studies are usually carried out as a pilot. Once there is some reassurance regarding likely effects, the numbers of patients and duration of therapy can be increased. The numbers of patients involved may vary from fewer than 50 to a few hundred at the end of a phase II programme.

It is quite possible that patients with the disease for which the drug is being investigated will differ in their tolerance and handling of the drug in comparison with healthy subjects. This may be related to the pathology (e.g. more permeable blood-brain barrier in multiple sclerosis) or concomitant medication (e.g. enzyme induction by concomitant anticonvulsant therapy).

Whilst the patient numbers are usually too small to provide definitive information on the correct dose and tolerance, the phase II studies should identify a suitable dose schedule, give an estimate of clinical efficacy in relation to drug plasma concentration and provide information on dose-related adverse effects. The alert investigator may determine even at this early stage some unforeseen property, beneficial or otherwise.

Phase II (and phase III) studies require a Clinical Trials Exemption (CTX) or Clinical Trial Certificate (CTC). In the UK, most drug development is conducted under the CTX scheme [9]. The granting of a CTX or CTC is some reassurance to the investigator and Research Ethics Committee that there has been an independent review of the safety testing and quality of the product but does not imply the ethics of the protocol has been subject to review [9]. Research Ethics Committees, both local and multi-centre, have a fundamental role in drug research in the UK.

Phase III

Once there is evidence of efficacy and an acceptable safety profile, albeit in a limited population, phase III studies are conducted to confirm whether or not a drug is effective for a particular indication and to provide close monitoring of possible adverse effects. Whereas phase II studies are typically exploratory into therapeutic efficacy, phase III studies are designed to confirm that a drug is safe and effective for use in the intended indication and recipient population [12,13]. These studies are usually multi-centre double-blind randomised and controlled. The control is usually the best treatment available (the standard treatment) or, if there is no known effective treatment, a placebo. Phase III studies provide comparative data, often from hundreds of patients, not only to obtain regulatory approval for marketing of the drug but also to establish the best dosing regimen and the advantages and disadvantages of the drug in comparison with alternative treatments [14,15].

During this stage 1000 to 5000 patients will usually be involved in clinical studies. Exposure of a greater number of patients to the drug provides the opportunity for less frequent adverse events to be reported and investigated. From these large formal studies in a more heterogeneous population, it is often possible to discern those factors which predispose to toxicity. Population pharmacokinetic studies can be completed. During this stage, particular populations such as subjects with renal impairment, hepatic impairment and the elderly may be studied to determine whether dose modification is necessary. Drug interaction studies will also be performed. If the drug is to be used chronically, e.g. as an anti-convulsant, at least 100 patients will need to be exposed for 1 year. During this stage, long-term animal testing (especially carcinogenicity studies) will have been completed and reported.

Product Licence Application

At the end of phase III a marketing application will be made. In the UK this may be a direct product licence application to the Medicines Control Agency or via a centralised licensing procedure through the European Medicines Evaluation Agency (EMEA). All biotechnology products must be considered by the latter.

All information concerning the drug with world-wide adverse event data are collated. Key documents include a summary of product characteristics (SPC) and clinical expert reports. There are three self-contained reports in which the experts (pharmaceutical, pharmacotoxological and clinical) evaluate the investigations and give an opinion in the light of current scientific knowledge [16,17]. An application may involve more than 300 kg of paper. A marketing authorisation (product licence) is granted if the licensing authority is satisfied the product is sufficiently effective, safe and of good quality. Relative efficacy in comparison with established treatments and cost are currently specifically excluded from the approval process in the UK, but risk/benefit ratio is considered.

Phase IV

Phase IV studies are performed after drug approval and relate to the approved indication [12]. They evaluate efficacy and safety, usually in comparison with an established therapy. If a different indication from that/those in the original licence is proposed, a new marketing application will be necessary which may warrant further phase I, II and III studies even though the drug is licensed.

When a product licence is granted, the median number of subjects in the safety database for successful applications to the MCA in the years 1987 to 1989 was 1480 [18]. Following approval, most drugs will be prescribed to a much more heterogeneous and larger population. To identify rare but severe idiosyncratic adverse events and particular patient characteristics that may predispose to drug toxicity requires rigorous reporting and evaluation of adverse events. Currently, there is the voluntary yellow card system in the UK which relies on spontaneous reporting.

Other methods of value in post-marketing surveillance include case–control studies, cohort studies, prescription event monitoring (PEM) and record linkage with population databases. Unfortunately, it is likely that only a fraction of all important reactions are notified [19].

References

1. Inglis B. A history of medicine. London: Weidenfeld and Nicholson, 1965.
2. Walker SR. The innovative pharmaceutical industry. a history of research in creating the right environment for drug discovery. Quay Publishing, 1991.
3. Baber NS, Smith RN. Clinical trials. In: Griffen JP, O'Grady J, Wells FO, editors. Textbook of pharmaceutical medicine, 2nd ed. Belfast: Queen's University, 1994.

4. Masi, et al. New drug development in the United States from 1963 to 1994. Clin Pharmacol Ther, 1994;55:609–622.

5. Anon. Testing, testing. The Economist, 1 Feb 1997.

6. Padfield JM. Making drugs into medicines. In: Burley DM, Clarke JM, Lasagna L, editors. Pharmaceutical medicine, 2nd ed. London: Edward Arnold, 1993.

7. Parkinson C, McAuslane N, Lumley C, Walker S. The timing of toxicological studies to support clinical trials. Proceedings of a CMR Discussion Meeting, May 1994. Dordrecht: Kluwer Academic, 1994.

8. Non-clinical safety studies for the conduct of human clinical trials for pharmaceuticals. Fourth international conference on harmonisation, July 1997.

9. Guidelines on the practice of ethics committees in medical research involving human subjects, 3rd ed. London: The Royal College of Physicians, August 1996.

10. American Society of Clinical Oncology. Critical role of phase I clinical trials in cancer treatment, J Clin Oncol 1997;15:853–859.

11. Mant TGK, Spector RG. Phase I studies and pharmacokinetics. In: Lloyd J, Raven A, editors. ACRPI handbook of clinical research. Edinburgh: Churchill Medical, 1994.

12. ICH harmonised tripartite guideline, general considerations for clinical trials. ICH,1997.

13. Sheiner LB. Learning versus confirming in clinical drug development. Clin Pharmacol Ther 1997;61:275–291.

14. Halbert GW. Pharmaceutical development. In: Griffin JB, O'Grady J, Wells FO, editors. Textbook of pharmaceutical medicine, 2nd ed. Belfast: Queen's University, 1994.

15. Burley DM, Lasagna L. Clinical trials. In: Burley DM, Clarke JM, Lasagna L, editors. Pharmaceutical medicine, 2nd ed. London: Edward Arnold, 1993.

16. Jefferys DB, Jones G. The regulation of medicines in the UK. In: Griffin JB, O'Grady J, Wells FO, editors. Textbook of pharmaceutical medicine, 2nd edition. Belfast: Queen's University, 1994.

17. Farrell FG. Drug regulation in the 1990s. In: Lloyd J, Raven A, editors. ACRPI handbook of clinical research. Edinburgh: Churchill Medical, 1994.

18. Rawlins MD, Jeffreys, DB. Study of United Kingdom product licence applications containing new active substances, 1987–89. BMJ 1991;302:223–225.

19. Ferner RE. Newly licensed drugs. BMJ 1996;313:1157–1158.

6. Drug Regulatory Requirements in the United Kingdom and Europe

D.B. Jeffreys

Introduction

Drug regulation in both the UK and in Europe began following the Thalidomide disaster in the early 1960s. Prior to this a pharmaceutical company could undertake clinical trials without obtaining official approval and could market a product once the manufacturer was satisfied with the data which had been obtained. The only official controls came through the various poison control measures and through the Therapeutic Substances Act which set out requirements for controlling the standardisation of biological products such as insulin.

Interestingly, as Dr R.D. Mann records in his book *Modern Drug Use* [1], a Select Committee had considered formal drug regulation in the UK in 1914 and had recommended the introduction of such a system. Perchance this report was issued on 4 August 1914, the day that the First World War broke out. No action was therefore taken and thus at the time of the thalidomide disaster there were no formal requirements and no pre-approval needed for the launch of a drug. The thalidomide disaster changed all this.

In 1964 a voluntary scheme to control the introduction of new medicinal products was introduced, with the Committee on the Safety of Drugs being established by the Department of Health. In 1968 the Medicines Act was enacted which progressively came into force by 1971. At the same time the then six members of the Common Market enacted the first Pharmaceutical Directive 65/65 which bears very close similarity to the UK Medicines Act. Interestingly the pharmaceutical quality of medicines was much more tightly controlled through the operation of the pharmacopoeias. The British Pharmacopoeia can trace its origins back to the reign of James I when it was issued as the London Pharmacopoeia. The present British Pharmacopoeia was introduced in 1863 and remains an important element of drug control. More recently the European Pharmacopoeia has assumed much greater importance.

The Medicines Act of 1968 introduced regulation and controls on the development of a medicine through clinical trials and upon the manufacture, supply and distribution of medicines. Under the legislation a pharmaceutical company has to apply for an authorisation to undertake a clinical trial and to be authorised to manufacture a drug. In addition, before a product can be authorised a comprehensive development programme has to be undertaken which is then critically assessed, with a licence being needed before the product can be placed on the market. The Medicines Act established the Medicines Commission and the so-called Section 4 Advisory Committees, the most well known of which is the Committee on the Safety of Medicines (the CSM). The responsibility for authorising a new medicine lies with the health ministers of the UK who comprise the so-called Licensing Authority.

Drug regulation has undergone major changes since 1968. The developments in the UK have been closely interwoven with the development of the internal market in pharmaceuticals and the introduction of the so-called Future System for the pan-European control of medicines in 1995.

This chapter will consider the current regulation of medicinal products in the UK and Europe, particularly from the position of those undertaking clinical trials on drugs in the field of neurology. It will also look at some of the recent developments and those which are likely to influence the conduct of clinical trials in the near future.

The Current Regulation of Medicines in the UK and Europe

Drug regulation has come a long way since the introduction of the Medicines Act in 1968. There is now an extensive corpus of European Community law which is interwoven with the UK Medicines Act. Since December 1995 a new system of control of medicines in Europe also exists which is increasingly influencing both the development of new drugs and their control. The responsibility for medicines licensing within the UK lies with health ministers who comprise the so-called Licensing Authority. The executive function of medicines control is undertaken by the Medicines Control Agency (the MCA) which is a Next Steps Agency for the Department of Health.

The MCA was established in 1989. Previously the regulation had been effected by the Medicines Division of the Department of Health. Following an external review it was decided to set up an Agency which became an executive body in 1991. This chapter will describe how the MCA operates and how it works with the CSM and the Medicines Commission. The involvement of the European institutions and the new system will also be described.

Control of Clinical Trials

Phase I, or volunteer studies, are not controlled by legislation in the UK although they are controlled in some other European countries. This is likely to change as a result of a new European Clinical Trials Directive which will be implemented by 2002. The control in the UK is currently through self-regulation and through the operation of the Local Research Ethics Committees. Two formal reviews were undertaken in the mid-1980s of phase I trial controls in the UK. These concluded that self-regulation was satisfactory and that formal government control would not produce added safety for the public.

Any clinical trial undertaken in a patient in the UK is controlled under the Medicines Act. The vast majority of clinical trials are controlled through the CTX (or Clinical Trial Exemption Scheme) [2]. This system was introduced in 1981 to speed up the approval of clinical trials in the UK. The scheme is now seen as a model for the control of clinical trials and has been emulated in many other countries. It operates whereby an applicant or manufacturer will supply a summary of the data available and the MCA will make its decision in defined time limits on the summary data. Frequently approval will be sought for a very limited additional study and then subsequently additional quality and pre-clinical safety data will be submitted to allow expansion of the trials. Adverse reactions and adverse events have to be reported to the MCA for drugs under trial and these are closely monitored by staff of the

Agency. Should significant safety problems emerge, then the trial can be restricted or closed by the Agency.

In March 1996 the CTX scheme was further refined with the introduction of a new guideline (MAL 4) [2]. This simplified some aspects of the scheme and introduced the concept of the clinical usage guideline. It means that a manufacturer can now set wider parameters taking account of the available pre-clinical data. The requirement for the additional approval for new studies has also been simplified. The result is that the drug development can proceed along agreed parameters provided adequate pre-clinical supporting data are available. Approximately 250 new substances are approved for trials each year through the UK CTX scheme. In addition the Agency will receive almost 2000 requests for additions and variations to trials. These are all now handled through a state-of-the art computer system, the assessments being undertaken on screen. Currently there are proposals from the European Commission to bring forward a directive on the control of clinical trials and on the implementation of good clinical practice across the European Union, and this is under consideration by the EU Member States. The possible extent of these proposals and their implications are uncertain at present but could have significant effects on clinical trial development in Europe.

Good Clinical Practice

The concept of good clinical practice (GCP) and indeed the current Committee on Proprietary Medicinal Products (CPMP) guideline [3] is seen as a major advance. The current guidance defines the conduct expected of those undertaking clinical trials and the responsibilities of the investigators and of the sponsor company. In Europe the guideline lays the responsibilities on the sponsor. This is somewhat different from the control point in the United States. Thus the European system expects that the sponsor will ensure the quality of the data through appropriate monitoring and quality assurance procedures. The European authorities will inspect and control the activities of the sponsor. Increasingly GCP compliance units are being established by Member States. They are undertaking voluntary inspections and giving approval certificates to sponsors. These inspections will become statutory with the implementation of the EC Clinical Trials Directive. On occasions they may also be undertaking a quality assurance audit of major or pivotal clinical studies. All investigators should be familiar with the GCP guidelines and ensure that they are being followed. The important element of these is the policy on the retention of records to allow the verification of source data.

Investigator-Sponsored Clinical Trials

Many clinical trials are organised and conducted solely by clinicians or under the auspices of medical charities. If a sponsor pharmaceutical company is not directly involved in such trials then these are controlled through the Doctors and Dentists Exemption Scheme [4], often referred to as the DDX scheme. Here the lead investigator will apply to the MCA for permission to undertake the investigation. He or she will provide brief details of the protocol and a statement that a pharmaceutical company is not involved in funding or organisation of the study. In these circumstances the responsibility for the conduct of the trial lies with the investigator and any other supporting organisation. The majority of requests to the MCA for such trials concern small investigations but some requests will come from professional societies or from medical charities and may involve large-scale investigations. Some of these will be on already marketed products and may be comparative studies for the assessment of a new indication of the medicine.

The Role and Responsibilities of the Regulatory Authorities

It is important for investigators to understand the role and responsibilities of the regulatory authorities. These are determined by the relevant legislation, increasingly the European directives. Where there is an area not covered by the directives, then these would be addressed by the natural drug laws such as the UK Medicines Act. The prime function of the regulatory authority is to assess the quality, safety and efficacy of all medicinal products before granting a marketing authorisation. A product may not be marketed unless such an authorisation is given. In determining whether a medicine can be licensed the authority has to be satisfied the medicine is of satisfactory quality and that the safety of the product's proposed indication is appropriate. The authority also has to be satisfied that the efficacy of the clinical indication has been established. Thus the prime function of the regulatory authority is to assess the risk to benefit ratio for the new medicine.

The responsibilities of the authorities go much wider than just the initial assessment. The determination of the quality also involves inspection of the manufacturing facilities and the licensing of the manufacturer. Furthermore, samples of the new medicine may be analysed before marketing and in the UK samples will be taken from the marketplace after authorisation, to assess whether product continues to comply with the specifications set out in the licence.

At the time of granting an authorisation, approximately 1100 patients will have been involved in the clinical trials to determine the efficacy of the medicine [5,6]. A slightly higher number of patients may be evaluable for safety but in a recent study the median number evaluable for safety was only 1480. This means that rare adverse reactions are unlikely to be identified during the development programme. Moreover, given the low frequency of such rare reactions, there is little to be gained by expanding the size of the initial development programme. Thus there is an increasing emphasis on the role of post-marketing surveillance. In addition there is a very important role to be played by the spontaneous adverse reaction reporting schemes. One of the leading such schemes is the Yellow Card system in the UK, whereby all doctors are asked to report adverse reactions on new medicines and unexpected and serious adverse reactions on older medicines to the CSM and the MCA. This reporting scheme provides an essential alert mechanism and has been responsible for identifying many post-marketing problems over its 30 years of operation. In addition the regulatory authorities have a role in the approval and monitoring of clinical trials. The regulatory authority is also responsible for monitoring the advertising and promotion of medicinal products.

Guidance and Guidelines During Development

The regulatory authorities have an important role both in offering guidance and in issuing guidelines to assist the pharmaceutical industry in the development of new drugs. The MCA in the UK has offered extensive advice to pharmaceutical companies and this was described in the 1994/95 Annual Report of the Agency[7]. This advice was previously more concerned with the regulatory aspects of drug development but recently more advice is being given on the emerging consensus for new development issues and on statistical matters. This advice is not formalised as it is through the Food and Drug Administration procedure in the United States, and the resources for such advice are still rather limited.

Currently there are initiatives through Europe to offer dialogue and advice to pharmaceutical companies for major new medicines. This advice is channelled through the CPMP whose functions will be described later in this chapter. The notion here is to offer European advice to companies, recognising that such medicines are being developed for the European market and are likely to be submitted through the new Community procedures [8].

A large number of guidelines have now been produced by the CPMP. There are more than 200 such guidelines, covering a significant number of drug development issues. When a new subject is identified, a concept paper will be issued to all interested parties. Following this a working party will produce an initial document which is then issued for a period of informal consultation. Then a more formal document will be developed which will be issued for a 6 month consultation period before its final adoption. The guidelines fall into two broad categories. The first are the horizontal guidelines which address general matters relevant across a range of products. Examples of such guidelines relevant to the field of neurology are those concerning statistical issues, drug development in the elderly, drug development in children, the development of sustained release preparations and good clinical practice. The second category of guidelines addresses specific product areas. Thus in the field of neurology there is a guideline on the development of drugs for the treatment of epilepsy and for drugs for the treatment of dementia.

The guidelines serve to reflect the consensus view from the regulatory authorities as to the requirements necessary to obtain a marketing authorisation. In 1991 the International Conference on Harmonisation (ICH) was established [9]. This Conference has been co-sponsored by the Japanese, American and European regulatory authorities, along with the pharmaceutical industry associations from the three regions. The object was to explore and then to harmonise guidelines across the three regions, thus reducing the cost and expediting the approval of new drugs world-wide. The procedure has proved to be successful and a significant number of international guidelines have now been approved. These have concentrated more on the general or horizontal issues and to date none has addressed specific problems in the field of neurology.

Current Issues in Drug Development

In the field of neurology, drugs appear to be currently investigated either in acute intervention such as the management of stroke, or are for long-term use. Examples here are in the fields of multiple sclerosis, dementia, epilepsy, motor neurone disease and Parkinson's disease. Indeed, the neurological field is

one of the most active in current drug development. The demonstration of short-term efficacy and short-term safety is usually well addressed. The more difficult matter is to determine the true safety profile and to establish long-term efficacy. It is important that clearly defined and agreed endpoints are used in such long-term trials. Although comparative efficacy is not a criterion for authorisation, comparative safety is an important matter. Moreover, regulatory authorities are looking for clinically meaningful benefit from drugs and wish to have long-terms efficacy data available.

In the past it was a requirement that two independent pivotal studies were needed. This requirement has been relaxed in the era of the multi-centre, multi-national trial. Nevertheless it is important that the trials are conducted to avoid centre bias and to allow, if possible, a retrospective, centre-by-centre analysis to confirm the validity of the efficacy findings in the study as a whole. In such trials rigid adherence to the protocol is essential. An important debate in these studies is the determination of the statistical response, whether this should be by intention-to-treat analysis or by a last-result-carried-forward analysis. In designing such studies the pharmaceutical company should be clear as to the indication which would be sought in the data sheet or summary of product characteristics.

One important matter which remains unresolved is that of the adequate dose determination. This is perhaps the most difficult issue for the pharmaceutical industry and drug regulators. Experience over many years has shown how difficult it is adequately to determine the dose of a new medicine. Indeed, on very few occasions has the true dose been fully defined at the time of authorisation. Much of this difficulty derives from the population of patients in which new drugs are investigated. The regulatory authorities wish to see a drug investigated in a population which is representative of those who will be receiving the drug in normal use. All too often the populations studied are younger, fitter and receiving fewer concomitant medications. All of this is scientifically justified in producing a clear result but can lead to difficulties later. In these circumstances the regulator is faced with the difficult decision as to how much can be extrapolated from the study population. If such representative populations are used, much important data concerning drug interactions will also be available.

The issue of dose response has been a major topic in the ICH process. A fuller review of the current position is set out in the chapter "Dose Response Information to Support Drug Regulation" in the proceedings of the Third International Conference on Harmonisation published in 1996 [9]. This chapter is worthy of study because it sets out the various approaches to establishing and then confirming the dose of drugs under clinical investigation. In particular the chapter discusses the uses of concentration-response data and the problems with titration designs. It is recognised that in some cases, notably where an early answer is essential, the titration to highest-tolerable-dose is acceptable. This approach often requires a minimum number of patients. However, it means that subsequently the dose may have to be adjusted from the analysis of further data or studies.

Parallel dose-response study designs using either placebo or placebo-controlled titration study designs are very effective in the development of drugs for conditions such as angina or hypertension but are usually unacceptable for use in life-threatening conditions. This issue may well be relevant to the development of drugs for acute intervention in the management of stroke. A number of specific study designs can be used to assess dose response. These include parallel dose response, cross-over dose response, forced titration and optional titration. It is important to recognise, however, that additional data should also be collected at all stages of the drug's development. Thus the use of population pharmacokinetics and of dosage enrichment designs may also assist the determination of the most appropriate dosing regimen to be identified.

Approval decisions are usually based on a consideration of the totality of information presented in the dossier.

Specific Issues in Drug Development in the Field of Neurology

Several of the drugs currently under investigation for neurological conditions are biotechnology products which may elicit the development of neutralising antibodies. This further emphasises the need for long-term follow-up data, to assess both the impact on long-term safety and the potential for diminishing efficacy.

Once a drug has been approved through the new centralised procedure, a European Public Assessment Report (or EPAR) is issued by the CPMP and the European Medicines Evaluation Agency. This document describes how the authorisation was assessed and evaluated. It also gives an overview of the supporting database and highlights the discussions which led to the production of the Summary of Product Characteristics or datasheet. Thus it will be very helpful for those developing new drugs in particular fields to read the EPARs carefully and

to understand the emerging regulatory consensus and the approaches being adopted. The EPAR can either be obtained from the European Medicines Evaluation Agency (EMEA) or can be found on the homepage of the EMEA on the Internet. EPARs have so far been generated for Betaferon and for Riluzole. It may also be helpful to understand how an EPAR is produced and how it reflects the assessment process. Therefore readers may wish to refer to the document which has been generated by the CPMP and by the EMEA entitled *From Assessment Report to EPAR* [10].

There are two areas of major interest at present in the field of neurology which are in the public domain: the development of drugs for epilepsy and the development of drugs for the treatment of dementia. The CPMP produced a guideline in 1989 [11] setting out the issues and the criteria for the development of medicinal products for the treatment of epileptic disorders. This guideline draws heavily on a document produced by the International League Against Epilepsy which was published at the same time [12].

These documents highlight the studies necessary to the successful development of a new epileptic drug and give the requirement of the regulators. A paper in the *British Medical Journal* by Marson, Kadir and Chadwick [13] reviewed new anti-epileptic drugs and considered their efficacy and tolerability. In this paper the authors undertook a systematic review of published and unpublished randomised controlled trials of gabapentin, lamotrigine, tiagabine, topiramate, bigabatrin and zonisamid. This article highlights the difficulty of identifying the true position of newer agents in particular, as many are initially developed with trials as add-on treatments in patients with drug-resistant partial epilepsy. The article also highlights the issue of developing anti-epileptic drugs for children. This is part of a wider debate on how data can be extrapolated from adults to children.

In the area of dementia several guidelines have been developed. These highlight the selection and criteria for recruiting patients for trials. They also address in detail the criteria of defining efficacy, in particular noting the necessity of identifying improvement in the three domains of cognition, activities of daily living and overall clinical response (global assessment). The CPMP draft guideline also sets out a possible general strategy for drug development and addresses issues such as enrichment design, adjustment for prognostic variables and the handling of concomitant treatments [14]. It is important that those developing drugs for use in dementia or undertaking studies are familiar with the guidelines and any subsequent amendments.

Production of the Dossier

The Notice to Applicants issued by the European Commission describes how the dossier has to be assembled both for a new drug application and for an abridged or abbreviated file [15]. The dossier serves many functions. It provides a history of the drug development, it brings together in one place the totality of the data on the drug and it is the resource document against which the assessment process will be undertaken. The dossier is also required to give a full summary of the data. The latter is increasingly important, given that many dossiers now exceed 300 volumes and some exceed 600 volumes. Increasingly, modern technology is being used to assist the assembly and the submission of these large files.

It is important in such a complex process not to lose sight of the prime objective of the dossier. This is to bring to the regulator all the pertinent data presented to demonstrate the safety and the efficacy of the drug in the proposed indications. The dossier therefore needs to be focused and to substantiate the claims being proposed in the summary of product characteristics. The summary of product characteristics should be written not to promote the drug but rather to reflect the available data and to allow the safe usage of the drug by clinicians and by the patients. It is also important that the dossier reflects the studies undertaken on the product proposed for marketing. If there have been changes in the manufacture or in the final specification of the product then this can undermine the validity of the clinical trials if they have been undertaken on a different product. At the very least there will be a requirement for bridging studies to show that the changes in formulation have not invalidated the clinical studies. This may be a problem for drugs being investigated in neurology if they are derived from biotechnology processes. Finally, the dossier is meant to provide the regulator with the reassurance of the safety of the drug in clinical studies and a reassurance that the drug will be safe when exposed to a much larger population.

The Clinical Expert Report

The Clinical Expert Report is a very important document in the European dossier. The expert report is a critical analysis undertaken by either an internal or an external expert of the company which is meant to highlight the strengths of the drug development programme and to analyse critically the data in the dossier, presenting the issues relevant to the approval process for the regulatory authority. The expert report is not meant to be a summary, rather the report should critically analyse the dossier and discuss potential downsides of the medicinal product. The expert report should pay particular attention to the proposed summary of product characteristics. The expert is required to look across the entire efficacy database and to reflect upon the global analysis of safety which has been produced. Within the report there is an additional section for a statement on the compliance of the sponsor and of the studies with the principles of good clinical practice. The expert reports form a valuable part of the dossier submitted throughout Europe. The documents should also be seen as an opportunity for the company to describe the development of the drug and the problems which have been addressed during the development phase. The expert report should be considered as part of a continuing process throughout the development of the drug, rather than a bureaucratic requirement for a document to be produced at the end of the development. Thus many now refer to the "expert report process". A more detailed discussion on the role and the functions of the clinical expert can be found in *The Textbook of Pharmaceutical Medicine* [16]. The importance of the expert report has been enhanced with the introduction of the new authorisation procedures within the European Union.

The Assessment Process

It is important for those developing new drugs and also for those writing expert reports to have an understanding of the assessment process and the requirements of the regulator. In late 1994 the European Member States adopted a guideline which for the first time codified the assessment process across Europe [17]. This document describes not only the way in which an assessment is to be undertaken but also the report which is exchanged between Member States. In most regulatory authorities major new drugs will be assessed by the staff of the national agency and also be considered by independent advisory committees. In the UK all new active substances submitted through the national or the mutual recognition procedures are assessed by the staff of the MCA. A team will be brought together for the assessment of each new drug, comprising a pharmacist (or biotechnology expert), a toxicologist, a physician and a statistician. They will analyse the dossier in depth and will produce a detailed report which will summarise the data and also give a critical analysis. There are obvious similarities here between the tasks being undertaken within the regulatory authority and those which are expected of the external clinical expert in the report required from the company. This is no accident and indeed the clinical expert report from the applicant's experts is designed to facilitate the work of the internal reviewers. The summarisation of the dossier is necessary so that a freestanding report can be prepared which is then able to be discussed in depth by the independent advisory bodies.

In the UK the CSM consists of independent experts drawn from the fields of academia, clinical medicine, toxicology, pharmacy, biotechnology and epidemiology. The independent committees bring an important element of quality assurance to the regulatory process and also mean that each new drug is scrutinised by a wide number of experts and, in particular, those who have up-to-date knowledge in the area of therapeutics for which the drug will be used. In recent years the CSM has established an external panel of experts to assist in the consideration of more specialised applications [18]. The UK system allows an appeal against a provisional decision made by the CSM and a second appeal to the more senior body, the Medicines Commission. This two-stage appeal process is unique in Europe. In most other authorities there is only a single appeal, which is back to the first body which gave the original view.

Once a medicine has been licensed, much further development work may take place. Indeed, in recent years many applicants have chosen to introduce a new medicine with a specialist indication and have then sought to extend the use of the drug through either a line extension or variations. Line extensions and variations constitute a significant further workload for the regulatory authorities. The UK MCA will receive in excess of 13 000 variations per year. The majority of these will be for pharmaceutical or manufacturing changes, but an increasing proportion are for the introduction of new indications or modifications to the summary of product characteristics. To support such a complex procedure the UK MCA has invested heavily in a major IT system which allows for the on-screen assessment of new drug applications and for the on-screen approval of the authorisation.

The Single European Community Licensing System

Over the last decade a new system for the approval of medicines has been evolving within Europe. During this time a multi-state and a so-called concertation procedure were established. Both of these sought to introduce a supranational route for licensing within Europe but neither gave a binding opinion

and the final decision on whether a drug should be approved or not remained with the national competent authorities. With the drive to complete the internal market and particularly to conclude the internal market in pharmaceuticals, a new system was introduced from 1 January 1995. It is important for those developing drugs and interested in clinical trials to have a knowledge of this new system. The remainder of this chapter will therefore consider the new authorisation procedures.

From 1 January 1995, two new routes for drug authorisations were introduced. These were the centralised system and the so-called decentralised or mutual recognition system. The latter was made optional from 1995 but became compulsory from 1 January 1998. At that time it will be seen that a single Community system has been produced with two manifestations: one the centralised system and the other the mutual recognition system.

The Centralised System

The centralised system operates whereby an applicant can submit a dossier to the European Medicines Evaluation Agency (the EMEA), which is located in Docklands in London. This agency acts as a coordinating centre for the Member States and provides logistical support for a scientific advisory committee drawn from the Member States which is called the CPMP (or the Committee on Proprietary Medicinal Products). The centralised procedure is mandatory for all products of biotechnology, for example betainterferons for the treatment of multiple sclerosis, and is also available optionally for any new active substance or for a major therapeutic advance. In this context riluzole was approved through the centralised procedure. Once the application has been submitted, two teams of assessors are appointed – so-called rapporteur and co-rapporteur teams. These are drawn from two of the Member State authorities. These teams will assess the dossier and produce an assessment report. In doing so they will usually seek advice from their national advisory committees. Their assessment report will then be referred to the CPMP member, who will consider the report and bring the views of the other 15 Member States to the deliberations. The European Economic Area countries, Iceland and Norway, have become members of the CPMP from 1 January 2000. The European Committee will then decide whether the drug is approvable or not approvable and whether there are objections and issues which need to be resolved.

If there are issues to be resolved then the clock can be stopped to allow the company to respond. Once the applicant has responded then a further evaluation of the response data will be made by the rapporteur and co-rapporteur and then the Committee will give its opinion. Should this be a negative opinion the company has a right of appeal back to the CPMP. If the opinion is positive the Summary of Product Characteristics (SPC) will be agreed and the opinion will then be made binding across all Member States. This is done by the European Commission, which acts as the licensing authority for the new procedure. The approval involves a role for the Member States through a so-called Standing Committee, with the final authorisation being granted by the European Commission.

When a drug is authorised through the centralised procedure the SPC will be identical in all the Member States and in all 11 languages in the European Union. Furthermore the Patient Information Leaflets and the labels will also be identical. Any subsequent variations or any matters of pharmacovigilance to do with the product are also discussed through the new procedure and action taken by the European Commission. However, the monitoring of pharmacovigilance of such products remains the responsibility of the Member States.

Thus it can be seen that this procedure, although called the centralised system, operates in a decentralised manner. The EMEA acts as a coordinating centre. The assessment work is done by the Member States and the deliberations take place between the Member States. It is likely that many of the major new drugs in the field of neurology will be authorised through this new procedure. Indeed there have already been several important new medicines in the field of neurology which have come through this system.

Mutual Recognition Procedures

The mutual recognition procedure is an equally important part of the system. Indeed it became the major route for licensing medicines throughout Europe from 1 January 1998. It was decided that mutual recognition should be introduced in a phased manner over 3 years. The procedure operates whereby an applicant obtains authorisation in the first country, known as the Reference Member State (RMS), and then seeks to extend the licence into other Member States via the process of mutual recognition. This means that the first country supplies it initial assessment report to the other Member States, so-called Concerned Member States (CMS). This report is supplied at the request of the applicant. The CMSs have up to 90 calendar days during which to assess the dossier and raise any serious public health objections. Other more minor objections may be

raised in the initial period of the 90 days but are expected to be resolved through dialogue and clarification.

Any serious public health objections must be raised by day 90. If such objections are raised then the matter is referred to arbitration by the CPMP. To assist in this arbitration the CPMP will appoint one or two Member States to act as rapporteurs. They will assess the issue in dispute and the company then may submit further data. The Committee will consider the matter and give its opinion. This opinion is then made binding on all Member States through the same decision-making process as is used for centralised applications. This involves a standing committee of the Member States with the final decision being taken by the European Commission.

Previously an applicant could invoke the mutual recognition procedure after obtaining a first authorisation. From 1 January 1998 this has remained the preferred route. If an applicant submits dossiers in two or more Member States, then as soon as one country grants the authorisation the other applications are immediately transferred into the mutual recognition system.

Figures 6.1 and 6.2 illustrate how both centralised and mutual recognition procedures operate. The article in the *European Journal of Clinical Pharmacology* from which the diagrams are taken describes the procedures in more detail [19].

The system also involves the coordination of national inspections and national pharmacovigilance. A significant innovation of the centralised procedure is the production of the European Public Assessment Report (EPAR). This document describes the assessment of new drug application and provides a publicly available statement as to why the product was licensed and the issues which were faced during the approval process. It can be regarded as the equivalent of the former Summary Basis of Approval documents issued by the FDA in the USA.

Conclusion

Drug regulation in Europe has changed dramatically over the last 30 years. At the same time there have been huge advances in the development of new medicines, particularly with the introduction of biotechnology products. The future holds the promise of further major developments in the field of neurology and the probable impact of gene technology. We can also expect to see the benefits from recent advances in molecular biology. This will call for greater dialogue between the regulators and the pharmaceutical industry. In the field of neurology many advances are occurring in areas where previously no treat-

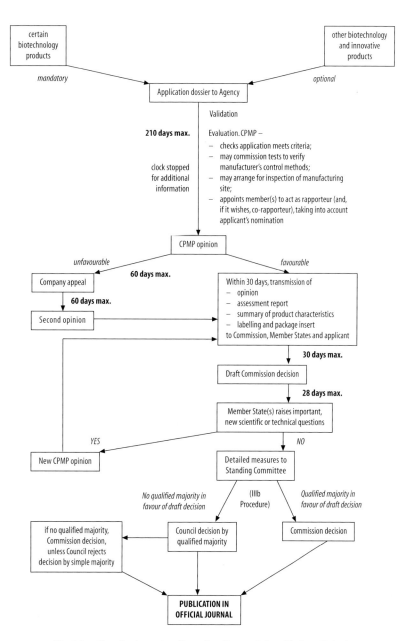

Fig. 6.1. Centralised procedure. (Reproduced by permission of Springer-Verlag.)

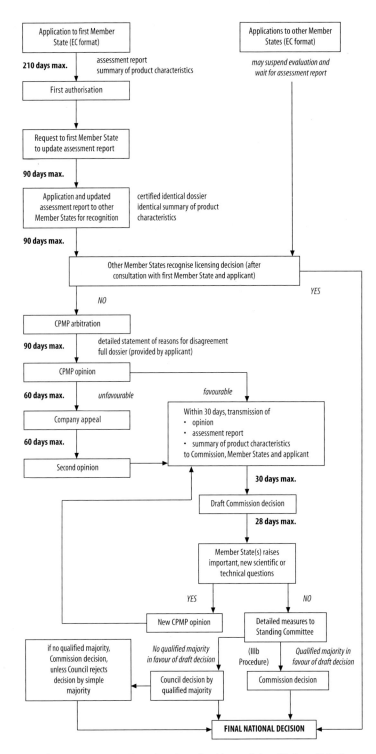

Fig. 6.2.   Decentralised procedure. (Reproduced by permission of Springer-Verlag.)

ments existed. In these areas it will be important that long-term efficacy and safety are fully determined. Research into treatment of neurological disease appears to be one of the most active areas and is one where close cooperation between the regulators and the regulated are likely to produce major benefits.

References

1. Mann RD. Modern drug use, chapter 8. Leicester: MTP Press, 1984.
2. Guideline notes on applications for clinical trials certificates and clinical trials exemptions (MAL 4), revised 1996.
3. Good clinical practice for trials in medicinal products in the EC. In: The rules governing medicinal products in the EC, vol III 1996. Addendum III/9104/90 EN.
4. A guide to the provisions affecting doctors and dentists. MAL 30. London: HMSO, 1985.
5. Rawlins MD, Jefferys DB. Study of the UK product licence applications containing new active substances, 1987–89. BMJ 1991;302:233–235.
6. Rawlins MD, Jefferys DB. UK product licence applications involving new active substances, 1987–89: their fate after appeal. J Clin Pharmacol 1993;35:599–602.
7. Annual report and accounts. MCA 1994/95. London: HMSO, 1995.
8. Scientific advice to be given by the CPMP for innovative medicinal products. EMEA/SOP/002/95/Final.
9. D'Arcy PF, Harran DWG, editors. Proceedings of the third international conference on harmonisation 1995. Belfast: Queen's University Belfast, 1996.
10. Centralised procedure: from assessment report to EPAR EMEA/SOP/005/95/Final.
11. Medicinal products for the treatment of epileptic disorders. In: The rules governing medicinal products in the European Union, vol III, 1996:537–543.
12. Guidelines for the clinical evaluation of antiepileptic drugs: International League Against Epilepsy. Epilepsia 1989;30: 400–408.
13. Marson AG, Kadir ZA, Chadwick DW. New antiepileptic drugs: a systematic review of their efficacy and tolerability. BMJ 1996;313:1169–1174.
14. Note for guidance on medicinal products in the treatment of Alzheimer's disease IX 1997.
15. Commission of the European Community The rules governing medicinal products in the EC, vol II, Notice to applicants, 1994.
16. Mann RD, Rawlins MD, Auty RM, editors. Textbook of pharmaceutical medicine. London: Parthenon, 1993: chapter 15.
17. The EC assessment report guideline. CPMP III/5447. 1994.
18. Annual report of the Medicines Commission. London: HMSO, 1995.
19. Jefferys DB, Jones KH. EMEA and the new pharmaceutical procedures for Europe. Eur J Clin Pharmcol 1995;47:471–476.

Sources of Information

Information on the centralised procedure including copies of the European Public Assessment Reports (EPARS) and draft guidelines and consultations are available on the EMEA website: *http://www.eudra.org/EMEA.html*

Copies of final guidelines are available on the European Commission pharmaceuticals website: *http://pharmacos.eudra.org* whilst further information on the mutual recognition procedure can be obtained from the Heads of Agencies mutual recognition website: *http://heads,medagencies.org*

Information on the UK Medicines Control Agency can be obtained from its website: *www.open.gov.uk/mca/home.htm*

7. Drug Regulatory Requirements in the United States

P. Leber

The American System of Drug Product Regulation

Under the requirements of the Federal Food, Drug and Cosmetic (FD&C) Act, enacted in 1938, a new drug product may not be marketed (distributed in inter-state commerce) unless it is the subject of an approved New Drug Application (NDA). The requirement for an NDA is the linchpin of the federal system of pre-market clearance of new drug products that operates within the United States.

The Congress established a system of pre-market clearance with the intent that it would eliminate forever the risk that a new drug could be distributed in the United States before it had undergone sufficient testing to ensure it would be "safe for use" under the conditions of use recommended in its labeling. Congress did not act out of concern about some theoretical, unrealized risk to the public health, but in the aftermath of a tragedy [1] in which more than 100 persons suffered needless and painful deaths as a direct consequence of a commercial drug sponsor's reckless decision to market a new sulfonamide antibiotic solubilized in diethylene glycol, a potent renal toxin. Ironically, the sponsor, a well-established ethical pharmaceutical house, had tested the product for appearance, fragrance, and palatability, but not for safety.

The federal system of drug regulation, although modified in a number of important ways since its creation, still operates, at least in regard to its basic mechanisms, pretty much as it did when it was first devised. A sponsor seeking to market a new drug, having conducted all tests reasonably applicable to determine whether or not the drug meets the requirements of the Act, submits an NDA containing full reports of the results of those tests to the Food and Drug Administration (FDA).

The FDA, the agency within the executive branch of America's tripartite federal government that bears responsibility for enforcement of the Act, is obliged to review a sponsor's NDA and to approve it, unless upon review, the agency's staff, among them clinicians, pharmacologists, statisticians, determine that the application fails to show that the drug product for which the application has been submitted meets the requirements of the Act.

The Efficacy Requirements

The requirements of the 1938 Act were devised to ensure that all marketed drug products would be competently made, manufactured to reasonable specifications of purity, and safe for use when administered as recommended under the conditions of use described in their labeling (the latter, importantly, could not be false or misleading in any particular). The Act stood silent on the matter of efficacy, however. Indeed, it was not until 1962 that the Act was amended to require that marketed drugs not only be "safe for use" but "effective in use" under the conditions of use recommended in their approved labeling.

It is noteworthy, especially because it stands in stark contrast to almost all other requirements of the Act which are presented primarily in terms of Congressional aims or intents (i.e., that all reasonably applicable tests have been performed to show the drug is safe) that the kind/quality of evidence necessary to document a drug's effectiveness in use is described in relatively explicit detail. Specifically, the Act requires that an NDA be disapproved if, upon review, the agency determines that there is a lack of substantial evidence of the product's effectiveness in use. The Act defines "substantial evidence" as:

> evidence consisting of adequate and well controlled investigations, including clinical investigations, by experts qualified by scientific training and

experience to evaluate the effectiveness of the drug involved, on the basis of which it could fairly and responsibly be concluded by such experts that the drug will have the effect it purports or is represented to have under the conditions of use prescribed, recommended, or suggested . . . in [its] labeling . . .

The critical thrust of the definition is that the determination of effectiveness must turn on evidence adduced in valid clinical experiments. Although the definition makes clear reference to experts and their judgment, it does so only to explicate the qualities of the evidence adduced in adequate and controlled investigations that would allow the evidence to be deemed probative. Thus, before they can conclude that a drug has been shown to be effective in use, agency officials must make a determination that the evidence adduced in more than one valid clinical experiment is such that it would allow a fair-minded and informed expert to conclude "fairly and responsibly" from the results of adequate and well-controlled clinical investigations that the drug product has the beneficial therapeutic actions its sponsor claims it does. The fact that one or more individual experts might, for any number of other reasons, including clinical experience, logic, results of experiments in animals, or sanguine expectations, deem the drug to be effective is, in the absence of the necessary findings from adequate and well-controlled investigations, irrelevant.

The Attributes of an Adequate and Well-Controlled Clinical Investigation

The Act's definition of substantial evidence, although clear as to the source of the evidence that may be deemed probative in effectiveness determinations, is, however, essentially bereft of practical details regarding the nature, design, and conduct of the adequate and well-controlled clinical investigations that sponsors are expected to conduct to adduce the evidence necessary to gain approval of their products.

This is not unusual. Federal laws typically provide but a broad outline of Congressional intent because Congress cannot reasonably view itself as a source of technical expertise. Accordingly, Congress delegates to the executive branch agency responsible for the administration of an Act, authority to promulgate the technical regulations required for an Act's efficient day-to-day enforcement.

An agency's regulations are developed through a process known as "notice and comment" rule making. Briefly, the agency responsible for the enforcement of an Act publishes in the Federal Register (FR) a draft of the set of rules it proposes to issue (i.e., the "notice" part of notice and comment rule making). A period then ensues during which comments may be submitted. Once the comment period ends, the agency involved evaluates the comments submitted and, in good faith, revises the proposed rule as appropriate. Depending upon the number and nature of the comments received, the agency may either re-propose a new draft of the rule for further comment, or may issue a final version of the rule. Once a rule becomes final, it is included in the US Code of Federal Regulations (CFR); these codified regulations are tantamount to law and their requirements are binding upon both the agency and all parties subject to the requirements of an Act.

The federal regulations that apply to the clinical investigation of unapproved new drugs appear in the Code at 21 CFR 312; those that address the new drug approval process appear at 21 CFR 314.

It is important to appreciate that the scope and nature of the requirements set forth in federal regulations are constrained not only by the explicit requirements of federal law but by what legal authorities term "congressional intent." For example, if the interpretation of a section of some federal law is arguable or obscure, those responsible for its enforcement are obliged to interpret the section in regard to what they discern is/was the intent of Congress in drafting that particular section. "Congressional intent" can often be surmised from congressional documents, hearing reports, etc. When there is no clear written legislative history on a point, legal authorities are obliged to determine what "Congress, in its wisdom," probably intended.

The federal regulations that explicate the attributes of adequate and well-controlled clinical investigations [21 CFR 314.126] are a product of notice and comment rule of the kind just described. Thus, the principles of trial design and conduct described in the agency's regulations are those the agency, taking into consideration comments offered by the regulated industry, academia, constituency groups and consumer organizations among others, determined are necessary to meet the requirements of the FD&C Act. In considering the validity of the strategies and approaches taken by the FDA, one must be mindful that the agency can neither require more, nor accept less, than the FD&C Act demands.

Issues and Considerations Affecting the Design of Controlled Clinical Trials Employed in the Assessment of Neurological Drug Products

An adequate and well-controlled clinical investigation is one which by design and conduct is capable of adducing valid and reliable evidence that will contribute to the body of evidence upon which a regulatory assessment of a product's effectiveness in use must turn. An adequate and well-controlled clinical investigation is intended, therefore, to provide an empirical estimate of a drug's effect that is both fair and minimally biased in regard to the specific sample of patients being evaluated in the clinical trial.

Choice of the Patient Sample

Agency regulations require that substantial evidence of effectiveness of a new drug be gained in clinical investigations that enroll patients suffering from the condition for which the drug will be proffered as a treatment, if marketed. There is no expectation, however, that the samples studied be representative of the population of patients with the disease in the way that statistical theories of sampling would demand if the goal were to generate an estimate of a drug's expected effect in the population of potential users. To the contrary, as to the nature of the patients studied in clinical trials, FDA regulations (21 CFR 314.126[b][3]) require only that: "The method of selection of subjects provides adequate assurance that they have the disease or condition being studied, or evidence of susceptibility and exposure to the condition against which prophylaxis is directed."

Controlled clinical trials conducted to evaluate new drugs, accordingly, typically recruit what the author describes as "samples of convenience," so called because they are comprised of individuals chosen almost entirely to suit the needs and interests of the investigator and/or sponsor involved.

The agency's willingness to evaluate the efficacy of new drug products in controlled investigations employing such sampling practices is often challenged because such studies cannot reasonably be claimed to provide a reliable and valid estimate of a drug's typical expected effect in the population. While the criticism that the quantitative estimate of the magnitude of a drug's treatment effect adduced from the typical controlled clinical drug study cannot be legitimately generalized to the population as a whole is correct, it is important to appreciate that the criticism is largely irrelevant from a regulatory perspective. The Act requires only that a drug be shown to be effective as claimed in its labeling; accordingly as long as the evidence adduced is such that it would allow an expert with experience in managing patients with the disease being treated to conclude from the evidence that the drug has the therapeutic effect claimed, the evidence, its limited external validity notwithstanding, must be deemed substantial.

To be clear, the results of effectiveness trials are often put to other uses (as a basis for devising directions for the use of the product, to gain insight into whether sex, race, or other factors, among them age, genetic makeup, etc., exert a substantive influence on realized estimates of the drug's effects, both desired and untoward, etc.), but, from a strictly epistemological perspective, no one has ever claimed that results of effectiveness trials conducted to establish the effectiveness of drugs provide a robust and reliable estimate of a drug's expected therapeutic effect in the population to which it will be administered upon marketing.

It is important, too, to recognize that those who decry the limited external validity of controlled trials conducted with new drugs regularly fail to offer any practical and, more critically, valid alternative to the regulatory approach. To the contrary, the alternatives typically proposed are entirely untrustworthy. Evidence about drug effects obtained in open studies or case series, even if published in the archival medical literature, are notoriously unreliable and misleading. Reports based on controlled trials conducted by individual academic investigators are certainly no more representative than the typical multiclinic study conducted by commercial sponsors, and, worse, tend to be based on very small numbers of subjects. Perhaps the most unreliable among all alternatives offered are proposals to rely upon the findings of so called "outcomes" research, in which drug effects are estimated from differences observed among the outcomes of patients who are determined (e.g., record linkage) to have been prescribed different treatments for what is taken (typically based on some nominal coding in a data base) to be the same medical conditions, complaint or illness. "Outcomes" research has many enthusiastic proponents who note that it not only costs far less to conduct than traditional randomized controlled trials, but, because it is based on information gained from large numbers of real patients who suffer from diverse manifestations of the illness treated, provides, unlike randomized controlled trials, externally valid results. This is patent nonsense.

Admittedly, the external validity of a randomized controlled clinical study is limited, but, if conducted correctly, its results are at least internally valid. Outcomes research of the sort described, in contrast, can claim no kind of formal validity whatsoever, a truth evident to anyone who has ever bothered to contemplate the multiplicity of factors beyond pharmacological treatment that affect clinical outcome. Indeed, this very kind of confounding is the reason why a rational assessment of a physician's competence cannot turn solely on the outcomes of the patients in his care, but must consider the nature of the patients taken into care.

It is not that the regulatory system prefers to rely upon estimates that have limited external validity; the problem is that there is no practical way to test new drugs in patients that are representative of the population in the statistical sense. Moreover, even if it were possible, there would be little advantage in doing so.

Could random, or stratified random, sampling be used in drug testing? In theory, of course it could, but it would make commercial drug development far more expensive and time-consuming than it currently is. Perhaps even more important, one needs to consider carefully the question as to what use or uses an unbiased estimate of the mean effect of a drug treatment in the population would be put.

The notion of effect size, although of some utility statistically (e.g., in estimating sample sizes for power calculation, it is customary to use, as a measure of "effect size," the ratio of the numerical value of the expected difference on the outcome measure to the standard deviation of that outcome in the population), has little, if any, real-world meaning.

Indeed, the very concept of a population-based estimate of a drug's effect in patients with a given disease is illusory because the diagnostic process in much of medicine, and certainly in neurology, cannot be relied upon to capture samples of patients that are biologically homogeneous. The neurologic nosology, in particular, is still largely taxonomic, grouping patients into diagnostic categories on the basis of a seemingly common phenotype (shared signs, symptoms, test findings, and clinical course). Phenotypic homogeneity cannot guarantee genotypic homogeneity, however. As a consequence, almost any sample of patients, even one that appears phenotypically homogeneous (and few are, on close examination, ever truly homogeneous), seems certain to consist of a mixture of subjects for whom a single estimate of treatment effect size is largely uninformative.

From a strictly mathematical point of view, of course, it is always possible to construct a single overall average estimate of a drug's effect given (1) the identity and proportional representation of each homogeneous subset in the population and (2) an estimate of the drug's effect within each of these homogeneous subsets. If, arguendo, the field of neurology had the capacity to identify these homogeneous subgroups, however, it is not in the least clear to what practical use a single overall estimate of the effect of any drug averaged across all these subgroups groups would serve, at least for medical or regulatory purposes. The goal of clinical pharmacology and therapeutics is to individualize treatment recommendations as much as possible. For regulatory work, the primary aim is to determine whether or not the drug has the effects its labeling claims it does. Thus, for both clinical and drug regulatory purposes, an estimate of an average treatment effect of a drug is rather like an estimate of the average size of fruit: estimable, but of little practical utility. Admittedly, an estimate of the average size of a drug's effect might be useful for some non-clinical purpose. A health care provider organization, for example, might, for financial reasons, want to limit the number of products in its official formulary. Accordingly, the provider might elect to choose among competing products within a given area of therapeutics on the basis of each drug's reported average effect size much as a careful homemaker might want to choose which supermarket to patronize on the basis of the average size of fruit sold. Incidentally, whether or not it would be wise to use average size of the entity measured as a means to select supermarkets, let alone drug products, is another highly arguable question. The author's point is that the kind of quantitative estimates one requires turn upon the purpose one has; what is useful in one area of endeavor (e.g., cost curtailment) may be totally inappropriate in another (e.g., choice of a drug for clinical use).

Outcome Measures: Content

An adequate and well-controlled clinical investigation, beyond enrolling appropriate subjects, must employ measures of outcome that will be accepted among experts in a field as capable of capturing, in a substantively meaningful fashion, the therapeutic benefits of the investigational drug being evaluated.

In some areas of therapeutics, certain measures of outcome have, over time, achieved widespread acceptance among experts as suitable for such use. Typically, this obtains when a therapeutic drug class is well established (e.g., outcome measures used to assess anti-epileptic, anti-parkinsonian, anti-spastic effects). Incidentally, there is no intent to suggest that these widely accepted measures have ideal properties. To the contrary, most can be improved upon; the point is that their use is accepted and is unlikely to provoke controversy among experts. In other areas, especially those involving the development of treatments for conditions lacking known effective treatments, there is likely to be no widely recognized measure and, in such instances, there is always a risk that a difference in an outcome measure favorable to the investigational drug will not have the impact that those conducting the study intend it to have.

Sponsors are, accordingly, well advised to consider their choice of outcome measures carefully, seeking the advice of experts knowledgeable both in the nature of disease and in the history of prior efforts to develop treatments for its management. If the results of a study in such an area are likely to be advanced in support of a regulatory claim, the author strongly recommends that the sponsor consult with the appropriate FDA review division about its plans.

Incidentally, although current Investigational New Drug (IND) regulations only require sponsors holding INDs to submit a protocol to their IND file for a clinical study prior to its initiation, the agency is still willing to offer comments about a study. To take advantage of this guidance, however, the sponsor must allow the agency sufficient lead time to review a clinical trial proposal.

Outcome Measures: Form

The Act has no preference as to the means used to obtain a quantitative measures of a drug's effects; either counts or continuous measures or both may be employed. Similarly, those who conduct a trial are free to choose the domain of measurement that best serves their purpose; an estimate of a drug's effect may, accordingly, be derived from a difference in the time taken to reach some critical event or from a difference in symptom intensity or behavioral performance at some arbitrary point in time after treatment is begun.

As noted previously, because of the sampling methods employed, the absolute magnitude of the estimated effect is not of primary regulatory importance. What counts is whether or not the estimate relied upon can be deemed by experts to be a valid and fair measure of the drug's effect fairly obtained. Agency regulations, accordingly, emphasize the importance of sponsors employing methods of trial design and conduct that will permit the agency to rely upon the results of the trial as a source probative evidence.

The Choice of a Control: An Epistemological and Ethical Conundrum

Estimates of a drug's therapeutic effect useful in regulatory drug assessment are typically derived from a comparison of outcomes attained among patients treated with the drug and one or more appropriate control conditions. Although the agency's regulations recognize five types of adequate and well-controlled trials that may be employed to obtain valid estimates of drug effect (i.e., historical, no-treatment, active, placebo and graded dose), only the latter three of these designs permit blind evaluation of outcomes among samples of patients concurrently randomized to the treatments of interest.

Ordinarily, unless the treatment effect of a drug is so constant and so large (relative to the natural variation in the illness/condition treated) that it cannot reasonably and responsibly be attributed to anything but the action of the drug (e.g., general anesthetic), sponsors will be well advised to employ a study design that relies upon a showing of the superiority of the experimental treatment over the control condition, whatever it may be, as the basis for documenting their product's effectiveness in use.

In some areas of neurological therapeutics, in particular those where effective treatments are available, for example, epilepsy, there has been considerable reluctance to carry out studies employing designs that turn on showing a between-treatment difference. No doubt investigators have their reasons, among them the practical considerations involving the ease of subject recruitment and the moral disquiet posed by any experimental design that requires the randomization of a sick patient either to placebo or to a less than fully potent dose of a standard drug used as an active control.

The author finds these objections understandable, but not especially persuasive. Although the failure to find a difference between an investigational treatment and a standard control is not incompatible with a conclusion that the former is equivalent to the latter, it is not proof of that possibility. In particular, the failure to find a difference in an experiment may have nothing whatsoever to do with the potential effect of either treatment. The reason is that a finding of no difference in an experiment is a null finding, and a null finding has no unique interpretation.

In contrast, a study that documents the superiority of an experimental agent over a standard control condition virtually compels the analyst to conclude the drug is effective, provided, of course, that the difference cannot be ascribed to fraud, bias or chance, each of which is an alternative explanation for the finding [2].

As to the "ethical" objections raised to designs intended to show a difference, the author has long found them less than compelling [3], but acknowledges that they pose dilemmas for all. If no effective or truly effective treatment exists for a condition, it is hard to argue persuasively that a physician violates his or her obligation to a patient by agreeing to allow him or her to participate in an experiment in which he or she may be randomized to placebo rather than to some investigational treatment of uncertain efficacy and safety. In such circumstances, the investigational drug, being pharmacologically active, may well do the individual patient more harm than good [3], but this possibility, admittedly, is rarely given much weight by either desperate patients or the practitioners caring for them. To the contrary, the mere existence of a hypothesis that an investigational drug may have a beneficial effect is often sufficient to persuade some physicians that they must administer the drug to patients in their care, especially when the disease affecting the patient is serious and lacks a known effective treatment.

The issue is not easily resolved because tensions exist between the interests and desires of the individual patient and those of society as a whole. The desire of a patient to have immediate, unrestricted access to any and all new treatments is totally understandable. Society, however, has a compelling interest in determining whether or not an investigational drug is effective in use and safe for use prior to allowing its wide-scale marketing. The conundrum is that society cannot obtain the information required to distinguish effective from ineffective drugs without subjecting each new drug to testing in adequate and well-controlled clinical trials, and to do so it must limit access to investigational new drugs. Not surprisingly, there is no simple and clear solution that will fully serve the interests and desires of all the parties involved. Resolution of the conundrum will not be easy because our democratic society holds the view that it is, war and other public emergencies excepted, not only obliged to treat all equally before the law, but to prevent unreasonable and unfair infringements upon the rights and interests of individual citizens. Our society has largely foresworn, in particular, the utilitarian argument that would allow it to ignore the rights of a few in order to serve the overall interests of the many.

It bears emphasis, however, that no individual patient in our society, no matter how ill or desperate, has an automatic and unquestioned legal right of immediate access to any and all experimental agents or treatments that might conceivably be helpful to him or her. To the contrary, investigational drugs are, for the most part, not only private property but are private property that the FD&C Act requires not be distributed save for investigational purposes.

An individual in our society who seeks access to something (product or service) is ordinarily obliged to pay for that access with money, goods or services.

How is a patient to pay for access to an investigational drug that is not legally marketed? While we do not ordinarily think of the process in these terms, patients gain access to experimental drugs by agreeing to participate in randomized controlled clinical trials. In truth, patients do not really gain access to an investigational drug, at least not immediately, but to the opportunity to be randomized to the drug (i.e., they in a sense purchase, by agreeing to participate in a study, a lottery ticket that ordinarily carries a 1 in 2 chance of winning.)

Compelling patients seeking investigational drugs to submit to randomization to gain access may be seen as coercive to some, but the author is among those who would dispute that characterization as being unfair. Being asked to pay a price for something that has no established value is no way equivalent to being compelled by physical force or threat of deprivation of goods and materials essential to survival (e.g., food, clothing, shelter, etc.) to act against one's own interests.

To be fair, the process is only equitable and defensible as long as all who seek access to an investigational drug are required to follow the same rules. It would be morally condemnable to force some patients to run the gauntlet of randomization while others were being given immediate, non-randomized access to the same drug for the asking. Indeed, this is why, when randomized clinical studies with a drug are under way, the author finds the granting of so-called compassionate use INDs to individual patients to be so morally troubling.

When an investigational drug is being developed as a potential alternative to already available treatments, the issues are further complicated. How is it possible once an effective treatment exists, critics of randomized controlled trials ask, to randomize a patient to placebo? Are we not, by dint of the Declaration of Helsinki, obliged to assign every patient, including those assigned to the control condition, the best available treatment? But, if it is improper to deny a patient immediate access to the treatment known to be best for him, how can any patient ever be randomized to a pharmacologically active treatment of unknown utility and safety? In sum, if we were to take the tenets voiced at Helsinki literally, would we not have to foreswear the conduct of all randomized trials once an effective treatment was marketed (or widely available)?

Accordingly, the author personally advocates that with the possible exception of early phase I trials, clinical experiments evaluating experimental treatments for neurological illness should regularly employ randomization as the means to assign treatments. Ideally, randomization would remain as the only route providing access to the investigational drug until such time that a formal determination was made that there was sufficient evidence to support the use of the drug under a treatment use protocol (i.e., treatment IND).

Trial Conduct and Censoring

Poor execution can undermine the acceptance of a study as a source of "substantial evidence" no matter how well conceived and thought out its experimental design. Failure to adhere to, even failure to document that there was, in fact, adherence to, the requirements of a protocol, may render a trial's results unacceptable. To be clear, a certain level of non-compliance or deviation is tolerated, even expected, in the best conducted of clinical trials. At some point, however, the extent of non-compliance and/or deviation from protocol requirements will make what would have otherwise been a potential source of valid evidence, unacceptable. Where that point lies is determined, ad hoc, by those who rely upon the results of the study to make a regulatory determination.

Ordinarily, an experienced investigator can, with careful planning and due diligence, carry out a clinical investigation that conforms to what the typical agency reviewer would require to find a study an acceptable source of evidence that speaks validly to a drug's effectiveness in use. Ensuring that the method of randomization is valid, that treatment assignment is properly and effectively blinded, that subjects comply with treatment assignments, that raters employ assessment procedures as required, that ratings are done in a timely fashion, etc., are but a few of the matters to which good clinical trialists attend.

Unfortunately, there are phenomena beyond the effective control of the investigator that can occur during the course of a clinical trial that can affect its validity and interpretation (e.g., the introduction of a new treatment, reports of adverse events). Perhaps most vexing within this category is censoring, that is, the premature loss of randomized subjects from a study prior to their scheduled time of completion.

Censoring, to be clear, is only a potential threat because it may occur only to a minimal extent or, if to a greater degree, randomly in a manner that in no way alters the accuracy of the estimate of treatment effect adduced, although the loss of subjects will invariably cause the estimate provided to lose precision. Unfortunately, there is no way to know, with certainty, whether or not a censoring mechanism is in some manner linked to the potential outcome status of those censored. If this kind of censoring does occur, the nominal results of a study may not accurately reflect the true performance of the drug. For example, if the adverse effects of a drug selectively cause the sickest patients with the poorest prognosis to discontinue treatment, an analysis of a study based on the subset of patients surviving to its end (i.e., a so-called completer's or observed cases analysis) will be biased in favor of the investigational drug.

Not surprisingly, therefore, the extent of censoring, and the factors that might account for it, are a major focus of the regulatory assessment of controlled clinical trials. To facilitate the analysis of the impact of censoring, the agency encourages sponsors to collect information on the status of censored subjects at the same point in secular time that they would have been assessed had they remained in a trial, even if such subjects are receiving treatments not allowed and/or intended under the study protocol. The goal is not to obtain an estimate of treatment effect, but to gain some insight into the nature of the patients censored (i.e., are they characterized by some identifiable attribute affecting outcome).

Analysis of Clinical Trial Results

Estimates of treatment effect used in regulatory drug assessment are obtained typically from between-subject randomized designs (e.g., patients are randomized concurrently, that is in parallel, to one of several treatments). Under certain circumstances, so-called within-subject (i.e., cross-over) designs are used. In every case, including even those "experiments" that rely on comparisons with historical controls, the estimate of treatment effect derives from a comparison between what is observed during exposure to the drug as compared with what is (was) observed in the absence of that exposure.

It is evident, therefore, that realized estimates of drug effect must vary from one experiment to the next, not only as function of random error of measurement but as a consequence of systematic differences in the samples of patients studied and the specific conditions under which experiments are conducted – additional reasons, incidentally, why estimates of effect size of drugs generated in different experiments may not be reliably compared.

The realized estimate of a drug's effect is often affected by the time at which the effect is measured. If a disease condition improves spontaneously (as in cluster headache), an outcome assessment made too late after onset may fail to detect an effect because too many of the patients in the control group have recovered by the time the comparison is made. If response after initiation of treatment is delayed (a feature of both antipsychotic and antidepressant treatment), an experiment may fail to document the efficacy of an effective drug because outcome is assessed too soon after treatment initiation to be detected.

In still other situations, the effect of a drug may actually vary non-linearly with time. In such circumstances, the realized value of the effect would depend upon the duration of the experiment (e.g., rising to a maximum and then declining). Similarly, the stage in a disease at which a drug is evaluated for efficacy may have similar effects on the estimate (e.g., the response to L-dopa therapy in early versus advanced Parkinson's disease).

How the treatment effect is expressed may also be important. To illustrate, consider a hypothetical drug that totally blocks the progression of a degenerative neurological disease. When the effect is estimated from the differences observed in the mean changes from baseline for the groups being compared, the duration of the study is a major factor controlling its magnitude. If, in contrast, the effect is based on differences in the mean "slope" of deterioration, and the slope for an individual patient is both characteristic and reasonably constant over a prolonged period of time, the duration of the study should not affect the size of the estimate.

In sum, as noted earlier, the regulatory issue is not how large the estimates of an effect are in absolute terms, but whether or not the effect estimated can be deemed, responsibly and fairly, by an informed expert to provide legitimate support for a conclusion that the drug is effective as claimed. It is taken as a given that no difference could be deemed to meet this standard if it were not statistically significant (i.e., too large to be explained by chance alone). In sum, a difference can be statistically but not clinically significant, but it is impossible for a difference to be clinically significant if it is not statistically significant.

Because statistical significance is so critical, it is not uncommon, regrettably, for those analyzing trials to report results as achieving statistical significance (i.e., the p value reported is <0.05, two-tailed) when, in fact, the result is only nominally significant. The problem arises when the p value reported is not what it is represented to be, that is, a statement of the risk of observing the experimental results under the null of no treatment effect. Failing to adjust the size of the test (i.e., significance level) following interim looks at emerging trial results, multiple looks at several different endpoints, multiple methods of analysis applied to the same data, etc., are but a few of the practices that are problematic. Analyses reported as significant that arise from "data conditioned" comparisons are especially troubling. Data

dredging takes many forms; it may involve tests made on subsets (identified post hoc) of the patients randomized in an experiment or it may involve the use of a statistical model for data analysis that employs a set of covariates (explanatory variables) chosen, after the fact. In either case, the p value reported has little, if anything, to do with the probability of observing the reported results under the null hypothesis.

Safety

No biologically active drug substance is likely to be entirely free of some risk. Accordingly, the notion that any drug is "safe for use" is a relative one. A regulatory determination that a drug has been shown to be "safe for use" is, therefore, more aptly characterized as a conclusion that the documented benefits of the drug's use outweigh the risks known to be associated with that use under the conditions of use recommended in the drug product's approved labeling [4]. One must be mindful that a determination of this kind is not only subjective but arguable.

Subjective or not, a responsible assessment of risk and benefit is only possible if the harms that are likely to be associated with the use of a drug under the conditions of use recommended are both identified and well characterized. Accordingly, a major thrust of most pre-marketing drug development programs is devoted to gaining experience with the drug in as many patients as possible for as long as possible under the conditions of use that will be recommended in product labeling.

Not all subjects exposed to the drug during its pre-market testing may provide meaningful information; observations reported on subjects exposed only briefly to the drug (i.e., in phase I, in PK studies, etc.), or exposed to doses well below those being recommended may offer little useful information. Even subjects treated with appropriate doses under conditions of use recommended may not serve as a reliable sources of clinical data, however, if that experience is inadequately monitored and/or ascertained. It is important, in this regard, to be mindful that every patient on treatment who is lost to follow-up (i.e., censored) may be a patient who suffered grievous harm as a consequence of exposure to the drug.

While tight clinical and laboratory surveillance ordinarily provides useful information about drug-associated risk, surveillance in the absence of an experimental structure (control group) cannot distinguish drug-associated from drug-induced adverse clinical and laboratory events. As a consequence, at the time a typical new drug is first approved for marketing, the quality of information available about its risks of use is of mixed quality.

Evidence from controlled trials, provides reliable data on drug-caused risk that occurs at a relatively high incidence (e.g., 5–10% or so). Open clinical experience serves, largely, to put a cap on the upper limit of risks not seen. To illustrate, to ensure that a risk occurring in as few as 1 in every 400 to 500 patients or so exposed to the drug will have been seen at least once, more than 1500 patients have to be followed under conditions similar to those in which the drug will be used once marketed.

Events occurring in a smaller proportion of treated patients are likely to be missed, however. To illustrate, if no catastrophic events are reported in a drug development cohort of 1500 patients, there is still a 5% chance that some catastrophic event not seen even once during the drug's testing will occur regularly in 1 of every 500 patients subsequently treated with the drug. If the risk of suffering the event is greater in some subset of the population that is not proportionally represented in the drug development cohort (e.g., patients at the extremes of age, those with serious medical illness, those taking certain drugs), events occurring at even greater frequency in the overall population may also fail to be detected.

Although the proportion of subjects exposed that is likely to be harmed may seem low from the perspective of any individual patient, the proportion is very high from a public health perspective. A catastrophic event occurring in 1/10 000 patients, for example, can have devastating consequences if a drug is widely used, yet the chance of detecting a risk of such a small magnitude during premarketing development is virtually non-existent. The discovery, during the first year of its marketing, that felbamate caused aplastic anemia is a classic illustration of the problem in the area of neurological therapeutics.

Labeling and Directions for Use

Ultimately, the goal of a drug development program is to gain approval to market a new drug under the conditions of use recommended in its approved product labeling.

To a large extent, if the goals of the sponsor are reasonable, and the development program well thought out, and a drug is both effective and not unreasonably unsafe for use, it is a relatively straightforward task to use the information developed in the course of a drug development program to craft labeling for a drug that is informative about its intrinsic properties (chemical structure, pharmacologic activities, pharmacokinetics, etc.), its clinical use or uses, and adequately describes the risks that accompany that use. Good product labeling, importantly, not only provides reliable information about the regimen and dose best used to gain the drug's effects with minimum risk, but provides information that allows the prescriber to make an informed judgment about whether or not the product is a reasonable choice for a particular patient.

Once a drug product is marketed, new information concerning the drug that becomes available is, by requirement of the FD&C Act, incorporated into product labeling. The goal, of course, is to ensure that drug product labeling provides an up-to-date, authoritative compilation of information bearing on the product's safety and effectiveness in use.

It is important to be mindful, however, that a substantive proportion of what appears in drug product labeling is, despite the efforts expended by sponsor and regulator, both pre- and post-marketing, necessarily uncertain, reflecting information gained under conditions that preclude both causal and quantitative assessment.

Summary

The system of federal drug regulation in the United States is intended, among other goals, to ensure that marketed drugs are safe for use, effective in use, and not misleadingly labeled as to their benefits and risks. The strength of the American drug regulatory system lies in its insistence that the safety and efficacy of a marked drug be demonstrated in bona fide experiments conducted with human subjects who suffer from the condition that is the intended target of treatment.

The chapter reviews highlights of the system's requirements as they are currently applied to the development of new drug products intended for use in the management of neurological disease. The reader should be mindful that the standards a democratic society imposes are always subject to revision. This is an especially important point to bear in mind in regard to the American domestic drug regulatory system which has, not surprisingly, its critics as well as admirers. The author, again not surprisingly, numbers himself among the latter. In his view, were it not for the FDA's enforcement of the FD&C Act as currently construed, much of the armamentarium would consist of ineffective and unsafe drugs that, paraphrasing the words of Oliver Wendell Holmes, Sr. would best serve mankind if they were sent to the bottom of the sea, although that solution would not be so good for the fishes [5].

References

1. Jackson CO. Doctor Massengill's elixir. In: Food and drug legislation in the new deal. Princeton, NJ: Princeton University Press, 1970.

2. Leber P. Hazards of inference: the active control investigation. Epilepsia 1989;30 (Suppl 1): S57–63.

3. Leber P. Is there an alternative to the randomized controlled trial? Psychopharmacol Bull 1991;27:3–8.

4. Leber P. Postmarketing surveillance of adverse drug effects. In: Lieberman Kane, editors. Adverse effects of psychotropic drugs. New York: Guilford Press, 1992.

5. Holmes OW. Medical essays, 1842–1882 (Boston, 1891). Cited in: Young JH. Pure food: securing the federal Food Drugs Act of 1906. Princeton, NJ: Princeton University Press, 1989.

8. Quality Control and Data Monitoring: A Guide to Good Clinical Practice

L. Brown

Introduction

It is essential that clinical trials are carried out to the highest standards to ensure that the rights and confidentiality of patients are protected and the data are accurate and credible. Guidance for quality control procedures and data monitoring for clinical trials has evolved through the development of Good Clinical Practice (GCP) standards. There are many GCP guidelines used in the world, which has resulted in many different standards of GCP being followed. In recent years the regulatory authorities and their corresponding pharmaceutical industries in Europe, Japan and the USA have been trying to harmonise the requirements for developing and marketing drugs, which includes harmonising the requirements for GCP. A harmonised guideline for GCP was issued in 1996 for implementation in Europe from 17 January 1997.

This chapter describes the physician's GCP responsibilities for carrying out clinical trials to this new GCP standard. Practical advice on how to implement these requirements, including a template for consent forms, is given. An overview of the development of GCP is provided, commonly used terms are defined and recent findings concerning physicians' compliance with GCP are reviewed.

In 1991 the European Community issued a Directive (91/507/EEC) [1] which stipulates that all phases of clinical research performed in Europe should be undertaken in accordance with GCP. Many European countries have implemented this Directive as law. A more comprehensive Directive specifically concerning clinical trials and GCP is in preparation and is expected to become law in the European Union during the next few years. The issuing of GCP guidelines and Directives has a major impact on how clinical trials are carried out by pharmaceutical companies and physicians (such as neurologists) participating in these studies. Since GCP should apply to all clinical studies that are intended to be submitted to regulatory authorities [8], it should apply to neurologists carrying out trials sponsored by pharmaceutical companies. The principles of GCP may also be applied to other clinical studies such as neurologists carrying out their own research. Whoever initiates the trial, it should be performed to GCP standard. These GCP standards apply to all therapeutic areas. Neurologists participating in pharmaceutical studies will need to comply strictly with GCP requirements. However, when carrying out their own research, in practice, it is unlikely that physicians will adhere to all aspects of GCP. In recent years the standard of GCP of many physicians' own research has increased considerably and is likely to continue to do so. Eventually, the GCP standards used may even be the same as those achieved by pharmaceutical companies.

Development of Good Clinical Practice

Following numerous events which have cast doubt on the validity of the results of clinical trials and concerns at how patients have been treated, clinical trials are now subject to great scrutiny and standards of GCP have evolved.

The origins of GCP are to be found in concerns regarding serious abuses of vulnerable human subjects. For example, in the 1950s vulnerable subjects such as prisoners, disabled people and pregnant women, without consent, took part in studies where they were exposed to radioactive substances [2]. Also at this time, poor black Americans with syphilis were denied treatment so that the natural course of the disease could be followed, even though syphilis was easily treatable [3]. Such unethical behaviour led to the World Medical Association producing the Declaration of Helsinki, which was adopted at the

18th World Medical assembly in 1964. The principles in this document form the basis of GCP.

The Declaration of Helsinki has been amended four times, most recently in 1996 at the 48th World Medical Assembly in South Africa*. The Declaration of Helsinki is the basis of the guidelines for carrying out biomedical research by the pharmaceutical industry and academic medicine. It is concerned with patient protection as exemplified by obtaining consent and having an ethics review of clinical research. The aim of the Declaration of Helsinki is for "the medical doctor to safeguard the health of the people. His or her knowledge and conscience are dedicated to the fulfilment of this mission". Ethics review is a very important component of patient protection.

The principles laid down by the World Medical Association demanded that clinical research must contain the following: good science, sound animal experiments, morally responsible investigators, reasonable risk for subjects, respect for privacy, willingness to stop for hazards, integrity in reporting and informed consent. These principles are still true of GCP today.

In 1962 the thalidomide tragedy resulted in at least 8000 children being born and surviving with severe birth defects in 46 countries. It is thought that as many as twice this number died at birth as a result of their mothers having taken thalidomide [4]. The pharmaceutical company which supplied this drug did not fully assess the adverse events reported. This case led to the development of legislation throughout the world and the introduction of GCP.

The USA took the lead in introducing GCP, because of deficiencies in carrying out clinical research, concerns regarding abuses to vulnerable patients, cases of fraud and drug tragedies such as thalidomide.

A precursor to the introduction of GCP was the development of a regulatory framework and in particular the Food, Drug and Cosmetic Act in the USA. The regulations and guidelines governing clinical trials carried out in the USA have evolved over many decades. The original Food and Drug Act became law in 1906 and required drugs to meet official requirements of strength and purity. There were no requirements concerning safety. It took a major tragedy in 1937 in the USA when "Elixir Sulfanilamide" was linked to over 100 deaths, mainly in children, to change this. The deaths were caused by diethylene glycol (anti-freeze) which was used as a solvent in the "Elixir". As a result, the Federal Food,

Drug and Cosmetic Act was passed in 1938 requiring safety to be assessed before a drug could be licensed [5].

The US Food and Drug Administration (FDA) has authority to inspect the sponsor's and physician's facilities and records to ensure they are carrying out their responsibilities. In the 1970s the General Accounting Office (GAO) of the FDA published two highly critical reports (in 1973 and 1976) concerning the FDA's inspections [6]. The 1976 report concluded: "As a result of inadequate monitoring of sponsors and clinical investigators, FDA lacks assurance that human test subjects are adequately protected and that the data upon which marketing approval is based is accurate and reliable." Several cases of fraud were detected at this time and this resulted in an intensified inspection [3].

Further efforts were made by the FDA to improve the situation at this time by publishing proposed regulations in the Federal Register. The FDA proposals were:

- Proposed Establishment of Regulations on Obligations of Sponsors and Monitors – Fed Reg 42, 49612 (1977)
- Proposed Obligations of Clinical Investigators of Regulated Articles – Fed Reg 43, 35210 (1978)
- Proposed Standards for Institutional Review Boards for Clinical Investigations – Fed Reg 43, 35186 (1978). This was withdrawn and reproposed as Protection of Human Subjects – Fed Reg 44, 47688 (1979).

Although these proposals were not called GCP guidelines, they contained the elements of GCP and are frequently described as the first GCP guidelines. The USA went on to issue several guidelines and information sheets which are concerned with GCP.

In the mid-1980s GCP guidelines and regulations based on the original FDA proposals, but amended to reflect local requirements and cultures, were developed. Guidelines now exist in many countries and regions including Scandinavia, the European Union, Japan and Australia and national legislation exists in some countries such as France, Germany and Italy.

The European Union's (EU) Committee for Proprietary Medicinal Products GCP guidelines were published in July 1990 and took effect from July 1991. The EU Commission Directive 91/507/EEC, mentioned earlier, was issued on 19 July 1991 and provides a legal basis for GCP with effect from January 1992. Since that time it has provided a standard for carrying out clinical research in the EU and has attempted to harmonise GCP in the Member States.

---

* Following completion of this chapter a new draft of the Declaration of Helsinki was issued in 2000.

A large number of GCP guidelines and regulations now exist. Although there are similarities between them, the lack of consistency was recognised as a weakness for efficient drug development. The International Conference on Harmonisation (ICH) was to overcome the different standards of GCP by producing a single GCP guideline, the ICH GCP guideline.

International GCP

ICH is a unique initiative which brings together the regulatory authorities and the pharmaceutical industries of Europe, Japan and the USA to harmonise the technical requirements for pharmaceutical registration. ICH addresses all the key aspects of drug development including GCP. The aim of ICH GCP is to provide a unified international standard to facilitate the mutual acceptance of clinical data by the regulatory authorities in different countries. GCP is one of the major topics addressed by ICH. The finalised ICH GCP guideline may be the most influential GCP initiative to harmonise GCP between the European Community, Japan and the USA. It was finalised on the 1 May 1996 [7].

The guideline was approved on the 17 July 1996 by the Committee for Proprietary Medicinal Products (CPMP), the European Community's body responsible for coordinating regulation of GCP and implemented on 17 January 1997. Clinical trials carried out in Europe from this date should comply with the ICH GCP guideline. Japan has also implemented the guideline. Although the FDA have issued it as an official guideline, there are no plans to incorporate it into US legislation.

Commonly Used GCP Terms

The following are commonly used terms in clinical research which physicians are likely to come across. The definitions are those given in the ICH GCP guideline [8].

Audit. A systematic and independent examination of trial-related activities and documents to determine whether the trial activities were conducted and the data were recorded, analysed and accurately reported, according to the protocol, sponsor's standard operating procedures, GCP and applicable regulatory requirements.

Case Report Form (CRF). A printed, optical or electronic document designed to record all the protocol-required information to be reported to the sponsor on each trial subject.

Contract Research Organisation (CRO). A person or an organisation contracted by the sponsor to perform one or more of a sponsor's trial-related duties and functions.

Clinical Trial/Study. Any investigation in human subjects intended to discover or verify the clinical, pharmacological and/or other pharmacodynamic effects of an investigational product(s), and/or to identify any adverse reactions to an investigational product(s), and/or to study absorption, distribution, metabolism and excretion of an investigational product(s) with the object of ascertaining its safety and/or efficacy.

Ethics Committee (Independent Ethics Committee). An independent body (a review board or a committee, institutional, regional, national or supranational), constituted of medical/scientific professionals and non-medical/non-scientific members, whose responsibility it is to ensure the protection of the rights, safety and well-being of human subjects involved in a trial and to provide public assurance of that protection by, among other things, reviewing and approving/providing favourable opinion on the trial protocol, the suitability of the investigator(s), facilities and the methods and materials to be used in obtaining and documenting informed consent of the trial subjects.

Good Clinical Practice (GCP). A standard for the design, conduct, performance, monitoring, auditing, recording, analysis and reporting of clinical trials that provides assurance that the data and reported results are credible and accurate and that the rights, integrity and confidentiality of trial subjects are protected.

Inspection. Regulatory authority(ies) conducting an official review of documents, facilities, records and any other resources that are deemed by the authority(ies) to be related to the clinical trial and that may be located at the site of the trial, at the sponsor's and/or contract research organisation's facilities, or at other establishments deemed appropriate by the regulatory authority(ies).

Institutional Review Board (IRB). An independent body constituted of medical, scientific and non-scientific members whose responsibility is to ensure the protection of the rights, safety and well-being of human subjects involved in a trial by, among other things, reviewing, approving and providing continuing review of the trial protocol and amendments and of the methods and material to be used in obtaining and documenting informed consent of the trial subjects.

Investigator. A person responsible for the conduct of the clinical trial at a trial site. If a trial is conducted by a team of individuals at a trial site, the investigator is the responsible leader of the team and may be called the principal investigator.

Investigator Brochure. A compilation of the clinical and non-clinical data on the investigational product(s) which are relevant to the study of the investigational product(s) in human subjects.

Monitoring. The act of overseeing the progress of a clinical trial and of ensuring that it is conducted, recorded and reported in accordance with the protocol, Standard Operating Procedures, GCP and the applicable regulatory requirements.

Protocol. A document that describes the objective(s), design, methodology, statistical considerations and organisation of a trial. The protocol usually also gives the background and rationale for the trial, but these could be provided in other protocol reference documents.

Protocol Amendment. A written description of a change(s) to or formal clarification of a protocol.

Quality Assurance (QA). All those planned and systematic actions that are established to ensure that the trial is performed and the data are generated, documented (recorded) and reported in compliance with GCP and the applicable regulatory requirements.

Quality Control (QC). The operational techniques and activities undertaken within the quality assurance system to verify that their requirements for quality of the trial-related activities have been fulfilled.

Sponsor. An individual, company, institution, or organisation which takes responsibility for the initiation, management, and/or financing of a clinical trial.

Source Documents. Original documents, data and records (e.g. hospital records, clinical and office charts, laboratory notes, pharmacy dispensing records, recorded data from automated instruments, radiographs, subject files).

Principles of GCP: General Guidance for Carrying Out Trials

The ICH GCP guideline contains a detailed list of 13 principles of GCP [8] which gives general instructions for carrying out clinical trials to GCP:

1. Clinical trials should be conducted in accordance with ethics principles that have their origin in the Declaration of Helsinki and that are consistent with GCP and the applicable regulatory requirements(s).
2. Before a trial is initiated foreseeable risks and inconveniences should be weighed against the anticipated benefit for the individual trial subject and society. A trial should be initiated and continued only if the anticipated benefits justify the risks.
3. The rights, safety and well-being of the trial subjects are the most important considerations and should prevail over the interests of science and society.
4. The available non-clinical and clinical information on an investigational product should be adequate to support the proposed clinical trial.
5. Clinical trials should be scientifically sound and described in a clear, detailed protocol.
6. A trial should be conducted in compliance with the protocol that has received prior institutional review board IRB/IEC approval/favourable opinion.
7. The medical care given to and medical decisions made on behalf of, subjects should always be the responsibility of a qualified physician or, when appropriate, of a qualified dentist.
8. Each individual involved in conducting a trial should be qualified by education, training and experience to perform his or her respective task(s).
9. Freely given informed consent should be obtained from every subject prior to clinical trial participation.
10. All clinical trial information should be recorded, handled and stored in a way that allows its accurate reporting, interpretation and verification.
11. The confidentiality of records that could identify subjects should be protected, respecting the privacy and confidentiality rules in accordance with the applicable regulatory requirement(s).
12. Investigational products should be manufactured, handled and stored in accordance with applicable good manufacturing practice. They should be used in accordance with the approved protocol.
13. Systems with procedures that ensure the quality of every aspect of the trial should be implemented.

Investigator's Responsibilities

The responsibilities of physicians (i.e. investigators) and practical suggestions for carrying out these responsibilities are described. The responsibilities are those listed in the ICH GCP guideline and/or are what is current practice. Since most of these are required by other GCP guidelines in current use, most of these duties should be familiar to physicians who have participated in trials, especially trials organised by pharmaceutical companies.

Investigator Qualifications and Delegation of Activities

The investigator should be adequately qualified to meet the applicable regulatory requirements to carry out the study and should provide evidence of such qualifications on an up-to-date curriculum vitae (CV). For trials in neurology an investigator would normally be medically qualified, have experience in the neurological speciality of the trial and previous experience in clinical research. To show that the CV is current it is advisable to sign and date the CV to the effect that it is not more than a year old at the time the study starts.

The investigator should have sufficient time to carry out the trial within the time agreed with the sponsor and adequate facilities to carry out the trial. In many cases the investigator will have other staff available to perform some duties for the trial.

The CVs of all investigators at each centre should be available. Some pharmaceutical companies (i.e. sponsors) will also ask for the CVs of other non-medically qualified personnel involved with the study at the site, such as research nurses, study site coordinators and pharmacists.

The investigator should maintain a list of persons to whom the investigator has delegated trial-related duties, for example which doctors at the study site will be taking informed consent, who will be completing the CRFs and handling study administration. It is advisable for such a list to have the name, signature, initials, trial-related duty and qualifications of each person and a comment on what training they have received to show that they have been appropriately informed of the study (for example that they attended the study set-up meeting with the sponsor representative). The investigator should have documentary evidence that all persons assisting in the trial are adequately informed about the protocol, the study drug (or device), and their trial-related duties.

Properties of the Study Drug

The investigator should be thoroughly familiar with the study drug. Where the study is carried out by a pharmaceutical company, the company will supply an investigator brochure which will contain relevant information about the pharmacokinetics, pharmacodynamics, results of animal studies and results of previous clinical trials. Information will also be in the protocol and other information such as data sheets may be provided.

Ethics Approval

All studies must have written approval from an ethics committee. In most European countries these are called ethics committees; in the USA and Japan they are called institutional review boards (IRBs). The term ethics committee will be used throughout this chapter, although the requirements equally apply to IRBs. The role of an ethics committee is to review the safety, integrity and human rights of patients or volunteers who participate in trials. According to the ICH GCP guideline an ethics committee should be made up of at least five members, at least one of whom should be a lay person and at least one of whom should be independent of the trial site/institution. Investigators who are members of ethics committees must not vote on studies in which they are participating.

The information the investigator should submit to the ethics committee for approval should include the following:

- protocol and any amendments;
- investigator brochure or other appropriate information on the study drug;
- CRF (if applicable – this is not often submitted);
- informed consent information including informed consent forms and any other information given to patients;
- patient recruitment information (e.g advertisements);
- details of patient compensation for participating in the study (if any);
- details of patient travel expenses;
- any other information requested by the ethics committee.

The investigator should to keep a copy of the submission made to the ethics committee and all correspondence with the ethics committee. To identify the documents reviewed by the ethics committee, the version number and date of the documents should be recorded and retained with the study documents filed at the study site. The sponsor will need a copy of the submission to the ethics committee, which should specify what documents have been reviewed by the ethics committee as well as the review/approval letter from the ethics committee. The sponsor will also want a copy of the names of the members of the ethics committee who attended the meeting at which the protocol was reviewed and a copy of the ethics committee's working procedures.

If the investigator brochure is updated during the trial, the investigator should provide the ethics committee with the updated version. To provide evidence that the investigator has carried out this, and any other responsibility, it is advisable that the investigator documents it by keeping a copy of a covering letter provided with the investigator brochure to the ethics committee, or by writing a file note.

Patient Recruitment

The success of any study depends on the recruitment of an adequate number of suitable patients. The investigator should be able to estimate the number of patients he or she will be able to recruit in the agreed recruitment period. Before the start of the study, investigators should be able to provide retrospective data on the number of patients who would have satisfied the proposed entry criteria recently, to help with the accuracy of this estimate.

Informed Consent

Obtaining consent from a study patient to participate in a study is one of the most important tasks an investigator must carry out. A patient may only enter a study when consent has been given.

Although obtaining informed consent is the responsibility of the investigator, frequently this may be delegated to other physicians involved with the patient's care. The investigator should ensure that these doctors have a good understanding of the study and have read the protocol. The ICH GCP guideline states "The investigator, or a person designated by the investigator, should fully inform the subject . . . " This has been interpreted as suggesting that obtaining informed consent may be delegated to a person designated by the investigator, such as a nurse. Nurses frequently take consent in the USA (although it is not specified in any USA GCP requirements); it is not standard practice in Europe or Japan and may cause problems because some nurses may feel pressurised into persuading patients to participate in trials. Also, it is inconsistent with the Declaration of Helsinki, which states that physicians should obtain consent from subjects. Nurses involved with the study may provide helpful information about the study to the patient, but it is preferable that a physician takes the patient's consent. The explanation of the study given to the patient should be provided both verbally and in writing. The patient should be given a copy of the written information to keep.

The patient or the patient's legally acceptable representative should be given sufficient time and opportunity to ask questions about the study in order to decide whether or not to participate in the study. The patient and the person taking consent should both sign and personally date the consent form.

If a patient or the patient's legally acceptable representative is unable to read the informed consent information, an independent witness should witness the consent.

Before a patient takes part in a study, the written informed consent form should be signed and personally dated by the patient or the patient's legally acceptable representative and by the person who carried out the informed consent procedure, which should preferably be the investigator or a physician helping the investigator with the study.

The ICH GCP guideline allows for consent in an emergency situation, for example head injury, where it may not be possible to obtain pre-trial consent. However, as soon as possible the patient and/or their legally acceptable representative must be informed of the situation, and consent to continue treatment in the study should be obtained. These circumstances should be described in the protocol and approved by the ethics committee.

The written information to be given to patients is normally an information sheet which is separate from a consent form or a combined information consent form. For trials carried out by a pharmaceutical company, particularly in Europe, the written information will usually be prepared by the pharmaceutical company. There is a comprehensive list of 20 items listed in the ICH GCP guideline to include in the written information to be given to patients. These are:

Information about the consent procedure

- Circumstances and/or reasons the subject will stop participation in the trial.
- An explanation that participation is voluntary and the subject may withdraw at any time.

Information about the study

- An explanation that the study is a research procedure.
- Purpose of the trial.
- A description of the study medications and the probability of the patient being assigned to each medication.
- A description of the study procedures including invasive procedures.
- Subject's responsibilities (i.e. what is expected of the patient concerning their participation – for example that they must take the study drug at the appropriate times).

- Alternative medications or procedures.
- Aspects of the study that are experimental.
- The length of time the patients will participate in the study.
- The number of subjects (approximately) who will participate in the trial.

Information about the risks/benefits

- The possible foreseeable risks or inconveniences.
- The expected benefits; if there are none this should be stated.
- Compensation and/or treatment available in the event of injury related to the trial.
- Payment details, if any.
- Anticipated expenses, if any.
- An undertaking that subjects will be informed of any new information that is relevant to the subject's willingness to continue in the trial.

Other

- An explanation that the signing of informed consent authorises access to the patient's notes by appropriate sponsor personnel, ethics committees and regulatory authority(ies).
- An undertaking that participation of the patient will be kept confidential.
- Details of who to contact for further information about the trial.

A suggested consent form based on that recommended by the Royal College of Physicians [9] is given in Fig. 8.1. The information form/information sheet must be in the language which is understandable to the patient.

A new UK standardised format for the patient information sheet and written informed consent form was published in 1999 by the UK working party for Patient Information and Informed Consent [12]. The format is described in Fig. 8.2.

Informing the Subject's Primary Care Physician

The investigator should inform the subject's primary physician of the subject's participation in the trial, if the subject has a primary physician. Often the sponsor will provide a standard letter for the investigator to send to primary physicians.

Study Drug

The investigator is responsible for ensuring that records are kept regarding receipt of study drugs from the sponsor, appropriate secure storage of study drug, for ensuring that accurate dispensing records are kept and that unused drug is returned to the sponsor or occasionally for destroying unused drug. In hospital studies these activities are normally delegated to a pharmacist.

Drug accountability is an important part of the study and records of the study drug given to each subject and returned must be kept. For studies sponsored by a pharmaceutical company the monitor will discuss what is required with the investigator, the pharmacist and other personnel at the study site involved with handling, storing and control of study drug supplies. At monitoring visits the monitor will ensure that the correct procedures are being followed. An example of a drug dispensing form in given in Fig. 8.3.

Code Breaking

If the study is double-blind, the sponsor will provide the investigator with sealed individual subject randomisation envelopes or something similar with instructions for breaking the code in an emergency. Investigators should not break the code unless absolutely necessary. Randomisation codes should only be opened when treatment for an adverse event is dependent on knowing what study drug was administered or when the study is stopped because of safety. The investigator should only break the randomisation code in an emergency in accordance with the protocol. If the study is unblinded by the investigator, the investigator should promptly document and explain to the sponsor the circumstances for unblinding the study. At the end of the study the monitor will collect the randomisation code envelopes.

Recording Data and Monitoring the Study

It is the investigator's responsibility to ensure that data recorded in the CRF is accurate, complete, legible and recorded in a timely manner. Entries made in a CRF which are changed or corrected should be dated, initialled, and if the reason for the correction is not clear, an explanation given. This applies to paper and electronic CRFs. The sponsor should provide guidance to the investigator and/or the investigator's designated representative on how to make corrections to CRFs. The investigator should consider the following when completing CRFs:

- Use a black ball-point pen.
- Tick the box where appropriate.
- Complete all sections.
- Write comment or figure, where appropriate.
- Do not use correcting fluids.

Title of study ....

Have you read the Patient Information Sheet?   YES/NO

Have you received satisfactory answers to all your questions?   YES/NO

Have you received enough information about the study?   YES/NO

Have you received a copy of the written information for you to keep? YES/NO

Who have you spoken to? Name(s)

Do you understand that you are free to withdraw from the study:

    At any time?   YES/NO
    Without giving a reason?   YES/NO
    Without affecting your future medical care?   YES/NO

Do you understand and agree to authorised representatives of either the sponsor of the
study or government regulatory authorities reviewing your medical records on the
understanding that your confidentiality will be respected and you will not be identified
in any report?   YES/NO

Patient Signature ....   Date ....
Name ....

Signature of person taking consent ....   Date ....
Name ....

Signature of witness ....   Date ....

Fig. 8.1.   Recommended consent form. Adapted from [9].

- Correct data by striking through the incorrect value with a single line, enter the new data alongside, initial and date and give a reason for any change which is not obvious.
- Sign the CRF as instructed (for example, at the end of each visit and at the end of the CRF) to certify the data are correct and accurate.

The study monitor, who may be a science graduate, qualified nurse or person otherwise medically qualified, is often called a "Clinical Research Associate" and is responsible for ensuring that the investigator and the sponsor carry out their responsibilities.

The monitor is normally the main contact the investigator has with the sponsor. The monitor may be employed directly by the sponsor or, as is very common these days, may work for a contract research organisation on behalf of the sponsor. The monitor will usually visit the site (normally called "monitoring") before, during and at the end of the study.

At each visit during the study the monitor will want to discuss the progress of the study, review the CRFs and check the data with the source documents and will usually check the study drug storage facility and associated documentation. It is most helpful if

1 STUDY TITLE

Is the title self explanatory to a lay person? If not, a simplified title should be included.

2 INVITATION PARAGRAPH

This should explain that the patient is being asked to take part in a research study. The following is a typical example:

"You are being invited to take part in a research study. Before you decide it is important for you to understand why the research is being done and what it will involve. Please take time to read the following information carefully and discuss it with friends, relatives and your GP if you wish. Ask us if there is anything that is not clear or if you would like more information. Take time to decide whether or not you wish to take part.

"Consumers for Ethics in Research (CERES) publish a leaflet entitled Medical Research and You. This leaflet gives more information about medical research and looks at some questions you may want to ask. A copy may be obtained from CERES, PO Box 1365, London N16 0BW. Thank you for reading this."

3 WHAT IS THE PURPOSE OF THE STUDY?

The background and aim of the study should be given here. Also mention the duration of the study.

4 WHY HAVE I BEEN CHOSEN?

You should explain how the patient was chosen and how many other patients will be studied.

5 DO I HAVE TO TAKE PART?

You should explain that taking part in the research is entirely voluntary. You could use the following paragraph:

"It is up to you to decide whether or not to take part. If you do decide to take part you will be given this information sheet to keep and be asked to sign a consent form. If you decide to take part you are still free to withdraw at any time and without giving a reason. This will not affect the standard of care you receive."

6 WHAT WILL HAPPEN TO ME IF I TAKE PART?

You should say how long the patient will be involved in the research, how long the research will last (if this is different), how often they will need to visit a clinic (if this is appropriate) and how long these visits will be. You should explain if the patient will need to visit the GP (or clinic) more often than for his/her usual treatment and

if travel expenses are available. What exactly will happen e.g. blood tests, x-rays, interviews etc.? Whenever possible you should draw a simple flowchart or plan indicating what will happen at each visit. What are the patient's responsibilities? Set down clearly what you expect of them.

You should set out simply the research methods you intend to use; the following simple definitions may help:

• *Randomised trial:*
Sometimes because we do not know which way of treating patients is best, we need to make comparisons. People will be put into groups and then compared. The groups are selected by a computer which has no information about the individual, i.e. by chance. Patients in each group then have a different treatment and these are compared.

You should tell the patients what chance they have of getting the study drug/treatment e.g. a one in four chance.

• *Blind trial:*
In a blind trial you will not know which treatment group you are in. If the trial is a double blind trial, neither you nor your doctor will know in which treatment group you are (although, if your doctor needs to find out he/she can do so).

• *Crossover trial:*
In a crossover trial the groups each have the different treatments in turn. There may be a break between treatments so that the first drugs are cleared from your body before you start the new treatment.

• *Placebo:*
A placebo is a dummy treatment such as a pill which looks like the real thing but is not. It contains no active ingredient.

7 WHAT DO I HAVE TO DO?

Are there any lifestyle restrictions? You should tell the patient if there are any dietary restrictions. Can the patient drive/drink/take part in sport? Can the patient continue to take their regular medication? Should the patient refrain from giving blood? What happens if the patient becomes pregnant?

Explain (if appropriate) that the patient should take the medication regularly.

8 WHAT IS THE DRUG OR PROCEDURE THAT IS BEING TESTED?

You should include a short description of the drug or device and give the stage of development.

You should also state the dosage of the drug and method of administration. Patients entered into drug trials should be given a card (similar to a credit card) with details of the trial they are in. They should be asked to carry it at all times.

9 WHAT ARE THE ALTERNATIVES FOR DIAGNOSIS OR TREATMENT?

For therapeutic research the patient should be told what other treatments are available.

10 WHAT ARE THE SIDE EFFECTS TO TAKING PART?

For any new drug or procedure you should explain to the patients the possible side effects. If they suffer these or any other symptoms they should report them next time you meet. You should also give them a contact name and number to phone if they become in any way concerned.

The known side effects should be listed in terms the patient will clearly understand (e.g. "damage to the heart" rather than "cardiotoxicity": "abnormal liver tests" rather than "raised liver enzymes"). For any relatively new drug it should be explained that there may be unknown side effects.

11 WHAT ARE THE DISADVANTAGES AND RISKS OF TAKING PART?

For studies where there could be harm to an unborn child if the patient were pregnant or became pregnant during the study, the following (or similar) should be said:

"It is possible that if the treatment is given to a pregnant woman it will harm the unborn child. Pregnant women must not therefore take part in this study, neither should women who plan to become pregnant during the study. Women who are at risk of pregnancy may be asked to have a pregnancy test before taking part to exclude the possibility of pregnancy. Women who could become pregnant must use an effective contraceptive during the course of this study. Any woman who finds that she has become pregnant while taking part in the study should immediately tell her research doctor."

Use the pregnancy statement carefully. In certain circumstances (e.g. terminal illness) it would be inappropriate and insensitive to bring up pregnancy.

There should also be an appropriate warning and advice for men if the treatment could damage sperm which might therefore lead to a risk of a damage foetus.

Fig. 8.2. Consent form from UK Working Party (1999).

If future insurance status could be affected by taking part this should be stated. If the patients have private medical insurance you should ask them to check with the company before agreeing to take part in the trial. They will need to do this to ensure that their participation will not affect their medical insurance.

You should state what happens if you find a condition of which the patient was previously unaware. Is it treatable? What are you going to do with this information? What might be uncovered (e.g. high blood pressure, HIV+ status)?

12 WHAT ARE THE BENEFITS OF TAKING PART?

Where there is no intended clinical benefit to the patient from taking part in the trial this should be stated clearly.

It is important not to exaggerate the possible benefits to the particular patient during the course of the study, e.g. by saying they will be given extra attention. This could be seen as coercive. It would be reasonable to say something like:

"We hope that both/all the treatments will help you. However, this cannot be guaranteed. The information we get from this study may help us to treat future patients will [name of condition] better."

13 WHAT IF NEW INFORMATION BECOMES AVAILABLE?

If additional information becomes available during the course of the research you will need to tell the patient about this. You could use the following:

"Sometimes during the course of a research project, new information becomes available about the treatment/drug that is being studied. If this happens, your research doctor will tell you about it and discuss with you whether you want to continue in the study. If you decide to withdraw your research doctor will make arrangements for your care to continue. If you decide to continue in the study you will be asked to sign an updated consent form.

"Also, on receiving new information your research doctor might consider it to be in your best interests to withdraw you from the study. He/she will explain the reasons and arrange for your care to continue."

14 WHAT HAPPENS WHEN THE RESEARCH STUDY STOPS?

If the treatment will not be available after the research finishes this should be explained to the patient. You should also explain to them what treatment will be available instead. Occasionally the

company sponsoring the research may halt the study. If this is the case the reasons should be explained to the patient.

15 WHAT IF SOMETHING GOES WRONG?

You should inform patients how complaints will be handled and what redress may be available. Is there a procedure in place? You will need to distinguish between complaints from patients as to their treatment by members of staff (doctors, nurses etc.) and something serious which occurs during or following their participation in the trial i.e. a reportable serious adverse event.

Where there are no Association of the British Pharmaceutical Industry (ABPI) or other no-fault compensation arrangements, and the study carries risk of physical or significant psychological harm, the following (or similar) should be said:

"If you are harmed by taking part in this research project, there are no special compensation arrangements. If you are harmed due to someone's negligence, then you may have grounds for a legal action but you may have to pay for it. Regardless of this, if you wish to complain about any aspect of the way you have been approached or treated during the course of this study, the normal National Health Service complaints mechanisms may be available to you."

Where there are ABPI or other no-fault compensation arrangements the following (or similar) should be included:

"Compensation for any injury caused by taking part in this study will be in accordance with the guidelines of the Association of the British Pharmaceutical Industry (ABPI). Broadly speaking the ABPI guidelines recommend that the 'sponsor', without legal commitment, should compensate you without you having to prove that it is at fault. This applies in cases where it is likely that such injury results from giving any new drug or any other procedure carried out in accordance with the protocol for the study. The 'sponsor' will not compensate you where such injury results from any procedure carried out which is not in accordance with the protocol for the study. Your right at law to claim compensation for injury where you can prove negligence is not affected. Copies of these guidelines are available on request."

16 WILL MY TAKING PART IN THIS STUDY BE KEPT CONFIDENTIAL?

You will need to obtain the patient's permission to allow restricted access to their medical records and to the information

collected about them in the course of the study. You should explain that all information collected about them will be kept strictly confidential. A suggested form of words for drug company sponsored research is:

"If you consent to take part in the research any of your medical records may be inspected by the company sponsoring (and/or the company organising) the research for purposes of analysing the results. They may also be looked at by people from the company and from regulatory authorities to check that the study is being carried out correctly. Your name, however; will not be disclosed outside the hospital/GP surgery."

or for other research:

"All information which is collected about you during the course of the research will be kept strictly confidential. Any information about you which leaves the hospital/surgery will have your name and address removed so that you cannot be recognised from it."

You should explain that for studies not being conducted by a GP, the patient's own GP will be notified of their participation in the trial. This should include other medical practitioners not involved in the research who may be treating the patient. You should seek the patient's agreement to this. In some instances agreement from the patient that their GP can be informed is a precondition of entering the trial.

17 WHAT WILL HAPPEN TO THE RESULTS OF THE RESEARCH STUDY?

You should be able to tell the patients what will happen to the results of the research. When are the results likely to be published? Where can they obtain a copy of the published results? Will they be told which arm of the study they were in? You might add that they will not be identified in any report/publication.

18 WHO IS ORGANISING AND FUNDING THE RESEARCH?

The answer should include the organisation or company sponsoring or funding the research (e.g. Medical Research Council, pharmaceutical company, charity, academic institution).

The patient should be told whether the doctor conducting the research is being paid for including and looking after the patient in the study. This refers to payment other than that to cover necessary expenses such as laboratory tests arranged locally by the researcher, or the costs of a research nurse. You could say:

Fig. 8.2. (*Continued*)

"*The sponsors of this study will pay [name of hospital department/research fund] for including you in this study*" or "*Your doctor will be paid for including you in this study.*"

19 WHO HAS REVIEWED THE STUDY?

You may wish to give the name of the Research Ethics Committee(s) which reviewed the study (you do not however have to list the members of the Committee).

20 CONTACT FOR FURTHER INFORMATION

You should give the patient a contact point for further information. This can be your name or that of another doctor/nurse involved in the study.

Remember to thank your patient for taking part in this study!

The patient information sheet should be dated and given a version number.

The Patient Information Sheet should state that the patient will be given a copy of the information sheet and a signed consent form to keep.

Fig. 8.2.   (*Continued*)

Study title: ....

Protocol no.: ....

Drug name: ....

Investigator name: ....   Centre no.: ....

Subject no.	Amount dispensed	Dispensed by (initials)	Date dispensed ----/----/----	Date returned ----/----/----

I confirm that the above is an accurate record for the dispensing of the study drug

Investigator or pharmacist signature: ....   Date: ....

Name: ....

Position: ....

Fig. 8.3.   Dispensing form.

the investigator can provide a quiet room for the monitor to carry out this work. The monitor usually likes to meet the investigator and/or other relevant staff at the start of the day and at the end of the day to discuss any queries concerning data in the CRFs.

The investigator should ensure that any important contacts between the sponsor and the site are documented in the study file. For example, if the investigator is reporting a serious adverse event to the sponsor there should be a paper trail available for inspection by auditors and regulatory inspectors if needed.

The investigator is required to comment on the clinical significance of abnormal laboratory values. Often the laboratory report will have highlighted the out-of-range values to help the investigator with this requirement. The CRF should contain a space for comments by the investigator on clinically significant abnormal values.

Direct Access to Source Documents

Data recorded in the CRF which are derived from source documents should be consistent with the source documents. The monitor will compare the data recorded in the CRF against the source documents.

The investigator/institution and trial subject should agree in writing that monitors, auditors and regulatory inspectors be given "direct access to the subject's original records". The "back to back method" or "interview method" is no longer acceptable. In the USA direct access has been preferred by the FDA for some time. However, in Europe this has caused problems in some member states where direct access has sometimes been difficult, for example in Germany, Italy and the Netherlands and it has also been difficult in Japan where until recently the law allowed only medical personnel direct access to patient notes. Also in Japan patients often look after their own notes.

Adverse Event Reporting

Instructions for reporting adverse events should be described in the protocol. The investigator must inform the sponsor immediately of adverse events that are serious and/or unexpected. Sponsors normally have a special serious adverse event form which must be completed and sent to the sponsor as soon as possible. The investigator should usually inform the ethics committee of this type of event. The sponsor will inform the relevant regulatory authorities and other investigator sites if applicable.

Most regulatory authorities require specific information about serious and/or unexpected adverse events to be reported, all or the following items may be asked for:

- reporter's details (name and address);
- protocol number and title;
- date of receipt of report by the sponsor;
- reporting method;
- drug and, if known, formulation and dose;
- route of administration;
- details of the patient (initials, study number, age, sex);
- nature of the event including date of onset, duration, resolution, supportive laboratory data and concomitant treatment;
- investigator classification of severity, drug relationship;
- action taken;
- progress of follow-up (e.g. hospitalised, outpatient, resolution).

Definitions

Adverse Event. Any untoward medical happening (clinical or laboratory) experienced by the patient administered the study drug which does not necessarily have a causal relationship with the study drug.

Serious Adverse Event. An event characterised by any of the following:

- results in death;
- is life-threatening;
- requires inpatient hospitalisation or prolongs hospitalisation;
- results in persistent or significant disability/ incapacity;
- leads to congenital anomaly/birth defect;
- cancer is usually included in this definition by the regulatory authorities in the USA.

Unexpected Adverse Event. An event which is not identified in nature, severity or frequency in the investigator brochure, current data sheet or international product document.

For deaths, the investigator should supply the sponsor and the ethics committee with any additional information requested, such as autopsy reports.

All adverse events which occur during the study must be recorded in the CRF.

Keeping Study Document

It is essential that the investigator has a study file. This is often called the investigator trial file and may be inspected by auditors and/or regulatory authorities. The ICH GCP describes a list of 50 or so documents which are the minimum that will allow evaluation of the conduct of a trial and the quality of the data produced to comply with GCP. Most of the documents will be filed by both the sponsor and investigator in the trial file. Documents filed at the trial site should include the following:

- copy of the signed protocol and any amendments;
- ethics committee approval;
- signature list to document the signatures and initials of all persons authorised to make entries and corrections on CRFs;
- CRFs;
- consent forms;
- information about the study drug;
- list identifying patients who are screened to the study;
- list of patients entered to the study identified by trial number;
- confidential patient list identifying patients;
- general correspondence.

These documents should be retained until at least 2 years after the last approval of a marketing application and until there are no further applications in progress or being considered. It is the responsibility of the sponsor to inform the investigator when the 2 years have elapsed. Since in most cases it is difficult for the sponsor to predict when the two years will have been reached, many sponsors in Europe ask investigators to archive documents for at least 15 years, which was the time period specified in the previously used European GCP guideline.

If the investigator does not have sufficient space (which is usually the case) to store documents such as CRFs, the sponsor will normally organise off-site archiving on the investigator's behalf. In Europe, if the sponsor organises storage of documents on behalf of the investigator, the sponsor will ask the investigator to keep a confidential patient identification list for 15 years and for patient data and other source documents to be kept for as long as the hospital or general practice allows.

It is advisable that investigators discuss the potential problems of archiving study data with the sponsor before the study starts, so that arrangements are agreed early on.

Clinical Report(s)

At the end of the study, even if it is stopped prematurely, the sponsor must analyse the study and prepare a final clinical report. The investigator would normally review the final report and sign it to confirm agreement with the content. In a multicentre trial the Principal Investigator may sign the report on behalf of all the investigators.

Upon completion of the study, the investigator should inform the ethics committee and provide them with a summary of the study's outcome. The investigator should also provide the ethics committee with written summaries of the study's progress, at least annually, or more frequently if required. It is likely that the sponsor will provide the investigator with the summaries and progress reports to pass on to the ethics committee. This information is normally provided by the pharmaceutical company to pass onto the ethics committee.

The investigator should also inform the sponsor and ethics committee about any changes which would significantly affect the study or increase the risk to patients.

Premature Ending or Suspension of the Study

If the trial is prematurely ended or suspended, the investigator should promptly inform study patients, the sponsor and the ethics committee. A detailed written explanation should be provided to the sponsor and the ethics committee.

Audits and Inspections

As part of the quality assurance procedures, it is now common for investigators to be audited by quality assurance personnel from sponsors (or an independent auditor) to ensure that the study complies with GCP. Regulatory authorities may also inspect data from studies. The regulatory authority in the USA, the FDA, regularly carries out inspections in the USA and in Europe. Most European authorities have introduced inspection systems.

Audits or inspections usually involve a visit to the investigator site to check the study documentation, including the study file, for completeness and to ensure that the data have been recorded accurately in the CRFs and can be verified in the patient notes or other source documents.

In Europe the sponsor will give the investigator notice of the audit/inspection to enable him or her to arrange to have the study documentation available and all relevant personnel present whom the auditors/inspectors may also need to meet (e.g. support staff to the investigator, pharmacy and laboratories). The study monitor will often be present at the audit/inspection.

It is not usually necessary for the investigator to be present throughout the entire audit. However, the investigator should be available to answer questions and be present at the end of the audit/inspection, when the auditor/inspector will normally provide the investigator with some feedback of the findings.

FDA Inspections

Investigator Inspections in the USA

Between 1977 and 1994 the FDA carried out more than 3000 routine inspections and over 650 for-cause inspections in the USA) [10]. The four most common deficiencies were inadequate patient consent forms, protocol non-adherence, inadequate and inaccurate records and inadequate drug accountability.

Consent deficiencies observed by the inspections at investigator sites included:

- identification of person(s) the subject could contact to ask questions regarding research, rights and injury;
- incomplete description of research procedure (e.g. failure to mention certain laboratory tests);
- incomplete confidentiality statement (i.e. failure to explain to the subjects that the fda may have access

to their clinical records, including, when necessary, the subject's name);
- incomplete description of compensation and treatment for research-related injury;
- incomplete description of alternative treatments.

Findings of more than 3700 FDA inspections between January 1977 and January 1996 reported the following 10 most common areas of non-compliance [11]:

1. not providing all the elements of informed consent in the subject consent information (53%);
2. non-adherence to protocol (30%);
3. inadequate or inaccurate records (25%);
4. inadequate drug accountability (20%);
5. irb problems (12%);
6. problems with availability of records (3%);
7. failure to list sub-investigators or failure to document their suitability (3%);
8. failure to obtain patient consent (1%);
9. inappropriate payment to subjects (1%);
10. inappropriate follow-up of adverse reactions (1%).

Although investigators generally carry out trials well, minor compliance problems are common. Improved management and better adherence to GCP regulations is needed to overcome the above non-compliance problems.

FDA Inspections Outside the USA

From 1980 the FDA started to inspect studies carried out in foreign countries. By September 1993, nearly 90 inspections had been carried out in almost 20 different countries, mainly in Europe or Canada. Deficiencies found included: inadequate communication of some investigator responsibilities by the USA sponsor; incomplete consent forms; unused study drug not returned from the study site; CRFs not collected; and legal difficulties resulting from differences between countries.

Conclusion

The investigator's GCP responsibilities described in this chapter illustrate the large amount of time and effort that is needed to take part in clinical research. Investigators should be fully aware of these trial requirements before deciding to carry out a clinical trial. Performing trials requires great care, attention and organisation, particularly regarding the documentation produced during the study. However, GCP provides investigators and sponsors with procedures on how to carry out clinical trials to ensure that patients are fully protected and the results are accurate and credible.

References

1. European Commission Directive 91\507\EEC. Commission Directive of 19 July 1991 modifying the Annex to Council Directive 75\318\EEC on the approximation of the laws of Member States relating to analytical, pharmacotoxicological and clinical standards and protocols in respect of the testing of medicinal products. Luxembourg: Office for Official Publications of the EC, 1991.
2. Horace. Good clinical practice in Europe. Scrip Report. BS 693. 4th ed. Richmond, Surrey, UK: PJB Publications, 1994.
3. Pilgrim G. Regulatory authority for good clinical practice. Scrip Report. Good clinical practice in the USA. BS 703. 3rd ed. Richmond, Surrey, UK: PJB Publications, 1994:9–14.
4. Poy E. Audit of clinical studies. In: Lloyd J & Raven A, (eds) ACRPI handbook of clinical research, 2nd ed, London: Churchill Medical Communications, 1994:419.
5. Piasecki S. Introduction to good clinical practice. Scrip Report. Good clinical practice in the USA. BS 703. 3rd ed. Richmond, Surrey, UK: PJB Publications, 1994:1–7.
6. Farrell F. Drug regulation in the 1990s. In: Lloyd J & Raven A (eds) ACRPI handbook of clinical research. 2nd ed. London: Churchill Medical Communications, 1994:23–59.
7. Brown L. ICH GCP and its worldwide implementation. Good Clin Practice J, 1996;3(4):6–10.
8. ICH Harmonised tripartite guideline. Guideline for good clinical practice, 1996.
9. Royal College of Physicians. Guidelines on the practice of ethics committees in medical research involving human subjects, London: Royal College of Physicians, 1990.
10. Duncan D. Clinical investigator programs: discussion paper. Annex III. Scrip Report. Good clinical practice in Europe. BS 693. 4th ed. Richmond, Surrey, UK: PJB Publications, 1994.
11. Lisook A. FDA lists 10 danger zones for trial non-compliance. Clin. Trials Advisor 1996;12:22–23.
12. UK Working Party for Patient Information and Informed Consent, The UK Standard Format for Patient Information sheets and written Informed Consent 1999.

9. Statistical Issues in Clinical Trials in Neurology

S. Senn

Introduction

It would be impossible in the space of one brief chapter to provide the reader with even a basic education in medical statistics. It will be assumed, therefore, that the reader already has considerable familiarity with descriptive and inferential statistics and, in addition to knowing about means, medians, variances and standard deviations, has encountered the general framework of hypothesis tests, confidence intervals and so forth and particular applications of them for both continuous and binary outcomes. Suitable texts, in order of increasing difficulty, are those of Campbell and Machin [1], Altman [2] and Fisher and Van Belle [3]. For general advice on clinical trials Pocock [4] or, at a more advanced level, Piantadosi [5] are extremely useful. However, the science of medical statistics is developing rapidly and it may be useful for the trialist to have some overview of the current status and developing trends. This is all that will be attempted in this chapter. More extensive coverage of various statistical issues affecting drug development will be found in Senn [6]. The European Statistical Guideline [7] and International Conference on Harmonisation E9 Guideline are also extremely useful as reminders regarding points which should be covered in any analysis plan.

Design of Trials

Parallel Group Trials

The simplest form of clinical trial is the parallel group trial, which has been defined as "a trial in which patients are allocated to a treatment (or sometimes a combination or sequence of treatments) with the purpose of studying differences between these treatments (or combination or sequence of treatments)" [6]. This type of trial is generally suitable for all conditions and treatments. Its main drawbacks are that it requires relatively many patients compared with the main rival design, the cross-over, and that it does not permit the study of individual response to treatment.

In double-blind trials, allocation of treatment has generally been by randomised pre-prepared treatment packs. If, however, the trial is not blinded it may be preferable to run a procedure of central telephone randomisation. If prognostic covariates are being fitted, then a randomised trial is not fully efficient and some form of dynamic balancing of prognostic factors may be valuable. However, for even moderately large trials a randomised design is very nearly fully efficient and the extra inconvenience may not justify such balance. On the other hand recent technological developments mean that such telephone allocation is now much easier than before. If such dynamic balance is employed then the algorithm of Atkinson [8] is superior to that of Taves [9] and Pocock and Simon [10].

Where such dynamic balance is not used, it is common to randomise in blocks. For example, in a trial comparing two treatments A and B for epilepsy it might be decided to use a block size of 12. By this device, every 12 patients would consist of 6 treated with A and 6 treated with B, the sequence of treatments being otherwise unpredictable. Other things being equal, an even allocation of patients to both treatments being compared is most efficient. On the other hand large blocks contribute to maintaining blinding in the trial. (The cloak and dagger manoeuvre of using small block sizes and not publishing the fact in the protocol is a foolish attempt at subterfuge which should be eschewed in any serious approach to designing clinical trials.) Trialists commonly use blocks that are too small, small blocks showing little advantage over large ones in terms of balance. A useful approach is to use blocks which are at least as large as the expected number of patients in the smallest centre.

Cross-over Trials

> A trial in which patients are allocated to sequences of treatments with the purpose of studying differences between individual treatments. The simplest common example is of a placebo controlled trial of an active treatment in which patients are allocated at random either to the sequence "placebo followed by active" or to the sequence "active followed by placebo". [6]

Cross-over trials are not suitable for studying all conditions and treatments: the former must be chronic and the effects of the latter must be reversible. Thus, for example, multiple sclerosis, stroke and motor neurone disease are unsuitable for study through cross-over trials, whereas epilepsy and migraine may be.

The main advantage of cross-over trials is their efficiency: where they are possible, far fewer patients will be needed than for a corresponding parallel group trial. On the other hand, they are vulnerable to the presence of carry-over and their analysis can be difficult. As a result of a paper by Freeman [11], medical statisticians working on the methodology of cross-over trials have now abandoned the so-called two-stage procedure [12,13]. The reader should be warned, however, that general introductory textbooks on medical statistics are still being written which recommend this biased procedure. In fact, most introductory textbooks cannot be trusted as regards the advice given on this issue. Advice on analysing cross-over trials will be found in Senn [14].

n-of-1 Trials

Cross-over trials are supremely useful for studying individual response to treatment. Where an individual patient is given repeated randomised allocations of the treatments under study, this is sometimes referred to as an n-of-1 trial. A series of n-of-1 trials is really a form of multi-period cross-over [6]. If a random effects model is used for analysis (see below), individual response to treatment may be identified. This potential is sadly under-exploited in drug development.

Dose Escalation Studies

It is often ethically desirable, especially in dose-finding for a new treatment, to treat patients with gradually increasing doses rather than, as would be the case in a cross-over trial, to have some patients starting on the highest dose in addition to some starting on the lowest. If the same sequence is used for every patient, blinding in such trials is not possible. The results will also be vulnerable to trend

effects. One solution is to have a randomly intervening placebo as, say, in a design using the sequences:

P D1 D2 D3
D1 P D2 D3
D1 D2 P D3
D1 D2 D3 P.

Here D1, D2, D3 are lowest, middle and highest doses of treatment and P is a placebo. Patients would be allocated at random (and usually blocked in equal number) to one of the four sequences.

Such ethical designs impose a price in efficiency. If the trend effect is eliminated, the dose escalation study, for example would require nearly twice as many patients as a suitable cross-over design [6] which might use sequences arranged in a Latin square for example:

P D1 D2 D3
D1 P D3 D2
D3 D2 P D1
D2 D3 D1 P.

If some patients fail to reach the highest dose in a dose escalation study because of satisfactory response at lower doses, then no *simple* analysis of the data is valid. For example, the comparison of mean responses at each dose will tend to disadvantage the highest dose since only the more refractory cases will proceed to the highest dose. On the other hand, an analysis of completers only will bias in favour of the highest dose since these are patients who have, by definition, failed on lower doses.

Uncontrolled Studies

Uncontrolled studies should be avoided if at all possible. They are vulnerable to trend effects in patients and observers, to prejudiced judgement and to regression to the mean [15]. The price of carrying out an uncontrolled study is complex mathematical modelling and most trialists are unable or unwilling to pay it.

Sequential Trials

Trials in which the number of patients to be treated is not determined beforehand but termination of the trial is based upon results to data are known as sequential trials. This name refers to the fact that they are analysed sequentially (on a number of occasions) and not to the fact that patients are recruited sequentially, this being a common feature of most trials.

Such trials require somewhat different approaches to analysis. Within the frequentist (or classical) approach to analysing clinical trials, the stopping rule for the trial can have a strong impact on the way it is analysed. Within the Bayesian framework this impact is much less. (Indeed it is sometimes claimed that there is no impact at all.) Nevertheless, whatever approach to analysis is used, organisation of such trials is a complicated matter and there is an enormous body of literature not only on their analysis but also on their conduct, the duties of monitoring committees, etc. A classic text is Whitehead [16]. An elementary introduction covering a number of issues is given in Senn [6], chapter 19.

Equivalence Trials

It may be advantageous to be able to offer patients and their physicians a choice of roughly comparable treatments. Treatments that are similar in terms of average effects may differ for given patients. Patients may gradually develop a tolerance to some treatments and have to be offered others. Some patients may have side effects with some drugs and other patients with others. These are all reasons why variety in equivalence may be valuable.

At one time, trialists used to claim equivalence by dint of failing to find a difference. This is now realised to be inadequate. The modern approach is to calculate confidence intervals for the treatment difference and see that these exclude "practical inferiority" of the new treatment.

There is now an extensive theory of such trials. A particular application is in bioequivalence studies where, for example, a generic manufacturer attempts to show equivalence to a brand name product by comparing concentration time profiles in the blood for the two products.

Reviews of many statistical issues involved in such trials are given in chapters 15 and 22 of Senn [6].

The Importance of Pharmacokinetics

Pharmacokinetics, together with statistics, can claim to be one of the threads that runs throughout drug development. The difference between a successful and a failed treatment is often a matter of finding the correct dose. The more successfully pharmacokinetics (PK) and pharmacodynamic (PD) response are modelled, the greater the chances of moving successfully from one step of developing a treatment to another. For example from moving from single-dose studies to multiple-dose studies knowledge of PK time profiles and dose proportionality is crucial. Statisticians have been guilty in the past of ignoring PK and PD [17,18]. This is particularly true of approaches to modelling carry-over for the cross-over trial [14].

General Design Considerations

It is of course important to establish the number of patients that should be studied in a trial. There are now a number of statistical packages that assist the trialist in this task and which will, when provided with a presumed variance of the response and a clinically relevant difference, calculate the number of patients that should be studied to achieve a target power for a given significance level. Such packages will provide answers for a number of different types of outcome and some will even produce statements for inclusion in a trial protocol. Nevertheless, they will not cover more complex designs and cases where many prognostic variables are being used. An experienced statistician will be able to adapt the input to such packages appropriately to deal with such cases.

Other matters that require extreme care and attention and for which statistical considerations are relevant include: (1) Choice of comparator(s); (2) the basic design – parallel or cross-over and so forth; (3) treatment structure for factorial and dose-finding trials; (4) the choice of outcome measure; (5) the timing of measurements, particularly if treatments with different regimes are being compared; (6) treatment allocation including randomisation and blocking; (7) approaches to blinding; (8) wash-out periods, especially in cross-over trials; (9) duration of treatment; (10) selection of patients; (11) screening and run-in periods.

As regards the latter, placebo run-ins, although popular, should be avoided as they raise ethical problems regarding the deception of patients [19]. If necessary an active treatment may be given in the run-in period, unless onset of action is to be studied, in which case the alternative of no treatment at all should be considered.

Analysis
Common Pitfalls

The most common pitfall in analysis is to consult the statistician too late, which is to say, at the time the trial is to be analysed rather than when it is planned. This is now largely a thing of the past within the pharmaceutical industry and indeed the Good Clinical Practice Guidelines of the European Union [20] now require that a qualified medical statistician be involved in all stages of the trial. Unfortunately standards outside the industry are not so high and many of the features now taken for granted within it, such as pre-specified analysis, blinded review of data, analysis by qualified personnel, monitoring and quality assurance, are often absent. Obviously it is unreasonable to expect the private investigator to match the resources of a drug development sponsor; nevertheless a simple consultation with a statistician at the beginning of planning a trial is often a feasible and valuable action.

All standard statistical analyses of clinical trials make an assumption about independence that applics at some level or other. The most serious of common mistakes made is falsely to assume that independence applies at a level at which it does not. For example, many trials have a repeated measures structure in which n patients are measured at k visits. To treat the nk observations as though they were independent is a serious mistake.

A related common error is to fail to take account of the basic design structure of the trial: for example to analyse a cross-over trial using techniques appropriate to a matched pairs or, more seriously, parallel group design. Multi-centre trials are common and it is usually advisable to allow for the centre effect in the analysis. This is commonplace within the pharmaceutical industry but somewhat rarer outside.

A particularly egregious error in this connection is to fail to take account at all of the fact that one has run a clinical trial. Unfortunately, the medical literature is littered with papers in which separate comparisons with baseline have been performed within each treatment group but no direct comparison with control is given. If, however, such comparison to baseline is at all valid, then the control group is not needed. If the control group is necessary for valid conclusions, however, then the only relevant statistics are those which compare treatment with control and the comparison with baseline is irrelevant. If journal editors were to ban such comparisons with baseline there would be far fewer "significant" results from clinical trials but much in the way of clarity would be gained.

A number of leading journals now require that treatment estimates and confidence intervals be provided in addition to the results of significance tests. This is a welcome development. Note that certain parametric procedures more readily lend themselves to the production of treatment estimates and confidence intervals. Nevertheless, many of the non-parametric procedures also have corresponding estimation approaches and these are currently under-utilised. For example, in association with a Mann–Whitney–Wilcoxon rank sum test a Hodges–Lehmann estimator together with confidence intervals can be produced [21].

Different types of outcome call for different approaches to analysis. Some useful techniques will be considered under relevant headings below.

Types of Measurement

Continuous Data

Continuous data are those that arise as a result of measurement rather than counting. Survival times are a form of continuous measure but require highly specialised treatment and are considered under a separate heading below. "Standard" continuous measures, although not rare, are less common in neurology than in some other indications such as (say) asthma, where all the most commonly used measurements are continuous.

By far the most useful techniques for analysing continuous data are those based on the so-called *general linear model*. These assume that the response (possibly suitably transformed) that a patient shows can be expressed as a weighted sum of various (possibly transformed) prognostic scores including treatment and an error term which is approximately Normally distributed. Two-sample and matched pairs *t*-tests, analysis of variance and covariance and multiple regression are all examples of this general form of analysis.

A standard alternative approach where there are fears concerning the Normality assumption is to use a non-parametric procedure [21]. For example the Wilcoxon–Mann–Whitney rank sum approach is a popular alternative to the two-sample *t*-test. Where the data are in strata, say as in a multi-centre trial, the van Elteren [22] test is commonly used within the pharmaceutical industry. The general power of the general linear model compared with non-parametric alternatives, however, means that one should think carefully before abandoning the former approach. It is important to realise the following: (1) It is only the error terms in the model on which the requirement for (approximate) Normality is placed. The original data do not need to be Normally distributed. (2) The adequacy of this assumption can only be tested by fitting the linear model in question. (3) It is often worth searching for a suitable transformation. (4) The usual consequence of departure from Normality is loss of power rather than an increase in the type I error rate. (5) Non-parametric approaches that do not include valuable prognostic factors may themselves lose considerable power. (6) Given the choice between reflecting the basic structure of the trial but ignoring some distributional difficulties with the data on the one hand, or performing a non-parametric analysis but ignoring the structure of the trial on the other, the former is nearly always preferable to the latter.

It is also interesting to note that statisticians who use non-parametric procedures often do so in a way that contradicts one of the standard arguments for them, namely that they are a form of *randomisation test*. For example, nearly all parallel group trials are blocked using sub-centre blocks. However, it is most unusual for statisticians to include the block in the analysis. If the van Elteren test is used, stratification is likely to be by centre and not by block. Thus the randomisation as performed is *not* reflected in the analysis.

Binary Data

The most common modern approach to binary data amongst medical statisticians is to use *logistic regression*. Suppose, for example, that at the end of a trial of epilepsy, patients are classified either as having had no seizures or as having had at least one seizure. A possible approach is to model the probability of no seizure (p) as a function of various prognostic factors, including treatment, via a form of regression model. Because p must lie between 0 and 1 but any straight line is unbounded, it is useful to have a transformation which is not so bounded. One possibility is to model the so-called *logit*, $\log\{p/(1 - p)\}$. Whereas the probability lies between 0 and 1, the logit lies between plus and minus infinity. This approach is called logistic regression. Using such a form of regression ensures that all predicted probabilities lie within the possible range of 0 and 1.

Of course, in elementary statistics courses, the student is introduced to the analysis of such data using either the Pearson–Fisher chi-square statistic or Fisher's exact test applied to simple fourfold frequency tables of the sort in Table 9.1.

Such procedures, however, like their corresponding tables, do not include prognostic information on the patients and such information may be very valuable. Although there are approaches, such as that of Mantel and Haenszel [23], which generalise the chi-square analysis to more complex structures, logistic regression is more flexible and suitable when many covariates are available, especially if these covariates are continuous.

Both logistic regression and the general linear model are special case of *generalised* linear models (the terminology is rather confusing!) and a third such case, *Poisson regression*, is considered below.

Frequencies

A more discriminating use of the seizure data in the previous example would have been to analyse the actual numbers suffered by each patient rather than dichotomising. (In fact, in general, dichotomising data is an excellent way to throw information away and is a very bad habit that should be avoided.) The simplest of distributions which is suitable for describing such frequency data is the Poisson distribution and a form of regression model based upon it is Poisson regression.

The basic assumption behind Poisson regression is that any two patients with exactly the same modelled covariate values will have the same expected frequency of events. For example, if the outcome were seizures in epilepsy and the modelled covariates were observed number of seizures during the run-in period and treatment given, then the model states that any two individuals having the same treatment will have the same expected seizure rate if their rates in the run in period were the same. This assumption is most unlikely to be guaranteed in practice because, usually not all relevant covariates will have been identified, some of them will be imperfectly measured or subject to random variability (as for example seizures in the run in period) and in any case apparently very similar patients may in fact be different.

In practice, then, so-called *extra-Poisson* variation is likely to be present. This can be dealt with most simply by a suitable rescaling of standards errors [24]. More complex approaches require the use of random effect models.

Ordered Categorical Data

By ordered categorical data are meant data which arise from rating scales with a discrete number of possible values. An example is the Hoehn and Yar [25] scale for Parkinson's disease which has five points. There are two common faults in analysing ordered categorical data from clinical trials. The first is to reduce an n point scale to a dichotomy and then analyse the resulting 2×2 table, using, for example, a chi-square on one degree of freedom. Because fine distinctions in the original data are coarsened, this is wasteful. The second fault is even worse. This is to analyse the original $2 \times n$ table as though it were a contingency data with unordered categories, for example using a chi-square with $n - 1$ degrees of freedom. This approach involves a considerable loss of power and gives the same answer if the columns of the table are permuted (in other words if the information on ordering is destroyed).

Within the pharmaceutical industry it is now common to analyse such data using logistic regres-

Table 9.1. Example of a fourfold frequency table

	No seizure	At least one seizure	Total
Treated	a	b	a + b
Control	c	d	c + d
Total	a + c	b + d	a + b + c + d

sion for ordered categorical data [26]. This is now implemented in all major statistical packages.

Survival Analysis

Even if death is not the endpoint of a clinical trial, survival analysis may be an appropriate tool. For example, the survival in question can be a time until the next event of interest such as the time until next seizure in epilepsy, time to assisted ventilation for motor neurone diseases or time to reach a particular point on the Hoehn and Yar [25] scale in Parkinson's disease.

A particular feature of such data is that they are often *censored*. That is to say that, by the time of usual follow-up for such a trial, many patients will not yet have reached the "failure" point. For such patients a minimum survival time rather than an exact survival time is available. The fact that this is so means that special considerations are needed for analysing such data.

Since the seminal paper by Cox [27] introducing the *proportional hazards model*, there has been extensive methodological interest in analysing survival data and hundreds of articles and at least 20 books have been written on this topic. A good introductory text is that of Marubini and Valsecchi [28]. Major statistical packages such as Genstat, Splus and SAS, permit modelling of survival data.

Repeated Measures

Repeated measurement of the same outcome over time is a common feature of many clinical trials and represents both a challenge and an opportunity. Common approaches are: (1) reducing the measures to a summary measure per patient and then analysing these; (2) independent analysis at each time point; (3) the so-called split-plot or repeated measures analysis of variance; (4) multivariate analysis of variance (MANOVA) [29,30]; (5) hierarchical, including random "growth curve" models.

The first approach is a simple and robust way of dealing with the problem. It loses in efficiency somewhat compared with the fourth approach in some cases, especially if there is incomplete information on some patients. The second approach is generally valid but shifts difficulties from analysis to interpretation. Multiplicity is an awkward and unwanted feature when it comes to interpretation and most statisticians will seek to avoid it. The third approach is very popular in the psychological literature but is, in fact, a misuse of the split-plot methodology. Either conservative adjustments must be made or strong assumptions are necessary. In any case it makes no use of the temporal aspect of the data since any permutation of the time points would produce the same answer. This latter criticism also applies to

MANOVA, which lands an answer in the trialist's lap but leaves the trialist struggling for the question. The fifth approach is the one with the greatest potential but is also the most difficult to implement. There is, however, at least one computer package devoted to this particular topic and such models are now much easier to implement than before.

Random Effect Models

Such random growth curve models are really examples of random effect models. It is assumed that the effect of treatment over time will not be exactly the same for each patient and that the results of patients on the same treatment will differ as a result of genuine differences in response. (Even if the true response were the same due to measurement error and random variability within patients the observed response would differ.)

There is increasing interest in such models, particularly in the context of combining results from a number of trials (meta-analysis). However, they can also be appropriate for analysing clinical trials and are particularly appropriate for analysing series of n-of-1 trials. It is to be expected that there will be a great increase in the use of such models in the future.

Use of Baselines and Other Covariates

The modern approach to the analysis of clinical trials reflects that in applied statistics generally, the emphasis is on modelling. Where professional statisticians are involved in the analysis of clinical trials, as in the pharmaceutical industry or in large publicly funded clinical trials, models with prognostic covariates in addition to the treatment allocated are the norm.

A common example is using baseline information. Elsewhere, a standard, but inefficient device, is to use an analysis of the so-called change scores: the differences between the values for the patients at outcome and baseline. A more efficient approach, however, is to fit the baseline in an analysis of covariance. (If this is done it makes no difference whether original values or change scores are used as the outcome measure.) There seems to be an extraordinary resistance in the general medical literature, however, to using analysis of covariance and the inefficient change score approach persists, despite the fact that analysis of covariance is nearly 70 years old as a technique and has been easily available in computer packages for at least quarter of a century.

A foolish, but regrettably common, use of baselines and demographic factors is to demonstrate that the groups are "comparable", in particular by means of a significance test. However, if one has randomised, it is known in advance that over all randomisations the groups are comparable and that for a given randomisation they are not. The challenge is to use prognostic information, not to find excuses for ignoring it [31].

Use of prognostic information generally leads to much more powerful analyses, and a consequent reduction in the number of patients needed to reach a conclusion of a given precision. There is surely no excuse in the modern approach to clinical trials for failing to exploit this.

Current and Future Developments

In this section I consider some modern developments in statistics which may be of interest to trialists working in neurology.

Bayesian Approaches

Bayesian statistics has been defined as follows:

> An approach to statistics named for Thomas Bayes (1701–1761) and which has the following features. (1) A subjective interpretation is given to probability. (2) It is accepted that one may talk of the probability of hypotheses being true and of parameters having particular values. (3) *Prior probabilities* are assigned on a personal basis to hypotheses or to parameter values. (4) These probabilities are updated in the light of evidence to become *posterior probabilities* in a way which is described by Bayes theorem. (5) Only the prior probability and the data actually obtained are directly relevant to the assessment of the posterior probability. (Data which might have been obtained but weren't, play no direct role. (6) As a consequence of point 3, the resulting answer is valid only for the person for whom it is calculated. [6]

The Bayesian approach to data analysis has many features that make it philosophically attractive. Until recently, however, it was difficult to implement for all but the most simple data structures. Recent advances in numerical approaches to calculating posterior probability distributions through simulation, together with rapidly increasing computer power [32], have meant that this is no longer the case and more and more medical statisticians are exploring Bayesian approaches to analysing clinical trials. A good introduction to the strength and scope of Bayesian approaches is given in the book edited by Berry and Stangl [33].

Hierarchical Generalised Linear Models

Ordinary linear regression is a modelling approach in statistics that was implemented very early on in statistical packages. Linear regression models consist of linear predictors (the signal) which are functions of various explanatory variables (prognostic factors in the context of medical statistics) and a single Normal error term (the noise). Such models are often referred to as *general linear models*.

An extremely influential paper by Nelder and Wedderburn [34] generalised ordinary regression by allowing for different types of error term. They introduced a very flexible family of models, *generalised linear models*, and a fitting algorithm. Logistic regression, Poisson regression and standard linear regression are all special cases of generalised linear models. A program, GLIM, was developed to fit such models and nowadays many other statistical packages such as Genstat, SAS and SPlus include software for fitting such models.

Another very obvious generalisation of ordinary linear regression is to allow different types of normal random error terms. For example, in modelling the response over a number of trials for the purpose of meta-analysis, we might like to allow for difference between patients within trials and also for random differences between the effects of the same treatment from trial to trial.

If both generalisations are made, then we have what Lee and Nelder [35] have called *hierarchical generalised linear models*. These look set to become extremely important tools for statistical analysis, including that of clinical trials, and they will shortly be incorporated in Genstat.

The Bootstrap

Student's original paper of 1908 [36] which introduced the *t*-test was revolutionary for one particular reason. An ingenious statistical trick meant that, given the assumption of Normality, a statistic could be produced for testing hypotheses about the mean that did not depend on the unknown population variance. Prior to Student's revolution, a test was used which was valid given that the population variance was known. In practice, of course, it was not known and the sample variance was substituted instead, the statistician hoping that, provided the sample size was large enough, no harm would come of this sleight of hand.

Student's test did, however, rely on the distribution of the original data being Normal. In 1973, Efron, building on earlier ideas by Quenouille and Tukey, introduced a statistical procedure, the bootstrap, which from one point of view may be regarded as taking Student's step one stage further [37]. The step is to regard the sample distribution as being a first approximation of the population distribution and then to sample repeatedly with replacement from this. In this way an empirical approximation of the distribution which the test statistic might exhibit under repeated sampling can be built up.

The bootstrap is a flexible technique of considerable general applicability. It is not uncontroversial. Nevertheless, it is being used increasingly in the analysis of clinical trials.

Wavelets

Wavelets are a very flexible modern approach to signal processing [38]. They have already been applied with considerable success to the analysis of electrocardiographic data and no doubt further applications for signal processing in connection with medical data will be found for them. They thus extend the options for the statistician in the way in which, for example, a patient's individual data may be summarised for the purpose of further analysis using the summary measures approach.

Neural Networks

Given the name of this statistical technique, it could hardly be ignored in a book on neurology. Neural networks are a flexible tool for modelling complex data-structures where some connections between inputs and outputs are hidden. Some critics maintain that they are *too* flexible in that two data modellers fitting ostensibly the same neural network would come to different conclusions. Others have claimed that similar results can be obtained with existing statistical tools such as logistic regression and that neural networks are therefore unnecessary. Nevertheless, the development of this field is worth watching.

Conclusion

Statistics is a vigorous discipline that continues to develop rapidly. Such development brings new opportunities for planning and analysing clinical trials. The better the tools we use for analysing trials, the fewer mistakes we shall make in doing so. We shall also be able to come to reliable conclusions with fewer patients. Just as the trialist has a duty to current patients to use the best of treatments, there is an ethical imperative on the trialist in regard to future patients to use the best of tools in studying the effects of treatment.

References

1. Campbell M, Machin D. Medical statistics: a commonsense approach. New York: Wiley, 1990.
2. Altman D. Practical statistics for medical research. London: Chapman and Hall, 1991.
3. Fisher LD, Van Belle G. Biostatistics for the health sciences. New York: Wiley, 1993.
4. Pocock SJ. Clinical trials: a practical approach. Chichester: Wiley, 1982.
5. Piantadosi S. Clinical trials: a methodologic perspective. New York: Wiley, 1997.
6. Senn SJ. Statistical issues in drug development. Chichester: Wiley, 1997.
7. CPMP Working Party on Efficacy of Medicinal Products. Biostatistical methodology in clinical trials in applications for marketing authorizations for medicinal purposes. Stat Med 1995;14:1659–1682.
8. Atkinson A. Optimum biased coin designs for sequential clinical trials with prognostic factors. Biometrika 1982;69: 61–67.
9. Taves DR. Minimization: a new method of assigning patients to treatment and control groups. Clin Pharmacol Ther 1974; 15:443–453.
10. Pocock SJ, Simon R. Sequential assignment with balancing for prognostic factors in the controlled clinical trial. Biometrics 1975;31:103–115.
11. Freeman PR. The performance of the two-stage analysis of two-treatment, two-period cross-over trials. Stat Med 1989;8: 1421–1432.
12. Grizzle JE. The two-period change over design and its use in clinical trials. Biometrics 1965;21:467–480.
13. Hills M, Armitage P. The two-period cross-over clinical trial. Br J Clin Pharmacol 1979;8:7–20.
14. Senn SJ. Cross-over trials in clinical research. Chichester: Wiley, 1993.
15. Stigler S. Regression towards the mean, historically considered. Stat Methods Med Res 1997;6:103–114.
16. Whitehead JA. The design and analysis of sequential clinical trials, revised 2nd edn. Chichester: Wiley, 1997.
17. Sheiner L. The intellectual health of clinical drug evaluation. Clin Pharmacol Ther 1991;50:4–9.
18. Senn SJ. Statisticians and pharmacokineticists: what can they learn from each other? In: Aarens et al., editors. COST B1 Medicine: the population approach: measuring and managing variability in response, concentration and dose. Brussels: European Commission.
19. Senn SJ. Are placebo run ins justified? BMJ 1997;314: 1191–1193.
20. CPMP (Committee for Proprietary Medicinal Products). Good clinical practice for trials on medicinal products in the European Community. Office for Official Publications of the European Community. Reproduced in: Good clinical practices, US EEC & Nordic Versions. Charlottesville, VA: Pharmaceutical Research Associates, 1990.
21. Sprent P. Applied nonparametric statistical methods. London: Chapman and Hall, 1989.
22. van Elteren PH. On the combination of independent two-sample tests of Wlicoxon. Bulletin Inst Int Stat 1960;37: 351–361.
23. Mantel N, Haenszel W. Statistical aspects of the analysis of data from retrospective studies of diseases. J Nat Cancer Inst 1959; 22:741–748.
24. McCullagh P, Nelder JA. Generalized linear models. 2nd ed. New York: Chapman and Hall, 1988.
25. Hoehn MM, Yahr MD. Parkinsonism: onset, progression and mortality. Neurology 1967;17:424–442.
26. McCullagh P. Regression models for ordinal data. J R Stat Soc B 1980;42:109–142.
27. Cox DR. Regression models and life tables. J R Stat Soc B 1972; 34:187–220.
28. Marubini E, Valsecchi MG. Analysing survival data from clinical trials and observational studies. Chichester: Wiley, 1994.

29. Finney D. Repeated measurements: what is measured and what repeats? Stat Med 1990;9:639–644.

30. Finney D. Temporal or spatial repetition. J Ind Soc Agric Stat 1996;49:11–20.

31. Senn SJ. Base logic: baseline balance in randomized clinical trials. Clin Res Regul Affairs 1995;12:171–182.

32. Gamerman D. Markov chain Monte Carlo. London: Chapman and Hall, 1997.

33. Berry D, Stangl D, editors. Bayesian biostatistics. New York: Dekker, 1996.

34. Nelder JA, Wedderburn RWM. Generalised linear models. J R Stat Soc A 1972;135:370–384.

35. Lee Y, Nelder JA. Hierarchical generalized linear models [with discussion]. J R Stat Soc B 1996;58:619–678.

36. "Student". The problem error of a mean. Biometrika 1908;6: 1–25.

37. Efron B. The jackknife, the bootstrap and other resampling plans. Philadelphia: SIAM, 1982.

38. Chui CK. Wavelets: a mathematical tool for signal analysis. Philadelphia: SIAM, 1997.

10. Analysis of Results: Statistical Principles

D. Hoberman and J.T. Sahlroot

Introduction

Human beings are anything but homogeneous experimental units. No matter how rigorous the effort to restrict a pool of patient candidates for a controlled clinical trial, even an effective treatment accounts for only a small portion of the resulting range and variability of clinical measurements. In other words, there is usually a lot of "noise" in the data. Ultimately, a mass of data must be condensed into quantities (statistics) which can be used to determine whether or not there is a signal of efficacy amongst the noise. Often the statistical challenge is to design a trial so that a chosen statistic will produce the greatest chance of detecting a true difference between treatments (power) while simultaneously limiting the chance of falsely concluding that there is a difference when there is none (type I error). For any given trial, the "p value" of a statistical test estimates the probability of a statistic at least as large as that found in the trial *under the assumption that the treatment and control are indistinguishable as measured* (null hypothesis). If the p value falls below a given threshold of improbability (α-level) under the assumption of no treatment effect, we are led to conclude that the lack of a treatment effect is implausible. For example, the finding of a large difference between the sample means in the trial would suggest that the original assumption of no difference between the populations was wrong. If the difference is large enough compared with a measure of noise in the trial (i.e., the p value is less than α), we then say that the test is "statistically significant". Conventionally, α is set at 5%, or a 1 in 20 chance (over repeated similarly designed trials) of arriving at the false conclusion that the treatment is effective when, in fact, it is not. Rather than depend upon a probability model of the actual state of nature, an alternative strategy is to gather evidence which may serve to *contradict an assumed state of nature, e.g., no treatment effect.*

Statistical Versus Clinical Significance

The ability of statistical theory to accommodate widely divergent sources of data does not guarantee a useful result for the clinician; hence the confusing statement "statistically but not clinically significant." Statistical reasoning often stops short of reconciling the tension between the clinical interpretation of a "meaningful clinical response" and the statistical detection of a *de minimus* difference between the distributions of two populations. For example, McFarland [1] states that "Endpoint analysis of treatment trials in MS has often used, incorrectly, the difference between EDSS mean scores of the treatment groups or, correctly, a comparison of the numbers of patients improving or worsening using the Expanded Disability Status Score (EDSS) changes." He goes on to advocate, instead, the use of survival analysis which compares the time it takes to reach, say, an EDSS grade of 7. Going further, Kurtzke [2] states that rating scales are often problematic: "Since the numbers used are not true numbers [i.e., they are ordinal at best], the use of parametric tests (e.g. tests of means or of variance of means) seems inappropriate, since such tests require not only a real number system but also a mathematical distribution that must be approximated for the test's validity. This is a fortiori even more the case when subscales are added together for an overall single score." Nonetheless, Kurtzke is denying validity to statistical procedures in this setting. Regardless of how unin-

Dr. Hoberman and Dr. Sahlroot are with the Food and Drug Administration, Rockville, Maryland. However, this chapter was written by the authors in their private capacity. No official support or endorsement by the Food and Drug Administration is intended or should be inferred.

terpretable the difference between average scores of rating scales may be in any practical sense, statistical tests are very forgiving. For all practical purposes, they are valid for distinguishing one group's distribution of scores from another's, no matter how they were generated. *For if there is one common methodology in clinical trials of neurological treatments, it is the rating scale.* Furthermore, the summation of several subscales may even make the statistical test more powerful than if only one or two scales had been used. Admittedly, the ability to detect *some* evidence of efficacy using a *total* score can often complicate the search for the truly affected constituent clinical domains. In addition, the *composition* of the scale can determine its clinical interpretation: the separate tasks comprising the cognitive portion of the Alzheimer's Disease Activity Scale (ADAS-Cog), for example, may be of less interest than the components of the Appel scale used in summarizing the degree of deficit due to amyotrophic lateral sclerosis. It is as though the difference between the means of two treatments on a mutidimensional rating scale needs to be projected onto a prism which will separate the blended domains into useful constituent parts. This is difficult to do. Usually, the effort to separate the spurious from the real in this situation involves a discussion of "multiple endpoints" (illustrated below in the section on Parkinson's disease).

Inferences from clinical trials require valid analytic methods and clinical outcomes of interest. This chapter will begin with descriptions of designs, clinical outcomes and analyses of clinical trials in neurology. They are then placed in the context of specific neurological studies involving Alzheimer's disease, amyotrophic lateral sclerosis (ALS), multiple sclerosis, stroke, Parkinson's disease and epilepsy.

Similarities Among Trials in Neurology

Because the forms of clinical endpoints for many neurological conditions are similar, common statistical techniques are often used. Trials in both multiple sclerosis and epilepsy employ a patient's *frequency of event* (sometimes expressed as a *rate*, i.e., frequency per unit time) as the unit of observation. Both Alzheimer's and Parkinson's disease trials may use a patient's *average score on a multi-item measurement scale* (the Alzheimer's Disease Assessment Scale (ADAS) and Unified Parkinson's Disease Rating Scale (UPDRS)). Trials in cerebrovascular disease often use *ordinal scales* (Barthel, Rankin, NIH and/or Glasgow scales) indicating the patient's level of

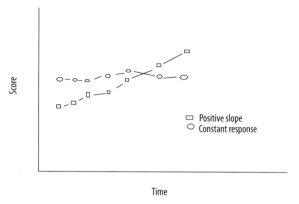

Fig. 10.1. Two possible patterns of a patient's repeated observations over several measurements.

neurological function. For ALS, the clinical observation can consist of a *composite score of laboratory measurements* (the Tufts Quantitative Neuromuscular Examination (TQNE)) depicting various muscle strength and pulmonary function, or a more general *multi-scale questionnaire* that consists of several subscales of general functioning (Norris or Appel scale). Note that the *forms* of the endpoints in these examples do not dictate unique statistical methodologies. By design, virtually all of these trials produce repeated observations on each patient over time, usually weekly or monthly. The choice of methodology depends upon the question under consideration. If the issue centers upon the average response over time, each patient's data may be averaged over time as the analytic unit (an example of a simple repeated measures analysis) or, alternatively, regard "rate of change" (slope) as the primary unit (Fig. 10.1).

In the latter case, for example, one can fit straight lines to each individual's ADAS scores in an Alzheimer trial and then compare the average slopes of the treatment groups. Alternatively, if only the *last* observation on each patient is used (Last Observation Carried Forward or LOCF), the analysis will usually compare the averages of those single observations or their differences from baseline. The "best" choice depends upon a combination of factors: (1) If the clinical question is specific enough actually to specify rate of change as the issue of interest, then the direction, if not the specific measure of rate of change, is clear. For example, in a *progressive* neurological disease, where individuals' clinical scores are anticipated to change in a monotonic pattern over time, an analysis which uses all information on study will almost certainly be preferable to one that uses only the last observation. The rectangles in Fig. 10.1 illustrate such a case. (2) If, on the other hand, the emphasis is on choosing that analysis which will maximize the chance of finding *some* difference between the treatments, but not necessarily one that is well defined in terms of either a quantifiable "treatment effect" or time course of effect, it is wise to take advantage of anticipated patterns of the data as a guide to the most powerful analyses [3].

Trials Using Repeated Measures

Two problems are encountered immediately by statistical analyses of trials designed to collect several observations on patients at scheduled intervals: (1) the choice of a summary measure for patients over time and (2) missing data as a result of premature withdrawal from the study (right censoring). Reasons for termination include adverse events and lack of efficacy, and they will most likely cause problems with the interpretation of *any* analysis. It is, in this context, important to distinguish between three types of *bias*. The first could be classified as *administrative* bias: by the way a study is conducted (e.g., perhaps through the unblinding of investigators), patients randomized to drug may systematically be placed at a clinical advantage over those randomized to placebo. The second could be called *attrition* bias and occurs when the differential patterns and/or condition of dropouts affect the comparison of treatments. If a drug, for instance, induces side effects but is generally effective, patients who drop out due to adverse effects may fail to contribute favorable information about the effectiveness of the drug. The third form of bias could be called *statistical*. In this case, a statistical model has been used to describe distributions of the data in both treatment arms. The model can be as simple as "two samples that come from populations which are each normally (bell-shaped) distributed with possibly different means μ_1 and μ_2." The important feature of the model under discussion is that it contains a parameter which stands for the "treatment effect." Here, the parameter would be $\mu_1 - \mu_2$. Deciding whether the drug is different from placebo as *defined by the model*, rests upon estimating this parameter. Due to such influences as dropouts and an inaccurate statistical model, the estimates may be biased in the sense that, on average over repeated similar trials, the estimate produced from the model does not estimate the parameter that is assumed to apply to the population of interest. It misses its target.

Last Observation Carried Forward (LOCF)

The purpose of the trial may be to decide whether or not the therapy is effective *at the end of a prespeci-*

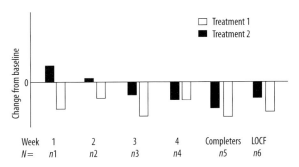

Fig. 10.2. The trial is 5 weeks long. The *bars* show the average change from baseline for each distinct cohort whose last observation is at week *X*, for patients who complete 5 weeks, and the result (LOCF) of combining all the data.

fied duration of treatment. Clearly, carrying forward the last clinical observation noted on a subject is an arbitrary way to assure a patient's inclusion in the analysis. LOCF is really a misnomer since the last observations on patients may fall far short of the ability to answer a question about the drug after the planned duration of exposure. Only if patients drop out of the trial completely at random would the analysis not be contaminated with attrition bias. Nonetheless, even when statistical bias exists, the direction of the trend may be such as to argue for the effectiveness of the drug. If, for example, placebo patients drop out more frequently and/or are sicker than patients on therapy who drop out at the same time, one could argue that an analysis including only the patients' last observation validly answers the question: "Is there something different about the distributions of observations that would point to the efficacy of the drug?" One useful graph is a bar chart showing the means of clinical observations for cohorts of *dropouts* in each treatment group by clinic visit (Fig. 10.2). The figure indicates the effect of carrying forward scores of dropouts together with the means of observations for the "completers" to produce the end result – namely, the LOCF means. For studies in which mortality occurs, some convention such as assigning the "worst score" on a clinical scale may be reasonable. However, see the discussion below on the treacherous use of LOCF when mortality is a common event during a trial.

Inevitably, questions arise about the efficacy of the drug in completers (i.e., patients who have taken assigned therapy for the trial's planned duration). Certain essential issues must be considered. First, given the potential problems that arise from multiple causes of censoring, a statistical analysis which produces a valid *p* value is still one which includes all randomized patients. Furthermore, since completers are a subset of those originally randomized, there is no guarantee that the distributions of prognostic factors are similar among the completers or dropouts in the treatment groups. The comparison of groups may therefore contain a systematic bias. Still another issue may involve a numerical difference between two groups that may not be statistically significant owing partly to fewer patients than anticipated. Finally, in the event that the analyst believes the two groups of completers to be different, the population for whom the result should be applied may not be clear. Compared with patients who drop out, those who complete trials could be less sick or simply more determined to finish. Thus *external*, in addition to *internal*, validity may be questioned.

It must be acknowledged that using the last observation on trial (editorial note: the expression "last observation carried forward" should be summarily abandoned) is fraught with problems and in no way is to be advocated when a statistically "unbiased" estimate of treatment effect is paramount. It is up to the collaborative efforts of the clinician and analyst to decide whether or not a potentially useful pattern such as that found in Fig. 10.2 has sufficient biological plausibility to be exploited by using the last observation on study. Such a case may occur when the lack of discernable longitudinal patterns (among dropouts, completers or both) suggest that *bona fide* longitudinal analyses (disussed in the following section) do not apply or may have to cope with so much noise in the data as to be inefficient compared to other methods. As far as dropouts are concerned, information which could possibly differentiate *biologically* between the dropout subgroup in one treatment group as opposed to another is usually never available. In the absence of evidence to the contrary, "treatment failure" or "lack of efficacy" is usually regarded as a homogenous phenomenon among the randomized treatment groups.

Longitudinal Analyses

We have seen that an LOCF analysis may be useful in detecting an omnibus difference between treatment groups in settings in which there are substantial numbers of dropouts. However, when there is some anticipation that the time course of repeated observations will follow some pattern, a test making use of all the data collected on each individual will more likely detect a difference than one using only the last observation. If, for example, observations are expected to remain stable after a relatively short period of study, a simple option would be to use the average of a patient's observations over time as the unit of analysis. Frison and Pocock [4] compare the properties of various simple statistics derived

from repeated measures. On the other hand, if observations are expected to increase or decrease over time, some form of rate of change analysis might be appropriate.

There are at least two basic approaches to assessing differences in rate of change: (1) a model of the population slopes, and (2) the repeated measures analysis of variance (rm ANOVA), both of which can take advantage of the covariance structure of the repeated observations over time. In other words, the degree to which each individual's scores remain consistently above or below the mean for the rest of the individuals at each time point can provide information useful a difference between the treatment groups. Both approaches to longitudinal analysis use mathematical models to describe the evolution of observations over time. However, a major difference between them is that the "population slope" analysis assumes that the slopes are a random sample from a population (random effect), whereas rm ANOVA often treats any effect as "fixed", i.e. any inference from the data applies only to the experimental situation at hand. The resulting difference in the specifications of the models results in different covariance structures describing the covariance of the observations among the observation times. See below. This discussion implies that longitudinal analyses can be very useful in cases with missing data or patients who leave the study. Other approaches for handling dropouts in longitudinal trials are discussed in Heyting et al. [5] and Brown [6] and in Chapter 13.

A model for the rate of change of a population usually assumes that a patient's time trajectory for some measure approximates a straight line. It is reasonable, but not necessary, to assume that each patient's true slope is itself a random variable (random slope model) [7,8]. The simplest analysis comparing two groups fits a "least squares" (unweighted) line to each patient and uses a t-test or ANOVA that ignores the number of observations contributed by each patient. There are several ways to try to reduce the standard error (noise) of the treatment difference. One is simply to weight each patient's slope by the number of observations taken on each patient [9]. In the spirit of standard theory, more sophisticated methods incorporate the covariance of the observations between different visits as weights applied to the observations [10,11] as in rm ANOVA.

The foregoing analyses are straightforward as long as dropouts are randomly distributed in time. Otherwise, if patients' slopes tend to depend upon the time of dropout (often called "informative censoring") and/or different rates of dropout occur between the groups, a careful examination of the reasons for dropping out and the relation between slope and the time of dropout should be made in order to assess the degree to which these factors affect the estimated difference between the groups. Some authors discuss ways to incorporate information about informative censoring into the analysis. Some authors [12] propose specifying a (usually) unverifiable model of the censoring pattern over time. Another group [13] stratifies patients by the "final visit" (after which they no longer participate in the trial). Using stratum-specific weights to compute a weighted average slope for each treatment group, one can then subtract the two averages to generate a treatment difference. However, one needs to be very careful about the question under consideration. If the question asks: "Does either approach estimate a difference between drug and placebo in the absence of dropping out, as would likely be the case in general public use?" the answer is "probably no". These models may not estimate a parameter which applies to the general population. They *do* generate estimates which are appropriate for treatment differences found in repetitions of similar trials. Consequently, when dropouts occur in a clinical trial in a manner which is related to the clinical endpoint under study, an optimal estimate of pure treatment effect may not exist. Nevertheless, the approach that stratifies by dropout pattern is easy to reproduce and understand. In addition, it allows straightforward inspection of the differences between groups with respect to the relationship of efficacy to patterns of censoring.

Assessing Clinical Endpoints in the Presence of Mortality

As an example of a trial particularly vulnerable to misinterpretation, consider one which uses both clinical measurements and mortality as endpoints. Although this is not usually a problem in studies involving a disease such as Alzheimer's disease because of relatively low mortality and little or no expectation that a drug will actually prolong life, ALS trials are especially vulnerable. Mortality is obviously a form of censoring with respect to measurements of other clinical outcomes; often the event of death is related to clinical measurement(s) such as functional scores on a rating scale. It is possible that a comparison of the slopes (of scores) between treated and placebo groups can produce a statistically significant difference, albeit no difference whatsoever exists between the groups with respect to the LOCF on the clinical scale. For if the drug is effective in slowing mortality, placebo patients will tend to die earlier than patients on drug. Consequently, scores carried forward for placebo patients may be

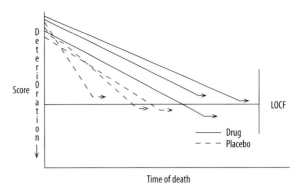

Fig. 10.3. Contrast between group comparisons of slopes versus average of LOCF in the presence of a trend in mortality favorable to the drug.

"as good" or "better" than those carried forward for patients on drug whose clinical condition has longer to deteriorate during extended survival (Fig. 10.3). The result is that, unless one can clearly determine that the decline in the clinical condition contributed significantly to the deaths, the difference in slopes may simply be a reflection of different patterns of mortality generated by other domains of clinical deterioration not captured by the clinical scale used.

In short, the interpretation of clinical scores in the presence of substantial mortality is an unsolved problem. If the primary endpoint is death, then the problem may be suppressed. On the other hand, if clinical functioning is also relevant, mysteries may persist as in the case of the trials of riluzole for ALS in which a mortality benefit was found with disappointing results on functional endpoints (see section below on Amyotrophic Lateral Sclerosis.

Categorical Data Analyses

Virtually all large-scale trials for neurological diseases have the investigator rate each patient's final clinical disposition (Investigator's Global Assessment) or a specific clinical condition (e.g., Rankin scale) on a scale with 5–7 points. If there is a placebo group and one treatment group, the number of patients who are observed in each category can be displayed in a $2 \times k$ table, where k is the number of categories on the ordinal scale as follows:

	Category						
	1	2	3	4	5	6	7
Placebo:	n_{11}	n_{12}	n_{13}	n_{14}	n_{15}	n_{16}	n_{17}
Drug :	n_{21}	n_{22}	n_{23}	n_{24}	n_{25}	n_{26}	n_{27}

The purpose of the statistical analysis is to decide whether the distribution of counts (n_{ij}) found in the trial reflect samples from different underlying distributions. Even more than that: if they are different, the difference may reflect a general shift of the distribution in the active treatment group toward more favorable scores. The most popular test for this purpose is a version of the Cochran–Mantel–Haenszel (CMH) test which takes advantage of the fact that the scale is ordinal (i.e., there is an order relation of categories across columns with respect to clinical condition). The analyst must first decide on a set of scores to assign to each category. The analysis then compares the mean category scores for each treatment group. Since different inferences could be drawn, depending on the scores chosen, it is important that the investigator specify the scores beforehand and not use the data post hoc to search for a set of scores which produces statistical significance. The most popular scores are either the integers used in the table (1, 2, 3, 4, 5, 6, 7) or "ridit" scores, which produce essentially the same result as a Wilcoxon rank sum test. (Note that there are inherently many ties since there are only several possible scores.) In the event that there is prior information about where along the distribution of scores the distributions may differ (e.g., the higher or lower end of the scale), scores can then be chosen a priori to maximize the chance of finding a statistically significant difference when in fact there is a true difference. Lesaffre et al. [14] provide a general discussion of sample size calculations for ordered categories using the Barthel Index from a stroke trial.

An alternative to comparing mean scores using the CMH test is the "proportional odds" analysis [15]. Rather than assigning scores to categories, the latter makes a provisional assumption that the odds of a random patient in one treatment group scoring less than or equal to a given number (clinical condition) on the scale is K times that of a random patient from another group. Moreover, this same proportionality factor K is the same regardless of the given number on the scale. Should the odds not be proportional in this strict sense, the test would still be valid, but its ability to distinguish the groups would likely be less than if they were proportional. Note that the proportional odds assumption builds in the general shift in distribution discussed earlier whereas the CMH analysis does not. In addition, since the proportional odds test is a special case of multivariate logistic regression, important covariates can be incorporated through standard logistic model methodology.

Survival Analysis

Mortality is often an endpoint in trials involving stroke and ALS. Mortality experience in two groups

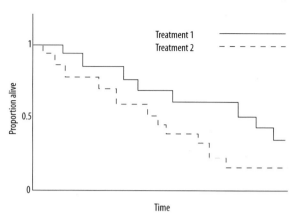

Fig. 10.4. Kaplan–Meier plot of survival.

can be contrasted simply by comparing the proportions of patients still alive at the end of the prescribed follow-up time. Usually, however, there are reasons for adopting methods that take into account patients' variable time on study due to death, dropout, or curtailed follow-up times resulting from the termination of the study. By using more information than merely the proportion of the sample who remain alive, the hope is that a comparison of the distributions of times-to-event will have more power. As long as the pattern of dropouts is not related to distribution of death, the interpretation of results will be straightforward.

The basic structure of survival experience is the Kaplan–Meier plot of the probability of remaining alive (through time T) against T [16,17] (Fig. 10.4).

This graph takes into account the progressive loss of patients by deleting them from subsequent risk sets (i.e., the cohorts of patients who are alive and therefore "at risk" for death just before time T). For example, assume that 20 patients begin the trial. If a patient dies at 5 weeks, then the probability of surviving beyond 5 weeks is $1 - 1/20$. Now assume a patient is lost to follow-up at 6 weeks and another one dies at 7 weeks. The probability of surviving beyond 7 weeks is equal to $(1 - 1/20) \times (1 - 1/18)$, i.e., the probability of survival through 5 weeks *times* the probability of surviving through 7 weeks, *given* that one survives through 5 weeks. The denominator 18 at 7 weeks is derived by subtracting one previous death and one previous censored observation from the original 20. The fractions 1/20 and 1/18 represent the estimated *hazards* at their respective death times. The process of recursive multiplication, using these hazards at each time of death, continues through the last time of death. The hazards themselves then take a prominent role. The sequence of hazards over time in each group can be thought to estimate the groups' respective underlying continuous *hazard functions*. If the ratio of one hazard function to another is constant over time, the hazards are called *proportional*. Otherwise, they may vary in relation to each other, and even cross each other from time to time. It is important to emphasize that even if the hazard functions cross, the survival curves themselves do not necessarily cross. An example of this phenomenon follows in the discussion of ALS trials.

The object of survival analysis is to determine whether or not any manifest difference between the Kaplan–Meier plots for treatment groups is due to chance more than a limited percentage (usually 5%) of the time. There are basically two approaches for comparing Kaplan–Meier plots. One (e.g., Kolmogorov–Smirnov) compares the plots directly by calculating the maximum difference between the curves over the course of the study. If this number is large enough, we conclude that the underlying population distributions are different. The nearly universal method, however, does not compare the curves directly but rather in terms of the hazard functions which, as we have seen, determine the Kaplan–Meier plots. The most commonly used statistical test to compare the distributions of death over time is the "logrank" statistic. Let us postulate two groups, 1 and 2. We may focus our attention on one of the groups, say group 1. Each time a patient dies, we ask: "If the probability of death were the same for all patients at risk in each treatment group (i.e., if there were no effect of treatment), what would be the difference between the number of patients in group 1 who actually died at time T (usually 0 or 1) and the number expected to die?" The statistic accumulates this information over all death times. If, assuming no treatment effect, we find that the *actual* number of deaths in group 1 is discrepant enough from the *expected* number, the result will be statistically significant, and we will conclude that the hypothesis of no treatment effect is implausible. This test is particularly sensitive to departures from no treatment effect when the hazards are proportional. The corresponding pattern in the survival curves shows separation predominantly at the later times of the distributions. However, if the hazard functions cross, indicating that, during some time intervals, placebo patients tend to die faster than those on drug and vice versa during other intervals, the logrank statistic will lose the ability to detect a difference by cancelling itself out over the course of the entire follow-up period. Covariates can be incorporated into the analysis to increase power beyond that of the logrank test or simply to assess the influence of baseline covariates through Cox proportional hazards regression. This model structures each factor or covariate as having a multiplicative influence on an arbitrary hazard which is assumed to be a function of time, only. An alternative to the Cox model separates patients into a few important covariate *strata* in order to perform a "stratified logrank" test. This technique of combining logrank tests over strata attempts to use much of the information in the Cox model in a conceptually simpler manner. Another popular statistic is the version of the Wilcoxon rank sum test applied to censored data. Often called the Wilcoxon–Gehan test, it tests the hypothesis that a random survival time from one group has no greater chance of being larger or smaller than a random survival time from another group. Like the logrank test, the sensitivity of this test is vulnerable to crossing hazards; unlike the former, it is particularly sensitive to earlier departures of the survival curves.

Multiple Endpoints

Since clinical trials in neurological conditions obtain totals or subtotals of a clinical scale with several components, they collect multiple endpoints. Whenever treatment comparisons are made on more than one endpoint using a nominal significance level of 5%, there is a risk that a false positive may occur for at least one endpoint more than 5% of the time. In other words, if similar trials were repeated, an ineffective treatment would be found to be statistically significant for at least one endpoint in more than 5% of the trials. The Bonferroni adjustment provides the easiest way to test more than one hypothesis in a family, while at the same time guaranteeing that no null hypothesis within the family is wrongly rejected more than 5% of the time. It requires the nominal type I error for each tested endpoint to be $0.05/k$, where k is the number of hypotheses in the family. When k is only moderately large, the chance of finding *any* statistical significance among the hypotheses diminishes considerably. More powerful alternatives reside in the class of procedures which begin with an overall or global test to determine whether or not at least one hypothesis can be rejected. If the global test is rejected, tests can be performed using *closed testing* procedures [18,19] based on rejecting a hypothesis of interest only if all sets of the null hypotheses it contains have been rejected. Lehmacher et al. [20] recommend O'Brien's OLS procedure [21] for testing a set of hypotheses when the directionality of the treatment differences is expected to be in the same direction over all the endpoints in a set.

Alzheimer's Disease

Trials evaluating therapies in Alzheimer's disease often depend on measurements of (1) cognitive functioning (e.g., the "cognitive" section of the Alzheimer's Disease Assessment Scale, ADAS-Cog), and (2) the clinician's judgment of improvement, which may include information gathered from a family member or guardian. The ADAS-Cog battery usually consists of 11 items whose total score lies between 0 and 70; the higher the number, the greater the cognitive deficit. The ADAS-Cog is a fine enough scale that the patients' total scores on the 11 items in trials of moderate size can be regarded as "continuous" rather than "categorical" for analytical purposes. This means that the analyst can at least anticipate that the distribution of total scores in each group is not grossly different from a Normal distribution. The global measure of improvement typically runs from 1 (markedly improved) to 4 (no change) to 7 (markedly worse). There are at least four elementary approaches to the analysis:

(1) To determine whether the average ADAS-Cog score has declined from the baseline score more in the treatment group than the control group after a specified treatment duration (*change from baseline LOCF*). The difference between a patient's last observation and his or her baseline score is the unit of analysis. Use of the "change from baseline" will reduce noise to some extent as long as the correlation between baseline and on-study score is positive and substantial. If there is only one clinical center, a *t*-test or Wilcoxon rank sum test would be appropriate. If the trial is multicenter, then a two-way analysis of variance (ANOVA) using centers as blocks or Wilcoxon tests combined over centers would be appropriate.

(2) To determine whether the average score *on study* has declined more in the treatment than in the control group after a specified duration (*absolute LOCF score*). The same methodology could be applied to the LOCF score for each patient. An alternative would be analysis of covariance in which a relationship between the baseline and final scores (i.e., final = a + b × baseline) can reduce the estimate of noise mentioned in the Introduction, thus increasing the chance of finding a statistically significant difference between the groups when the drug is in fact different from placebo.

(3) To determine whether the distributions of scores *averaged over evaluations* (visits) differ for the groups. One could simply average the scores for each patient over the patient's visits and apply any of the above methods as appropriate.

(4) To determine whether slopes of *straight line fits* of the data on each patient are distributed differently for the groups. Any analysis as presented in number (1) would be appropriate.

Knapp et al. [22] conducted a 30-week trial which randomized 663 Alzheimer's patients to one of

Table 10.1. Results of a trial of tacrine in Alzheimer's disease

	Intent to Treat		Evaluable Completers	
	CIBI	ADAS-Cog	CIBI	ADAS-Cog
Dose-Response trend	0.03	0.004	0.001	0.001
Regimen 2 vs pbo	0.33	0.20	0.20	0.11
Regimen 3 vs pbo	0.04	0.008	0.13	0.11
Regimen 4 vs pbo	0.04	0.002	0.002	0.001

three forced titrations of tacrine (Cognex, Warner-Lambert) or placebo: regimen 1 was placebo; regimen 2, 40 mg/day × 6 weeks followed by 80 mg/day × 24 weeks; regimen 3, 40 mg/day × 6 weeks, then 80 mg/day × 6 weeks, then 120 mg/day × 18 weeks; regimen 4, 40 mg/day × 6 weeks, then 80 mg/day × 6 weeks, then 120 mg/day × 6 weeks, then 160 mg/day × 12 weeks. Dropouts were numerous with 58% withdrawing before week 30, 75% of these due to adverse effects; patients on tacrine tended to have marked ALT elevations. In Table 10.1, the first two columns display the *p* values for the CIBI (a 7-point scale of Clinician Interview-Based Impression) and ADAS-Cog for the 653 patients who had at least one post-baseline observation. The authors performed, but did not report, an LOCF analysis; instead, they provided a "retrieved dropout" analysis in which patients who had withdrawn early were evaluated at what would have been their 30-week assessment. The third and fourth columns display results for the 263 patients who completed the study and were deemed "evaluable", namely patients who did not violate compliance standards in the protocol.

The results for ADAS-Cog were derived from an analysis of variance of the actual scores at 30 weeks; results for the CIBI, from a CMH analysis using ridit scores. Differences from placebo ranged from 2 to 5 points on the ADAS-Cog and from 0.2 to 0.5 points on the CIBI, depending on the data set and treatment regimen. Regimen 4 produced the largest treatment differences. In general, these results present a case for the effectiveness of tacrine, clearly at 160 mg/day. However, there are some points worth mentioning for the general case:

(1) There is no assessment for the effects of dropouts or analysis which takes into account all the data over time for each patient.

(2) The term "dose-response trend" is, in general, ambiguous unless the investigator makes clear whether or not the placebo group was included in the analysis. If included, "dose-response" might be misleading since the term could imply that efficacy increases with the dose of drug when in fact the drug

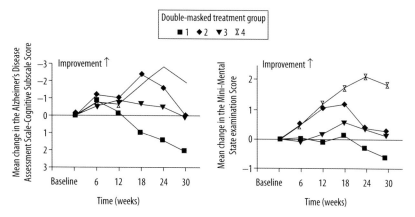

Fig. 10.5. Mean change from baseline in Alzheimer's Disease Assessment Scale-Cognitive subscale (*left*) and Mini-Mental State Examination (*right*) for week 30 evaluable patients. Reproduced with permission from [22].

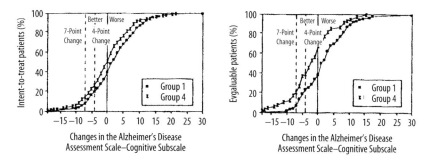

Fig. 10.6. Changes in Alzheimer's Disease Assessment Scale-Cognitive subscale score from baseline at week 30 for intent-to-treat patients (*left*) and evaluable patients (*right*). Reproduced with permission from [22].

is simply different from placebo while no order relation exists between efficacy and dose. All doses could be equally effective relative to placebo.

(3) In a trial which proposes to compare more than one treatment with control, some provision should be made to ensure that false positives do not arise simply because numerous tests were conducted. The authors in the above study do not state whether one was specified in the protocol.

The left-hand plot in Fig. 10.5 displays the group means (ADAS-Cog) of evaluable completers over time for each treatment group. It is always important to make sure that the set of patients who contribute to each time-wise mean is well defined. Time-wise group means, including *all* patients who happen to be in the trial at that time, would blind the effect of dropouts. These do not identify the profile of any well-defined cohort of patients.

Figure 10.6 offers a useful example for summarizing continuous data. Shown are the *empirical distribution functions* of the placebo and high-dose groups at the end of 30 weeks. The horizontal axis

depicts the range of changes from baseline ADAS-Cog while the vertical axis depicts the fraction of values that are less than or equal to a chosen value on the horizontal axis. Since positive values on the horizontal axis represent clinical worsening, a displacement of the curve for the active treatment group to the left of the placebo's indicates a favorable profile for the active treatment. For example, for the intent to treat sample ($n = 653$), approximately 50% of the patients on regimen 4 improved or did not change from baseline, whereas 50% of the placebo patients had values less than 2–3 points in the direction of deterioration. The graph for the evaluable completers indicates a slightly larger difference between the groups.

Amyotrophic Lateral Sclerosis

Disability due to amyotrophic lateral sclerosis (ALS) often leads relatively soon to premature death. Consequently, mortality is an important endpoint along with several measures of clinical function, including vital capacity, muscle function and activities of daily living. Examples of functional scales are the Norris and Appel scales containing separate physician ratings for respiratory and muscle function. The Tufts Quantitative Neuromuscular Exams (TQNE) [23] measure pulmonary function, bulbar function, timed hand activities, isometric arm strength and isometric leg strength. For each patient, the raw score on each domain is standardized by subtracting the mean of some reference group (typically the baseline average of all the patients) and then dividing the difference by the estimated standard deviation of that group. The intention is to force measurements of different quantitative scales (e.g. pulmonary function and time hand activities) onto a common scale. The five standardized scores are then averaged to produce the patient's *megascore*, which positions the patient's overall functioning relative to a group mean. Munsat et al. [24] examined the natural history of megascores and found that they decline over time in a linear fashion. A standard straight line fit to a patient's data often provides an excellent approximation to the decline of this composite measure over a course of up to 2 years. The properties of megascores have been studied in detail by Pradas et al. [25] for a cohort of 277 patients, half of whom had at least six megascores per patient for a median time of 10 months. This is reasonable with the caveat that results must be interpreted in the light of the pattern of deaths in the groups.

The rate of decline for symptomatic conditions has been studied in several randomized, double-blind, placebo-controlled clinical trials. In one [26] results of the TQNE slopes failed to show any effect of human growth hormone. In a 6-month multicenter study [27], patients taking 800 mg gabapentin t.i.d. tended to have slower rates of decline for the "arm" megascore (megaslopes) than patients taking placebo: -0.0035/day vs -0.0045/day ($p = 0.06$ using two-way ANOVA). This trial, in contrast to that of Andres et al. [23], used bilateral shoulder and elbow flexion and extension (eight measurements) rather than the 10 which included grip strength of both hands as well. Two other trials, testing insulin-like growth factor (IGF-1), used three functions of the Appel score which combines functional and respiratory measurements: (1) the unweighted slopes of the Appel scores, and (2) the time to treatment failure (reaching a score of 115 on the Appel score or a forced vital capacity of less than 39%), and (3) change from baseline of the average Appel score. (These trials of IGF-1 were discussed at a public FDA hearing on May 24, 1996.)

Lacomblez et al. [28] describe a study in which 959 ALS patients were randomized to placebo or one of three doses of riluzole (Rilutek, Rhone-Poulenc)

(50 mg/day, 100 mg/day, 200 mg/day). The primary endpoint was intubation- or tracheostomy-free survival with a comparison of the 100 mg/day group with placebo using the logrank test. Secondary endpoints included muscle strength, vital capacity, functional status and stiffness. Functional scales were analyzed by ANOVA. Slopes of unweighted least squares fitted lines to each patient measured the rate of change of muscle strength, limb and bulbar scores. The survival result (p value = 0.076) using the logrank test at 18 months illustrates the weakness of that statistic when crossing hazards occur. With 50% of the patients alive at the termination of the study, the Kaplan–Meier curves began to separate at about 3 months and appeared to be coming together again at 18 months. The reason for the convergence is that the estimates of the hazard functions (not shown in the paper) cross in the middle of the trial. Consequently, patients on placebo died faster during the first part of the trial, while those on riluzole died faster during the remaining part. This pattern reflects the fact that the logrank test was statistically significant earlier in the trial at 12 month. Although the Wilcoxon test too would have suffered from the crossing hazards, the p value would have been lower because of its greater sensitivity to the initial divergence of the curves starting at 3 months. Another consideration in many mortality trials (and this one in particular) is the substantial amount of censoring of patients alive at the end of the study. If there were a substantial number of patients who had been followed for only a short time by the end of the study follow-up, it is possible that the relative patterns of deaths between the groups would have changed substantially after further follow-up. Lastly, Lacomblez et al. [28] also used Cox regression incorporating clinical factors related to the rate of death. By incorporating these prognostic variables, the analysis was able to generate p values far less than the significance level of 5%.

Crossing hazards also occurred in the first trial of riluzole [29]. More intriguing, however, is the statistically significant result in favor of riluzole using slopes for deterioration of muscle strength. This conclusion is questionable in view of the increased possibility of a false positive over 5% among tests on several secondary endpoints. Nonetheless, whatever the treatment difference for muscle strength, it may have emerged from the confounding of slopes and the pattern of mortality depicted in Fig. 8.3. The LOCF comparison of average muscle scores showed no evidence of effect, despite the authors' report of a p value of 0.028 in favor of riluzole's effect on rate of deterioration. This example at least raises the possibility that the differential pattern of deaths due to myriad influences induced this treatment difference.

Again, comparisons of average slopes cannot be made apart from a consideration of patterns and causes of death.

Multiple Sclerosis

Trials in multiple sclerosis often provide counts of exacerbations per patient and/or scores on functional scales such as the Kurtzke (EDSS) scores. Cladribine [30], for instance, has been studied using 24 pairs of patients, matched by age, sex, and severity of disease. For the EDSS, the analysis [31] first ranked the absolute paired differences for all 24 pairs at a given time point. By assessing these rankings for all time points, a vector of signed scores was constructed for each matched pair. By combining these scores over the time points of the trial, a statistic was then computed to assess how far from zero these differences diverged over the course of the trial. The EDSS and Scripps Neurological Rating Scale both produced statistically significant differences between cladribine and placebo.

Bornstein [32] randomized 50 patients to either copolymer-1 or placebo; 48 were matched by sex, number of exacerbations in the previous 2 years, and degree of disability as measured by the Kurtzke Scale. Kurtzke scores over the treatment period (2 years) were analyzed using both change from baseline and repeated measures. The latter was the more powerful test, probably because it analyzed the average of the patient's scores over time rather than the patient's last observation alone. The analysis conformed to a stable pattern of group means over time after about 3 months. The primary efficacy endpoint, however, was the proportion of exacerbation-free patients. This was an ambitious endpoint for a pilot study. The ability to find a statistically significant difference between two proportions can be less than an analysis of a continuous measure. In this case, the number of exacerbations per patient was clearly statistically significant, whereas the result for the proportion of exacerbation-free patients was less clear since statistical significance depended upon a small number of patients.

Matched data can be analyzed by either preserving or ignoring the identification of pairs. Preserving the pairs usually means that the treatment difference will be estimated by finding the difference between the scores within a matched pair. Although the overall difference is the same in either case, the estimate for the variance of the difference will not be. Counts of events can be analyzed using a *t*-test or two-way ANOVA in multicenter trials. However, because counts can often be extreme, an analysis based upon averages can be vulnerable to outliers,

giving rise to a distorted estimate for a treatment difference. Sometimes the logarithm of the count is taken as the unit of analysis in order to induce a distribution closer to normal. An alternative test in the matched-pair setting is the Wilcoxon signed rank test, which preserves the pairs but will not be as sensitive to outliers. For an unmatched analysis or cases in which patients are individually randomized, the Wilcoxon rank sum test would be appropriate. Other approaches attempt to model the counts according to a particular probabilistic process, such as Poisson, or make use of semi-parametric modelling. The problem with much of the literature on counts (or recurrent events) is the complicated nature of the recurrence process that may exist for each individual. This is most likely the reason that analyses of count data in clinical trials has remained elementary.

When comparing proportions for paired data, the standard analysis (McNemar's test) relies upon a count of the number of pairs in which the placebo patient has the attribute (or event of interest) and the matched drug patient does not, versus the number of pairs in which the opposite discordance occurs. Pairs in which both patients either do or do not have the event are ignored.

Parkinson's Disease

In general, patients who participate in trials in Parkinson's disease can be divided into two groups: those with early Parkinson's disease and those who exhibit "wearing off" phenomena associated with prolonged exposure to levadopa. The UPDRS and its subscales and/or the Hoehn and Yahr Scale have been used in trials of either subgroup. Patients with "wearing off" phenomena may also fill out daily diaries indicating the proportion of the day spent in ON and OFF time.

Just as with the ADAS-Cog for Alzheimer's disease or the EDSS for multiple sclerosis, treatment comparisons employing the UPDRS can be done by standard methods: patient rates of change, LOCF or repeated measures. Alternatively, DATATOP [33] used the UPDRS and time to the onset of disability prompting the clinical decision to begin administering levadopa to compare the effects of deprenyl and tocopherol in early Parkinson's disease using a full factorial design with placebo. It was found that the hazard ratio for time to levodopa rescue was 0.5 in favor of patients treated with deprenyl ($p < 0.001$) as opposed to those not taking deprenyl. The annual rate of decline in the total UPDRS was also found to be significantly different by analysis of variance. In addition, the authors report statistically significant p values for comparisons based on the Mental, Motor and Activities of Daily Living subscales. These sub-scales constitute *multiple endpoints* which require methods such as those mentioned earlier to control the false positive rate for the simultaneous testing of all hypotheses of interest. Since the *p* values in DATATOP were less than 0.001 using all subjects, any multiple testing procedure would conclude that patients treated with deprenyl benefited on all three subscales. Another trial in 55 early Parkinson patients [34] analyzed the change from baseline of the UPDRS Parts II (Activities of Daily Living) and III (Motor Examination) after 9 weeks. In a trial of 44 patients with motor fluctuations [35], cabergoline was compared with bromocriptine using the UPDRS and the average percentage of hours spent OFF and ON during each day over the 7 days preceding a hos-pital visit. Changes from baseline were computed by the difference between baseline and the average of patients scores over a stable dose period, thus utiliz-ing all available information on each patient in a simple manner. Analysis of variance was then em-ployed to analyze the changes.

Stroke

Several measurements of clinical outcome are typical in the assessment of drugs for stroke: mortality, total Barthel Index, Glasgow Outcome Scale (GDS), Rankin Scale, NIH Stroke Scale and the European Stroke Scale. The question is often whether the drug has affected functional outcome at the end of a pre-scribed follow-up period after treatment. The total Barthel score can be treated as continuous for prac-tical purposes or as ordered categories by appor-tioning ranges of the total score to ordered categories a priori. In some cases, the investigator will add the category "death" to one of these scales as the worst case, a convenience that allows for score to be "carried forward" to the end of the follow-up period. In addition, since death is part of the scale, the inves-tigator avoids the vexing problem of interpreting the results in the presence of censoring through death. For, if the patient's score is related to time of death and mortality is different between the treatment arms, an analysis of the scores will not be indepen-dent of the pattern of mortality. In other words, there will be no "pure treatment effect in the absence of mortality". If mortality is low enough to be only a minor factor, ANOVA can be performed on the total Barthel score and a CMH test or a proportional odds test can be used on the ordered categorical scale.

Inclusion of mortality on the scale, on the other hand, can complicate trial interpretation:

(1) It is possible that a therapy might prevent death but move a patient into a vegetative state. The distributions of clinical outcomes would be found to be statistically different, but the *pattern* of departure from no treatment effect may raise moral and clini-cal dilemmas. This problem can be alleviated by dichotomizing the scale so that "vegetative state" and "death" are in the same category.

(2) In the face of statistical significance, there may be some ambiguity about what has truly been demonstrated. Consider the following scenario of a trial that has enrolled enough patients to make a comparison of overall mortality meaningful – in other words, a trial in which there is a good chance of finding a statistically significant difference if in fact the drug has an effect on mortality. Let us sup-pose further that a "trend" in favor of the drug for mortality is found but the resulting *p* value is too high to conclude that the drug has an effect on mor-tality. Now assume that the distributions on the func-tional scale (including death) yield a statistically significant difference. The favorable trend on mor-tality will have some influence on the overall analy-sis of the functional scale. Moreover, it is possible that the distributions on the functional scales would not have been statistically different were "death" not included as an extreme category. The question then becomes: "Has the drug been found to affect func-tional status among those alive at the end of the trial in the context of the inconclusive result on overall mortality?"

A large trial using tissue plasminogen activator (t-PA) [36] used all four scales to define a patient as having "minimal or no neurological deficit": 95–100 on the Barthel Index, *or* less than or equal to 1 on either the NIHSS or Rankin Scale, *or* 1 on the Glasgow Outcome Scale. The study then compared the proportion of patients who achieved this status on t-PA and placebo at 3 months. Death before 3 months was assigned the worst score on the respec-tive scale. An LOCF rule was adopted for patients who did not have 3-month assessments. A global statistic assessing the effect of t-PA on the compo-site endpoint was derived from a logistic regression methodology [11,37]. Treatment comparisons on the univariate functional scales were done if the overall test was statistically significant; if so, a Mantel–Haenszel test was then used to compare the odds of minimal or no deficit on each scale.

The case of tirilazad administered for subarach-noid hemorrhage in which some positive results occurred in subgroups illustrates the need to attend to comparisons set forth a priori in the protocol. Kassel et al. [38] reported no statistical difference between any of the three doses and placebo on the primary endpoint, namely, incidence of clinical vasospasm. The *p* value of 0.048 for the 6 mg/kg per day group was not statistically significant due to the necessity of lowering the nominal type I error for each comparison against control. This should be done in order to guard against the probability of finding *at least one of these comparisons* significant more than 5% of the time when all doses are ineffective. In this case, the Bonferroni correction was applied so that each comparison with control was tested at the 0.0167 (0.05/3) level. Among several subgroup analyses on clinical outcome and mortality, the authors report a statistically significant result on a tertiary endpoint: the Glasgow Outcome Scale (GOS) at 3 months. Specifically, the proportion of patients in the tirilazad group with a "good outcome" was 63%, while that in the placebo group was 53% ($p = 0.01$). The benefit appeared to be limited to men (71% vs 47%, $p < 0.001$). No statistical evidence was obtained for women. The question is whether one can fairly state that these findings indicate that tirilazad is responsible for "an improvement in overall outcome", as stated by the authors. Any attempt at an answer requires knowing that (1) gender was one of many possible dimensions for subgrouping mentioned in the protocol and that (2) no plan was carried out to guard against spurious results when testing the five GOS categories together with all the other secondary and tertiary endpoints. In addition, the authors report the results of grouping the first two GOS categories as "favorable outcome", resulting in no statistical significance in men. The sobering nature of this example is brought into focus when we examine the results of a similarly designed trial of tirilazad. (Trials of tirilazad were discussed at a public FDA hearing on September 26, 1994.) When 6 mg/kg per day of the drug was compared with vehicle, not only was no significant difference seen between the groups when all patients were included (58% vs 61%, in favor of vehicle), but the percentage of *men* with "good outcome" was greater in the placebo group (58% vs 68%). Ultimately, the task of separating signal from noise in the first trial was made more difficult by the lack of statistical structure required for examining the myriad combinations of subgroups and endpoints. This case emphasizes the need for a full rendering of the relevant parts of the protocol so that the reader is fully aware of all investigations that may have taken place when secondary and tertiary endpoints are reported as statistically significant.

Epilepsy

The clinical manifestation of epilepsy is seizures, typically discrete countable events. Seizure data are usually summarized by a patient's seizure rate, or the average number of seizures per fixed time interval. Treatment group means are used as the basis for comparing efficacy between treatments. This approach has been criticized as, at the very least, naive [39]. One problem is whether or not a dropout's event rate calculated using the time he or she was in the trial would be similar to that calculated if he or she were to remain in the trial for its full duration. As discussed earlier, all the *caveats* using the last observation on trial apply. However, more information about the actual distribution of events within an individual may be useful for designing a more powerful study. For example, more sophisticated models have been proposed to take advantage of the recurrent nature of seizure data. The Poisson model, the most likely candidate, does not fit seizure data well due to overdispersion [39,40]. To improve the fit of the basic Poisson model, Hopkins et al. [39] modified the mean of the distribution. In one model, the expected number of seizures on day t (Poisson mean) is made a function of the number of seizures on day $(t − 1)$. In another, the authors formulate a two-state Markov model in which the Poisson mean varies stochastically between states. Both models allow for overdispersion and correlation between observations, but allow for inferences about drug effects only in a single patient. Thall and Lachin [41] proposed a nonparametric method for analyzing count data obtained at random intervals (e.g., visits). Also in this setting, Thall [42] proposed a mixed Poisson likelihood regression model in which each count is multiplied by a random subject effect that allows for extra-Poisson variation. The model utilizes covariate information and permits estimation and testing of the event rate. The Thall analyses are best suited for diseases in which the underlying event rate exhibits marked changes over time, usually not the case in a chronic condition such as epilepsy. Each of the models just described is statistically complicated, and can be misleading. Since one never knows the true model, it makes sense simply to compare mean seizure rates.

To increase efficiency, most analyses utilize baseline seizure information as well as on-treatment seizures. Let T be the on-treatment seizure rate, B the baseline seizure rate. Each subject's rate is calculated for the portion of the trial corresponding to their participation. The simple change from baseline $(B − T)$ is superior (i.e., has smaller variance) to the uncorrected seizure rate T if and only if the correlation $\rho\rho$ between B and T is at least 0.5 [43]. Temkin and Wilensky [44] found a correlation of 0.76 between seizure counts in the two periods of a crossover trial, and 0.80 between seizure counts in different time blocks. The ANCOVA of T with B as covariate is even more efficient than change from baseline [43]. Performing the ANCOVA is equivalent to using the ANOVA with an endpoint, $\rho B − T$, whose variance is never greater than the variance of $B - T$. Other endpoints encountered in epilepsy clinical trials are percentage change from baseline ($[B - T]/T$) and response ratio ($[B - T]/[B + T]$). These endpoints each have their own strengths and weaknesses [45].

The endpoints discussed above are usually analyzed statistically using tests based on the normal distribution, such as the simple t-test, ANOVA or ANCOVA. The analyst must, however, first evaluate the consistency of the data with normality. If the data are not Normally distributed – and in epilepsy they often are not – the endpoint can be transformed or truncated, though neither approach is guaranteed to normalize the data. Furthermore, the search for the perfect transformation may inflate the probability of the type I error if the analyst conducts the search with an eye toward minimizing the p value. Nonparametric analyses based on ranks, such as the Wilcoxon and Friedman tests, are valid for any distribution and are more efficient than Normal-based tests in the presence of a few large observations. The rank-transform method is a popular approach which applies standard parametric models found in software packages to the rank-transformed data [46]. Many sponsors circumvent the normality issue entirely, choosing instead to categorize the response and use categorical statistical methods. For example, percent seizure rate reductions might be converted to the following ordered categories: (1) $\geq$50%, (2) $\geq$25% and <50%, (3) $\geq$0% and <25%, (4) $\geq$–25% and <0 and (5) <–25%. This exercise is generally self-defeating; the cutoffs are artificial from a clinical standpoint, and the information lost by chopping up a continuous measure into discrete units produces a less efficient endpoint.

The discussion above is relevant to standard designs of investigational drugs, which are placebo-controlled, add-on trials of fixed duration with 8–12 week baselines and 12–16 week on-treatment durations. Add-on trials, in which the therapy of interest or placebo is added to the patient's previous antiepileptic regimen, have evolved primarily to satisfy ethical concerns. In add-on trials, patients will receive some therapy to permit at least partial control of their seizures. The test drug or placebo will then be added to this background medication. This design suffers from a number of limitations, however, most especially the "plateau effect" which arises when patients are already at maximally tolerated dosages of other antiepileptic drugs. Problems include increased toxicity, decreased sensitivity, and difficulty of interpretation in the presence of drug interactions [47]. Van Belle and Tempkin [48] point out that even attempts to control the background drug's serum level may not guarantee an interpretable add-on trial.

New monotherapy designs counter some of the criticisms levelled at add-on designs while still addressing ethical concerns. These designs permit the use of a placebo or low-dose active control.[1] Standard efficacy variables based on seizure frequency during a fixed time interval are not applicable to these designs [49]. Instead, monotherapy designs use endpoints which limit a subject's exposure to placebo or ineffective treatment while enabling efficacy comparisons. The endpoint is fashioned so that a subject exits the trial after the occurrence of a prospectively designated number and/or type of seizures. Examples of such endpoints which have been used successfully in clinical trials include time-to-fourth-seizure [51] and time to "therapeutic failure" [52]. For the latter, a subject exits the trial (reaches the trial endpoint) when any of four exit criteria are satisfied: (1) a doubling of the mean monthly seizure frequency (from baseline), (2) a doubling of the highest 2-day seizure frequency (from baseline), (3) a single generalized tonic-clonic seizure (GTC) if GTCs were not present during the baseline period, or (4) a prolongation of generalized seizure duration deemed by the investigator to require intervention.

Efficacy data are analyzed by the usual survival-type methods, Cox proportional hazards regression or logrank. Categorical methods may also be applied, such as a chi-square analysis of the percentage of patients reaching therapeutic failure [52].

Some seizure events are not countable, as, for instance, so-called seizure flurries, seizure clusters and status epilepticus (SE). The epilepsy community has not reached a consensus about the quantification of uncountable events, although some have suggested using a measure based on "duration". One recent FDA submission of a drug for SE used the endpoint "cessation of SE within 10 minutes with continued cessation for 30 minutes following drug administration". Uncountable events may also occur in patients having countable seizures as their primary seizure type. Ideally, both countable and uncountable events should be combined in a single analysis, though there is no satisfactory method at this time.

Acknowledgements. I would like to express my gratitude to J. Todd Sahlroot, PhD. for his extensive contributions to the section on epilepsy, and to Paul Leber, MD, Russell Katz, MD, John Feeney, MD, and Richard Tresley, MD for their editorial comments.

---

[1] Monotherapy trials with an active control group should have as their goal the demonstration of superiority of the test drug to the control. Pledger [47], Pledger and Kramer [49] and Leber [50] discuss the inferential problems inherent in active control equivalence studies.

References

1. McFarland HF. In: Porter RJ, Schoenberg BS, editors. Controlled clinical trials in neurological disease. Boston: Kluwer Academic, 1990:333.

2. Kurtzke JF. In: Porter RJ, Schoenberg BS, editors. Controlled clinical trials in neurological disease. Boston: Kluwer Academic, 1990:15.

3. Salzburg DS. The use of restricted significance tests in clinical trials. New York: Springer, 1992: chapter 6.

4. Frison L, Pocock SJ. Repeated measures in clinical trials: analysis using mean summary statistics and its implications for design. Stat Med 1992;11:1685–1704.

5. Heyting A, Tolboom JTBM, Essers JGA. Statistical handling of drop-outs in longitudinal clinical trials. Stat Med 1992;11: 2043–2061.

6. Brown M. A test for the difference between two treatments in a continuous measure of outcome when there are dropouts. Controlled Clin Trials 1992;13:213–225.

7. Lefante JJ. The power to detect differences in average rates of change in longitudinal studies. Stat Med 1990;9:437–446.

8. Palta M, Cook T. Some considerations in the analysis of rates of change in longitudinal studies. Stat Med 1987;6:599–611.

9. Gumpertz M, Pantula SG. A simple approach to inference in random coefficient models. Am Stat 1989;43:203–209.

10. Laird NM, Ware JH. Random-effects models for longitudinal data. Biometrics 1982;38:963–974.

11. Liang K, Zeger SL. Longitudinal data analysis using generalized linear models. Biometrika 1986;73:13–22.

12. Wu MC, Carroll RJ. Estimation and comparison of changes in the presence of informative right censoring by modeling the censoring process. Biometrics 1988;44:175–188.

13. Wu MC, Bailey K. Analyzing changes in the presence of informative right censoring caused by death and withdrawal. Stat Med 1988;7:337–346.

14. Lesaffre E, Scheys I, Frohlich J, Bluhmki E. Calculation of power and sample size with bounded outcome scores. Stat Med 1993;12:1063–1078.

15. Whitehead J. Sample size calculations for ordered categorical data. Stat Med 1993;12:2257–2271.

16. Peto R, Pike MC, Armitage P, et al. Design and analysis of randomized clinical trials requiring prolonged observation on each patient: I. Br J Cancer 1976;34:585–612.

17. Peto R, Pike MC, Armitage P, et al. Design and analysis of randomized clinical trials requiring prolonged observation on each patient: II. Br J Cancer 1977;35:1–39.

18. Marcus R, Peritz E, Gabriel KR. On closed testing procedures with reference with special reference to analysis of variance. Biometrika 1976;63:655–660.

19. Bauer P. Multiple testing in clinical trials. Stat Med 1991; 10:871–890.

20. Lehmacher W, Wassmer G, Reitmeir P. Procedures for two-sample comparisons controlling the experiment-wise error rate. Biometrics 1991;47:511–521.

21. O'Brien PC. Procedures for comparing samples with multiple endpoints. Biometrics 1984;40:79–1087.

22. Knapp JK, Knopman DS, Solomon PR, Pendlebury WW, Davis CS, Gracon SI for the Tacrine Study Group. A 30-week randomized controlled trial of high-dose tacrine in patients with Alzheimer's disease. JAMA 1994;271:985–991.

23. Andres PL, Finison LJ, Conlon T, Thibodeau LM, Munsat TL. Use of composite scores (megascores) to measure deficit in amyotrophic lateral sclerosis. Neurology 1988;38:404–408.

24. Munsat TL, Andres PL, Finison L, Conlon T, Thibodeau L. The natural history of motorneuron loss in amyotrophic lateral sclerosis. Neurology 1988;38:409–413.

25. Pradas J, Finison L, Andres PL, Thornell B, Hollander D, Munsat TL. The natural history of amyotrophic lateral sclerosis and the use of natural history controls in therapeutic trials. Neurology 1993;43:751–755.

26. Smith RA, Melmed S, Sherman B, Frane J, Munsat TL, Festoff BW. Recombinant growth hormone treatment of amyotrophic lateral sclerosis. Muscle Nerve 1993;16:624–633.

27. Miller RG, Moore D, Young LA, Armon C, Barohn RJ, Bromberg MB, et al. Placebo-controlled trial of gabapentin in patients with amyotrophic lateral sclerosis. Neurology 1996;47:1383–1388.

28. Lacomblez L, Bensimon G, Leigh PN, Guillet P, Meininger V for the Amyotrophic Lateral Sclerosis/Riluzole Study Group II. Dose-ranging study of riluzole in amyotrophic lateral sclerosis. Lancet 1996;347:1425–1431.

29. Bensimon G, Lacomblez L, Meininger V and the ALS/Riluzile Study Group. A controlled trial of riluzole in amyotrophic lateral sclerosis. N Engl J Med 1994;330:585–591.

30. Sipe JC, Romine JS, Koziol JA, McMillan R, Zyroff J, Beutler E. Cladribine in treatment of chronic progressive multiple sclerosis. Lancet 1994;344:9–13.

31. Koziol JA, Maxwell DA. A distribution-free test for paired growth curve analyses with application to an animal tumour immunotherapy experiment. Stat Med 1982;1:83–89.

32. Bornstein M. A pilot trial of cop 1 in exacerbating-remitting multiple sclerosis. N Engl J Med 1987;317:408–414.

33. Parkinson Study Group. DATATOP: a multicenter controlled clinical trial in early Parkinson's disease. Arch Neurol 1989;46:1052–1060.

34. Hubble JP, Koller WC, Cutler NR, Sramek JJ, Friedman J, Goetz C, et al. Pramipexole in patients with early Parkinson's disease. Clin Neuropharmacol 1995;18:338–347.

35. Inzelberg R, Nisipeanu P, Rabey JM, Orlov E, Catz T, Kippervasser S, et al. Double-blind comparison of cabergoline and bromocriptine in Parkinson's disease patients with Motor fluctuations. Neurology 1996;47:785–788.

36. The National Institute of Neurological Disorders and Stroke rt-PTA Stroke Study Group (1995) Tissue plasminogen activator for acute ischemic stroke. N Engl J Med 1996;333: 1581–1587.

37. Dunlop DD. Regression for longitudinal data: a bridge from least squares regression. Am Stat 1994;48:299–303.

38. Kassel NF, Haley EC, Apperson-Hansen C, Alves WM and the Participants. Randomized, double-blind, vehicle-controlled trial of tirilazad mesylate in patients with aneurysmal subarachnoid hemorrhage: a cooperative study in Europe, Australia, and New Zealand. J Neurosurg 1996;84:221–228.

39. Hopkins A, Davies P, Dobson C. Mathematical models of patterns of seizures. Arch Neurol 1985;42:463–467.

40. Balish M, Albert PS, Theodore WH. Seizure frequency in intractable partial epilepsy: a statistical analysis. Epilepsia 1991;32:642–649.

41. Thall PF, Lachin JM. Analysis of recurrent events: nonparametric methods for random-interval count data. J Am Stat Assoc 1988;83:339–347.

42. Thall PF. Mixed Poisson likelihood regression models for longitudinal interval count data. Biometrics 1988;44:197–209.

43. Senn SJ. The use of baselines in clinical trials of bronchodilators. Stat Med 1989;8:1339–1350.

44. Temkin NR, Wilensky AJ. Cross-over studies: do the assumptions hold? Controlled Clin Trials 1980;1:167.

45. Pledger GW, Sahlroot JT. (1993) Ch. 15, Alternative analyses for antiepileptic drug trials. In: French JA, Dichter MA, Leppik IE, editors. New antiepileptic drug development: preclinical and clinical aspects. New York: Elsevier, 1980: chapter 15.

46. Conover WJ, Iman RI. Rank transformations as a bridge between parametric and nonparametric statistics. Am Stat 1981;35:124–133.

47. Pledger GW. Design issues in controlled clinical trials of investigational antiepileptic drugs: summary of an NINDS workshop. Unpublished manuscript, 1990.

48. Van Belle G, Temkin NR. Design strategies in the clinical evaluation of new anti-epileptic drugs. In: Pedley TA, Meldium B, editors. Recent advances in epilepsy, vol 1. Edinburgh: Churchill Livingstone, 1983: chapter 8.

49. Pledger GW, Kramer LD. Clinical trials of investigational antiepileptic drugs: monotherapy designs. Epilepsia 1991;32: 716–721.

50. Leber P. Hazards of inference: the active control investigation. Epilepsia 1989;30(Suppl 1):S57–S63.

51. Bourgeois BFD, Leppik IE, Sackellares JC, et al. Felbamate: a double-blind controlled trial in patients undergoing presurgical evaluation of partial seizures. Neurology 1993;43:693–696.

52. Sachdeo R, Kramer LD, Rosenberg A. Felbamate monotherapy: controlled trial in patients with partial onset seizures. Ann Neurol 1992;32:386–392.

11. Survival Analysis

R. Newson

Introduction

Survival analysis is defined as the analysis of survival time data. These data are time intervals, during which a patient is under observation. These time intervals start at a starting time (or starting point), and end at an end time (or end point). In a clinical trial, the starting time is usually the date on which a patient joined the trial. The end time is typically the death date of the patient or the end date of the trial, whichever is sooner. The intervening interval is usually referred to as a lifetime, even though the starting point is not often a birth date, and the end point is not always a death date.

Associated with each lifetime, there is usually also an indicator of the cause of termination. In any one analysis, termination causes are grouped into two classes. These are causes of clinical interest to that particular analysis, on the one hand, and other "uninteresting" causes, on the other. In a clinical trial setting, the cause of interest may be the death of a patient, and uninteresting causes include the end of the trial, and sometimes loss of the patient to follow-up because of emigration. Sometimes, however, the termination of interest may be a non-death event, such as attainment of a CD4 count below a certain level by an HIV-positive patient whose CD4 count is measured regularly. Alternatively, the cause of interest may be death by a certain cause, as specified on the death certificate, and deaths from other causes are considered uninteresting, as are non-death terminations. Lifetimes terminating from the cause of interest are often referred to, in shorthand, as deaths. If a lifetime terminates from an "uninteresting" cause, then it is said to be censored. During the lifetime, the patient is said to be at risk of dying (or, more accurately, of being observed to die).

The reason for referring to "uninteresting" end points as censorships arises from the conjecture that, had the censorship not taken place, then the lifetime might have been observed to end, at some later time, from the cause of interest. If the termination cause of interest is any death, and censoring arises from the end of the trial, then it can be assumed that all the patients will die eventually, and that each one has a "time due to die", which would be observed if only the trial could be funded for a long enough time. If the termination cause of interest is restricted to death by a particular cause, then that assumption is questionable, and the "time due to die from the cause of interest" may be assumed possibly to be infinitely far in the future. Similarly, it may be assumed that patients who died have a "time due to be censored", which, in a clinical trial setting, is the end date of the trial, if not sooner. However, the "time due to die" is not observed for censored lifetimes, and the "time due to be censored" is not observed for lifetimes ending from the cause of interest. Statisticians therefore often discuss survival methods without referring to either of these hypothetical quantities, and prefer to discuss only the lifetimes and terminations, which actually are observed. Each lifetime is a series of patient-days, each of which is viewed by statisticians as a "trial", in which the patient is said to be "at risk" of terminating from the cause of interest.

A set of survival data, therefore, is typically a table of data whose rows (or data points) correspond to lifetimes, and whose columns (or data variables) include a start time, an end time, and a discrete-valued variable denoting the cause of termination. The principal outcome variables are the termination date and the termination cause. Usually, the start date is subtracted from the end date to express the end date in days from randomisation. Other variables usually include a patient identification number. Typically, each lifetime belongs to a patient, and there is only one lifetime per patient. However, it is possible to carry out survival analysis where each patient may have several "lifetimes", as when the patients are epileptics and the "lifetimes" are intervals between successive epileptic attacks. Usually, there are other variables in the data set. Some of them are included in the analysis as predictor variables (also known as risk indicators), predicting the outcome. In a clinical trial, there are variables denoting which treatment is associated with each lifetime. However, there may be other predictors, even in a randomised clinical trial. For instance, it may be feared, especially in a small trial, that the organisers have been unlucky in their randomisation and allocated a disproportionate share of older people, or men, to treatment A and a disproportionate share of younger people, or women, to treatment B. Of course, it is best, if possible, to guard against this eventuality by grouping patients into strata such as age or sex groups, and randomising within each stratum. However, if this is not easy, or if the trial organisers are worried about a new candidate risk indicator that they did not think about at the design stage, then the trial may be "salvaged" at the analysis stage by including age, sex or other risk indicators in the analysis.

The remainder of this chapter is grouped under four main topics, as follows:

- An example data set, from a clinical trial of neurological treatments. This will be used to illustrate general points about survival methods.
- Methods for estimating the probability of survival to given times after the start point. These are based on the Kaplan–Meier curve.
- Methods for comparing death rates in different treatment groups. These include the logrank test, the Gehan test and the more informative Cox proportional hazards regression.
- Methods for comparing death rates in different treatment groups while adjusting for confounding variables. This is done using Cox proportional hazards regression with covariates.

Statistical analyses and production of graphics were all carried out using the Stata statistical package [1]. This contains probably the most comprehensive collection of survival analysis routines on the market, and is to be recommended.

An Example Data Set

Survival methods will be illustrated here by reference to data from a particular randomised controlled multi-centre clinical trial: the Scientific Pan-European Collaboration in ALS. It was carried out on 423 patients with amyotrophic lateral sclerosis (ALS), otherwise known as motor neuron disease. Two types of ALS were represented in these patients: bulbar ALS (220 patients) and non-bulbar ALS (203 patients). These two categories were used as strata. Within each stratum, patients were randomised

Table 11.1.   Patients in the Scientific Pan-European Collaboration in ALS

ALS type	Treatment	Patients	Deaths
Bulbar	A	106	34
	B	114	41
	Total	220	75
Non-bulbar	A	103	20
	B	100	17
	Total	203	37
Total	A	209	54
	B	214	58
	Total	423	112

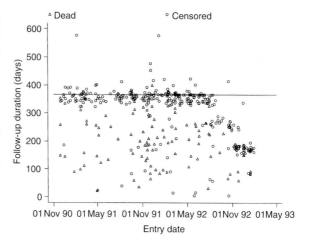

Fig. 11.1.   *Ordinate*: Follow-up time (days). *Abscissa*: Date of entry to the trial. Data points are patients (*triangles* for deaths, *circles* for censored lifetimes). *Reference line* represents a follow-up time of 1 year after entry.

to two possible treatments. These were treatment A (branched-chain amino acids) and treatment B (placebo). The distribution of patients between strata and treatments, and numbers of deaths in each category, are summarised in Table 11.1.

Figure 11.1 shows follow-up duration plotted against entry date for all the patients, with deaths distinguished from censored lifetimes. Note that most censored lifetimes are censored about a year after entry into the trial, but that those entering after the spring of 1992 seem to be censored prematurely by the fact that follow-up ceased in the spring of 1993, when not all of them had had a year of follow-up. Late entrants therefore spend fewer days being observed in the study, and at risk of being observed to die, than do early entrants. There are also a few patients, in all phases of the study, who are censored before their "allotted time" has expired, presumably due to dropout or emigration. In addition, a few patients, entering in the early phase of the study, are followed up for appreciably more than a year. Different patients may therefore have unequal opportunities of being observed to die, even if they are equally likely actually to die at a given number of days after entry. The methods of survival analysis are designed to correct for bias caused by this "inequality of opportunity" to die.

Estimating Survival Probabilities

Survival analysis methods are used for two main purposes. On the one hand, they are used to estimate the proportion of patients in a group who survive to a given time, assuming that none of them has been censored before that time. On the other hand, they are used to measure differences in death rate (and therefore survival probability) between groups, for instance between patients on different treatments. The first of these uses will be examined in this section.

Survival analysis is based on the assumption that each day spent in the study by a patient is a "trial", similar to a throw of a dice, in which the patient is at risk of terminating from the cause of interest. However, when estimating survival curves, we allow for the possibility that the risk might be different on different days after entry to the study. If the study has a very long follow-up, then the fact that the patients are getting older may make them more likely to die on the thousand-and-first day (given that they have survived for the first thousand days) than to die on the first day (given that they enter the study on day 0 and survive to the end of the day). On the other hand, for a shorter-term study on stroke recurrence in patients who are entered into the study because they have recently had a stroke, patients might be less likely to have a second stroke on the hundred and first day of observation (given that they have survived the previous hundred days without having one) than on the first day of observation (given that they survived to the end of day 0). Therefore, rather than comparing the termination rates per thousand person-days at risk between different treatment groups, we might find it more informative to compare probabilities of surviving for a certain amount of time (say 1 year in the ALS study, or 5 years in a long-term study on cancer therapies).

However, looking at Fig. 11.1, we can foresee problems calculating a 1-year survival probability, because so many patients are censored before a year of follow-up. We do not know which of these would have been observed to survive for a year of follow-up, given the chance, and which would have died. However, some late entrants died before the end of the study, and others survived, and the study organisers presumably did not go to the expense of collecting this information simply to waste it.

When estimating a survival probability, we define this probability as the proportion of patients that would have survived to a given time (say 1 year), assuming that there had been no censorship. To be able to do this, we must make assumptions about the times that the censored patients would have been observed to die, had they only been followed up for long enough. Normally, we assume that the "time due to die" is independent of the "time due to be censored", or at least conditionally independent within each treatment group and disease stratum. That is to say, it is assumed that, for each combination of treatment and disease (such as amino-acid-treated patients with bulbar ALS), the early-censored ones would have had the same lifetime distribution as the late-censored ones, had they not been censored so early. (The methods allow the possibility that some treatment groups tend to be censored earlier and die earlier than other treatment groups.)

If this assumption is reasonable, then we estimate survival probabilities using the Kaplan–Meier estimate [2]. This is described briefly in the Appendix, and in greater depth in [3], [1] and references from these sources.

For the example of the ALS trial, we refer to Table 11.2. For each treatment group, this gives the numbers of patients, the number observed to die before 366 days, the proportion *not* observed to die before 366 days (with 95% confidence limits), and the 366-day survival estimate (also with 95% confidence limits). Note that the 366-day survival estimates are

Table 11.2. Survival estimates (with 95% confidence limits) for the two treatment groups in the ALS trial

Treatment group	Patients	Deaths before 366 days	Proportion not dying after 366 days	366-day survival
A	209	53	0.75 (0.69, 0.81)	0.69 (0.61, 0.75)
B	214	58	0.73 (0.67, 0.79)	0.66 (0.58, 0.73)

a

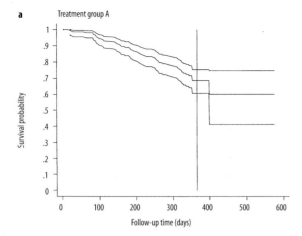

b

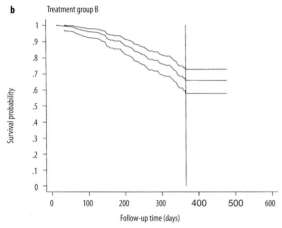

Fig. 11.2. a Survival function for patients on treatment *A*. *Ordinate*: Survival probability. *Abscissa*: Follow-up time (days). *Lines* are the Kaplan–Meier survival probability estimate and its upper and lower 95% confidence limits. *Reference line* represents 366 days after randomization. b Survival probability for patients on treatment *B*. Legend as for **a**.

lower than the corresponding proportions not observed to die after 366 days. This is because the survival estimates are corrected by estimating how many of the patients censored before 366 days would have been observed to die, had they been followed up for longer. This correction is carried out by assuming that, had the censored patients been followed up for longer, then they would have died at similar rates to patients in the same group who actually were followed up for longer.

The survival function estimates for the two treatment groups, over a fuller range of times after randomisation, are plotted against time (with 95% confidence limits) as Fig. 11.2. Note that the survival function descends in steps, each step corresponding to a death. The steps become larger at later times, because later deaths represent a loss of a greater pro-

portion of patients still alive than do earlier deaths. The fact that there are large steps in the survival function at later times therefore does not signify any tendency for the later deaths to occur in clusters, or epidemics. Similarly, the fact that the survival function at later times shows long periods of constancy does not imply that it is "bottoming out", or that no further deaths can be expected. These points are illustrated graphically by the inclusion of 95% confidence limits to the survival curve. Theses become wider at later times, implying greater uncertainty caused by the presence of fewer patients still alive and still under observation.

The questions remain as to whether we are justified in assuming independence of death and censorship within each group, and what (if anything) we can do about it if the assumption does not hold. The first question, in general, cannot be answered by data analysis, and this has been proven mathematically [4]. This is essentially because we do not observe any such quantity as "the time at which a patient would have died, had s/he not been censored", or "the time at which the patient would have been censored, had s/he not died". This problem is part of the general problem with missing data values, namely that the event of a data value being missing is not necessarily independent of the value that would have been observed had it not been missing.

The best we can do, therefore, is to design the trial so that we have good grounds for expecting censorship to be independent of death. If the main cause of censorship is the end of the trial, as seems to be the case with the ALS data, then there are good grounds for expecting "time due to die" to be (almost) independent of "time due to be censored", as long as there is (almost) no tendency for death rates to be different for patients recruited later in the duration of the trial, when the "time due to be censored" is sooner after recruitment (Fig. 11.1). There are greater problems with other causes of censorship, such as a patient breaking contact with the trial because he or she feels on the point of dying.

It is important to stress that the use of the Kaplan–Meier formula is *no substitute* for analysing the data by intention to treat. That is to say, the two groups being compared should be those randomised to each treatment, rather than those who continued with each treatment to the end of the trial. The two "treatments" being compared are then the *policies* of offering the two treatments, rather than the treatments themselves, with which the patient may or may not comply. (If one treatment is a placebo, then the corresponding policy would arguably be unethical, but we usually still want to know whether a more expensive alternative policy is worth the expense.) To carry out an intention-to-treat analysis, it is therefore necessary to monitor the outcome for all patients allocated to each treatment, and not only for patients who decided to continue with each treatment to the end of the trial. The alternative policy is known as on-treatment analysis, and compares only the two self-selected groups who chose to comply with the treatments to which they were randomised. If the treatments are compared by survival analysis, then an on-treatment comparison involves censoring the lifetimes of patients who dropped out from the trial at the times at which they dropped out, whereas an intention-to-treat comparison involves continuing the follow-up of such patients after they dropped out.

Intention-to-treat comparison is usually preferred for two reasons. Firstly, if a patient withdraws from a treatment because he or she cannot endure it any more, and then dies, then, for practical purposes, the treatment has failed, even if the patient might have survived had he or she been willing and able to endure it for longer. Secondly, patients who selectively refuse treatment A, after having been randomised to it, are likely to be different from patients randomised to treatment B, who would have taken treatment A had it been offered to them. For instance, in the case of the BCG vaccine against tuberculosis, there was reason to believe that people who did not co-operate with treatment were more at risk of tuberculosis than people who were more co-operative [5], whereas, in the case of Salk vaccine against polio, there was reason to believe that people who refused the vaccine were less at risk of paralytic polio than people not offered the vaccine [6]. (This is generally rationalised by assuming that refusers are less hygienic people than acceptors, and that being hygienic decreases the risk of tuberculosis but actually increases the risk of paralytic polio, because less hygienic people meet the virus for the first time at an earlier age, at which time it is more likely to cause lasting immunity without first causing paralytic polio.) Biases such as these will not always be removed by the routine practice of blinding, because patients may selectively refuse Treatment A because of side effects that cannot be hidden by blinding. Patients who do this may tend to be either more or less at risk than patients who persevere with Treatment A regardless of side effects, and this difference in risk may be unconnected with the effects of the treatment itself.

If the intention-to-treat principle is applied to survival analysis, then the outcome measure is survival (or otherwise) to a certain time after randomisation, and it is measured by monitoring all patients to the end of their allotted time with the trial, so the deaths will be recorded, whether or not each patient complied with the treatment to which he or she was randomized. If this is done, then refusal to comply with the treatment is eliminated from the list of causes of censorship. If the clinical trial takes place in Britain, and the clinically interesting end point is death, then this monitoring can sometimes be done by using the services of the National Health Service Central Registry (NHSCR). These are described in Peto et al. [3], and have been improved since then by computerisation.

Follow-up to the end of a patient's allotted duration may not be an option if a patient becomes censored by leaving the neighbourhood (or the country) altogether during the course of the trial. The cause of censorship may, of course, be correlated with subsequent mortality, either because it is mainly the healthier people who "get up and go", or (on the other hand) because people may return to the land of their birth specifically to die. This kind of censorship will almost inevitably lead to bias, and the best that can be done is usually to minimise it by choosing a study population that tends to stay in place. From Fig. 11.1, it appears (not surprisingly) that this is the case with the ALS patients studied here.

Comparison of Treatment Groups

The survival curves of Fig. 11.2 give a visual impression of the survival curves for each of the two treatment groups, but do not measure the difference between them. There are several ways of doing this. In general, however, the comparison to be used should be decided at the design phase and specified in the trial protocol, rather than decided at the analysis stage. This is because, if the comparison is chosen at the analysis stage, then members of the diverse skeptical public who read the trial report might conclude that the trial organisers have tried a number of comparison methods and chosen the one that gives them the answer that they most like to hear, or the one that gives the minimum p value. It is preferable that the public do not suspect this, especially if it is not true. (And, if it is true, then the p values and confidence limits quoted in the report will be lies.)

Ideally, a comparison between treatments should take the form of a confidence interval for a difference, or ratio, between two treatment-specific performance measures, which can be explained to a medical audience in words rather than equations. Confidence intervals are more informative than p values, as a p value measures how compatible the data are with the "null hypothesis" of no difference between treatments, whereas a confidence interval gives a range of hypotheses with which the data *are* compatible (see [7]).

One possibility is to compare the Kaplan–Meier survival probabilities for two groups at a standard

Table 11.3. Hazard ratios (treatment *A* versus treatment *B*) for the ALS trial, with 95% confidence limits

ALS type	Hazard ratio	Logrank *p* value	Gehan *p* value
All ALS	0.97 (0.67, 1.41)	0.8853	0.9871
Bulbar ALS	0.89 (0.57, 1.41)	0.6267	0.8232
Non-bulbar ALS	1.19 (0.62, 2.26)	0.6038	0.6087

reference time, say 366 days. The difference between the two survival probabilities can be estimated, and assigned confidence limits. The main objection to doing this is that any choice of a follow-up time at which to compare survival probabilities must be somewhat arbitrary, even if it is specified in the design protocol. (And, if it is not, then it will be very difficult indeed to convince the public that the trial organisers have analysed the data honestly.)

In the past, attempts have been made to compare mean or median lifetimes between groups. However, comparing means is not strictly possible in the presence of any appreciable amount of censorship, as information about the upper tails of the lifetime distribution does not exist. In a trial such as the ALS trial, where most patients do not die, there is not much information about the median lifetime either.

A standard solution is to compare death rates under the two treatments over the entire duration of the trial. This is the principle behind the logrank test [3] and the Cox proportional hazards model [1,8,9]. Theses are based on the concept of hazard rate. This is defined as the probability, per unit time, that a patient will terminate from the cause of interest, and is measured in units of "per cent per person-day" or something similar. The hazard rate itself will typically be a small fraction of a per cent per day, even for ALS patients, and is likely to vary with follow-up time in any case, because of patients ageing or recovering. However, the ratio of hazard rates in two treatment groups is easier to understand. It can be hypothesised that the hazard ratio between two treatment groups is constant over time, so that (for instance) the hazard rate under Treatment *A* may always be twice the hazard rate under Treatment *B*, although the two hazard rates themselves may both increase in parallel as the disease progresses to more advanced stages. The Cox proportional hazards model is used to estimate the hazard ratio between two treatment groups, assuming that the ratio is indeed constant over time, and to calculate confidence limits for that ratio.

In practice, there is no reason to believe that the hazard rate ratio between two treatment groups is exactly constant over time, although it simplifies life if group *A* has a consistently greater hazard rate than group *B* (or vice versa) throughout the follow-up. However, if the hazard rate ratio varies slightly, then it may still make sense to use the hazard rate ratio estimated by the Cox model formula, and to interpret it as a ratio between "appropriately weighted average" hazard rates over the follow-up time. If the treatment *A*/treatment *B* hazard ratio is greater than one, then we can say (informally) that, *on average*, treatment *A* is more hazardous. Simulation studies have shown that the Cox regression estimate of the hazard ratio is affected more by sampling error if the hazard rate ratio is not exactly constant [9]. These authors accordingly derived a corrected formula for calculating the confidence limits, taking this inconstancy into account. These corrected confidence limits are known as robust confidence limits, and can be calculated if the data are analysed using the Stata statistical package [1].

In the case of the ALS trial, the hazard ratios are presented in Table 11.3, with 95% confidence intervals. If both types of ALS (bulbar and non-bulbar) are taken together, then patients on treatment *A* die at 67%–141% of the rate observed in patients on treatment *B*. Therefore, the data are compatible with the null hypothesis that patients on the two treatments die at the same rate, but also with other possibilities, in which the death rate on treatment *A* is 2/3 to almost 3/2 of that on treatment *B*. Therefore, spectacular differences in death rate (such as a doubling or a halving) can be ruled out, but we have not "proved the null hypothesis". If we do the analysis separately on the bulbar and non-bulbar patients, then the conclusions are similar, but associated with wider confidence limits, because of smaller numbers of patients.

Table 11.3 also includes the results of two commonly used significance tests. The first, the logrank test, is the significance test corresponding to the Cox proportional hazards model, and tests the null hypothesis that the hazard rate ratio is constantly one. Its main advantage is that it is easy for non-statisticians to do without a computer [3]. The second is the Gehan test, which tests the hypothesis that, given a randomly chosen patients from each treatment group, the probability that the treatment *A* patient will be observed to survive the treatment *B* patient is equal to the probability that the treatment *B* patient will be observed to survive the treatment *A* patient. They are included partly for completeness, but mainly to demonstrate that *p* values are a lot less informative than confidence intervals. The *p* value for the logrank test is calculated assuming that the inter-treatment hazard rate ratio is constant, whereas the *p* value for the Gehan test is calculated without that assumption. For further details on these tests, see [3] and [1].

The above methods are used for comparing two treatments for which there is good reason to expect that, if one is less hazardous than the other "on average", then it will be less hazardous than the other (to a greater or lesser degree) for the duration of the trial. Sometimes, however, there is reason to expect that treatment A will be more hazardous than treatment B in the early phase of the trial but less hazardous than treatment B in the later phase of the trial. For instance, treatment A may be a bone marrow transplant for cancer, whereas treatment B may be the more orthodox chemotherapy. If this is the case, then there is an argument for using slightly more complicated statistics. For instance, we may decide to estimate an "early-phase hazard rate ratio" for the earlier part of the trial, and a "later-phase hazard rate ratio" for the later part of the trial. The Cox proportional hazards model allows us to do this. However, if, at the design phase of the trial, we suspect that there is such a trade-off between long-term benefits and short-term benefits, then we should make these concerns public when preparing the design protocol, and propose the more complicated analysis at that point. If, on the other hand, we design the study to discriminate between a uniform advantage for one treatment or the other, and then we analyse the study allowing for the possibility that one treatment is better in the short term and the other is better in the long term, then (human nature being what it is) the public will have good reason to suspect that we are "torturing the data" with a view to detecting a difference when none exists.

Adjusting for Confounding Factors

One patient, of course, may survive another for reasons other than a difference in treatment. Adjusting for confounding factors may improve our estimate of the inter-treatment hazard ratio for two reasons. The first is elimination of bias (affecting the position of the estimate), and the second is elimination of sampling error (affecting the width of the confidence limits). Bias is a danger mainly in small trials, where there is a high probability of being unlucky in randomisation, so that one treatment has been allocated the healthier patients. If we can identify risk indicators expected to predict which patients are more healthy (such as being young and female instead of old and male), then we can adjust for the effects of those risk indicators and correct for the bias. Sampling error is a problem for similar reasons, because sampling error in the distribution of confounding factors (such as age and sex) between

treatment groups may contribute to sampling error affecting the estimated between-treatment hazard ratio. If we measure the confounding factors for each group, then we can eliminate this contribution to the sampling variability, and thereby produce narrower confidence limits for the estimated inter-treatment hazard ratio.

The usual method for doing this involves Cox proportional hazards models. In this case, we use a more complicated version, estimating multiple hazard ratios corresponding to multiple risk factors. Different hazard ratios are assumed to combine multiplicatively. For instance, the hazard ratio of male smokers to female non-smokers in the same treatment group is typically expected to be equal to the male/female hazard ratio multiplied by the smoking/non-smoking hazard ratio. If we do not expect this multiplicative relationship to hold, then we must estimate additional parameters to describe this non-multiplicativeness (which statisticians refer to as "interaction"). For instance, we might estimate a baseline male/female hazard ratio for nonsmokers, a male-specific smoking/non-smoking hazard ratio and a female-specific smoking/non-smoking hazard ratio. The parameter of interest is still the (adjusted) inter-treatment hazard ratio (or even multiple inter-treatment hazard ratios for different groups such as men and women, if we think that inter-treatment hazard ratios may vary between groups). In general, the more patients and deaths there are, the more distinct hazard ratios can be estimated, and the narrower we can expect their confidence limits to be.

It should be stressed that, although adding a strong confounding factor to the regression model may narrow the confidence limits for the inter-treatment risk ratio, there is a countervailing tendency for confidence limits to be widened by the addition of extra parameters. Therefore, if a confounding factor is likely to have a hazard ratio close to one (corresponding to no effect at all), then including it in the model will widen confidence limits for the other hazard ratios, rather than narrow them. It follows that, if we think that treatment effect may not be exactly the same between subgroups, but that the treatment effects in different subgroups are probably of similar magnitude and direction, then it may make sense to estimate one inter-treatment hazard ratio for all subgroups, interpreted as an "appropriately weighted average treatment effect". It should also be stressed that the number of distinct treatment effects to measure, and the choice of confounders, should be decided before the data are analysed, and preferably documented in the trial protocol. This is because statistical methods are defined assuming that scientists first decide what effects they want to measure, and

Table 11.4. Cox regressions measuring inter-treatment hazard ratio adjusting for confounders

Group	Hazard ratio	Estimate (95% CI)
All ALS		
	Treatment (*A/B*)	1.10 (0.75, 1.61)
	Age (per year)	1.07 (1.05, 1.10)
	Sex (male/female)	1.58 (1.05, 2.37)
	Bulbar/non-bulbar	1.82 (1.21, 2.74)
Bulbar ALS		
	Treatment (*A/B*)	1.03 (0.64, 1.65)
	Age (per year)	1.06 (1.03, 1.10)
	Sex (male/female)	1.45 (0.90, 2.36)
Non-bulbar ALS		
	Treatment (*A/B*)	1.15 (0.59, 2.22)
	Age (per year)	1.10 (1.05, 1.14)
	Sex (male/female)	1.95 (0.89, 4.27)

then measure them. Researchers should *not* first measure a large number of candidate confounders and then attempt to find, by trial and error, a combination of these confounders which appears to explain the treatment effect after the fact.

In the case of the ALS trial, we might expect survival to be affected by age, sex and whether the patient has bulbar or non-bulbar ALS. (Baseline vital capacity might be an even better predictor, but I have no data on this.) Sex and ALS type are discrete binary variables, so including them in the model is straightforward. Age, however, is a continuous variable. If a continuous variable is included in a Cox regression without grouping, then the model assumes an exponential effect on the hazard rate, so that (for instance) each additional year of age multiplies the hazard rate by a constant amount. Including continuous variables in a Cox regression may therefore be a dangerous practice, as outlying values of the continuous variable will have disproportionate influence on the estimated hazard ratios, essentially because patients with very extreme values are assumed to have extremely high hazard rates, and, if they remain alive regardless, then the computer will adjust the values of the model parameters in unpredictable ways to account for this. However, in the special case of age, the assumption that death rates increase exponentially turns out to fit the data fairly well (at least as a first approximation), and spectacular outlying ages are rare (because very old people are eliminated by the exponentially increasing death rate) [10]. The exponential relationship between age and death rate is known as Gompertz's Law, and such deviations as are observed from it in real-life human populations appear consistent with the view that humans are a mixture of Gompertz subpopulations, differing from

each other because of variation in risk factors other than age. Including age at entry as a continuous variable in a Cox model is therefore a standard procedure, seldom queried by statisticians, and we will follow it here. Note that, although patients become older during the trial, they all become older at the same rate, so, if hazard rate increases by the same "per cent per year" for all patients, then hazard ratios between patients entering at different ages will stay constant over the trial. The patients in this trial are aged from 25 to 78 years at entry, with a mean age of 58.04.

Table 11.4 shows a simple Cox regression analysis, first on all patients, then separately on the bulbar and non-bulbar ALS groups. All analyses measure the hazard ratio of treatment *A* to treatment *B*, adjusting for age, sex and (in the pooled analysis) the bulbar/non-bulbar distinction. The pooled analysis has the narrowest confidence intervals, being based on the greatest number of patients. The hazard ratio for age is a multiplicative factor per year of age, and we see that death rates in these patients increase with age by 7% per year (with confidence limits from 5% to 10% per year). Men over 35 years old typically suffer death rates increasing by no more than 4% per year [10], so these patients seem to age faster than the general population. Men die at a rate 58% greater than women of the same age and with the same variant of ALS on the same treatment, and the confidence interval allows a relative excess of 5% to 137%. Bulbar ALS patients die 21% to 174% faster than comparable non-bulbar ALS patients. However, although all these confounders are statistically and clinically significant, adjusting for them does not greatly change the conclusion regarding the hazard ratio between treatments *A* and *B*. The data still rule out a spectacular difference (doubling, halving or more) in either direction, but allow treatment *A* to be associated with death rates 25% less to 61% greater than those under treatment *B*.

Analyses for the bulbar and non-bulbar groups are also included, in case bulbar and non-bulbar ALS are different diseases with different responses to treatment. However, the results are similar to those of the combined analysis, except that the confidence limits are slightly wider, so gender differences are not statistically significant in each group taken alone.

Many variations are possible on the theme of Cox proportional hazards regression. For instance, is possible to divide the patients into strata for the purpose of the analysis. If this is done, the assumption that hazard rate ratios stay constant over the follow-up time is relaxed for pairs of patients in different strata, and a constant hazard ratio between treatments is estimated for all pairs of patients on different treatments in the same stratum. Also, it is possible for some of the effects of predictors (treatments or confounders) to be time-dependent, so that (for instance) the hazard ratio between two treatments in the first month of the trial is allowed to be different from the hazard ratio between the same treatments later in the trial.

Appendix. The Kaplan–Meier Survival Estimate

We note that, to survive for a given amount of time (say a year), a patient must survive through all the 365 (or 366) days comprising that year. It follows that the probability that a patient is still alive at some time in day 366 of his or her follow-up is equal to

$$S_{366} = C_1 \times C_2 \times \ldots \times C_{365}$$

where each C_j, for values of j from 1 to 365, is the *conditional* probability that the patient survives through day j, *given that* he or she has entered day j after having survived through days 1 to $j-1$. (We assume that the day on which the patient entered the trial is day 0 for that particular patient.) The key to estimating the survivor probability S_{366} is therefore to estimate the component conditional probabilities C_1 to C_{365}, and to multiply them together. For the jth day, we estimate C_j as

$$\hat{C}_j = \frac{(n_j - d_j)}{n_j}$$

where n_j is the number of patients who enter the jth days of their respective follow-up periods (having survived through days 1 to $j-1$ without having either died or been censored), and d_j is the number of patients observed to die on the jth day of follow-up. (That is to say, n_{100} does not include patients who are censored on days 1 to 99.)

The estimated probability of entering day 366 of follow-up is therefore expressed as

$$\hat{S}_{366} = \hat{C}_1 \times \hat{C}_2 \times \ldots \times \hat{C}_{365}$$

Even more complicated formulae are used to calculate confidence limits around the survival estimates for each group. Readers who want to go into the mathematics more deeply can refer to references [1], [3] or even [2].

Acknowledgement. The author gratefully thanks Dr. A. Goonetilleke of Newcastle Royal Infirmary and Dr. Tim Steiner of Imperial College Medical School for allowing him access to data from the Scientific Pan-European Collaboration on ALS.

References

1. Stata Corp. Stata statistical software release 6.0. College Station, TX: Stata Corporation, 1999.
2. Kaplan EL, Meier P. Nonparametric estimation from incomplete observations. J Am Stat Assoc 1958;53:457–481.
3. Peto R, Pike C, Armitage P, Breslow NE, Cox DR, Howard SV, et al. Design and analysis of clinical trials requiring prolonged observation of each patient. II. Analysis and examples. Br J Cancer 1977;35:1–39.
4. Tsiatis A. A nonidentifiability aspect of the problem of competing risks. Proc Nat Acad Sci USA 1975;72:20–22.
5. Hill AB. Statistical methods in clinical and preventive medicine. Edinburgh: Churchill-Livingstone, 1962.
6. Meier P. The biggest health experiment ever: the 1954 field trial of the Salk poliomyelitis vaccine. In: Tanur JM, et al., editors. Statistics: a guide to the biological and health sciences. San Francisco: Holden-Day, 1977.
7. Gardner MJ, Altman DG. Statistics with confidence. London: British Medical Association, 1989.
8. Cox DR. Regression models and life tables (with discussion). J R Stat Soc Ser B 1972;34:187–220.
9. Lin DY, Wei LJ. The robust inference for the Cox proportional hazards model. J Am Stat Assoc 1989;84:1074–1078.
10. Kalbfleisch JD, Prentice RL. The statistical analysis of failure time data. New York: Wiley, 1980.

12. The Intention-to-Treat Principle for Clinical Trials

M.J. Schell, M.A. McBride, C. Gennings and G.G. Koch

The Randomized Clinical Trial and Randomization

The major objective of the randomized clinical trial is to obtain information about the relative efficacy of the treatments involved [1]. It is randomization that distinguishes the controlled clinical trial from other forms of medical research. During the 1920s, R. A. Fisher developed the concept of randomization as a method of assigning "treatments" to blocks or plots of land in agricultural experiments [2]. Sir Austin Bradford Hill, considered by many to be the father of the randomized clinical trial [3], later applied the concepts of randomization to the field of medicine during the 1940s. Hill's viewpoint, which now has wide acceptance, was that randomized clinical trials are necessary for the valid assessment of therapeutic efficacy [4].

The use of the randomized clinical trial is advocated by many authors, for example, Byar [5]; Green [6]; Spodick [7] and Koch and Paquette [8]. These authors point out the benefits of randomized trials compared with retrospective studies or studies that use historical controls. One of these benefits is that time trends are much less problematic in randomized clinical trials, since changes which take place over time apply to both treatment groups equally. Examples of time trend changes include changes in the nature of the patient pool admitted to the study, diagnostic procedures and the nature of patient management. In addition, missing data and data errors are often less likely to occur in a randomized clinical trial. This can be due to the fact that the trial requires that a detailed protocol be written which specifies exactly what data are to be recorded. In a clinical trial, data forms are used to ensure that data are collected uniformly for each patient, and data monitoring can often correct problems shortly after they occur, rather than after the study has been completed, when it may be impossible to obtain needed information.

Randomization can usually be defined as a "procedure for assigning treatments to patients in such a way that all possible assignments of treatments to patients are equally likely within the constraints of the experimental design" [9], although more general forms with unequal probabilities are possible. The major advantages of using randomization in clinical trials are discussed by many authors [6,9–13] and are presented below.

Selection bias occurs whenever patients with differing prognoses have differing probabilities for receiving the treatments [14]. Randomization eliminates bias from the assignment of treatments since the patients will not be selected (consciously or not) to receive a particular form of therapy in the trial. In addition, in a randomized trial, the physician, patient or both can be blinded from knowing the true identity of any assigned treatment so as to avoid further bias throughout the course of the study.

Randomization can underlie the validity of statistical tests of significance used to compare treatments. The randomization process makes it possible to ascribe a probability distribution to the difference in response between treatment groups receiving equally effective treatments. Thus, we may assign significance levels and confidence limits to observed differences because randomization ensures that the unknown and uncontrollable sources of variability have comparable distributions between the groups. A significant difference between treatment groups implies that a more favorable outcome occurred in some treatment group(s) than would have been expected by random allocation of equally effective treatments to patients [9]. Without randomization we can obtain confidence limits and significance levels only by *assuming* a random distribution for the uncontrollable sources of variability [15], with this random mechanism being independent of how patients are assigned to treatment groups.

Randomization assures that the groups are balanced, on average, with regard to baseline covariates (or prognostic factors), whether these factors are known or unknown. This balance between treatment groups can also increase the efficiency of the analysis since the groups tend to be more internally similar and random variability between the treatment groups tends to be reduced [5]. Although this similarity does not imply that the groups will be identical, any comparison of the groups will be valid. This is because the p value obtained by performing a test of significance takes into account that such imbalances may occur. The p value is a measure of how likely it is a given difference in outcome would occur in the absence of any real treatment differences [5]. As Fisher [16] points out, randomization properly carried out "relieves the experimenter from the anxiety of considering and estimating the magnitude of the innumerable causes by which his data may be disturbed." This does not mean that important prognostic factors must be ignored; stratification and covariance adjustments are useful adjuncts to randomization but do not replace it [9].

Non-compliance and Intention-to-Treat Analysis

Randomized clinical trials generally involve intricate protocols and are usually large in scale. As a result, some patients inevitably fail to comply fully with the therapy regimen to which they were assigned. For example, some patients may simply feel that the therapy is not working and decide to discontinue its use, other patients may experience side effects and withdraw from the study, and still others may be unable to comply with an intense treatment schedule. Whenever patient non-compliance occurs, difficulties arise in trying to determine the effects of the treatments and the question of which patients to include in the analysis emerges. Although several methods of analysis have been proposed, the intention-to-treat (ITT) analysis, which analyzes *all* patients in the groups to which they were randomized regardless of compliance, has been suggested as the preferred method because it remains an unbiased approach to data analysis [11,17–19].

The ITT analysis involves including all patients in the analysis; no patients are excluded from the analysis based on compliance measures. The ITT procedure "actually compares the policy of using treatment A where possible with the policy of using treatment B where possible" [20]. If all patients are compliant, then comparing the two policies is equivalent to comparing the two treatments. If many patients deviate from the protocol, however, the analysis may carry little information about the true treatment differences, but much information about the practice of using the two treatments. The approach of comparing policies of intentions is appealing to many investigators since they may feel it to be a more realistic statement of the purpose of the investigation [20].

The Intention-to-Treat Principle

The randomized clinical trial has a well-deserved reputation for being at the pinnacle of medical science. Were patients or their physicians to select which of several treatment arms to enroll on, it would remain unclear whether treatment differences seen should be attributed to the treatments themselves or to differences between patients. Proper statistical inference on the relative merits of the treatments depends critically on randomization. Deliberate selection to a particular treatment arm by or for patients violates the randomization, thereby compromising the inference.

How does deliberate selection compromise statistical inference? Suppose physicians were to place patients on the treatment arm that they think would best benefit them. From a medical standpoint, this should be done. Randomized clinical trials are only appropriate when physicians are in "equipoise" [21], meaning that they truly do not have a strong belief about which treatment is best for the patient. If deliberate selections are made, it would not be clear whether a given treatment is truly better or whether the physician just had some "sixth sense" in choosing the patients who would uniquely benefit from the treatment.

Similarly patient selection bias can occur. In some unblind trials (for example, surgery vs drug treatment), patients may not like the treatment arm that they were assigned to. In placebo-controlled trials, side effects or lack of response on a particular arm may lead to a greater withdrawal rate in one arm than another. Suppose that all patients not receiving complete relief from symptoms withdraw from some trial. If only the patients completing the trial are compared, all treatment arms would appear to be completely efficacious. However, if one arm had no withdrawals while half the patients dropped out from another arm, the true efficacy rates could be quite different. Since patients who dropped out are informative for treatment comparisons, some way to include their experiences in the analysis is important. Some procedures for doing this are discussed later.

Randomized trials are designed to avoid the inferential difficulty caused by deliberative treatment selection. However, deliberative selection occurs in almost every randomized clinical trial. The ITT principle is that all randomized patients be analyzed on the treatment arm to which they were assigned. While this principle has proved confusing to many scientists, it is used to avoid the inferential pitfalls caused by deliberative selection.

While the ITT principle is simple, sometimes its application is not. We will describe formal applications of it as well as departures, using examples to illustrate the ideas.

Reasons for Trial Non-completion

Ineligible Subjects

One of the first issues involves subjects found to be ineligible after randomization. While the ITT principle formally states that subjects should be analyzed to the treatment arm assigned to, removing ineligible subjects from the analyzed population does not compromise statistical inference, as long as all subjects are equally scrutinized for eligibility. It appears that most statisticians argue that ineligible subjects can be removed from analysis [13,22–24], perhaps because the treatments being compared were not directly intended for them. However, such a policy should be written into the study protocol [13] and should be applied uniformly and without regard to the study outcome for the patients. This complication can happen when definitive diagnosis cannot be made until a laboratory or pathological investigation is performed, but treatment cannot be delayed. Continued treatment may be inappropriate once the patient is found to be ineligible. Nevertheless, further follow-up of these patients may still be of supportive interest to confirm lack of harm from the originally assigned treatments.

Withdrawals

We will use the term "withdrawal" to refer to patients who discontinue the randomly assigned treatment in the clinical trial due to some reason directly related to the clinical trial. Patients who find the requirements of remaining on treatment too burdensome, who become concerned because of some side effect, or are dissatisfied with the treatment efficacy for them are all examples of withdrawals. These patients have made a deliberative decision not to remain on trial and constitute a direct threat to the inference of the trial if they are not included. They are also patients for whom continued follow-up is often possible for the planned duration of the study. This additional information can be helpful for ITT analysis.

Dropouts

Patients sometimes drop out from treatment due to some life event that is not obviously related to the treatment arm they are on. Patients who move away, become pregnant or who are lost to follow-up are often in this group. If the events are truly unrelated to treatment outcome, a reasonable balance would be expected between study arms. However, researchers can rarely be sure that the reason for dropping out is truly unrelated. Thus, these subjects should be included in the analysis, but how to do so has inherent difficulties due to the unavailability of data after the subject drops out. Consequently, several reasonable approaches for computing values to dropouts often need to be considered and the robustness of the findings to the different choices is crucial to the overall assessment of the trial. Also, their retrieval (on an overall basis or a random subset) at the time of study completion can provide useful information about the extent to which dropping out is unrelated to treatment or ultimate outcome.

Physician Refusal

Sometimes physicians decide that the treatment arm the patient is randomized to is inappropriate for them. In such cases, the patient should not have been randomized in the first place. Some physicians will place patients on clinical trials but do not agree with all the eligibility criteria. When the patients with "questionable" eligibility criteria get placed on the "wrong" arm in an unblind clinical trial, the physician will pull them off protocol. We will call this situation physician refusal. Such a physician is not truly in "equipoise" for that clinical trial as a whole. Physician refusal is another deliberative selection event that compromises a clinical trial if the patient is not included in the analysis.

Patient Accounting

Gillings and Koch [23] stressed the importance of accounting for all patients who are screened for participation in a randomized clinical trial, placing them into defined subgroups. We recommend use of this accounting method when describing the findings of a clinical trial and as an aid to the statistical analysis.

The basic design of the clinical trial is assumed to be as follows: after an initial screening period, patients are randomized in a double-blind manner to two or more parallel treatment groups or crossover sequence groups, with careful follow-up at regular visits, say over a relatively short period of time.

All Patients Screened

Inference from randomized clinical trials depends on the principle of randomization, not random sampling from a population. Indeed, in many acute disease treatment trials, patients are enrolled shortly after diagnosis and not randomly chosen from a population of all such patients. Consequently, researchers may not see a compelling need to obtain background data on patients who are screened for a trial but do not participate.

However, inference from a trial is usually extended to the population of patients eligible for the trial even if a significant subpopulation did not participate in it. One way to have greater assurance that the inferential basis is sound for generalizability is to show that patients who were screened and "eligible" for the trial but not enrolled, often referred to as exclusions, do not differ significantly from those who do enroll. To check for possible differences, background or baseline characteristics are necessary.

All Patients Randomized

In most clinical trials, not all patients screened are actually enrolled in the trial and randomized to a treatment arm. Sometimes these patients fail one or more eligibility criteria. Since ineligible patients are not part of the population of interest, they are properly excluded from a comparison between treatments. However, screened patients who are eligible for a trial but fail to enroll in it can limit the generalizability of the trial, as mentioned earlier. Also, ineligible patients who are randomized can be excluded from primary analyses but merit assessment in supportive analyses.

All Patients Who Took at Least One Dose

One modification of the standard definition of ITT is to include all randomized patients who took at least one dose. In cases where treatment is begun right away, this may be no different from the patients who were randomized to the trial. If the trial is blind and the patient fortuitously never began therapy, no bias is introduced in excluding the patient from the analysis, although generalizability to the eligible population may be weakened. If the trial is unblind, however, bias may be introduced. Gillings and Koch [23] argue that as long as the proportion of randomized patients who do not take a single dose is minimal (<5%), they should be excluded from the ITT analysis. We would further require that the trial be adequately blinded before such exclusions are appropriate.

Gillings and Koch [23] also discuss a further modification of the population to patients who take treatment for a minimum time period. This modification has clinical appeal but can lead to statistical concerns about the comparability of the treatment groups and, consequently, the generalizability of the findings. Gillings and Koch felt that the clinical argument was more compelling as long as the trial is blinded and no more than 10% of the patients fail to reach the minimum time period.

All Patients with Any Follow-up

In most reasonably sized clinical trials, some patients fail to provide any follow-up data. Exclusion of such patients may lead to bias in the analysis as described earlier. Justification of the exclusion of patients with no follow-up data rests on the assumption that the excluded patients are dropouts, not withdrawals. To be comfortable with this assumption, we recommend the trial be blinded and that all such patients be unlikely to have an awareness of the treatment's efficacy or reaction to its side effects at the time of dropping out. In many trials, it may be quite difficult to defend the second assumption.

An alternative approach is to assign a value to the response of patients who fail to provide follow-up data. A very conservative approach for placebo-controlled trials is to allocate the worst possible outcome to patients in the test treatment group and the best possible outcome to patients in the placebo group. More commonly used approaches are to assign all non-completers the worst outcome, a common neutral outcome (such as the mean or median value) or a "carried-forward" outcome. How these values are applied depends on the primary endpoint, and is discussed in greater detail later.

Flow Chart of Counts of Patients

We recommend use of the flow chart in Table 12.1, derived from Gillings and Koch [23], to identify carefully the extent of information available on patients

Table 12.1. Flow chart to account for patients in a randomized trial

Population	Count
All patients screened	n_1
All patients randomized	n_2
All patients who took at least one dose	n_3
All patients who took at least one dose with any follow-up	n_4
Efficacy analyzable patients	n_5

Typically, $n_1 > n_2 > n_3 > n_4 > n_5$. Gillings and Koch [23] suggested that good trials should try to ensure that $n_4/n_2 > 0.95$ and that $n_5/n_4 > 0.80$.

in a randomized clinical trial. Note, however, that for many disease treatment trials (e.g., cancer), the number of patients screened is often not identified because of the complexity of the eligibility criteria and the nature of investigating a patient for a possible trial protocol.

The Efficacy Analyzable Population

The efficacy analyzable population, sometimes referred to as the "per protocol" population, is a subset of the ITT population. This is the population of patients, randomized to treatment, who reasonably adhered to all protocol conditions. The relative strictness of the "reasonably adherent" criterion is based on clinical considerations regarding how much adherence is sufficient to reasonably expect the patient to respond to the treatment.

The ITT Population

Depending on the assumptions we are willing to make, one of the populations described above will be taken as the ITT population. Some statisticians, including Fisher et al. [13], favor the "all patients randomized" (APR) population. Gillings and Koch [23] essentially favor going down the list as far as possible as long as at least 95% of the patients randomized are still in the resulting "modified intention-to-treat" (MITT) population. They add the additional twist that patients be allocated to the treatment received rather than the one to which they were randomized, assuming that the errors are rare and inadvertent. (Their advice does not apply to situations in which treatments are unblind and the subject deliberately takes the alternate treatment.) Lewis and Machin [24] weigh in somewhere between these two positions. The principal reason supporting the perspective of Gillings and Koch is that a significant finding for the "all patients randomized" population is only interpretable in terms of real treatment effects when such significance similarly applies to the MITT population. Otherwise, the APR population has fortuitously excessive influence from how the imperfect information from withdrawals and dropouts was included in the analysis. In this sense, the role of the MITT population is primary since convincing inference for it is always necessary, and the role of the APR population is logically supportive for the purpose of confirming the robustness of findings to the method of managing the imperfect information from non-completers. When such confirmation is not sufficient, its use provides an appropriate basis for overruling the findings from the MITT population because of their sensitivity to the exclusion of imperfect information.

Proper application of the ITT principle depends on many factors, including the type of primary outcome variable being studied, the type of study being conducted and the hypothesis being tested. We now describe types of each that we will consider here.

Type of Primary Outcome Variable

We will discuss four types of primary outcome variable: dichotomous, ordinal, continuous and survival time.

Dichotomous Outcome Variable

For many randomized trials, the outcome for a given patient is simply scored as success or failure. In this case, one application of the ITT principle is to count all analyzable patients who did not complete the trial as failures. To do so potentially underestimates the success rates of the treatment arms. However, since the trial experience may reflect future compliance rates even after one treatment arm is judged to be the best, it may estimate the response rate achievable in the population reasonably well. Another issue is that this method may tend to exaggerate the difference between treatments when the control group has more trial non-completers; examples for which this is often true include studies of pain relief or healing of ulcers [23]. In these situations, there is often interest in analyses that classify a fraction f of non-completers as successes. A potential range for the choice of f is from 0 to twice as large as the highest of the group-specific success rates, although other choices may be of interest as well. Lack of sensitivity of the findings to the choice of f would support the conclusions for treatment comparisons.

Ordinal Outcome Variable

Sometimes the primary outcome is categorized into more than two groups. For instance, response to pain medication may be scored as "improved", "no change" or "worse". In this case, analyzable subjects for whom evaluations are not available might be categorized as "worse". However, if this categorization made the difference between treatments appear larger, then a classification of non-completers as "no change" may be more relevant to judging the extent of treatment differences.

Continuous Outcome Variable

It is more problematic to assign scores to subjects who do not complete the randomized controlled trial when the outcome variable is continuous. There is no "worst" category to assign. Perhaps one could assign the worst value obtained by a patient who completes the trial to all patients who did not. However, depending on the number of non-completers, such assignment may perturb the distribution theory from which significance is being assessed. A strategy that surmounts these problems is to assign "worst ranks" to the trial non-completers and perform a nonparametric analysis. A cardiovascular study by Barst et al. [25] provides an example of this method for an aspect of exercise performance after 12 weeks of treatment.

In some clinical trials, multiple observations are made on the subjects over time. In these cases, early response measures can be used as the definitive response for patients who do not complete the trial. Gillings and Koch [23] define this method as "last observation carried forward" or LOCF. Examples illustrating this method are discussed by Davis and Koch [26], Gansky et al. [27] and Carraro et al. [28]. (Note that this method can also be applied to dichotomous or ordinal response variables.) Unfortunately, the LOCF method depends on the additional assumption that there is no marked time trend to the observations: that is, the measurements do not tend to go up or down over time. The LOCF method can be viewed as a simple application of modeling of missing data, which will be discussed below. It can sometimes be modified to account for time trends through nonparametric analyses for "last rank carried forward" or percentiles based on last rank.

Survival Outcome Variable

When the primary outcome is some time-to-event, where the event signifies failure, one can assign failure to the subject at the point at which they are off the protocol. On the other hand, if the event signifies success, one can censor them at some long time, past all the known events. Sometimes, however, continued follow-up for a primary outcome is often possible even though the patient is no longer participating in any other aspect of the study. If the patient received no treatment off the study which would be expected to delay the occurrence of an unfavorable event, we recommend giving trial non-completers an event at the time when the event occurred or at the time of last follow-up if they were lost to follow-up. Patients who continue to be followed and have not had the event remain censored.

Modeling Data for Trial Non-completers

The LOCF method is a simple way in which the response outcome variable can be modeled. This approach, however, makes important assumptions

that may not hold for a clinical trial. Suppose that patients with a rapidly degenerative disease are being studied. Early outcome measures could then be expected to be better than later measures. Trial non-completers may then have better scores than those who complete the study. In such a case, it might be better to model the data, using a regression model for variation over time than to carry observations forward (or to use rankings within visits to remove the effects of time and to carry their values forward). When modeling the outcome for non-completers, patient baseline covariates will often be used. Unfortunately, there is one covariate that definitely differs between completers and non-completers – that of completing the trial. Thus, when modeling to obtain estimates for the missing responses, there is an assumption that the "completion of trial" covariate is unrelated to the response – which begs the whole concern behind ITT in the first place.

If researchers choose to model the missing data, we suggest that it should be based on patient-specific baseline factors and not population- or completer-based factors. For example, if 40% of subjects who complete the study are responders, the researcher should not simply assign responder status to 40% of the non-completers.

Type of Study

Most of the discussion of intention-to-treat presented so far has presumed a parallel treatment groups design. We will discuss how the practical aspects of analysis need to be revised for use with a crossover design.

Parallel Groups Design

In a parallel groups trial, study subjects are randomized to two or more treatment groups. For this type of trial, we recommend two principal analyses: one on "all patients who took at least one dose" if the trial is adequately blinded or on "all patients randomized" if the trial is unblinded and the other being the "per protocol" analysis on the "efficacy analyzable" population. The rationale behind the "at least one dose" rule for blinded trials is that the mix of reasons for discontinuing a trial after having started some treatment are very possibly different and more likely to be associated with the treatment received than are the reasons for disenrolling from a trial before any treatment is received.

Crossover Design

In a crossover trial, patients are randomized to two or more treatment groups. After a period of time on the first treatment and often a "washout" period, the patients then receive some other treatment (additional treatments may follow as well). Consequently, one of the main advantages to crossover trials is that fewer patients are needed to achieve high power because they serve as their own controls. Serious analytical problems arise if many patients leave the trial prior to the second period, since it then becomes unclear what response should be given to treatments that were not even started. In this case a "period one" analysis is likely to be preferred to the planned crossover analysis. In practical terms, this converts a crossover trial into a parallel groups trial.

Crossover trials are often undertaken when the intersubject variability is expected to be much larger than the intrasubject variability. Consequently, a period one analysis is likely to have greatly reduced power compared with the planned trial. It is thus useful to block the randomization of crossover trials so that the period one distribution of treatment assignments matches the study design. For example, for a two-group crossover study of 16 patients, this would mean having exactly 8 patients taking each treatment in period one.

There are two ways in which missing data in a crossover trial could occur. The first is that patients drop out during the course of the study. These are patients who do not complete the treatment protocol due to some event that apparently is not related to the treatment (e.g., a patient moves out of the area). These patients can be excluded from the ITT sample, but only if the researcher feels very confident that their failure to complete the study was due to reasons unrelated to the study. One must keep in mind, however, that the exclusion of these patients may have significant impact on the power of the study. Thus, for this situation, one may choose to replace the patients with incomplete participation (or missing periods) by newly randomized subjects. Adding newly randomized patients may be particularly important when the number of dropouts is greater for one treatment than another, although caution concerning generalizability of findings and potential implications of carryover effects may be necessary in such cases.

A second cause for missing data may be patients who withdraw from the study because of some reason directly related to the clinical trial. These may be patients who successfully complete one or more periods of treatment but who experience significant side effects and are forced to withdraw from the protocol. Again, if a significant number of withdrawals are expected, a crossover design is probably not the most prudent choice of study design. Excluding these patients from the analysis would not be recommended, as this is likely to introduce bias and would violate the ITT principles. In this situation, the MITT

population of patients might be defined as those patients who receive treatment and provide some follow-up data within at least one period of the treatment sequence, according to the guidelines given previously. This is similar to the notion of including only patients who receive at least one dose in the parallel groups randomized trial. Methodology has been developed that allows patients with incomplete data to be included in the analysis of crossover trials [29,30]. These techniques rely on the assumption that missing data occur for reasons that are not related to the treatments or to the study and leaves missing data as missing. Sensitivity analyses can be conducted that include imputing values for those that are missing. One approach of interest would be to use only the complete first period data [24], realizing the power limitations of this type of analysis as discussed above. If the number of withdrawals is small, the decrease in power may be minimal and first period comparisons may be useful.

Alternatively, one can assign values to periods with missing data. For example, if the outcome is a binary response, one conservative application of the ITT principle is to assign failures to all those patients with incomplete data. Similarly, if the response is ordinal, those subjects with missing data could be categorized as "worse". Another alternative would be to apply the LOCF principle, i.e., if a patient responded successfully in the first period, assign a successful outcome to any subsequent periods with missing data. An illustration for such use of LOCF is given in Davis and Koch [26] for a crossover trial with four periods to compare a test treatment for migraine headaches with placebo. All of the approaches for assigning values to periods with missing data have limitations, particularly for studies where the treatments might have different carryover effects.

Type of Hypothesis

In an unblind parallel groups study, we recommended that two analyses ("as randomized" and "per protocol") be performed. These analyses apply to a single statistical hypothesis under, it is hoped, very similar assumptions and study samples. This situation, where multiple analyses are conducted under slightly varying assumptions, is referred to as *sensitivity analysis*. Statistical inference is easiest if all analyses conducted yield the same finding. When they differ, questions arise as to which one to prefer. The analysis favored in our case depends on the type of hypothesis being considered. We will consider two types here: a *superiority trial* and an *equivalence trial*.

In a superiority trial, one wishes to show the superiority of one treatment over the others. In this case, the "as randomized" analysis is likely to be conservative (and hence preferred), since the subjects who do not complete the trial are typically given the same value. Consequently, if the trial non-completers are roughly equal across the treatments, the "as randomized" trial is biased toward the null hypothesis. The non-completers are unbalanced, different values must sometimes be assigned to non-completers from different treatments in order to have a conservative analysis (e.g. carried forward values for the control group and less favorable values for the test treatment).

In an equivalence (or a non-inferiority) trial, where the goal is to demonstrate the equivalence of two or more treatments (or a non-inferiority of some treatment to others), this bias favors the alternative hypothesis; hence the "per protocol" analysis might be preferred. Alternatively, an ITT analysis could become more appealing for reasons of reduced bias if non-completers on the test treatment were assigned poorer outcomes than those on the control treatment, since any bias in this type of assignment would be against equivalence (or non-inferiority). For example, when the objective of analysis is to produce a confidence interval whose lower limit exceeds $-D$, a continuous outcome might have *last value* $-D$ assigned to non-completers on test treatment and *last value* assigned to non-completers on control treatment. Similarly, for a dichotomous outcome non-completers could be assigned a success rate of $P - D$ for the test treatment and P for the control treatment. In each of the cases above, sensitivity analyses could consider various choices of the amount to subtract from the last value (and/or P). For either type of trial, however, additional analyses are often, and should be, conducted before a final conclusion is reached.

Alternative Methods of Analysis

Although the ITT analysis, or pragmatic approach, yields statistically valid p values and provides an unbiased assessment of clinical trial results, some clinicians and statisticians are uncomfortable with the idea of including all patients in an analysis when non-compliance or a substantial amount of missing data occurs. As a result, several alternative methods have been proposed to account for non-compliance to study protocol [18,31]. These include: (1) "the censored method" where patients are censored at the time they switch to the other treatment or withdraw from the study; (2) "the transition method" where patients are transferred from one group to another when treatment changes in the analysis; (3) "the adherers only method" where all patients who

changed treatments are excluded from the analysis; and (4) "the treatment-received method" where patients are counted from the date of randomization as though they had been randomized to the treatment ultimately received. All of these methods can be biased in unknown ways because they compare groups that have not been randomized to their respective treatments.

Using data from the Veterans Administration Cooperative Study of Coronary Artery Bypass Surgery, the Coronary Drug Project group compared the ITT analysis with the four alternative methods [18,31] mentioned above. This study, conducted between 1972 and 1990, was a randomized clinical trial designed to compare the survival time of patients assigned to medical therapy with those assigned to bypass surgery. In this study, approximately 25% of patients randomized to medical therapy eventually switched to the surgery arm of the study. The authors illustrate the problems that arise when using each of the alternative methods to deal with the non-adherence to protocol and describe the impact of each method on the results.

As discussed by Peduzzi et al. [18], the treatment-received and adherers only methods can be the most misleading because of length-sampling bias. In their study, length-sampling bias refers to the bias resulting from the time patients waited to receive the bypass operation. For example, using the adherers only method, the entire survival experience of the large number of patients who switched from medical therapy to surgery is excluded (i.e., these patients had a median of 5 years of survival prior to surgery and this information is lost). Alternatively, for the treatment-received method, the survival experience of these same patients is attributed entirely to the surgical group, resulting in an even larger apparent survival benefit for the surgical group. The longer the period of follow-up, the greater the potential for bias, since more patients will have the opportunity to withdraw from treatment or switch treatments. As the number of patients who change treatments and the length of time to this change increases, the bias in these two methods can also be expected to increase. Lee et al. [32] further discuss the treatment-received method and point out the following reasons to avoid this approach. "One reason is the lack of confidence that the only difference between treatment groups is the intervention. A second is the problem of reduced sample size and consequent loss of power. A third is the loss of the basis for statistical significance testing. A fourth is the difficulty of creating an objective operational definition of actual treatment."

The censored and transition methods also have problems. Although they correct for length-sampling bias, other biases exist. The censored method assumes that the change in treatments is independent of outcome, i.e., that the patients who switched would have had the same survival experience as the adherers if they had remained on the originally assigned treatment. The transition method uses all the data from time of randomization to time to event, but it changes the randomized comparison to an observational one by reassigning patients. It can then no longer be assumed that the groups are balanced with respect to baseline values. The results of the censored and transition methods can differ substantially from the ITT analysis if the assumption of independence between the change in treatments and outcome is false.

These alternative methods suffer from biases, and may therefore suggest a treatment difference when no difference truly exists, or the analysis may fail to detect a treatment difference that does exist. The Coronary Drug Project Research group stated that analyses restricted to patients who complied with the assigned treatment regimen were "unreliable or misleading because of the manner in which patients are selected or select themselves into groups that are good or poor with respect to adherence or response" [18].

These methods are not designed to replace the ITT analysis, but to supplement it. The methods described here can provide useful information, but the researcher must use them with caution and realize the limitations of each.

Examples

Example 1: Parallel Trial with Protocol Violations

Miller et al. [33] and Lacomblez et al. [34] conducted a stratified, double-blind, randomized and placebo-controlled clinical trial of riluzole in patients with amyotrophic lateral sclerosis (ALS). Patients were stratified by whether their disease was in the bulbar musculature or limb muscles. Nine hundred and fifty-nine patients were randomized to daily treatment of placebo, or 50, 100 or 200 mg riluzole. The primary endpoint was the tracheostomy-free survival of placebo compared with 100 mg riluzole.

Lacomblez et al. [34] state that "the statistical analysis was based on intent to treat and included all randomized patients." They also note that 134 of 236 patients taking 100 mg riluzole, of whom 21 prematurely discontinued treatment, were alive at the end of the study and 122 of 242 placebo-treated patients, of whom 14 discontinued treatment, were alive at the

end of the study. "Patients who stopped treatment were followed up in the same way as patients who continued on trial medication and every assessment was included in the intention-to-treat analysis. For patients lost to follow-up, we sought information from relatives or the family physician, and documentary evidence of death or tracheostomy was obtained". In parallel trials, where patients are randomized to concurrent treatment arms, endpoints such as survival can often be completed for lost patients by using other sources. Of course this requires extra effort on the part of the study coordinators.

The protocol violations for the trial were carefully identified and are reproduced in Table 12.2. These included both violations of entry criteria and incorrect treatment received. Although thirty-five patients had at least one protocol violation, these patients were analyzed in the treatment arm to which they were randomized, thus emphasizing the policy of treatment more than the treatment actually received.

These protocol violations fall into several different categories. The first two involve randomization errors. The patient who was randomized twice was lost to follow-up at one center and was subsequently randomized to another group at another center. Perhaps only the data from the first center should be used. The patients randomized in the wrong stratum were incorrectly identified as having either limb-onset or bulbar-onset. They should probably be analyzed in the correct stratum but with the treatment as randomized. The next five protocol violations involve violations of entry criteria. These patients could be dropped as they either designate the patient

Table 12.2. Protocol violations for riluzole versus placebo trial

Causes of protocol violations	Placebo n = 242	Riluzole		
		50 mg n = 237	100 mg n = 236	200 mg n = 244
Randomized twice		1		1
Randomized in wrong stratum	2	1		
Age >75 years	1			
Disease duration >5 years	1			
Vital capacity <60% normal value	2	4	2	3
Entry criteria not assessed	2	2	4	1
Misdiagnosed case			1	2
Never took medication		1	2	
Took another patient's treatment		1	1	2
No. with at least one protocol violation	7	10	9	9

as having a condition different from that under study or not completely assessed. Since the trial was blinded, the patients who never took medication could also be dropped. Finally, it is not clear from the article why patients took another patient's treatment. If it was a deliberate choice, they should be analyzed in the treatment group to which they were randomized; if it was inadvert, they could be analyzed on the treatment arm that they received. While the number of formal protocol violations in this trial is relatively small, over 20% of the subjects ultimately dropped out. The primary analysis was a comparison of two survival curves, with the test statistic assuming that the distribution of dropout times is independent of the event times observed. The robustness of the findings of this study certainly depends upon the extent to which this assumption holds, as noted by Guiloff et al. [35].

Example 2: Parallel Trial with a Binary Endpoint

Goodkin et al. [36] reported on the use of low-dose oral methotrexate in chronic progressive multiple sclerosis in a randomized, double-blind, placebo-controlled, clinical trial. Sixty patients were randomized and followed for 2 years for treatment failure. The authors stated that "the analysis was done using only the 2-year treatment phase data in an intent-to-treat framework regardless of patient compliance."

Table 12.3 accounts for the patients randomized in the study. Fifty-one of 60 patients completed the trial since 7 patients stopped taking their drugs for the specified reasons and 2 were lost to follow-up. Of the 9 trial non-completers, 6 failed prior to discontinuation of treatment. The remaining 3 patients, all of

whom "stopped treatment" on the methotrexate arm, were "clinically stable when last seen at 5, 16, and 17 months." We believe that the authors considered these 3 patients as not failing treatment within 2 years even though they did not complete the trial. Conservatively, if these 3 patients are considered to be failures, the difference in the binomial proportions is only borderline significant ($p = 0.065$) compared with the analysis presented by the authors ($p = 0.011$).

Example 3: Parallel Trial with a Continuous Endpoint

Beck et al. [37] reported on the use of corticosteroids to treat optic neuritis. Four-hundred and fifty-seven patients with acute optic neuritis were randomly assigned to receive 14 days of treatment with oral prednisone, 3 days of intravenous methylprednisolone, followed by 11 days of oral prednisone or oral placebo. The primary outcome measures were visual field and contrast sensitivity, measured at 6 months after treatment. Univariate Wilcoxon rank-sum tests were performed on both primary endpoints to test for group differences between each steroid group and the placebo group. Overall, 438 of the 457 patients randomized (95.8%) completed the 6-month visit. The authors did not indicate any use of ITT principles in their analysis.

What would we have done? Nine patients who were randomized were later determined to be ineligible. We would exclude these patients to obtain the ITT sample ($n = 448$). Six patients dropped out during the treatment period, 2 patients dropped out between the end of the treatment period and the 6-month follow-up and 2 patients were unaccounted for. The efficacy analyzable population ($n = 438$) also

Table 12.3. Accounting of patients for the methotrexate versus placebo trial

Patient status	Number of Patients		
	Methotrexate	Placebo	Total
Randomized to treatment	31	29	60
Stopped treatment	5	2	7
Felt the drug was not working	3	1	4
Felt the study was "too much hassle"	1	0	1
Required conflicting antibiotic with study medication	0	1	1
Incidental ovarian malignancy after initiation of therapy	1	0	1
Lost to follow-up	2	0	2
Completed protocol	24	27	51
Number failing	16	24	40
	(52%)	(83%)	(67%)
Number failing (conservative count)	19	24	43
	(61%)	(83%)	(72%)

excludes these 10 patients and appears to be the group analyzed by the authors. Conservatively, the 10 patients in the ITT sample with missing data would be given the lowest ranks or, more neutrally, they could be given carried-forward ranks.

Example 4: Unblind Parallel Trial with Eligibility Criteria Redefined

Dahl et al. [38] reported on a study of 87 children and young adults with acute nonlymphocytic leukemia (ANLL) who were treated uniformly with an induction chemotherapy regimen which included daunorubicin, cytarabine, etoposide and azacytidine. Siblings of induction responders were to be HLA-typed. Patients with an HLA-matched sibling donor were to receive a bone marrow transplant, and the remaining responders were to receive sequential intensive chemotherapy for 12 months. Informed consent was obtained from all parents of the patients at the outset of the study.

Sixty-five of the 87 patients achieved response to the induction therapy. Of these, 15 had HLA-matched siblings and received a bone marrow transplant, 42 did not have HLA-matched siblings and received chemotherapy, 4 patients had HLA-matched siblings but did not receive a transplant and the siblings of 4 patients were not typed. ITT considerations apply to the last 8 patients described. Three of the patients who were not typed had medical complications (leukoencephalopathy, Duchenne's disease, and severe neuropathy). In the other case, the parents refused. Three patients who had HLA-matched siblings did not receive a transplant due to additional medical complications (congenital osteomyelitis, low body weight (7 kg) and very young age (10 months), and pulmonary *Aspergillus*) and the parents of a fourth patient refused the transplant.

In the paper, the authors (who included one of us (M.J.S.)) excluded the 4 patients who were not typed and analyzed the 4 who had HLA-matched siblings but were not transplanted as though they had received the transplant. A good case can be made, however, for excluding all patients from analysis except for the one with an HLA-matched sibling whose parents refused, as long as there were no patients in the chemotherapy arm for whom transplant would not have been a viable option (had a match been found). As described above, 6 of the patients who did not follow the protocol involved physician refusal. Three of them were caught prior to determining which arm the patient "belonged" on and consequently no bias results. The other three were identified only after HLA typing was done, although all three conditions were known before the

typing. If there were clear guidelines at the transplant center on which patients are unsuitable for transplant and were no such patients in the chemotherapy arm (with no HLA-matched sibling), then exclusion of the other three would also not lead to bias. The fact that such exclusions were not planned for a priori is unfortunate, but they should not force an analysis that is more likely to be biased. If such patients are excluded from analysis, it is clear that the statistical inference would be limited to the "transplantable patients".

Example 5: Crossover Trial

Pezzoli et al. [39] reported on a 6-month randomized, blinded crossover trial comparing pergolide with bromocriptine as an adjunct to levodopa, for the treatment of Parkinson's disease. "Patients underwent a 2-week pretreatment screening period and then were randomized to one of the treatment sequences: either pergolide followed by bromocriptine (PB) (35 patients) or bromocriptine followed by pergolide (BP) (33 patients)" for 12 weeks each. The primary endpoint was the aggregate score from the three parts of the New York University Parkinson's Disease Scale (NYUPDS), which assesses activities of daily living, quantifies the physical examination and assesses dyskinesias, dystonias and psychosis.

Of 68 patients, 59 completed the study. Of the 9 patients who did not complete the study, 1 was hospitalized due to rectal cancer (not drug related), 3 had minor adverse events (nausea, hypotension and fatigue) and 5 did not comply with treatment protocol. Two additional patients, who had protocol violations, were dropped from statistical evaluation.

Our definition of an ITT sample for a crossover trial consists of patients who received treatment and provided follow-up data for one or more outcomes within at least one period of the treatment sequence. In this study, 62 patients completed the first period (33 in the PB group and 29 in the BP group). These patients comprise the ITT sample for analysis. Of the 6 patients who did not complete the first period, 4 experienced adverse events (1 in the PB group and 3 in the BP group) and 2 were either treatment or protocol violators. The ITT sample may include patients with treatment violations if these occur in patients who complete at least one period of the study. Gillings and Koch [23] recommend that such violations should be kept to no more than 5% of the study sample by good study management and administrative procedures.

Three patients in the ITT sample had missing second period data (these patients were discontinued due to treatment violations). A mixed-effects model can be used to analyze data from a crossover study with incomplete data. For comparison, sensitivity analyses can be conducted that include imputing values for those that are missing. One approach to the sensitivity analyses is to give these patients the same NYUPDS score as observed in the first period, i.e., LOCF. This is a conservative approach because it assumes there is not a treatment effect. Because we imputed data in our main ITT analysis, we would perform sensitivity analyses to check for consistent results. Three suggested analyses are: (1) analysis with no missing data and no protocol violators ($n = 57$), (2) efficacy analyzable analysis (remove 2 protocol violators from ITT sample, assuming that these were violators of inclusion or exclusion criteria, $n = 60$), and (3) impute means for missing values in the ITT analysis ($n = 62$). If the conclusions drawn from these analyses are comparable to those made from the LOCF analysis, then the analyst may conclude that the imputation of missing data did not excessively affect the overall interpretation of the data.

References

1. Pocock SJ. Allocation of patients to treatment in clinical trials. Biometrics 1979;35:183–197.
2. Fisher RA. The arrangement of field experiments. J Minist Agr 1926;33.
3. Lachin JM. Statistical elements of the randomized clinical trial. In: Tygstrop N, Lachin JM and Juhl E, editors. The randomized clinical trial and therapeutic decisions. New York: Marcel Dekker, 1982:77–103.
4. Hill AB. Statistical methods in clinical and preventive medicine. Edinburgh: E and S Livingstone, 1962.
5. Byar DP. The necessity and justification of randomized clinical trials. In: Tagnon HJ, Staquet MJ, editors. Controversies in cancer: design of trials and treatment. New York: Masson, 1979:75–82.
6. Green SB. Patient heterogeneity and the need for randomized clinical trials. Control Clin Trials 1982;3:189–198.
7. Spodick DH. The randomized controlled clinical trial. Am J Med 1982;73:420–425.
8. Koch GG, Paquette DW. Design principles and statistical considerations in periodontal clinical trials. Ann Periodont 1997; 2:42–63.
9. Byar DP, Simon RM, Friedewald WT, Schlesselman JJ, DeMets DL, Ellenberg JH, et al. Randomized clinical trials: perspectives on some recent ideas. N Engl J Med 1976;295:74–80.
10. Simon R. Heterogeneity and standardization in clinical trials. In: Tagnon HJ, Staquet MJ, editors. Controversies in cancer: design of trials and treatment. New York: Masson, 1979:75–82.
11. Armitage P. The role of randomization in clinical trials. Stat Med 1982;1:345–352.
12. Petrie A. Why randomization is essential and why we do it. In: Tygstrop N, Lachin JM, Juhl E, editors. The randomized clinical trial and therapeutic decisions New York: Marcel Dekker, 1982:105–116.
13. Fisher LD, Dixon DO, Herson J, Frankowski RK, Hearron MS, Peace KE. Intention to treat in clinical trials. In: Peace KE, editor, Statistical issues in drug research and development.

14. Ellenberg SS. Studies to compare treatment regimens: the randomized clinical trial and alternative strategies. JAMA 1981;246:2481–2482.
15. Simon R. Randomized clinical trials and research strategy. Cancer Treat Rep 1982;66:1083–1087.
16. Fisher RA. The design of experiments. New York: Hafner, 1971.
17. Peto R, Pike MC, Armitage P, Breslow NE, Cox DR, Howard SV, et al. Design and analysis of randomized clinical trials requiring prolonged observation of each patient. I. Introduction and design. Br J Cancer 1976;34:585–612.
18. Peduzzi P, Detre K, Wittes J, Holford T. Intent-to-treat analysis and the problem of crossovers [with discussion]. J Thorac Cardiovasc Surg 1991;101:481–487.
19. Lavori PW. Clinical trials in psychiatry: should protocol deviation censor patient data? Neuropsychopharmacology 1992;6: 39–48.
20. Tsiatis AA. Analysis and interpretation of trial results: intent-to-treat analysis. J Acquir Immune Defic Syndr 1990;3:S120–S123.
21. Royall RM. Ethics and statistics in randomized clinical trials [with discussion]. Stat Sci 1991;6:52–88.
22. Gent M, Sackett DL. The qualification and disqualification of patients and events in long-term cardiovascular trials. Thromb Haemost 1979;41:123–134.
23. Gillings D, Koch G. The application of the principle of intention-to-treat to the analysis of clinical trials. Drug Inf J 1991; 25:411–424.
24. Lewis JA, Machin D. Intention to treat – who should use ITT? Br J Cancer 1993;68:647–650.
25. Barst RJ, et al. A comparison of continuous intravenous epoprostenol (prostacyclin) with conventional therapy for primary pulmonary hypertension. N Engl J Med 1996;334: 296–301.
26. Davis RL, Koch GG. Statistical considerations for design and analysis of a multiperiod crossover study to compare two treatments for migraine headache. J Biopharm Stat 1994;4: 312–346.
27. Gansky S, Koch GG, Wilson J. Statistical evaluation of relationships between analgesic dose and ordered ratings of pain relief over an eight-hour period. J Biopharm Stat 1994;4: 233–265.
28. Carraro JC, Raynaud JP, Koch GG, Chisholm GD, Silverio FD, Teillac P, et al. Comparison of phytotherapy (permixon) with finasteride in the treatment of benign prostate hyerplasis: a randomized international study of 1098 patients. Prostate 1996;29:231–240.
29. Diggle PJ, Liang K-Y, Zeger SL. Analysis of longitudinal data. New York: Oxford University Press, 1994.
30. Vonesh EF, Chinchilli VM. Linear and nonlinear models for the analysis of repeated measurements. New York: Marcel Dekker, 1977: chapter 4.
31. Peduzzi P, Wittes J, Detre K, Holford T. Analysis as-randomized and the problem of non-adherence: an example from the Veterans Affairs Randomized Trial of Coronary Artery Bypass Surgery. Stat Med 1993;12:1185–1195.
32. Lee YJ, Ellenburg JH, Hirtz DG, Nelson KB. Analysis of clinical trials by treatment actually received: is it really an option? Stat Med 1991;10:1595–1605.
33. Miller RG, Bouchard JP, Duquette P, Eisen A, Gelinas D, Harati Y, et al. Clinical trials of riluzole in patients with ALS. Neurology 1996;47(Suppl 2):S86–S89.
34. Lacomblez L, Bensimon G, Leigh PN, Guillet P, Meininger V, for the ALS/Riluzole Study Group. II. Dose-ranging study of riluzole in amyotrophic lateral sclerosis. Lancet 1996;347: 1425–1431.
35. Guiloff RJ, Goonetilleke A, Emami J. Riluzole and amyotrophic lateral sclerosis (letter). Lancet 1996;348:336–337.

New York: Marcel Dekker, 1990.

36. Goodkin DE, Rudick RA, Medendorp SV, Daughtry MM, Schwetz KM, Fischer J, et al. Low-dose (7.5mg) oral methotrexate reduces the rate of progression in chronic progressive multiple sclerosis. Ann Neurol 1995;37:30–40.

37. Beck WB, Cleary PA, Anderson MM, et al. A randomized, controlled trial of corticosteroids in the treatment of acute optic neuritis. N Engl J Med 1992;326(9):581–588.

38. Dahl GV, Kalwinsky DK, Mirro Jr J, Look T, Pui C-H, Murphy SB, et al. Allogenic bone marrow transplantation in a program of intensive sequential chemotherapy for children and young adults with acute nonlymphocytic leukemia in first remission. J Clin Oncol 1990;8:295–303.

39. Pezzoli G, Marrignoni E, Pacchetti C, Angeleri V, Lamberti P, Muratoria A, et al. A crossover, controlled study comparing pergolide with bromocriptine as an adjunct to levodopa for the treatment of Parkinson's disease. Neurology 1995;45(Suppl 3):S22–S27.

13. Statistical Analysis of Repeated-Measures Data with Drop-outs

R.J. Little

Introduction

Many clinical trials in neurology follow patients longitudinally over time, and measure clinical outcomes of interest repeatedly. A common problem that arises in this context is missing data caused by subjects dropping out prior to the end of the study. For earlier discussions of this topic, see Heyting et al. [1], Gornbein et al. [2], Little and Schenker [3] or Little [4]. This chapter reviews some approaches to statistical analysis when faced with this problem. I first discuss some simple approaches, including complete-case analyses that restrict attention to the cases that do not drop out. The latter are liable to yield biased answers when individuals that drop out differ systematically from those that remain in the study, as is often likely to be the case. I then discuss two more modern approaches that eliminate or reduce the bias of complete-case analysis by exploiting partial information on nonrespondents, namely maximum likelihood based on repeated-measures models, and multiple imputation. Methods are illustrated on an intent-to-treat analysis of data from a randomized clinical trial for tacrine in the treatment of Alzheimer's disease, reported in detail in Little and Yau [5].

The Data

I assume we have repeated-measures data, with some cases that drop out before the end of the study, and a set of fixed, baseline covariates. For subject i, let $y_i = (y_{i1}, \ldots, y_{ik})$ represent the set of repeated measures for the ith subject, some of which may be missing. Let $y_{obs,i}$ denote the observed values and $y_{mis,i}$ the missing values of y_i, and let x_i denote the set of fixed covariates included in the analysis, assumed fully observed. Figure 13.1 sketches the data pattern with $k = 4$ time points. For modeling the missing-data

mechanism it is convenient to introduce another variable, R_i, which indicates whether somebody drops out or not and, if they do, when. Let R_i take the value 0 for complete cases, and the value j if the subject drops out at the jth time point (Fig. 13.1). For simplicity we assume that subjects who drop out do not re-enter the study, although many of the methods discussed here can be extended to handle this more complex pattern.

Example 1. Drop-outs in a Dose-Titration Study of Tacrine for Alzheimer's Disease

As an illustrative example, I consider a double-blind, placebo-controlled, parallel group study for the treatment of Alzheimer's disease using the drug tacrine (Cognex, Warner-Lambert) [6]. After establishing eligibility and completing baseline assessments, patients were randomized to control and treatment groups, and a variety of cognitive measures were administered periodically up to 18 weeks from baseline (a second set of outcomes measured through 30 weeks after baseline is not considered here). For the 18-week study, subjects were randomized to three treatment groups: a placebo group, a low-dose group where patients were given a 40 mg/day dose of tacrine for 6 weeks and an 80 mg/day dose for weeks 7–18, and a high-dose group where patients were given a 40 mg/day dose for 6 weeks, an 80 mg/day dose for weeks 7–12 and 120 mg/day for weeks 13–18. The titration to higher doses of tacrine was used because potentially serious side effects on liver function dictated against initial administration of a high dose of the drug. Measures were taken at baseline and after weeks 6, 12, 16 and 18; we will focus here on data for a primary outcome measure, the Alzheimer's' Disease Assessment Scale, Cognitive component (ADAS-Cog) [7]. The covariates x_i consisted of times of measurement, baseline ADAS-Cog, treatment group and treatment site.

$$R \quad X \quad Y_1 \quad Y_2 \quad Y_3 \quad Y_4$$

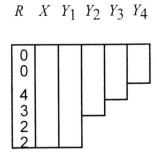

Fig. 13.1.   Schematic of a monotone missing data pattern, with rows representing cases, X representing covariates, $Y_1, \ldots, Y_4$ repeated measures at four time points, and Blocks representing data. R is the drop-out indicator.

Two types of drop-out occur in this trial – treatment drop-outs and analysis drop-outs, using the terminology of Meinert [8]. Analysis drop-outs arise when outcome data are not recorded because of loss to follow-up or other reasons, yielding a missing-data problem. Treatment drop-outs occur when subjects discontinue a treatment, because of side effects or lack of compliance. Treatment drop-outs are not necessarily analysis drop-outs, since follow-up data may continue to be recorded even though subjects are not longer on the assigned treatment. Conversely, analysis drop-outs may not be treatment drop-outs since subjects failing to have their outcomes recorded may still be on the assigned treatment.

In the tacrine study there were a substantial number of dose-related treatment drop-outs primarily due either to protocol rules, specifically an elevated liver function test, or to other reasons such as lack of compliance or various dose-related adverse events. In particular at week 18, 44 of the 184 subjects (24%) in the placebo group, 31 of the 61 subjects (51%) in the low-dose group and 244 of the 418 subjects (57%) in the high-dose group were no longer in the double-blind phase of the study. For simplicity, we confine attention here to the complete cases and drop-outs who yield a monotone missing-data pattern, omitting a small number of subjects who missed a visit but subsequently re-entered the study double-blind.

A basic assumption in all our methods is that each missing value hides a true underlying value that is meaningful for analysis. This may seem obvious but is not always the case. For subjects in example 1 who leave the study because they move to a different location, it makes sense to consider the ADAS-Cog score that would have been recorded if they had remained in the study. On the other hand if subjects had died during the course of the study, it is less clear whether it is meaningful to consider ADAS-Cog scores after time of death as missing values. Rather it may be more reasonable to treat death as a primary outcome and restrict the analysis of ADAS-Cog scores to indi-

viduals that are alive. A more complex missing-data problem arises when individuals leave the study for unknown reasons, which may include relocation or death.

Three Common Approaches to Missing Data

A simple way of dealing with missing data is complete-case (CC) analysis, also known as listwise deletion, where incomplete cases are discarded and standard analysis methods are applied to the complete cases. In many statistical packages this is the default analysis. The exclusion of incomplete cases represents a loss of information, but a more serious problem is that the complete cases are often a biased sample. For example, a subject in a longitudinal study may be more likely to avoid a treatment and drop out of a study because he or she felt the treatment was ineffective, which might be related to a poor value of an outcome measure. The size of the resulting bias depends on the degree to which respondents and nonrespondents differ on outcomes, the amount of missing data and the specifics of the analysis. In particular, the bias in estimating the mean of a variable is easily shown to be the difference in the means for complete and incomplete cases multiplied by the fraction of incomplete cases.

The degree of bias in CC analysis depends on the reasons why values are missing, and in particular whether these reasons relate to variables in the data set. Rubin [9] formalizes this idea by modeling the missing-data mechanism as the conditional distribution of R_i given x_i and y_i, say $p(R_i|x_i, y_i, \phi)$, where ϕ denotes unknown parameters. If missingness does not depend on the values of the outcome data y_i, missing or observed, that is:

$$p(R_i|x_i, y_i, \phi) = p(R_i|x_i, \phi) \quad \text{for all } y_i, \phi \quad (1)$$

then CC analysis yields valid inferences – in particular in clinical trials, estimates of treatment effects are not biased by restriction to complete cases. Little [10] calls mechanisms that satisfy Eq. (1) covariate-dependent. Mechanisms that depend on the time of measurement, the treatment arm or other covariates, fall into this category, provided drop-out does not depend on the outcome measures or, equivalently, drop-outs are a random sample of the original cases within categories formed by the covariates x_i.

A less restrictive assumption is that missingness depends on x_i and on outcome values $y_{obs,i}$ that are observed, and not on values $y_{mis,i}$ that are missing. That is:

$$p(R_i|x_i, y_i, \phi) = p(R_i|x_i, y_{obs,i}, \phi) \quad \text{for all } y_i, \phi \quad (2)$$

Following the terminology of Rubin [9], the missing data mechanism is then called missing at random (MAR). Murray and Findlay [11] provided an instructive example of MAR for data from a study of hypertensive drugs where the outcome was diastolic blood pressure. By protocol, the subject was no longer included in the study when the diastolic blood pressure became too high. This depends on the values of blood pressure, but blood pressure at the time of drop-out was observed before the subject dropped out. Hence the mechanism is MAR, because drop-out only depends on the observed part of y_i. CC analysis is valid when the missing-data mechanism is covariate-dependent, but is in general biased when the data are MAR, that is after conditioning on x_i, drop-out depends on values of y_i prior to drop-out.

A simple approach to incomplete data that retains the information in the incomplete cases is to impute or fill in the missing values. A common version of this approach in repeated-measures settings is last observation carried forward (LOCF) imputation, which imputes missing values with the last recorded observation for that individual (e.g. [12]). Clearly this method makes a very strong assumption about missing data: that the missing values in a case are all identical to the last observed value. In some settings this assumption may be plausible as an approximation, and the method is often considered to yield conservative estimates of treatment effects. In the tacrine example, patients with Alzheimer's disease typically experience a progressive decline in ADAS-Cog scores. Clearly LOCF imputation would be very misleading in such a setting since constancy of the level of LOCF values after drop-out is a very unlikely and favorable outcome. The important point is that LOCF, or any imputation method, is making assumptions about the predictive distribution of missing values that may or may not be reasonable, and that need to be assessed in the particular study setting.

Little and Su [13] proposed better methods for longitudinal imputation based on simple row and column fits. Another alternative to LOCF imputation is regression imputation, in which each missing value is replaced by an estimate of its conditional mean given the values of observed values. For example, in the case of univariate nonresponse with $Y_1, \ldots, Y_{k-1}$ fully observed and Y_k sometimes missing, the regression of Y_k on $Y_1, \ldots, Y_{k-1}$ is estimated from the complete cases, including interactions as needed, and the resulting prediction equation is used to impute the estimated conditional mean for each missing value of Y_k. For repeated-measures data with a monotone pattern, missing values can be filled in sequentially, with each missing value for each subject imputed by regression on the observed or previously imputed values for that subject. Iterative versions of this method lead (with some important adjustments) to maximum likelihood estimates under multivariate normality [14,15].

Although regression imputation incorporates information from the observed variables and yields best predictions of the missing values in the sense of mean squared error, imputations should be judged in terms of the quality of inferences about population parameters from the filled-in data. From this perspective, regression imputation leads to distorted estimates of quantities that are not linear in the data, such as percentiles, correlations and other measures of association, variances and other measures of variability. A solution to this problem is to use random draws rather than best predictions to preserve the distribution of variables in the filled-in data set. An example is *stochastic regression* imputation, in which each missing value is replaced by its regression prediction plus a random error with variance equal to the estimated residual variance. We apply a refinement of this approach to the tacrine data set in the section on multiple imputation below.

Even if imputation is based on an appropriate statistical model, people do not like the method since it seems to be inventing data. One way to view that is if you impute a missing value, the uncertainty from imputation is not taken into account in the analysis of the filled-in data set. Thus, statistical inferences will be distorted, in that standard errors of parameter estimates computed from the filled-in data will typically be too small, confidence intervals for parameters will not have their nominal coverage, and p values for testing null hypotheses will be too small. Large-sample results [16] show that for simple situations with 30% of the data missing, single imputation under the correct model results in nominal 90% confidence intervals having actual coverages below 80%. The inaccuracy of nominal levels is even more extreme in multiparameter testing problems. The section on multiple imputation discusses a refinement of imputation that addresses this problem.

An alternative approach to imputation that also avoids discarding the incomplete cases is to define a summary measure of the treatment effect for each individual based on the available data, and then carry out an analysis of the summary measure across individuals. A key issue is to define a suitable summary measure. In the tacrine example, three possible summary measures are:

(A) The change in ADAS-Cog score from baseline to last recorded measurement.
(B) The change in ADAS-Cog score from baseline to last recorded measurement divided by the time from baseline to last recorded measurement.
(C) The least squares slope of ADAS-Cog on time since baseline, calculated using the available data for each subject.

An analysis of the measure (A) is analogous to LOCF imputation, in that change to last recorded measurement equals time to last measurement when the last observation is carried forward. Hence this measure shares the unsatisfactory features of that method in the tacrine application. Options (B) and (C) are both measures of rate of ADAS-Cog change, with (C) having the advantage that intermediate recorded values are used to increase the precision of the estimated rate.

The summary measures for each individual can then be used to estimate treatment effects. For example the average rate of decline of ADAS-Cog computed using (B) or (C) might be compared between treatment groups using *t*-tests and associated confidence intervals for the difference in mean rates. This approach assumes that the rate of change of the ADAS-Cog score is linear, and that it remains a valid measure whether or not a subject drops out. The latter assumption may be unreasonable if dropout was associated with a change of treatment regimen, which has an impact on the subject's ADAS-Cog decline.

One feature of the summary-measures approach that is often overlooked is that the precision of the estimated summary measure varies according to the number of measurements. Specifically, in the tacrine example the rate of change is less precisely estimated for subjects who drop out early than for subjects who stay in the study, whether (B) or (C) is used as the estimate. Typically, this difference in precision is ignored in the statistical analysis, yielding distortions of standard errors and *p* values. The statistical resolution to the problem is to downweight summary measures from subjects with shorter intervals of measurement. However, the appropriate choice of weight depends on the relative size of intra-individual and inter-individual variation, and leads to complexities that negate the simplicity of the approach (see, for example, [2]).

In summary, complete-case analysis and imputation are not generally satisfactory approaches to statistical analysis of data with missing values, and the summary-measures approach also has weaknesses as usually employed. We now consider some better approaches to the missing-data problem.

Maximum Likelihood Estimation for Data with an Ignorable Missing-Data Mechanism

CC analysis and imputation achieve a rectangular data set by deleting the incomplete cases or filling in the gaps in the data set. There are other methods of analysis that do not require a rectangular data set, and hence can include all the data without deletion or imputation. The summary-measures approach is an example of such a method. Another example is estimation based on generalized estimating equations [17,18]. In this section we discuss a third approach, namely maximum likelihood, which is the basis of a number of recent statistical software packages for repeated-measures data with missing values [19,20]. These programs provide very flexible tools for statistical modeling of data with drop-outs.

Maximum likelihood is a statistical principle for inferences about parameters based on a statistical model. The model defines a probability distribution for the data indexed by unknown parameters; the likelihood function is simply this distribution regarded as a function of the unknown parameters. The estimates of the parameters are chosen to maximize the likelihood function, and hence can be interpreted as the values that make the data most likely. Standard errors of the estimates can also be computed from second derivatives of the likelihood function. For a discussion of maximum likelihood applied to missing data problems with many examples of models see [21].

The likelihood-based approach avoids imputation altogether by forming the likelihood function based on the incomplete data. Since this function can be complicated, maximizing often involves iterative computations, and tools such as the EM algorithm [21,22] can facilitate the computations. I shall not focus on the computational issues here.

For longitudinal data with unequal numbers of measurements across subjects, normally distributed outcomes and data missing at random, a wide range of problems can be tackled using the random-effects model:

$$(y_i|X_i, \beta_i) \sim N_k(X_{1i}\alpha + X_{2i}\beta_i, \Sigma)$$
$$\beta_i|X_i \sim N_q(0, \Gamma) \tag{3}$$

where $N_k(\alpha, B)$ denotes the *k*-variate Normal distribution with mean α covariance matrix B, X_{1i} is a known $(k \times p)$ design matrix containing fixed within-subject and between-subject covariates, with associated unknown $(p \times 1)$ parameter vector α, β_i is an unknown $(q \times 1)$ random-coefficient vector and X_{2i} is a known $(k \times q)$ matrix for modeling the random effects. Estimation for this model is discussed in Harville [23], Laird and Ware [24] and Jennrich and Schluchter [25], and maximum likelihood estimation is available in SAS Proc Mixed [20] or the BMDP program BMDP5V [19]. Maximum likelihood methods for ordinal data are provided in Hedeker [26].

Example 2 (Example 1 continued). Proc Mixed Analysis of Intent-to-Treat Effects of Tacrine

The first two rows of Table 13.1 show results of two analyses based on an application of the model (3) to estimate intent-to-treat effects of the treatments. Let z_{it} denote the ADAS-Cog score for subject i at time t, z_{i0} the ADAS-Cog score at baseline time 0, and $y_{it} = z_{it} - z_{i0}$ the change in ADAS-Cog score from baseline. The statistical model assumes the vector of measurements for subject i have a multivariate Normal distribution with covariance matrix Σ and mean ADAS-Cog score at time t given by the equation:

$$\mu_{it} = \beta_0 + \tau_t + \lambda_{s(i),t} + \alpha_t x_{i0} + \delta_{t1} r_{i1} + \delta_{t2} r_{i2} \quad (4)$$

where: β_0 is an intercept term, τ_t is an effect for time from baseline, $s(i)$ is the treatment site for subject i and $\lambda_{s(i),t}$ represents a site effect, α_t is a regression coefficient for the baseline ADAS-Cog score x_{i0}, r_{i1} takes the value 1 for an individual randomized to the low-dose group and zero otherwise, r_{i2} takes the value 1 for an individual randomized to the high-dose group and zero otherwise, and δ_{t1}, δ_{t2} represent intent-to-treat treatment effects at time t for the low-dose and high-dose groups, respectively.

This is an intent-to-treat analysis since the treatments are as randomized, and do not necessarily reflect dosages received. The row labeled (1A) in Table 13.1 shows estimates of δ_{41} and δ_{42}, the low- and high-dose treatment effects at week 18, and associated asymptotic standard errors, when this model is fitted to the complete cases, discarding drop-outs. The model was fitted by restricted maximum likelihood using SAS Proc Mixed. The results suggest significant effects of tacrine for both dosage levels, but with smaller effects for the higher dosage group. The row labeled (1B) shows the results from fitting the same model to all cases lying within the monotone data pattern, that is the complete cases and the drop-outs. The estimated treatment effect for the high-dose group is increased when the incomplete cases are included, and is now similar to the estimate for the low-dose group. Both treatment effects are highly statistically significant.

The model (3) for Proc Mixed does not include a distribution for the missing-data indicators, and yields a likelihood based on the joint distribution of y_i, β_i. The likelihood is often called the likelihood "ignoring the missing-data mechanism", or simply

Table 13.1. Summary of analyses of week 18 tacrine data

(I) Intent-to-treat restricted maximum likelihood estimates based on observed data, ignorable drop-out, unstructured covariance Matrix

Analysis	Treatment difference (SE)	80 mg/day p value	CI	Treatment difference (SE)	120 mg/day p value	CI
(1A) Complete cases	−3.584 (1.287)	0.0054	(−6.11, −1.06)	−2.236 (0.705)	0.0016	(−3.62, −0.85)
(1B) Monotone pattern	×3.673 (1.208)	0.0024	(−6.04, −1.30)	−3.436 (0.667)	0.0000	(−4.74, −2.13)

(II) Intent-to-treat analyses of data multiply imputed under alternative imputation models

Model	Multiple imputation	Treatment difference (SE)	80 mg/day p value	CI	Treatment difference (SE)	120 mg/day p value	CI
(2A) Continuing-dose	1	−3.486 (0.951)	0.0003	(−5.35, −1.62)	−4.146 (0.563)	0.0000	(−5.25, −3.04)
	2	−3.682 (0.876)	0.0000	(−5.40, −1.97)	−3.101 (0.518)	0.0000	(−4.12, −2.08)
	3	−3.142 (0.944)	0.0009	(−4.99, −1.29)	−3.567 (0.559)	0.0000	(−4.66, −2.47)
	4	−4.889 (0.908)	0.0000	(−6.67, −3.11)	−3.011 (0.538)	0.0000	(−4.07, −1.96)
	5	−4.633 (0.910)	0.0000	(−6.42, −2.85)	−3.395 (0.538)	0.0000	(−4.45, −2.34)
	6	−4.146 (0.920)	0.0000	(−5.95, −2.34)	−3.642 (0.545)	0.0000	(−4.71, −2.57)
	7	−5.239 (0.925)	0.0000	(−7.05, −3.43)	−3.255 (0.547)	0.0000	(−4.33, −2.18)
	8	−4.463 (0.933)	0.0000	(−6.29, −2.63)	−3.695 (0.552)	0.0000	(−4.78, −2.61)
	9	−4.511 (0.953)	0.0000	(−6.38, −2.64)	−3.762 (0.564)	0.0000	(−4.87, −2.66)
	10	−3.497 (0.899)	0.0001	(−5.26, −1.73)	−3.104 (0.532)	0.0000	(−4.15, −2.06)
	MI Inference	−4.169 (1.173)	0.0039	(−6.72, −1.62)	−3.468 (0.663)	0.0002	(−4.90, −2.04)
(3A) Zero-dose	MI Inference	−2.097 (1.087)	0.0734	(−4.42, 0.23)	−1.829 (0.688)	0.0203	(−3.32, −0.34)
(4A) Nearest-dose	MI Inference	−2.787 (1.097)	0.0230	(−5.13, −0.44)	−2.727 (0.656)	0.0010	(−4.13, −1.32)
(2B) Continuing-dose incl. follow-ups	MI Inference	−3.349 (1.020)	0.0032	(−5.46, −1.24)	−2.044 (0.597)	0.0020	(−3.27, −0.82)
(3B) Zero-dose incl. follow-ups	MI Inference	−2.466 (1.024)	0.0248	(−4.59, −0.34)	−1.489 (0.598)	0.0197	(−2.72, −0.26)
(4B) Nearest-dose incl. follow-ups	MI Inference	−2.658 (1.020)	0.0156	(−4.76, −0.55)	−1.649 (0.594)	0.0094	(−2.86, −0.44)
(3C) Zero-dose without adjustment	MI Inference	−1.906 (1.029)	0.0828	(−4.09, −0.28)	−0.941 (0.609)	0.1422	(−2.23, −0.35)

the "ignorable likelihood". Rubin [9] shows that maximum likelihood inference based on the ignorable likelihood is valid when the missing data are MAR, as discussed in the section Three Common Approaches to Missing Data above. That is, drop-out is allowed to depend on the covariates x_i and the observed values $y_{obs,i}$ of y_i, but cannot depend on the missing values $y_{mis,i}$ of y_i or the unobserved random effects β_i. A more technical condition concerning distinctness of the parameters of the complete-data model and the parameters of the model for the missing-data mechanism is required for ignorable maximum likelihood to be fully efficient, but MAR is the key condition in practice.

In our tacrine application, MAR means that drop-out at time t does not depend on unobserved outcomes at times $t' \geq t$, after controlling for the observed data up to time t and the regressors included in the model. This MAR assumption is highly questionable in our intent-to-treat analysis setting. The intent-to-treat analysis conditions on the treatment group to which the subject was randomized, specifically dummies r_{i1}, r_{i2} for low- and high-dose groups in the tacrine example, but the analysis does not condition on the actual treatments received, specifically the dosages of tacrine administered. Changes in treatment after an individual drops out are not reflected in the intent-to-treat treatment variable, which just indicates the treatment group to which an individual was originally randomized. Thus an intent-to-treat analysis of the observed data based on an MAR assumption does not model the effects of any changes in dose after drop-out, even when we know that they occurred. In the tacrine trial, subjects in the high-dose group who dropped out of the study because of liver enzyme elevations received reduced or zero doses after drop-out, but the MAR analysis treats them as though they still received the high-dose treatment, thus potentially overstating the intent-to-treat effect associated with the drug. Thus, a different analysis is needed.

Multiple Imputation

Rubin [27] introduced the idea of multiple imputation, which allows uncertainty from imputation to be taken into account in the analysis, and hence addresses the main weakness of the imputation method. A predictive distribution of plausible values is generated for each missing value, using a statistical model or some other procedure. We then impute not just one but a set of M (say $M = 10$) draws from the predictive distribution of the missing values, yielding M data sets with different draws plugged in for each of the missing values. We then apply the analysis to each of the M data sets and combine the

results in a simple way. In particular for scalar estimands, the multiple-imputation estimate is the average of the estimates from the M data sets, and the variance of the estimate is the average of the variances from the five data sets plus $1 + 1/M$ times the sample variance of the estimates over the M data sets (the factor $1 + 1/M$ is a small-M correction). The last quantity here estimates the contribution to the variance from imputation uncertainty, missed by single imputation methods. Rubin [27] justifies the approach more formally, and describes other forms of multiple-imputation inference. Often multiple imputation is not much more difficult than doing a single imputation – we must do the analysis M times at the end, but this is not a major burden with the high-speed computers that are now available. Most of the work of multiple imputation is in generating good predictive distributions for the missing values.

Example 3 (Example 2 continued). Multiple-Imputation Analysis of the Tacrine Data Set

We now use multiple imputation to improve on the analysis described in example 2. We multiply-impute values of the outcome after drop-out using an imputation model for the missing data that conditions on all relevant observed data, and in particular on information about treatments actually administered (as opposed to randomized). The intent-to-treat model (4) is then fitted to each of the M filled-in data sets. The results are combined using the multiple-imputation technology discussed in chapter 3 of Rubin [27].

The following as-treated imputation model was applied to the tacrine data set. As before, $y_i = (y_{i1}, \ldots, y_{iT})$ denotes the vector of repeated measures for subject i; in our application $T = 4$ and y_{it} represents the change in ADAS-Cog score between time t and baseline. The distribution of y_i given r_{i1}, r_{i2}, the actual dosage indicators $d_{it1}, d_{it2}, d_{it3}$ at time t, and other covariates is modeled as a normal linear regression with mean μ_{it} and variance σ_{tt}, where

$$\mu_{i1} = \beta_{01} + \alpha_1 x_{i0} + \lambda_{s(i),1} + \gamma_{11} d_{i11} + \gamma_{12} d_{i12} + \gamma_{13} d_{i13}$$

(5)

$$\mu_{it} = \beta_{0t} + \alpha_t x_{i0} + \gamma_{t1} d_{it1} + \gamma_{t2} d_{it2} + \gamma_{t3} d_{it3} + \sum_{j=1}^{t-1} \beta_{tj} y_{ij}$$

(6)

Here d_{it1}, d_{it2} represents indicators for the actual treatment for subject i at time t. That is, d_{it1} takes the value 1 for an actual 40 mg dose at time t and 0 otherwise, d_{it2} takes the value one for an actual 80 mg dose at time t and zero otherwise, d_{it3} takes the value one for an actual 120 mg dose at time t and zero otherwise, and γ_{t1}, γ_{t2}, γ_{t3} represent dose-specific treatment effects at time t. The coefficients $\{\beta_{tj}\}$ model the association of the outcome at time t with the values of outcomes at previous time points. The means are modeled as linear functions of the baseline score x_{i0} and site-specific effects, although the latter are included only for $t = 1$ since they added little predictive power to the regressions for later time points. The fact that indicators for the assigned dosages r_{i1}, r_{i2} are not included in the model implies that the distribution of outcomes depend on the treatments actually received rather than on the treatments randomized. This assumption is related to the "weak exclusion restriction of treatment assignment given treatment received" in Imbens and Rubin [28].

Multiple imputations based on this model were created sequentially, first filling in missing values of y_{i2} as draws from the predictive distribution of y_{i2} given y_{i1}, then filling in missing values of y_{i3} as draws from the predictive distribution of y_{i3} given observed or imputed values of y_{i1}, y_{i2} and so on. To account for uncertainty in parameter estimates, model parameters are first drawn from their posterior distribution and then missing values drawn from their predictive distribution conditional on the drawn parameters. Here, regression coefficients arising in these predictions were drawn from their posterior distributions based on the available data up to that time point, as is appropriate for the monotone missing-data pattern. Specifically, a residual variance was drawn as the residual sum of squares divided by a chi-squared deviate with residual degrees of freedom, and then regression coefficients were drawn as multivariate normal centered at their estimates, with covariance matrix given by the inverse of the design matrix multiplied by the drawn residual variance [27]. Programming of our methods was carried out using SAS macros [20]. An annotated listing of the SAS macro for the tacrine example is available in Dr. Little's World Wide Web home page: http://www.sph.umich.edu/~rlittle, and can be modified for other applications.

Since this imputation model conditions on the treatment information d_i, it requires information about nature of the treatment after drop-out. In some studies information about dose after drop-out may be unknown or unreliable. In the tacrine study an attempt was made to follow cases after drop-out, and dosage information was recorded. Dosage information might be used for imputations, although it could be argued that this limits the generalizability of the study to cases where similar dosage patterns are predicted in the real population; for example, it is questionable whether non-zero doses for tacrine should be allowed when imputing for control cases, even if

they actually occurred. Since there seems no obvious single answer to these questions, we carry out a sensitivity analysis of the tacrine data set, where imputations are obtained for a range of alternative assumptions about dose after drop-out.

The first assumption is that the subject continues on the same treatment as that immediately prior to drop-out. We call this the "continuing-dose" model. Subjects in the high-dose groups that drop out prior to the protocol dose increase are imputed to receive that increase. While this model is unrealistic in the tacrine example when drop-out is caused by the side effect, the analysis is interesting since it is the assumption implicit in an incomplete-data analysis based on an MAR model for the drop-out process, such as would be obtained from programs such as BMDPAM or SAS Proc Mixed. It might be expected to yield optimistic estimates of intent-to-treat treatment effects, if useful treatment effects exist and drop-outs in the treatment group in fact receive reduced doses after drop-out. Note that if treatment group "as randomized" is similar to treatment group "as treated", that is there is good compliance with the randomized treatment, then imputation under the continuing-dose model should yield similar estimates to the corresponding intent-to-treat analysis of the incomplete data assuming MAR, that is, the analysis in row (1B) of Table 10.1. Block (2A) of Table 10.1 shows the results of fitting the intent-to-treat model of Eqs. (5) and (6) to $M = 10$ data sets multiply imputed under this "continuing-dose" model. The multiple-imputation inference, summarized in the "MI Inference" row, shows estimates, standard errors, p values and confidence intervals computed using the methods summarized in example 1. The results are quite similar to the results in row (1B) for the ignorable intent-to-treat model fitted to the monotone incomplete data, illustrating that these two analyses make similar assumptions.

Our second assumption is that the subject reverts to the control treatment after drop-out, that is the placebo treatment in the tacrine example. We call this the "zero-dose" model. This analysis tends to minimize differences between treatment and control after drop-out, and hence might be expected to yield deflated estimates of intent-to-treat treatment effects. It may be argued that the zero-dose model is too conservative here, since the liver side-effect of tacrine is a often transient effect, and many who dropped out from this side-effect in fact resumed tacrine after a time. Analyses under the continuing-dose and zero-dose models plausibly bracket the actual effects of the treatments in this and other situations. Block (3A) shows the results of fitting the intent-to-treat model of Eqs. (1) and (2) to data sets multiply imputed under the zero-dose model. Note that the summary estimated treatment effects are half the size of the estimates under the continuing-dose model (−2.10 vs −4.17 for 80 mg, and −1.83 vs −3.47 for 120 mg). The effect for the 120 mg dose remains significant at the 5% level ($p = 0.02$), but the effect for the 80 mg dose no longer achieves statistical significance at the 5% level ($p = 0.07$). These results illustrate the more conservative nature of the intent-to-treat analysis based on the zero-dose model for this application.

Our final assumption is the "nearest-dose" model, where (a) cases in the control group are assigned a zero dose after drop-out, and (b) cases in the treatment groups are assigned a treatment-group dose (0, 40, 80 or 120 mg) that is closest to the actual recorded dose after drop-out, rounding up in the case of ties. The actual dose cannot be used here since the imputation model treats dosage as a categorical rather than a continuous variable. This model seems the most realistic for the tacrine example, although it is "counter-factual" in that some control cases took tacrine after drop-out. Estimated treatment effects for the nearest-dose model are shown in block (4A), and are −2.79 for 80 mg ($p = 0.02$), −2.73 for 120 mg ($p = 0.001$). These estimates, arguably the most realistic for the tacrine data set, lie between those for the zero-dose and continuing-dose models, reflecting predicted effects of reduced but non-zero tacrine doses after drop-out.

An important feature of the proposed analysis is that effects of treatment prior to drop-out are allowed to extend to effects after drop-out, via the estimates of the coefficients β_{tj} in the model (3.3). An excessively conservative analysis imputes the drop-outs in the treatment group like controls, ignoring carry-over effects of previous treatments. This approach can be illustrated by fitting our imputation model with the coefficients β_{tj} set to zero. Results are presented in block (3C) of Table 10.1, labeled "Zero-dose without adjustment". Note that the treatment effects are smaller than for the zero-dose model in block (3A), indicating that there is some predicted treatment gain for individuals who drop out before the end of the study and then receive a zero treatment dose. A fuller analysis of this data set, including analyses that make use of week 18 data for the retrieved drop-outs, is presented in Little and Yau [5].

An important assumption of the proposed imputation model is that the conditional distribution of outcomes after drop-out, given outcomes prior to drop-out, dose and other covariate information, is the same as the conditional distribution for cases continuing in the study. In the tacrine study there is essentially no information about the effects on outcome of switching to lower doses, so this assumption cannot be checked empirically. However, some

such assumption is needed to include the incomplete cases in the analysis, and the assumption adopted seems plausible.

The analysis of the tacrine data reflects our belief that there is often no single definitive intent-to-treat analysis for the repeated-measures problem considered. Any analysis requires assumptions about the dose after drop-out, and the choice of assumptions is subject to debate. Ideally, one should make assumptions that reflect how the drug will be used in the real world after the study, but knowledge about this will usually be sketchy at the clinical trial phase. Given this reality, an analysis that assesses sensitivity of answers to alternative assumptions, as in Table 10.1, may be the best option. The lack of a definitive intent-to-treat analysis has design implications for longitudinal clinical trials where drop-outs are likely. The tacrine trial attempted to collect information about dosages and outcomes after drop-out. While this information is often problematic because of its observational nature and the absence of blinding, it seems preferable to have it available for one or more of the sensitivity analyses.

A general advantage of multiple imputation over the maximum likelihood analysis of the previous section is that differences between the imputation and analysis model are readily accommodated. Here, the crucial difference is that the imputation model conditions on actual treatment (observed or imputed) rather than the treatment randomized. More generally, observed variables that improve the imputations should be included in the imputation model, even if they are not included in the final analysis model because they are not considered exogenous to the treatment.

Maximum Likelihood for Nonignorable Models

What if the missing data are not missing at random? Some new methods allow us to deal with situations where the data are not missing at random, by modeling the joint distribution of y_i, β_i, R_i [10,21,29]. There are two broad classes of models for this joint distribution. "Selection" models model the joint distribution as:

$$[y_i, \beta_i, R_i | X_i] = [y_i | X_i, \beta_i][\beta_i | X_i][R_i | X_i, y_i, \beta_i]$$
(7)

where parentheses represent distributions. "Pattern-mixture" models model the joint distribution as:

$$[y_i, \beta_i, R_i | X_i] = [y_i | X_i, \beta_i, R_i][\beta_i | X_i, R_i][R_i | X_i]$$
(8)

The first two components of the selection model (7) concern the joint distribution of y_i, β_i, and simply represent the model in the absence of any missing values, for example a model of the form (3). The third component of the selection model (7) concerns the distribution of R_i given y_i,β_i, and models the drop-out mechanism – that is, the probability of dropping out at a particular time as a function of other variables. There are many possible choices for this model, depending on the assumed reasons for drop-out. Nonignorable models are very hard to specify and vulnerable to model misspecification. We often do not have sufficient information to simultaneously estimate the parameters of the drop-out mechanism and the parameters of the complete data model. A useful approach in such situations is to do a sensitivity analysis to see how much the answers change for various assumptions about the drop-out mechanism.

In Little [10] two kinds of nonignorable drop-out are distinguished. The first is "outcome-dependent drop-out", where drop-out depends on y_i. In symbols:

$$[R_i | X_i, y_{obs,i}, y_{mis,i}, \beta_i] = [R_i | X_i, y_{obs,i}, y_{mis,i}] \quad (9)$$

For example, if the repeated measures are of pain and drop-out depends on the value of the pain variable at the time of drop-out, that would be outcome-dependent, because missingness then would depend on the (unobserved) value of Y at the time of drop-out. Another class of models assumes "random coefficient-dependent drop-out," where the probability of dropping out depends on the underlying random coefficients β_i. In symbols:

$$[R_i | X_i, y_i, \beta_i] = [R_i | X_i, \beta_i] \quad (10)$$

For example, one of the random coefficients may represent a slope. If people who have more rapid decline tend to drop out more frequently than those with less rapid decline, dropping out depends on this underlying, unobserved slope. Wu and Carroll [30] and Wu and Bailey [31] consider models for slope-dependent drop-out, using the term "informative censoring" to describe the drop-out mechanism. I prefer the term "random-coefficient dependent drop-out" since it is more explicit about the assumed form of the mechanism.

In summary, Eqs. (9) and (10) represent two kinds of missing-data models that are nonignorable: one where missingness depends on the missing components of Y_i, and one where missingness depends on underlying random effects. Both can be fitted, but we must determine the plausible mechanism in the particular setting. This is a substantive issue, and cannot usually be decided empirically using the data.

As mentioned earlier, there is another way to factor the joint distribution of y_i,β_i, R_i besides the selection models of the form of Eq. (7). Pattern-mixture models have the form given by Eq. (8). The main point about pattern-mixture models is that the distribution of y_i and β_i is conditioned on R_i, which means we are modeling in strata defined by the values of R_i, that is, the number of measurements. An advantage of this way of factoring the distribution is that this part of the model can usually be fit using standard software such as PROC MIXED [20], by simply including R_i as a covariate in the model for the distribution of the y_i values. Specification of the distribution of R_i given X_i in Eq. (8) allows us to combine the patterns, and derive inferences for the whole population. This requires some additional software, which is not yet available but should be soon. Just as there are selection models representing different mechanisms, there are also pattern-mixture models for alternative mechanisms. An advantage of the pattern-mixture modeling approach over selection models is that assumptions about the form of the missing-data mechanism are sometimes less specific in their parametric form, since they are incorporated in the model via parameter restrictions.

Example 4. Pattern-Mixture Models Applied to a Haloperidol Dosage Study for Schizophrenia

Little and Wang [32] present an example of a sensitivity analysis for a haloperidol dosage study for schizophrenia. It is difficult to determine a correct dosage of haloperidol, because if the dose is too high there are side effects whereas if the dose is too low the drug is not effective. The outcome variable is a rating scale for schizophrenia, BPRSS. With some simplification of the data, we have three repeated measures: BPRSS at baseline (Y_1), week 1 (Y_2) and week 4 (Y_3). The covariates consist of two dummy variables indicating each of the three dosages of haloperidol: 5, 10 and 20 mg. Some cases dropped out at week 4, and drop-out is differential across the treatment group because the higher the dose, the more people who dropped out. Overall, 29 of 65 dropped out, so the extent of missing data is high.

In the pattern-mixture model fit to these data, there are just two patterns of missing data: the cases with all the measurements, and the cases with Y_1,Y_2 observed and Y_3 missing. Within each pattern a separate multivariate-normal regression model is fit, with distinct means of Y for each dosage. Assumptions about the drop-out mechanism allow us to estimate the parameters for the incomplete pattern.

Specifically, it is assumed that the probability of dropping out at the third time point is a function of X and a linear combination $c_1Y_1 + c_2Y_2 + c_3Y_3$ of Y_1, Y_2, Y_3. The ability to estimate the coefficients c_1, c_2, c_3 together with the other model parameters is very limited, so instead models are fitted for a variety of assumed values of these coefficients, to assess sensitivity. In particular, estimates are displayed for the following models:

Ignorable model: $c_3 = 0$. In this model missingness depends only on Y_1, Y_2, which are fully observed, so the data are MAR.
Mechanism A: $(c_1, c_2, c_3) = (0.4, 0.4, 0.2)$.
Mechanism B: $(c_1, c_2, c_3) = (0.3, 0.3, 0.4)$.
Mechanism C: $(c_1, c_2, c_3) = (0.1, 0.1, 0.8)$.
Mechanism D: $(c_1, c_2, c_3) = (0, 0, 1)$.

When c_3 deviates from zero, there is a dependence of dropping out on the value Y_3 at the time of drop-out. Mechanism A is still quite close to MAR, because most of the dependence is on Y_1, Y_2. Mechanism D implies that the probability of dropping out depends only on the value Y_3 at the time of drop-out, not on previous values. This is the most extreme departure from MAR considered.

The results in Table 13.2 display treatment effects for the three dosage groups, defined as a difference between baseline in week 4, for the ignorable model and for the four choices of missing-data mechanisms A to D. The fact that conclusions do not differ markedly across these analyses suggests that results are relatively insensitive to the mechanism in this particular example.

This example is intended to convey the idea of a sensitivity analysis in a missing-data setting. Since we cannot estimate the missing-data mechanism very well, we look at a variety of plausible choices for the mechanism to see how much the answers change.

Table 13.2. Maximum likelihood estimates (standard errors) of the difference in the mean of BPRSS between baseline and week 4, for pattern-mixture models with a range of assumptions about the missing-data mechanism

	Treatment group		
	Dose 5	Dose 10	Dose 20
Sample size:	15	34	16
Missing fraction:	0.33	0.41	0.63
Ignorable model	3.291 (0.897)	4.087 (0.618)	6.463 (1.044)
Mechanism A	3.276 (0.898)	4.139 (0.621)	6.528 (1.048)
Mechanism B	3.251 (0.909)	4.184 (0.631)	6.610 (1.072)
Mechanism C	3.181 (0.945)	4.249 (0.663)	6.808 (1.155)
Mechanism D	3.140 (0.968)	4.268 (0.684)	6.913 (1.208)

Bayesian Simulation Methods

Maximum likelihood is most useful when sample sizes are large, since then the log-likelihood is nearly quadratic and can be summarized well using the ML estimate θ and its large sample variance–covariance matrix. When sample sizes are small, a useful alternative approach is to add a prior distribution for the parameters and compute the posterior distribution of the parameters of interest. For MAR models this posterior is:

$$p(\theta|Y_{obs}, M, X) \equiv p(\theta|Y_{obs}, X)$$
$$= \text{const.}\, p(\theta|X) \times f(Y_{obs}|X, \theta)$$

where $p(\theta|X)$ is the prior and $f(Y_{obs}|X, \theta)$ is the density of the observed data. Since the posterior distribution rarely has a simple analytic form for incomplete-data problems, simulation methods are often used to generate draws of θ from the posterior distribution $p(\theta|Y_{obs}, M, X)$.

For missing data problems where the likelihood can be factored into complete-data components, draws can be obtained directly from the complete-data posterior distributions and transformed back to the original parameters (Little and Rubin [21], chapter 6). In more complex problems, iterative algorithms such as data augmentation [33] and or the Gibbs' sampler [34] can be used to yield draws from the joint posterior distribution. For more information on these methods, see for example Gelman et al. [35] and Tanner [36].

These Bayesian simulation methods are closely related to multiple imputation, in that they involve drawing values of the missing data from their predictive distribution. In particular, Gilks et al. [37] discuss Gibbs' sampling algorithms for random-effects models appropriate for incomplete longitudinal data. Schafer [38] developed algorithms that use iterative Bayesian simulation to multiply impute rectangular data sets with arbitrary patterns of missing values when the missing-data mechanism is ignorable. The methods are applicable when the rows of the complete-data matrix can be modeled as independent observations from the multivariate Normal, multinomial loglinear and general location models. The BUGS computer program [39] can also be used for Bayesian analysis of longitudinal data. Little and Wang [32] present a Bayesian analysis of the data-set in example 2 that yields slightly larger and more realistic standard errors than the maximum likelihood analysis.

Conclusion

In summary, modeling the data and modeling the drop-out mechanism provides a general framework for considering missing data in repeated-measure studies. There are many possible mechanisms for drop-out. Drop-out might depend on covariates such as the treatment arm or age; it could depend on observed repeated-measures but not on missing variables (MAR); or it could depend on missing outcomes or on underlying unobserved variables (not MAR). We need to consider what is plausible in the substantive setting.

The data often provide limited information to distinguish among non-MAR alternatives. It is important to determine the reasons for drop-out and consider what mechanisms are plausible. One of the advantages of this modeling framework is that if we know and record some of the reasons people drop out, we can incorporate that into the model for the drop-out mechanism. Doing so could lead to better answers, particularly in cases where the data are not missing at random. But when little is known about the mechanism, we are often forced to do sensitivity analyses, because we lack the data to simultaneously estimate all the parameters.

Acknowledgements. This research benefited from collaborations with Don Rubin, Nat Schenker, Steven Wang and Linda Yau, and was supported by National Science Foundation Grant DMS 9408837 and by the Michigan Alzheimer's Research Center (NIH/NIA grant AG08671). I thank Parke Davis Pharmaceuticals for permission to use the tacrine data set, and Jim Mintz and Theodore Van Putten for permission to use the haloperidol data set.

References

1. Heyting A, Tolboom JTBM, Essers JGA. Statistical handling of drop-outs in longitudinal clinical trials. Stat Med 1992;11: 2043–2063.
2. Gornbein JG, Lazaro C, Little RJA. Incomplete data in repeated measures analysis. Stat Methods Med Res 1992;1:275–295.
3. Little RJA, Schenker N. Missing data. In: Arminger G, Clogg CC, Sobel ME, editors. Handbook for statistical modeling in the social and behavioral sciences. New York: Plenum Press, 1994:39–75.
4. Little RJA. Biostatistical analysis with missing data. In: Armitage P, Colton T, editors. Encyclopedia of biostatistics. New York: Wiley, 1997.
5. Little RJA, Yau L. Intent-to-treat analysis in longitudinal studies with drop-outs. Biometrics 1996;52:1324–1333.
6. Knapp MJ, Knopman DS, Solomon PR, Pendlebury WW, Davis CS, Gracon SI. A 30-week randomized controlled trial of high-dose tacrine in patients with Alzheimer's disease. JAMA 1994; 271:985–991.
7. Rosen WG, Mohs RC, Davis KL. A new rating scale for Alzheimer's disease. Am J Psychiatry 1984;141:1356–1364.
8. Meinert CL. Terminology: a plea for standardization. Controlled Clin Trials 1980;2:97–99.
9. Rubin DB. Inference and missing data. Biometrika 1976;63: 581–592.
10. Little RJA. Modeling the drop-out mechanism in longitudinal studies. J Am Stat Assoc 1995;90:1112–1121.
11. Murray GD, Findlay JG. Correcting for the bias caused by drop-outs in hypertension trials. Stat Med 1988;7:941–946.
12. Pocock SJ. Clinical trials: a practical approach. New York: Wiley.
13. Little RJA, Su HL. Item nonresponse in panel surveys. In: Panel Surveys, Kasprzyk D, Duncan G, Kalton G, Singh MP, editors. New York: Wiley, 1989:400–425.
14. Beale EML, Little RJA. Missing values in multivariate analysis. J R Stat Soc B 1975;37:129–145.
15. Orchard T, Woodbury MA. A missing information principle: theory and applications. In: Proceedings of the Sixth Berkeley Symposium on Mathematical Statistics and Probability vol 1. 1972:697–715.
16. Rubin DB, Schenker N. Multiple imputation for interval estimation from simple random samples with ignorable nonresponse. J Am Stat Assoc 1986;81:366–374.
17. Park T. A comparison of the generalized estimating equation approach with the maximum likelihood approach for repeated measurements, Stat Med 1993;12:1723–1732.
18. Robins J, Rotnitsky A, Zhao LP. Analysis of semiparametric regression models for repeated outcomes in the presence of missing data. J Am Stat Assoc 1995;90:106–121.
19. Dixon WJ. BMDP statistical software. Berkeley: University of California Press, 1988.
20. SAS. The mixed procedure. In: SAS/STAT software: changes and enhancements, release 6.07. Technical Report P-229. Cary: NC: SAS Institute, 1992: chap 16.
21. Little RJA, Rubin DB. Statistical analysis with missing data. New York: Wiley, 1987.
22. Dempster AP, Laird NM, Rubin DB. Maximum likelihood from incomplete data via the EM algorithm (with discussion). J R Stat Soc Ser B 1977;39:1–38.
23. Harville DA. Maximum likelihood approaches to variance component estimation and to related problems (with discussion), J Am Stat Assoc 1977;72:320–340.
24. Laird NM, Ware JH. Random-effects models for longitudinal data. Biometrics 1982;38:963–974.
25. Jennrich RI, Schluchter MD. Unbalanced repeated-measures models with structured covariance matrices. Biometrics 1986; 42:805–820.
26. Hedeker D. MIXOR: a Fortran program for mixed-effects ordinal probit and logistic regression. University of Illinois at Chicago: Prevention Research Center, 1993.
27. Rubin DB. Multiple imputation for nonresponse in surveys. New York: Wiley, 1987.
28. Imbens GW, Rubin DB. Bayesian inference for causal effects in randomized experiments with noncompliance. Ann Stat 1995;25:305–327.
29. Diggle P, Kenward MG. Informative dropout in longitudinal data analysis (with discussion). Appl Stat 1994;43:49–94.
30. Wu MC, Carroll RJ. Estimation and comparison of changes in the presence of informative right censoring by modeling the censoring process. Biometrics 1988;44:175–188.
31. Wu MC, Bailey KR. Estimation and comparison of changes in the presence of informative right censoring: conditional linear model. Biometrics 1989;45:939–955.
32. Little RJA, Wang Y-X. Pattern-mixture models for multivariate incomplete data with covariates. Biometrics 1996;52:98–111.

33. Tanner MA, Wong WH. The calculation of posterior distributions by data augmentation. J Am Stat Assoc 1987;82:528–550.

34. Geman S, Geman D. Stochastic relaxation, Gibbs' distributions and the Bayesian restoration of images. IEEE Trans Pattern Anal Machine Intell 1984;6:721–741.

35. Gelman A, Carlin JB, Stern HS, Rubin DB. Bayesian data analysis, 1st edn. New York: Chapman Hall, 1995.

36. Tanner MA. Tools for statistical inference: methods for the exploration of posterior distributions and likelihood functions. 3rd ed. New York: Springer, 1996.

37. Gilks WR, Wang CC, Yvonnet B, Coursaget P. Random-effects models for longitudinal data using Gibbs' sampling, Biometrics 1993;49:441–453.

38. Schafer JL. Analysis of incomplete multivariate data. London: Chapman & Hall, 1996.

39. Spiegelhalter D, Thomas A, Best N, Gilks W. BUGS: Bayesian Inference Using Gibbs' Sampling. Cambridge: MRC Biostatistics Unit, 1995.

14. The Role of Meta-analyses in Clinical Research: Uses and Limitations

L.A. Stewart

Introduction

Meta-analyses and systematic reviews are key elements in the objective and systematic evaluation of health care interventions. Their value is increasingly acknowledged by health care professionals, researchers and policy makers. Faced with unmanageable amounts of information, these groups require reliable summaries of research on which to base clinical and policy decisions [1] and to guide future research.

In the past, synthesising medical information has been the role of the review article, but there has been considerable criticism of this approach [2]. In contrast to reports of primary research, traditional narrative reviews rarely make their objectives and methods explicit and can represent little more than the subjective opinions of influential individuals. Reviewers are often in the difficult position of trying to evaluate conflicting or equivocal studies based on a qualitative and perhaps selective reading of the literature. Indeed, it has been suggested that "because reviewers have not used scientific methods, advice on some life-saving therapies has been delayed for more than a decade while other treatments have been recommended long after controlled research has shown them to be harmful" [3]. In contrast, systematic reviews use explicit methodology, aim to assess all relevant evidence objectively, and go to considerable lengths to achieve this [4]. Where appropriate, meta-analysis offers a quantitative means of combining this evidence.

A well-designed meta-analysis can be defined as an exhaustive, objective and systematic quantitative review of the best available evidence addressing a specific question. In practice, this means that most meta-analyses in medical research involve the summary and quantitative combination of the results of all relevant and suitably similar randomised trials.

Why We Need Meta-analyses

It is generally accepted that the best primary evidence on the effectiveness of health care interventions comes from the results of well-designed and conducted randomised controlled trials (RCTs). As in any scientific experiment, the observed effect in a clinical trial is composed of the true underlying effect plus the effect of both random and systematic error. Random error can never be eliminated, but can be minimised by evaluating the data from large numbers of patients. Systematic error or bias can arise through poor design or conduct of a study, and its effects can easily be as large or larger than the size of clinically important treatment effects [5].

Random Error

Individual RCTs are rarely large enough to detect moderate but potentially worthwhile differences between treatments. In most areas of medicine, major breakthroughs are rare and we may generally anticipate that new treatments will yield only modest improvements in outcome. Such benefits may, of course, be extremely important to individual patients and could, in common diseases, have considerable impact in public health. Assuming a baseline event rate of 50% for a standard therapy, then a typical two-arm trial with 400–500 patients is capable only of detecting benefits of a new treatment in excess of 15%, i.e. improving positive outcomes from 50% to 65% or more. To detect a 10% difference with reliability requires twice this number, while a 5% difference would require 3500 individuals. Unfortunately, few trials have recruited such large numbers of patients and for many practical and political reasons, trials of this size are not feasible in many circumstances.

In any group of small to moderately sized trials addressing similar questions, by chance alone a few may have demonstrated statistically significant positive or negative results, but most will be inconclusive. However, combining the results in a meta-analysis might give sufficient statistical power to answer the questions reliably. Importantly, the increased patient numbers also provide more reliable and precise estimates of the size of any observed effect, as the confidence intervals will be narrower. So, by including large numbers of patients, meta-analyses aim to reduce random error allowing us to make a more reliable assessment of whether a treatment works and if it does, the magnitude of any observed benefit; both of which are important in determining treatment policy.

Bias

Unfortunately it is all too common for those individual well-publicised trials, which have produced the most striking results, to be emphasised in both the primary and derivative medical literature. Perhaps the most important reason for performing systematic meta-analyses is to avoid this biased viewpoint and encourage conclusions on the relative merits of different treatments to be based on the results of *all* relevant trials. Additionally, the design, conduct, analysis and reporting of individual trials may be subject to many potential biases [6] which may be noted and possibly rectified in a well-designed meta-analysis.

The two main principles underlying meta-analysis are therefore to achieve sufficient statistical power to obtain reliable and precise results and to avoid bias and assess *all* the relevant evidence.

Principles of Meta-analysis

The fundamental assumption of any meta-analysis is that in a group of trials addressing similar questions, although the observed size of treatment effect may vary from trial to trial, the results are likely to be in same direction (although in a small number of cases this direction may be reversed by chance alone). It would be wrong to assume that the effect of a treatment in different patient populations, which may vary in a number of important characteristics, would be to produce exactly the same risk reduction. However, it is reasonable to assume that the net effect will tend to be in the same direction favouring one

or other treatment. Although the direction of effect may be obscured in an individual trial, when all the evidence is considered the benefit or detriment of treatment will be reflected in the overall pattern of individual trial results and the "summation" of these results will provide an estimate of the average treatment effect.

It is important to note that, in this summation, the only direct comparisons that are made are between patients in the respective arms of each trial and it is only the *results* of these individual within-trial comparisons which are combined.

Different Types of Meta-analysis

Although there are increasing numbers of papers published in the medical literature which describe themselves as meta-analyses, not all such projects are of a similar design, quality or validity. Just because a meta-analysis is based on large numbers of patients does not guarantee reliability and readers should critically appraise reports of meta-analyses in the same way that they would a clinical trial. There is a continuum in the effort that can be invested in a meta-analysis ranging from those based only on the information that can be readily extracted from the published literature, to those which aim to analyse updated individual patient data from all relevant trials, both published and unpublished.

All meta-analyses should be conducted objectively and systematically, and analyse all appropriate data in order to reduce bias. The meta-analyses that perhaps go to the greatest lengths to achieve this, and which might be regarded as a "gold standard" approach, involve the central collection, checking and analysis of individual patient data (IPD) [7]. However, meta-analyses which use aggregate data, either supplied directly by trialists or more frequently extracted from published reports, are less resource-intensive and more common. Although IPD meta-analyses are more time- and resource-intensive than other forms of systematic review, in some cases they may be the only way to obtain reliable answers from retrospective data.

There is evidence that meta-analyses based only on data extracted from published papers may give estimates of treatment effects and of their significance that are not confirmed when all the randomised evidence is re-analysed in an IPD meta-analysis [8–10]. For example, a comparison of the results of an IPD meta-analysis of platinum-based combination chemotherapy versus single-agent non-platinum drugs in advanced ovarian cancer [11] with a similar analysis using only data that could be extracted from the published papers, found that the IPD analysis gave less encouraging results [8].

The IPD meta-analysis was based on 11 trials and 1329 patients, whereas the analysis of published summary data included 8 trials and only 788 patients. The IPD had a median follow-up of $6^{1}/_{2}$ years whereas point estimates of survival at 30 months had to be used for the published summary data (the latest point in time for which survival data were available for all trials in the published reports). The published summary data favoured combination chemotherapy with an estimated improvement in survival at 30 months of 7.5%, which was marginally significant ($p = 0.027$). The IPD suggested only a 2.5% improvement which did not reach conventional levels of significance ($p = 0.30$). The differences were attributable to the effect of missing trials (those unpublished trials plus those which did not publish the required information), excluded patients, the point in time at which the aggregate data analyses were based, the method of analysis and also to the additional long-term follow-up which was available from the IPD. None of these factors was found to be very much more important than the others, rather they each contributed cumulatively to the difference. The analysis based on published summary data not only provided a statistically significant result but gave an estimated benefit which was 3 times larger than that suggested by the IPD. Given the poor prognosis for advanced ovarian cancer, when balanced against other factors such as toxicity and cost, the clinical interpretation of the results from the two approaches could well be different.

A major benefit of IPD is that it enables time-to-event analysis to be done which can be vital in illnesses where prolongation of survival is important, or where time to onset or recurrence of symptoms is more important than the simple count of presence or absence of symptoms at a specified point in time. The IPD approach is also the only practical way to carry out analyses to investigate whether any observed treatment effect is consistent across well-defined groups of patients (often termed sub-group analysis). Where trials have used different classifications or scales of measurement, IPD provides the opportunity to translate between scales and combine data which might not otherwise be feasible. It also allows detailed data checking to ensure consistency and quality of randomisation and follow-up. Importantly, it also means that up-to-date follow-up can be collected and thereby provides a valuable opportunity to look at longer-term outcomes.

Some additional advantages of direct collaboration with trialists, when collecting either IPD or summary data from source, is that this contact can result in more complete identification of relevant trials and better compliance in providing missing data. Discussions with the trialists during the project might also lead to a more balanced interpretation and wider endorsement and dissemination of the results and to better clarification of, and collaboration in, further research.

It will, of course, not always be necessary to go to the lengths of collecting IPD. For example, if we are interested in binary outcomes that are likely to occur relatively quickly after enrolment in a trial, where all relevant trials are published and data presented in a comprehensive and compatible way, then the most straightforward of meta-analyses based on data presented in trial publications is probably all that is required to obtain a reliable answer to the question posed. More usually unpublished trials will need to be assessed and trialists contacted to provide at least some additional summary data.

Whatever approach is taken – using data from publications, obtaining summary data directly from trialists or collecting IPD – it is vital that every effort is made to obtain all the relevant data and that appropriate methodology is used. Some of the most important methodological issues are discussed below.

Meta-analysis Methods

Include All Randomised Trials

It is now widely acknowledged that RCTs with statistically significant or striking results are more likely to be published than those with non-significant results, owing both to editorial policy and to the fact that investigators themselves do not submit negative studies for publication [12]. In consequence of such selective publication, the medical literature can represent a skewed or biased picture of all trials which have addressed similar issues. This bias towards the positive will be reflected in opinions and all forms of review based on the published literature alone and could lead to unjustified conclusions and subsequently to inappropriate decisions about patient care, health policy and future clinical research.

Although some would argue that unpublished data should not be included in a meta-analysis as it has not been subject to peer review and is therefore unreliable, this criticism can be circumvented by obtaining the trial protocol and by careful checking of the IPD or summary data supplied by the trialist. In fact, such checking is likely to be considerably more rigorous than is possible during peer review of a manuscript. Conversely it should be noted that publication of a well-written paper in a high-profile journal does not necessarily guarantee the quality of the actual data. Therefore to gain a balanced picture, it is important that all the randomised evidence is considered, irrespective of whether or not it is published. Clearly any meta-analysis of the published literature alone will always be at risk of publication bias.

There is good evidence that simple electronic bibliographic searching is currently poor at identifying RCTs [13]. Not only are positive trials more likely to be published than negative or inconclusive ones, but particularly striking results are perhaps more likely to be published in those English language [14] high-impact journals [15] indexed by bibliographic databases. Furthermore, such databases do not cover all medical journals: MEDLINE, for example, indexes only 3700 out of around 16 000 journals and indexing is not always accurate. To make full use of computerised databases it is important that efficient search strategies are employed [13] and inexperienced searchers should seek as much help as possible. Efforts are now in progress by the Cochrane Collaboration retrospectively to tag all RCTs and revise coding within MEDLINE to improve future identification of trials. In the meantime, most meta-analyses must additionally search appropriate journals and meeting abstracts by hand, consult trial registers and may also ask industry and experts in the field to help identify trials.

Include Only Randomised Trials

Randomised trials provide the best means of obtaining an unbiased and fair comparison between medical treatments and the problems associated with non-randomised studies are well documented [16]. Prospective allocation by a method that ensures that treatment assignment cannot be known in advance, ensures that individuals are not selected deliberately or unwittingly to receive a particular intervention. For example, a clinician with an understandable desire to see a benefit from a new treatment could perhaps subconsciously decide whether or not to enter a particular patient into a trial if they knew in advance to which treatment that patient would be allocated. The process of randomisation reduces the likelihood of systematic differences between patient groups because allocation is made according to the play of chance. In subsequent analysis, any observed differences should be due to differences in treatment and not to differences in the patient characteristics in the two groups. However, not all studies described in published reports as being randomised but without providing details of the method of allocation, can be assumed to be free

of bias in the allocation of treatment. It is not unusual to find out on further enquiry that "randomisation" has been done by birthdate, date of clinic visit or by alternate allocation, all of which could be biased. Even within RCTs, there is evidence that the method of concealment (how difficult it is to know or guess the next treatment to be allocated) is correlated with trial outcome, such that those trials with the most secure methods of randomisation give the least positive results [17].

Many meta-analyses are therefore restricted to "properly" randomised trials and any trials allocating treatment by quasi-random methods such as date of birth are excluded.

Include All and Only Randomised Patients

All patients who were randomised should be analysed and included in the meta-analysis. Any patients who were not randomised should be excluded. Unfortunately, not all RCTs follow this policy when reporting their results and patients can be excluded from published analysis for a number of reasons. Such exclusions, if related to treatment, could seriously bias the results, for example by excluding patients unable to tolerate the allocated therapy or follow the treatment schedule. Conversely, in some cases non-randomised patients may be included in published analyses if, for example, the RCT was preceded by a non-randomised pilot phase such that these early patients remain in the analyses. As IPD meta-analyses, or those collecting summary data from source, do not rely on the original analyses, excluded randomised patients can be reinstated in the analysis and any non-randomised patients removed from the dataset.

Analyses
Binary Data

The statistical techniques most frequently employed in meta-analyses are based on the Mantel–Haenszel method of combining data over a series of 2×2 contingency tables. Basically this involves comparing the observed and expected event rate on treatment and control within each trial and then combining the results of these individual trials.

There are a number of ways of doing this. The simplest, an example of which is shown in Box 14.1, makes use of the proportion of patients event-free at a given time point. For each individual trial the overall number of events within the study is used to calculate the expected number of events that would occur if there were no difference between the two

Box 14.1. Calculating an odds ratio: hypothetical example

Suppose there are four trials comparing treatment versus control and that the number of deaths on each arm of these trials are as below:

	Treatment	Control	P value
Trial A	29/67	39/72	0.20
Trial B	3/23	10/30	0.09
Trial C	7/39	11/28	0.05
Trial D	45/145	64/172	0.30

Individually, none of these trials shows a statistically significant difference between the number of deaths on the treatment and control arms. For trial A there are 67 patients on the treatment arm, of whom 29 have died. The expected number of deaths on treatment (E), $O - E$ value ($O - E$), variance (V) and odds ratio (OR) can be calculated as follows:

	Treatment	Control	Total
Dead	29	39	68 (D)
Alive	38	33	71
Total	67 (n_t)	72	139 (N)

$$E = (D/N)n_t \qquad O - E = 29 - 32.78$$
$$= (68/139)\, 67 \qquad\qquad = -3.78$$
$$= 32.78$$
$$\text{OR} = \exp(O - E/V) \qquad V = [E/(1 - n_t/N)\,(N - D)]/(N - 1)$$
$$= \exp(-3.78/8.74) \qquad\quad = [32.78(1 - 67/139)\,(139 - 68)]/138$$
$$= 0.65 \qquad\qquad\qquad = 8.74$$

Similar values can be calculated for trials B, C and D:

	$O - E$	Variance	Odds ratio
Trial A	−3.78	8.74	0.65
Trial B	−2.64	2.46	0.34
Trial C	−3.48	3.25	0.34
Trial D	−4.86	17.81	0.76

Combined or pooled OR can now be calculated as follows:

$$\text{OR} = \exp[\Sigma(O - E)/\Sigma\, V]$$
$$= \exp(-14.76/31.56)$$
$$= 0.63(95\%\ \text{CI}\ 0.45-0.89)^* \qquad 95\%\ \text{CI} = \exp[(\Sigma O - E/\Sigma V) + (1.96/(\sqrt{\Sigma\, V}))]$$

Although none of the individual trials in this hypothetical example showed a significant difference between treatments, the combined OR shows a conventionally significant survival in favour of treatment, with a 36% reduction in the odds of death for the treatment group patients.

arms of the trial. The difference between the actual observed (O) and the expected (E) number of events is then calculated for the treatment arm, giving the $O - E$ value. A negative $O - E$ value indicates that the treatment group has fared better than the control group, whilst a positive $O - E$ value indicates the opposite.

If the treatment has no effect then each individual $O - E$ could be either positive or negative and will differ only randomly from zero. Likewise the summated $O - E$ from all the studies will differ only randomly from zero if there is no difference between treatment and control. If, however, the treatment does have a beneficial effect then there will be a trend for individual $O - E$ values to be negative, and the overall summated value to be clearly so.

The $O - E$ and its variance can then be used to the calculate odds ratio (OR) for each trial. This OR gives the ratio of the odds of event or risk among the treatment group to the corresponding odds of event among the control group patients. An OR value of 1.0 represents equal risk or no difference between treatments, while a value of 0.5 indicates a halving of the chance of event measured for patients in the treatment arm. A pooled OR can be calculated by summing the individual $O - E$ and variance values in such a way that the pooled OR represents a weighted average of the individual ORs, where the individual trials which contain the most information (usually the largest trials) influence the estimate most.

Time-to-Event Data

A major advantage of collecting IPD is that it allows a more appropriate analysis of time-to-event data. Usually this involves running standard log rank analyses on individual trials and then combining the log rank $O - E$ and its variance to calculate a hazard ratio (HR).

Rather than summarising the overall number of events as in an OR, the HR makes use of the time (from randomisation) at which each individual event takes place and also uses information from patients who have not yet experienced the event (censored patients). In this way, the HR summarises the entire "survival" experience. The calculations follow through in exactly the same way as for calculation of an OR simply by substituting the log rank $O - E$ and variance for those calculated from the crude number

of events. These HRs represent the overall risk of failure on treatment as opposed to control. A HR of less than 1.0 favours treatment whereas a HR of more than 1.0 favours control. For example, when measuring survival, a HR of 0.8 indicates a 20% reduction in the overall risk of death when receiving treatment as compared with control. Such time-to-event analyses can be extremely important in chronic illness where either a prolongation of survival or time without evidence of disease or symptoms is anticipated.

Where IPD is not available, the provision of the results of log rank analyses by trialists also enables the calculation of HRs.

Where meta-analyses are based on published information, provided trials are sufficiently well reported, it may also be possible to estimate HRs from a variety of statistical summary measures rather than calculting ORs [18] as is usually done for this type of meta-analysis.

Graphical Representation of Meta-analyses

Results of meta-analyses are often presented as plots illustrating the HR (or OR) for each individual trial and for the overall combined results. An example of such a plot is shown in Fig. 14.1. The vertical line of equivalence drawn through unity indicates the point where there is no difference between treatment and control. Trials favouring treatment will have a HR of less than 1.0 and lie to the left-hand side of this line and those favouring control will fall on the right-

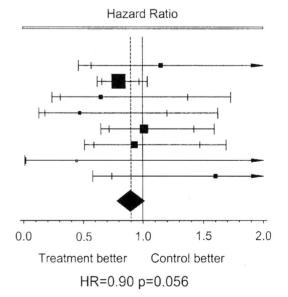

| | (no. events/no. entered) | | | |
	Treatment	Control	O-E	Variance
Trial A	17/18	15/18	1.08	7.91
Trial B	313/383	162/179	-22.01	98.21
Trial C	14/23	15/21	-2.99	6.93
Trial D	10/17	10/13	-3.27	4.29
Trial E	63/76	71/85	0.45	33.16
Trial F	37/57	39/73	-1.31	18.80
Trial G	1/3	1/2	-0.35	0.43
Trial H	15/20	12/20	3.07	6.49
Total	470/597	325/411	-25.32	176.23

HR=0.90 p=0.056

Fig. 14.1. Example hazard ratio (HR) plot. See text for further information.

hand side. Each individual trial is illustrated by a box drawn with a horizontal line and tick marks indicating the 95% and 99% confidence intervals. The size of the box is proportional to the amount of information in the trial such that the bigger the box, the bigger the trial. A trial reaches conventional levels of significance if the confidence intervals do not cross the equivalence line. The diamond at the bottom of the plot illustrates the combined results for all trials with the edges denoting the 95% confidence interval. An overall result reaches the conventional level of significance at the 5% level if the edge of the diamond does not cross the equivalence line. Trials are often ordered chronologically with the oldest trial at the top.

Statistical Issues in Meta-analysis

Fixed Versus Random Effect Model

The examples discussed above use the fixed effect model, which is the most straightforward and easiest to understand method of analysis. However, appropriate statistical methods are far from agreed, and some would argue that a random effect model is a more appropriate way to analyse the data.

In the simplest fixed effect model, as described above, the contribution of each trial to the combined estimate is proportional to the amount of information in it, with each trial weighted by its variance, which is an intuitively appealing scheme. However, in this approach only *within-trial* variability is considered and no allowance is made for any *between-trial* variability. Random effect models explicitly allow for between-trial variability by weighting trials by a combination of their own variance and the between-trial variance.

Where there is little between-trial variability, the random effect weighting will tend towards being the same as the weighting for the fixed effect model. If, however, there is significant between-trial variability, this will tend to dominate the weighting factor such that all trials will tend towards contributing equally towards the overall estimate and small trials may unduly influence the results. It is common to find that the estimates from the two approaches are similar, but in the presence of statistical heterogeneity the confidence interval for the random effects estimate will be much wider than the confidence interval for the fixed effect estimate.

There are strong proponents of both approaches. Those in favour of the random effect model argue that it formally allows for between-trial variability, and that the fixed effect approach unrealistically assumes a single effect across all trials and can overemphasise the result. Those in favour of the fixed effect approach argue that the random effect model is using a statistical model to address a clinical problem. In particular, it gives no insight into the source of between-trial variability.

Heterogeneity

There is of course clinical heterogeneity between trials, because of differing protocols, treatments and patients, and this will be true irrespective of whether any statistical test for heterogeneity is significant. If statistical heterogeneity is observed, then the possible reasons for this should be explored [19]. Perhaps the treatments are sufficiently different and can be split into less heterogeneous and more appropriate groups. If such a source of heterogeneity is found and trials can be subdivided according to the appropriate characteristic, separate analyses can be done. In fact, this may enable us to address questions such as which particular treatments perform best or which type of patients will benefit most. Indeed, it could be argued that modelling such heterogeneity using the random effect approach is effectively throwing away valuable information.

In the search for the clinical source of statistical heterogeneity, there is likely to be some post hoc reasoning in the explanation, so that only cautious conclusions should be drawn. Nevertheless, the aim should be to minimise statistical heterogeneity within a comparison, so that it becomes almost irrelevant which model is used. Heterogeneity can be investigated fully only when IPD are available, particularly when the endpoint is the time to an event. It is unlikely that in a meta-analysis based on data extracted from publications, all reasonable possible sources of heterogeneity can be investigated.

Subgroup Analyses

When assessing the role of any new treatment, an important additional question is whether the treatment is equally effective in well-defined subgroups of patients. For example, is the treatment more or less effective in males or females, or in old or young patients?

In general, the results of subgroup analyses can be very misleading owing to the high probability that any observed difference is due solely to chance [5]. For example, if 10 subgroup analyses are carried out, there is a 40% chance of finding at least one significant false-positive effect (5% significance level).

A well-known example of the problem associated with subgroup analysis is provided by an investigation based on the astrological birth sign of patients in a myocardial infarction trial involving 16 000 patients [5]. The trial found a reduction in the odds of death of 15% associated with the use of intravenous atenolol that was conventionally significant ($p < 0.05$). However, results of subgroup analyses showed a significant 48% benefit for Scorpios ($p < 0.04$), but a non-significant 12% benefit for all other star signs. Clearly, it would be extremely unwise to conclude from this that only those patients born between 24 October and 22 November should receive this particular treatment. However, similar conclusions for clinical factors such as age, sex or type of disease based on exploratory analyses are often reported for trials that fail to show any overall treatment difference.

Subgroup analyses are likely to be particularly unreliable in situations where no overall effect of treatment has been observed. In this case, if one subgroup exhibits a particularly positive effect of treatment, then another subgroup has to have a counteracting negative effect. For example, if a trial that showed no overall effect found a strikingly positive effect in women, then men must conversely show a strikingly detrimental effect. Although possible, real differences in direction of effect would be rare. Significant results of subgroup analyses are perhaps more plausible in cases where an overall benefit of treatment has been observed. In this case the difference between subgroups is in size rather than direction. It may be reasonable, for example, that women receive a larger benefit and men a smaller benefit from the treatment under investigation. Nevertheless, as in the birth sign example, even in such situations subgroup analysis can be very misleading.

Provided that data have been collected uniformly across studies, a meta-analysis of all trials may achieve sufficient power in each subgroup to permit a more reliable assessment of whether the effect is, in fact, larger (or smaller) for any particular type of patient. Although still potentially misleading, subgroup analysis within the context of a meta-analysis may be the only reliable way of performing such exploratory investigations.

Example of Subgroup Analysis in Meta-analysis

An IPD meta-analysis of thoracic radiotherapy for small-cell lung cancer [20] showed an overall benefit of combined radiotherapy and chemotherapy over chemotherapy alone ($p = 0.001$), equivalent to a 14% reduction in the mortality rate. In addition they found a significant trend ($p = 0.01$) towards a larger

proportional effect of radiotherapy on the mortality of younger patients than older ones.

The relative risk of death in the treated group ranged from 0.72 for patients younger than 55 years to 1.07 for patients older than 70 years, with a very clear pattern of a decreasing benefit of radiotherapy across the five increasing age categories that were investigated. Although the authors suggested that the smaller effect of treatment in older patients could be explained by toxicity, they were sensibly cautious in interpreting the result of this subgroup analysis.

The Cochrane Collaboration

In 1972, Archie Cochrane published a monograph [21] suggesting that because health care resources would always be limited, they should be used to provide equitably those forms of treatment which had been shown by properly designed evaluation to be effective. He also noted the problem that even though it may have been published, valid evidence about the effects of health care is not always readily available for those who need it.

The Cochrane Collaboration therefore grew from the idea that limited resources should be used to provide health care interventions that have been shown to be effective by properly controlled research and from the need for systematic, up-to-date reviews of such treatment. Since the opening of the first Cochrane Centre in Oxford in 1992, the Collaboration has grown to become an international network of health professionals, consumers and researchers working together using the principles of systematic review and evidence-based medicine to address unresolved health problems. The aim of this collaboration is to prepare, maintain and disseminate systematic reviews of all aspects of health care, based largely, though not exclusively on the results of RCTs. However, this will take time. Approximately a million RCTs have been published and it is likely to take at least 20 years to catch up and reach a stable state where new primary research can be easily assimilated into existing systematic reviews of previous research [22].

The results of this international research effort are published as the Cochrane Library in CD/disk format [23] and over the Internet. Results of completed systematic reviews and protocols of ongoing reviews are published alongside other information including a database of RCTs. For example, a simple electronic search of 2000 Issue 1 using the term "neurology" yielded 100 citations to completed Cochrane reviews and 80 protocols. Citations to a further 19 entries in the database of abstracts of reviews of effectiveness (DARE) – an ancillary database of critical abstracts of systematic reviews completed by other groups – and 1781 entries in the Cochrane Collaboration controlled trials register were also identified.

Examples of Meta-analyses in Neurology

Corticosteroids in Acute Traumatic Brain Injury

Traumatic brain injury is a major cause of ill health worldwide, causing premature death and disability such that even a small reduction in mortality or morbidity could be important in terms of public health. A number of randomised trials of corticosteroids in the treatment of head injury have been published with apparently conflicting findings. In consequence, there is no established consensus concerning the use of such treatment and a recent UK survey found that corticosteroids were used in just under half the intensive care units surveyed [24]. A systematic review was therefore undertaken by the Cochrane Collaboration Brain and Spinal Cord Injury Group [25], the main aim of which was to quantify the effectiveness of corticosteroids in reducing mortality and morbidity in individuals with acute traumatic brain injury.

Standard Cochrane Collaboration methods of review were used. Optimal searching of electronic databases was supplemented by handsearching numerous journals and publication reference lists and by asking all identified trialists to provide details of any additional published or unpublished trials. Trials were eligible for inclusion in the systematic review provided they were indeed RCTs; trials using quasi-random methods of allocation were excluded. The experimental intervention was corticosteroids administered in any dose by any route for any duration started within 7 days of injury and trials were included irrespective of any other treatments used. Data were extracted from trial publications, supplemented where necessary by additional information from those trialists with whom the reviewers were able to establish contact.

A total of 19 trials which met the inclusion criteria were identified, including 2 unpublished trials. Data were available from 17 trials including 2295 participants. Data were not available from one unpublished trial and for another the author could not be traced. Mortality data were available from 16 trials, all but one of which showed inconclusive results. The confidence intervals for the individual trials, eight of which favoured the use of corticosteroids and seven of which favoured no corticosteroids, were wide. The

pooled odds ratio for the risk of death was 0.96 (95% CI 0.85–1.08), indicating a trend in favour of corticosteroids but one which does not achieve conventional levels of significance (Fig. 14.2). For the 9 trials that reported death or severe disability the pooled relative risk was 1.01 (95% CI 0.91–1.11). For infections the pooled relative risk was 0.94 (95% CI 0.74–1.16) and for the 9 trials reporting gastrointestinal bleeding 1.11 (95% CI 0.54–2.26). The reviewers concluded that there remains considerable uncertainty concerning the use of corticosteroids in acute traumatic brain injury and that large RCTs are required. Further details of this systematic review can be found on the Cochrane Library.

High-Grade Gliomas

Malignant gliomas are amongst the most devastating of cancers, frequently producing profound and progressive disability leading to death. They are difficult to diagnose and challenging to treat. There are two peaks of incidence: one in childhood and the other at around 50–60 years of age [26]. These tumours are therefore a major cause of mortality in a relatively young population and improving survival by even a moderate amount could potentially result in many years of life saved.

Complete surgical resection of high-grade glioma is difficult without causing severe neurological damage, and thus standard treatment generally consists of cytoreductive surgery followed by radiotherapy. However, prognosis remains poor with a median survival of 9 months and only 5–10% of patients surviving to 2 years [27]. Consequently, there has been increasing interest in the use of adjuvant chemotherapy, with research focusing mostly on the use of nitrosoureas, which are used because they are lipid soluble and cross the putative "blood–brain barrier".

Eighteen randomised trials have been conducted in which surgery plus radiotherapy has been compared with the same standard treatment plus cytotoxic chemotherapy in adult patients with high-grade glioma. In total these trials account for over 3500 patients. Individually, these trials have shown inconclusive and conflicting results, and despite this considerable research effort there is currently no clear consensus on whether adjuvant chemotherapy improves survival of patients with high-grade glioma. It is therefore uncertain whether such treatment should have a routine role in clinical practice.

The majority of trials have been relatively small and many have randomised between multiple treatment arms. Most recruited fewer than 150 patients per arm, whereas more than 600 per arm would need to be randomised to reliably detect a 5% improve-

Review:Corticosteroids for acute traumatic brain injury
Comparison: Any steroid administered in any dose against no steroid
Outcome: Death at end of follow up period

Study	Expt n/N	Ctrl n/N	Peto OR (95%CI Fixed)	Peto OR (95%CI Fixed)
Alexander 1972	16 / 55	22 / 55		0.62 [0.28,1.36]
Braakman 1983	44 / 81	47 / 80		0.84 [0.45,1.56]
Chacon 1987	1 / 5	0 / 5		7.39 [0.15,372.41]
Cooper 1979	26 / 49	13 / 27		1.21 [0.48,3.09]
Dearden 1986	33 / 68	21 / 62		1.82 [0.91,3.65]
Faupel 1976	16 / 67	16 / 28		0.23 [0.09,0.58]
Gaab 1994	19 / 133	21 / 136		0.91 [0.47,1.79]
Giannotta 1984	34 / 72	7 / 16		1.15 [0.39,3.38]
Grumme 1995	38 / 175	49 / 195		0.83 [0.51,1.34]
Hernesniemi 1979	35 / 81	36 / 83		0.99 [0.54,1.84]
Pitts 1980	114 / 201	38 / 74		1.24 [0.73,2.12]
Ransohoff 1972	9 / 17	13 / 18		0.45 [0.12,1.73]
Saul 1981	8 / 50	9 / 50		0.87 [0.31,2.45]
Stubbs 1989	13 / 98	5 / 54		1.46 [0.53,4.08]
Zagara 1987	4 / 12	4 / 12		1.00 [0.19,5.27]
xZarate 1995	0 / 30	0 / 30		Not Estimable
Total (95%CI)	410 / 1194	301 / 925		0.93 [0.76,1.14]

Chi-square 18.29 (df=14) Z=0.68

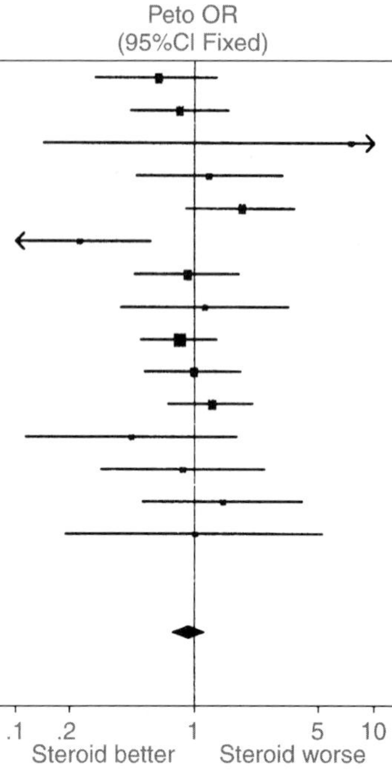

.1   .2   1   5   10
Steroid better   Steroid worse

Fig. 14.2.   Corticosteroids in acute traumatic brain injury: odds ratio (OR) survival plot. Reprinted from the Cochrane Library [22].

ment in survival from 10% to 15% (90% power, 5% significance level). Although each individual trial may not have sufficient numbers of patients to detect moderate survival benefits with reliability, the combination of the results of these trials in a meta-analysis might give sufficient statistical power to help decide whether chemotherapy is beneficial in the treatment of this disease.

Two meta-analyses based on summary data from trial publications have been published. However, these suffer from a number of limitations and potential biases. The first [28], published in 1987 and based on data from eight trials (including one "randomised" by birthdate) concluded that there was evidence that single-agent nitrosourea improved survival of high-grade glioma patients by a small amount. The second [29], published in 1993 and based on data from 16 trials (including one "randomised" by birthdate, one which used alternate allocation, one which did not include a no-chemotherapy arm, and one double-counted trial which reported the contribution of a single institution to a multi-centre trial which was also included), concluded that chemotherapy is advantageous and should be considered as part of standard therapy for patients with malignant glioma.

Although encouraging, these studies must be interpreted cautiously. As discussed above, meta-analyses based on published summary data can give different results from those based on updated IPD and it is extremely important that any systematic review or meta-analysis is based on as much of the relevant evidence as possible.

An additional six randomised trials including almost 1400 patients that were not included in the more recent of these studies have been conducted. Many of the analyses reported in trial publications excluded considerable numbers of patients (on average approximately 10–15%) which could potentially introduce bias to any meta-analysis based only on the published data.

An IPD meta-analysis was therefore initiated by the British Medical Research Council Cancer Trials Office and conducted on behalf of The Glioma Meta-analysis Trialists' group to investigate this question. Preliminary results [30] based on information from 10 trials, 2368 patients and 2106 deaths suggest that there is a 16% reduction in the risk of death associated with using chemotherapy (HR = 0.84, 95% CI 0.77–0.92, P = 0.0001). This is equivalent to a 5% increase in 2-year survival, increasing survival from 15% to 20%. As these results are based on only 70% of the worldwide randomised evidence, they should be interpreted cautiously. Final analyses (based on 85% of the worldwide evidence) which are currently ongoing should provide a reliable answer to this important question.

Conclusions

Systematic reviews and meta-analyses formally appraise and, where appropriate, combine the results of trials that have considered similar questions, to reduce the potential influence of both random error and bias, and to establish more reliably whether there is a real difference between treatments. This can be done in a relatively short period of time compared with initiating new prospective studies and, given that in many cases there may already be sufficient evidence to resolve therapeutic issues, it could be considered scientifically inappropriate and unethical not to carry out a formal systematic review of existing information before embarking upon a new prospective study.

The overall results of a well-conducted systematic meta-analysis provide the most reliable and least biased summary of the average effect of a treatment on some endpoints. This is probably the best available evidence to guide treatment policy for future patients. However, issues such as the clinical relevance, appropriate extrapolation to individual patients, toxicity and implications on quality of life and cost of the treatment cannot easily be addressed within a meta-analysis. Currently, these have to be assessed in detailed local, regional or perhaps national studies. In this sense the meta-analysis acts only as one, although essential, source of information.

The issue of what benefit is clinically worthwhile is clearly a subjective decision, likely to be influenced by factors such as the country, speciality of the clinician, patient-specific factors, quality of life considerations and the cost of the new treatment. For example, it is quite likely because of cultural differences that clinicians in the USA would accept a much smaller benefit to use toxic treatments than clinicians in the UK [31]. In some countries the cost of some new therapies may be so prohibitive that it is impossible to give a new treatment unless the observed effect is enormous, which is very unlikely.

When interpreting the results of any meta-analysis it is important to remember that neither individual trials nor meta-analyses can provide prescriptions on how individual patients should be treated. The estimated average treatment effect is, however, an essential piece of information to be considered alongside other factors such as toxicity, cost, patient preference and quality of life by both patients and doctors when making individual treatment choices.

In summary, there are very many advantages of systematic review and meta-analysis. The process enables us to take a more global perspective, as the value of any individual study depends on how well it fits with or expands other work as well as its own intrinsic properties [32]. Not only are the power and precision of estimating effect and risk improved and the influence of bias limited by adopting appropriate methodology, but we can also assess whether findings are consistent and can be generalised across different populations, settings and treatment variations [1].

However, it is important that this powerful tool is neither used nor interpreted blindly. We must not allow ourselves to be fooled by the apparent authority of numbers but critically appraise the quality and value of the evidence on which any systematic review or meta-analysis is based and ensure that the methodology used is appropriate. In this way we can obtain valuable answers to unresolved questions and establish baselines on which future research can be built.

Acknowledgements. I am grateful to Mahesh Parmar and Jayne Tierney for their valuable comments and to Linda Baulk for typing this chapter.

References

1. Mulrow C. Rationale for systematic reviews. BMJ 1994;309:597–599.
2. Mulrow C. The medical review article: state of the science. Ann Intern Med 1987;106:485–488.
3. Antman EM, Lau J, Kupelnick B, Mosteller F, Chalmers TGA. Comparison of results of meta-analyses and randomised controlled trials and recommendations of clinical experts. JAMA 1992;268:240–248.
4. Chalmers I, Enkin M, Keirse JNC. Preparing and updating systematic reviews of randomised controlled trials of health care. Milbank Q 1993;71:411–433.
5. Collins R, Grey R, Godwin J, Peto R. Avoidance of large biases and large random error in the assessment of moderate treatment effects: The need for systematic overviews. Stats in Med 1987;6:245–250.
6. Stewart LA, Parmar MKB. Bias in the analysis and reporting of randomised controlled trials. Int J Tech Assess Health Care 1996;12:264–275.
7. Stewart LA, Clarke MJ. Practical methodology of meta-analyses (overviews) using updated individual patient data. Stat Med 1995;14:2057–2079.
8. Stewart LA, Parmar MKB. Meta-analysis of the literature or of individual patient data: Is there a difference? Lancet 1993;341:418–422.
9. Pignon JP, Arriagada R. Meta-analysis. Lancet 1993;311:964–965.
10. Jeng GT, Scott JR, Burmeister LF. A comparison of meta-analytic results using literature vs individual patient data:

paternal cell immunisation for recurrent miscarriage. JAMA 1995;274:830–836.

11. Advanced Ovarian Cancer Trialists' Group. Chemotherapy in advanced ovarian cancer: an overview of randomised clinical trials. BMJ 1991;303:884–893.

12. Dickersin K, Min YI, Meinert CK. Factors influencing publication of research results. JAMA 1992;267:374–378.

13. Dickersin K, Scherer R, Lefebvre C. Identification of relevant studies for systematic review. BMJ 1994;309:1286–1291.

14. Egger M, Zellweger-Zahner T, Schneier M, Junker C, Lengeler C, Antes G. Language bias in randomised controlled trials published in English and German. Lancet 1997;350:326–329.

15. Easterbrook PJ, Berlin JA, Gopalan R, Matthews DR. Publication bias in clinical research. Lancet 1991;337:867–872.

16. Pocock SJ. Clinical trials: a practical approach. New York, John Wiley & Sons. 1993.

17. Schultz KF, Chalmers I, Haynes RG, Altman DG. Empirical evidence of bias: Dimensions of methodological quality associated with estimates of treatment effects in controlled trials. JAMA 1994;273:1408–1412.

18. Parmar MKB, Torri V, Stewart LA. Extracting summary statistics to perform meta-analyses of the published literature for survival endpoints. Statistics in medicine 1998;17:2815–2834.

19. Thompson S. Why sources of heterogeneity in meta-analysis should be investigated. BMJ 1994;309:1351–1355.

20. Pignon JP, Arriagada R, Ihde D, et al. A meta-analysis of thoracic radiotherapy for small-cell lung cancer. N Engl J Med 1992;327:1618–1624.

21. Cochrane AL. Effectiveness and efficiency: random reflections on health services. London: Nuffield Provincial Hospitals Trust. 1972.

22. Chalmers I, Haynes B. Reporting, updating and reporting systematic reviews of the effects of heath care. BMJ 1994;309:862–5.

23. The Cochrane Library (database on disk and CD Rom). The Cochrane Collaboration. Oxford: Update Software, 2000 (updated quarterly).

24. Jeevaratnam DR, Menon DK. Survey of intensive care of severely head injured patients in the United Kingdom. BMJ 1996;312:944–947.

25. Alderon P, Roberts I. Corticosteroids in acute traumatic brain injury. In: The Cochrane Library, Issue 1, 2000. Oxford: Update Software.

26. Souhami R, Tobias J. Cancer and its management, 2nd edition. Oxford: Blackwell Scientific, 1995.

27. Bleehen NM, Stenning SP. A Medical Research Council trial of two radiotherapy doses in the treatment of grades 3 and 4 astrocytoma. Br J Cancer 1991;64:769–774.

28. Stenning SP, Freedman LS, Bleehen NM. An overview of published results from randomised studies of nitrosureas in primary high grade malignant glioma. Br J Cancer 1987;56:86–90.

29. Fine HA, Dear KBG, Loeffler JS, et al. Meta-analysis of radiation therapy with and without adjuvant chemotherapy for malignant gliomas in adults. Cancer 1993;71:2585–2597.

30. Stewart LA, Burdett S, Souhami RL, for the Glioma Meta-analysis Trialists' Group. Chemotherapy high-grade glioma: A meta-analysis using individual patient data from randomised clinical trials. Proceedings of the American Society of Clinical Oncology 2000;19:650.

31. Parmar MKB, Ungerleider R, Simon R. Assessing whether to perform a confirmatory randomized trial? J Natl Cancer Inst 1996;88:1641–1645.

32. Cooper HM. The integrative research review: a systematic approach. Beverly Hills, CA: Sage Publications. 1984.

PART II

Diseases

15. Outcome Variables in Dementia Trials: Conceptual and Practical Issues

A.D. Lawrence and B.J. Sahakian

Introduction

The aim of this chapter is to determine the roles of different assessment methods (including neuropsychological tests, psychiatric rating scales, global clinical scales and functional scales) in evaluating treatments for dementia, most especially Alzheimer's disease (AD), with emphasis on neuropsychological assessment in trials of drugs designed to treat cognitive symptoms. We begin with a brief overview of issues in the diagnosis of dementia. We then review the desirable characteristics of instruments for evaluating dementia treatments, followed by a discussion of specific cognitive and other assessment instruments along with data on the extent to which they meet certain desirable validity, reliability and practicality criteria we detail below.

Dementia: Nosological Issues

Dementia is "an acquired syndrome of decline in memory and other cognitive functions sufficient to affect daily life in an alert patient" [1]. There have been significant advances in dementia diagnosis since the term first came into use in the seventeenth and eighteenth centuries [2]. However, inconsistent operational definitions have resulted in confusion in the nosological system. Four major criteria have been used to define both types (e.g. AD vs Huntington's disease) and subtypes (e.g. different variants of AD and frontal lobe dementia) of dementia. These are: (i) site of the maximum structural changes in the brain; (ii) histopathology; (iii) clinical symptomatology; and (iv) aetiology [3]. Of these, location of major pathology in the brain has been the most frequently used scheme to classify the dementias. Dementias such as AD which are considered to affect the cortical mantle most significantly have been labelled "cortical dementias",

which have been further subdivided into frontal, central and posterior dementias [4]. Disorders such as Huntington's disease, on the other hand, are classified as subcortical dementias, since the major pathology is in subcortical regions [4]. However, this system of classification has come in for heavy criticism, not least because of the lack of specificity in such a distinction. For example, the major neurotransmitter lesion in AD is subcortical, whilst Huntington's disease patients have been shown to have considerable cortical pathology, even in relatively early stages of the disease. Classifications via histopathology, clinical symptomatology and aetiology have also been subjected to much criticism [3,5,6].

At present, then, there is no integrated nosological system for the classification of dementia. This lack of a comprehensive dementia nosology does not alter the fact that diagnoses of the dementias are required for both clinical treatment and research protocols. Stuss and Levine [3] suggest that a convergence of classification criteria is necessary for improved dementia diagnosis. This suggestion is echoed by the proposals of the International Working Group on Harmonization of Dementia Drug Guidelines [7]. They propose that diagnosis of dementia should go through several phases, which would act as a series of progressively finer filters. The initial phase, conducted on the basis of evaluation of clinical symptoms and medical history, would include almost everyone who meets the criteria for dementia. The next phase would add a number of clinical tests to improve specificity and reduce false positives. Subsequent levels of evaluation would include structural and/or functional imaging, and genetic markers, which would further categorise patients for particular purposes. No single criterion at present can provide diagnostic certainty. However, evidence converging from multiple sources greatly increases the specificity and stability of prediction [3,7].

Assessment Issues

Because cognitive decline is the defining symptom of dementia, objective assessment of the cognitive functions impaired in dementia is central to diagnosis, patient selection and assessment of treatment efficacy [8]. Recently developed regulatory guidelines for the development of cognition-enhancing agents mandate that any such agent be superior to placebo on two types of measures: (i) a performance-based measure of cognitive function and (ii) an independent clinician-rated measure of global severity. This "dual outcome" approach was adopted to ensure that any approved anti-dementia agent would improve the core cognitive symptoms of dementia and that such improvements would be large enough to be of clinical significance. These "dual outcome" guidelines have been adopted in both the United States and the European Community [9,10].

Theoretical and Empirical Issues in the Development and Use of Assessment Tools

Clinical cognitive neuroscience has emerged within recent times as an important clinical science [11], and one of the major contributions of the discipline has been the development of standardised cognitive test instruments. However, the properties by which to judge the utility of a particular cognitive test battery as an outcome measure in clinical trials are still much contested. Traditionally, the psychometric constructs of reliability and validity have been the criteria by which any such instrument was to be judged. There are no single indices of "validity" or "reliability". It is not true that a test has inherent "validity", a test which is valid under one set of conditions may not be valid under another set of conditions. "Validity" can be broken down into three main types: content validity, criterion validity and construct validity [12–14] (see also Chapter 2).

Content Validity

Content validity is concerned with whether the instrument in question adequately probes the specific domain(s) one requires. Arguments about the content validity of instruments are thus inextricably linked with theories about what one is trying to measure, and hence there are no empirical measures of content validity [12–14].

Criterion Validity

Criterion validity determines whether a measure discriminates between individuals who are known to differ on a marker external to the measure itself. Criterion validity is often presented in terms of the sensitivity and specificity of the measure in question. The sensitivity of a measure is defined as the proportion of positive cases correctly identified, the specificity is the proportion of negative cases identified. Sensitivity and specificity are not fixed values, but will depend on the cut-off score of a particular measure. Receiver operating characteristic (ROC) curves are plots of the sensitivity (true positive rate) of a particular measure versus the false positive rate (100% − specificity). ROC curves can be used to determine the impact of selecting a particular cut-off score on the sensitivity and specificity of a measure, and can aid in determining the efficiency of different tests to discriminate between cases [12–14].

Construct Validity

Construct validity relates to the theoretical underpinnings of a test, and is evaluated by demonstrating that certain explanatory constructs account for performance on a test. The most important factor in construct validity is thus the explicitness of the theory behind the test in question. To have good construct validity, there must be a strong, well-articulated theoretical rationale underpinning measure, and there must be evidence of a consistent pattern of findings over a whole range of studies [12–14].

Reliability

The reliability of an instruments is concerned with the replicability of measurement. Test–retest reliability is established by administering the test to two groups of subjects at different time points, and correlating the scores obtained. A low test–retest reliability does not necessarily imply that a measure is poor, but that it is sensitive to a number of factors. For example, measures of "executive" function often have poor test–retest reliability, but this may be important information for theories of executive function [15]. If tests do have low test–retest reliability, then it is important to have alternative, equivalent forms of the test available.

Another form of reliability is the internal consistency of a measure, which relates to the reproducibility of measurement across different items within a test. There are a number of internal consistency measures available, all of which are obtained by intercorrelating subjects' scores on individual items within a test.

A number of assessment tools, most especially clinician-rated interview-based methods, cannot be assessed using the above measures. In this case, reliability can be assessed by comparing the ratings of two independent observers (usually by computing some form of correlation coefficient) to determine the extent to which they agree in their observations [12–14].

Extensions to the Standard Psychometric Approach

In several important recent articles, it has been strongly argued that the psychometric constructs of "validity" and "reliability" are insufficient criteria by which to judge the utility of cognitive test instruments in special populations, such as the elderly [16,17]. For example, Mohs [16] and Demonet et al. [18] have argued that, in addition to meeting criteria for validity and reliability, cognitive instruments must also meet certain "practicality" or "pragmatic" criteria, such as being brief enough to be well tolerated by patients.

The most thorough review of criteria that any cognitive test battery designed for use in clinical trials should fulfil has been provided by Milberg [17]. In this paper, Milberg strongly makes the case that the relative merits of any cognitive test instrument represent a compromise between the various demands of psychometry and practicality. Milberg argues that the properties of assessment techniques will be increasingly shaped not simply by advances in cognitive neuroscience theory, but by the forces of demographics and economics. With advances in medical technology and public health policy increasing the expected life span of people in industrialised nations, the incidence and prevalence of late-life disorders of cognition increased dramatically in the latter half of the twentieth century, and are expected to continue rising well into the present century [17]. Thus, more individuals will require the assessment of cognitive functions, while resources available for health care are becoming increasingly limited. Milberg [17] makes the argument that these circumstances demand that cognitive assessment techniques are designed to be as efficient as possible, where efficiency is defined as the ratio of "useful" information obtained to time/cost. Thus, in addition to the traditional concepts of validity and reliability, efficiency is an important criterion by which cognitive assessment instruments should be judged.

Milberg also laments the lack of a theoretical context behind the use of most cognitive assessment batteries. He claims that the developers/users of clinical assessment tools have been mainly concerned with criterion validity rather than interpretative/theoretical (i.e. content/construct validity) issues. For example, a great many neuropsychological assessment tools, such as the Wechsler Adult Intelligence Scale, were not designed to be tests of neural function per se, but have been appropriated by neuropsychologists for such a purpose. Further, other measures such as the Halstead–Reitan Battery have their origins in outdated anti-localistationist theories of neural function, but have persisted in use because of their validity as measures sensitive to "organic brain dysfunction". Such tests do not reflect clinically relevant theoretical advances in our understanding of psychological processes such as, for example, memory systems [19] and executive or control processes [20]. Thus, the sensitivity and specificity of an assessment tool to the presence of brain damage are not enough to ensure that an instrument is constructed in an optimally interpretable fashion, or that the levels of sensitivity and specificity obtained have been obtained in a maximally efficient manner. Similar arguments have been made by Cipolotti and Warrington [21], who state that "Before approaching a neuropsychological assessment it is necessary to have a theoretical structure on which to base and interpret the different levels of disturbance that can arise as a result of cerebral damage".

The dominant paradigm [22] in neuropsychology and cognitive neuroscience today is the localisationist paradigm. Although not without its critics [23,24], it is broadly accepted that there is a high degree of functional specialisation in the brain, and that brain damage can selectively disrupt some components of the cognitive system. Furthermore, it is accepted that broad functions such as memory, language and attention can be broken down into more basic processing elements (what has been called the "modularity approach to the analysis of complex skills") [21] and that these more basic elements are candidate descriptions for neural function. Although the precise natures of these basic cognitive functions are not resolved, there is sufficient consensus within the literature to inform clinical assessment practice. Even a division into such seemingly procrustean categories as language, memory, visual and space perception, attention, and executive function would be a useful starting point. Within each broad domain, tasks should be constructed that reflect the current understanding of underlying psychological processes. For example, memory measures should allow separation of encoding/retrieval/monitoring functions and assess separate information-domains (e.g. spatial/visual); measures of attention should assess selective, divided and sustained attention, etc. This type of specificity in assessment tools is particularly important because of the increasing recognition that dementia is not a unitary syndrome within or across aetiologies: even though broad patterns can be distinguished, patients with similar underlying pathologies may vary widely in the neural distribution of the causative lesion and hence in the behavioural manifestations of those lesions [3,25]. It is vital that cognitive assessment tools are sensitive to such biological and cognitive variability.

Although some clinicians might argue that such cognitive specificity is of little clinical relevance, this may not be the case. There is emerging evidence to suggest that domain-specific measures are better predictors of activities of daily living than are global measures of cognitive severity, and determining with specificity which areas of cognitive dysfunction strongly predict impaired day-to-day functioning will be of importance in informing patient management and rehabilitation strategies [25–27].

In addition to these efficiency and content/construct validity criteria, Mohr [16], Milberg [17] and Demonet et al. [18] have argued that certain "practicality" criteria are important when assessing measures that are applied to patients with dementia. Perhaps the most important of these is that the tests are brief enough to avoid fatigue effects, and enjoyable so that patients do not become frustrated or distressed during testing.

In classic psychometric theory, a measure's reliability is assessed in three ways: internal consistency (e.g. split-half reliability), temporal stability (test–retest) or inter-rate reliability [12–14]. However, internal consistency measures may be affected by patient fatigue, distractibility and mood, and measurements of temporal stability may be limited due to diurnal variations in symptoms, and because symptom severity changes over time. It has therefore been argued that the reliability of cognitive assessment tools to be used in clinical trials of dementia be determined within the clinical context in which the measure is being used. The goal should be to "optimise reliability as it empirically affects test validity and efficiency" [17].

A final feature of tests judged to be important by Milberg [17] is that tasks should cover a wide range of ability whilst avoiding ceiling effects in young, healthy individuals and floor effects in the dementing elderly.

The above considerations led Milberg [17] to propose the following seven criteria by which any cognitive assessment tool for use in dementing individuals be judged.

1. *Neuropathological sensitivity/specificity*: The ability to distinguish patients who show evidence from independent biological markers (e.g. neuroimaging/genetic data) of a particular neuropathological entity.
2. *Cognitive domain specificity*: Measures should be relatively homogeneous and designed to assess different cognitive domains. The choice of these domains should be justified on both biological and psychological grounds.
3. *Construct or process specificity*: Tasks should assess empirically and theoretically justified variables that reflect the information processing demands specific to each domain. The tasks should reflect the most recent understanding of cognitive processes.
4. *Functional specificity*: Tasks should be relevant to a patient's daily functional abilities.
5. *Contextually appropriate reliability*: Reliability for a given measure should be estimated for the clinical population and within the assessment context the task is likely to appear. Task length may be titrated to optimise the reliability of a measure as it will actually be used.
6. *Age-appropriate item difficulty*: The tasks should be appropriate in form and difficulty level for healthy adults in the age range of the patients being assessed.
7. *Efficiency*: The test should be as brief as possible given the constraints outlined above.

These requirements for cognitive assessment batteries had been presaged somewhat by the work of Ferris [28] on psychological testing in dementia patients. Although his arguments are somewhat less specific than those of Milberg, he reached somewhat similar conclusions regarding the requirements for psychological testing in dementia. His requirements are:

1. Sampling of the full range of relevant cognitive functions.
2. Sensitivity to deficits of ageing and dementia.
3. Sensitivity to longitudinal change.
4. Difficulty range appropriate to the severity of dementia in the patient sample.
5. Equivalent forms for repeated administration.
6. Reasonable duration (e.g. less than 1 hour).
7. Sensitivity to treatment effects.
8. Good reliability.
9. Good validity (relation to brain pathology or activities of daily living symptoms).

These lists raise important issues for clinicians to consider, and any test battery that satisfied all of these constraints would certainly be admirable. However, it would be wrong to dismiss a battery simply on the grounds that it fails to satisfy all of Milberg's or Ferris's criteria. Test batteries should be evaluated with respect to the question the clinician wants to answer with them.

In addition to the criteria set out by Milberg and Ferris, which are applicable to all clinical trials involving cognitive assessment as an outcome variable, the International Working Group on Harmonization of Dementia Drug Guidelines [29] has produced a position paper on the use of objective psychometric tests as outcome measures in clinical trials of AD. Below we provide a summary of their recommendations.

International Working Group on Harmonization of Dementia Drug Guidelines Recommendations

Recently the International Working Group on Harmonization of Dementia Drug Guidelines has made the following recommendations regarding the use of objective psychometric tests as outcome measures in AD clinical trials:

Psychometric Criteria. Test characteristics should include: validity (the instrument must measure the intended disease-relevant cognitive functions); reliability (test–retest; inter/intra-rater if subjectively scored); appropriate sensitivity (absence of ceiling/floor effects, taking into account anticipated decline over duration of trial); availability of longitudinal data; information on practice effects; availability of equivalent forms.

Cognitive Domains That Should Be Assessed. Recommended cognitive domains for AD trials should include memory, attention, processing speed, visuospatial function, praxis, language, executive function and abstraction.

Assessment of Multiple Versus Single Domains. It is not a requirement to assess and show improvement in multiple cognitive domains provided that it is one of the major cognitive domains impaired in AD (e.g. memory, attention), and that improvement is also seen on a clinician-rated measure of global change or activities of daily living measure, demonstrating the clinical meaningfulness of the cognitive effect. However, in a pivotal clinical trial, targeting of a specific cognitive domain for assessment must be specified a priori in the study protocol, rather then being justified on a post hoc basis.

Relevance of Stage of Drug Development for the Cognitive Measures Selected. A single comprehensive measure such as the ADAS (see below) is adequate for phase III trials, but more detailed cognitive testing is appropriate in early phase II trials when the nature of the drug's activity is uncertain, in order to allow selection of an optimal test battery for phase III trials.

Computerised Testing. The Working Group commented that computerised testing can have distinct advantages for clinical trials. For example, task information is presented in a standard format; and recording of responses is done automatically and with great precision, without bias. Thus, session-to-session and cross-site variability is minimised. It was recommended that before being used in major clinical trials, extensive assessment of a computerised battery's validity, reliability and utility must be made. In addition certain hardware/software requirements were recomended. It was recommended that responses be made via button-press or touch-screen input, not keyboard input; appropriate performance-feedback be given; accurate timing routines be used; presentation of information be constructed so that it is clearly visible to the patient; and security of automatically recorded data files be ensured. The Working Group concluded that such computerised batteries be used in tandem with established outcome measures (e.g. the ADAS) in order to determine the relative sensitivity/utility of such a computerised cognitive battery.

Cognitive Assessments for Special Patient Subgroups. Special cognitive measures are needed when trials are to be conducted with specific patient subgroups, such as patients with severe AD or "at-risk" individuals with high genetic risk for dementia, in order to avoid floor and ceiling effects. Similar non-AD dementias such as Huntington's disease and Lewy Body dementia require specialised assessment procedures.

Cross-cultural Studies and Language Translation. Multinational clinical trials require the use of culturally appropriate instruments. These should not be literal translations of existing tests: when translations are made, revalidation of the translation is required to ensure that construct validity has been maintained. The translation process should involve both the test developers and a group of experts in the field to give advice concerning adaptation to specific national populations.

Standardisation Versus Diversity. It was suggested that adoption of a single outcome measure (e.g. the ADAS), although useful in helping to standardise the determination of effect size and facilitating comparisons across studies and treatments, would be too rigid and ultimately be counterproductive for progress in the field of dementia research. The Working Group "endorse an evolutionary process in which cognitive assessment moves forward as the field moves forward" [29].

It can be clearly seen that the Working Group's recommendations [29] and Milberg's [17] criteria overlap to a considerable extent. We will use the Working Group's recommendations together with Milberg's criteria, to assess the cognitive test batteries now used as outcome measures for clinical trials in dementia. We will not cover all the batteries that have been used, such as the WAIS, which are not currently in common usage for clinical trials in dementia. Reviews of such instruments as outcome measures can be found in Mohr [16] and Milberg [17].

Comparison of Available Instruments and Batteries

Instruments for assessing cognitive function in dementia can be classified into two broad categories [16,28,29]; (i) Global cognitive assessment tools, which use performance subtests to assess a variety of relevant cognitive symptoms and provide a total score that represents a composite index of the magnitude of cognitive impairment. These instruments are generally used to confirm the presence of dementia, to select cases for research protocols and to monitor change in clinical trials. (ii) Objective neuropsychological/psychometric tests. These tests are useful in documenting significant decline in cognitive function, determining patterns of cognitive function, evaluating the rate and manner of cognitive decline, and assessing treatment effects. The greater breadth and sensitivity of these tests in comparison with more global scales makes objective psychometric tests especially useful in early clinical trials when the nature and effect size of a new drug are not fully known.

Table 15.1 lists the assessment instruments currently in use for clinical trials in dementia.

Table 15.1. Assessment instruments currently in use for clinical trials in dementia

Domain	Instrument	Reference
Global cognitive assessment tools	MMSE	30
	BIMC	33
	CAMCOG	34
	ADAS	36
	DRS	38
Objective psychometric tests	SKT	39
	MODA	40
	CERAD	42
	CANTAB	43
	CDR	58
	NYU	61
	MAC	63
Global severity scales	CDR	69
	GDS	70
Global change scales	ADCS-CGIC	72
	CIBI	73
Behavioural symptoms	BEHAVE-AD	79
	CERAD-BRSD	80
	CMAI	81

Global Cognitive Assessment Tools

The Mini-Mental State Examination (MMSE)

The classic and most widely used cognitive outcome measure in dementia trials is the Mini-Mental State Examination (MMSE) [30]. This instrument assesses orientation, recall, praxis, calculation and language with a score range of 0 (maximal impairment) to 30 (no impairment), and usually takes 10–15 minutes to administer. Although the MMSE is designed to produce a global score for rating cognitive status, it contains some tasks which could be classified as "domain it specific". The major strengths of the MMSE are that is quick and easy to administer, is within the capabilities of older adults, and yields a single summary score that can be used as the primary cognitive outcome measure for a clinical trial. Its major weaknesses are that it is too brief, so that separate cognitive domains are not assessed thoroughly or systematically, nor do they reflect conceptual details of the particular domains in question. For example, the tasks assessing memory cannot be separated into encoding/retrieval components. Thus the subcomponents of the MMSE do not easily lend themselves to being assessed as independent cognitive functions, although this has been attempted [31]. The MMSE is also not particularly sensitive to the early stages of dementia and to changes in mental status in individuals with high pre-morbid IQ levels [17]. Scores on the MMSE have been shown to be strongly influenced by education, background and linguistic capabilities [32]. Furthermore, the MMSE has no alternative forms, resulting in enhanced susceptibility to practice effects.

Another source of variability in MMSE scores relates to the version being used. In the nominally equivalent MMSE items relating to "mental control" there are 5 points out of a possible maximum of 30 for which the examiner is given the option of either assessing the subject's ability to subtract serial sevens from 100, or alternatively, to spell the word "WORLD" in reverse. In fact, performance on these two tasks is only weakly correlated [32]. In addition, using a spelling test has considerable problems when developing cross-cultural forms of the MMSE [32].

Blessed Test of Information, Memory, and Concentration (BIMC)

The Blessed Test of Information, Memory, and Concentration (BIMC) [33] is another brief mental status test which assesses primarily orientation and memory. Most investigators use an adaptation of this test with 27 items and a total score ranging from 0 (no impairment) to 33 (maximal impairment). Its major strengths are again its brevity, and its known correlation with biological markers of disease pathology [33]. In addition, extensive longitudinal data are available. Its weaknesses are similar to those of the MMSE.

Cambridge Cognitive Examination (CAMCOG)

The Cambridge Cognitive Examination (CAMCOG) is the cognitive assessment section of CAMDEX, the Cambridge Mental Disorders of the Elderly Examination [34]. The CAMCOG is a brief neuropsychological battery designed to assess the range of cognitive functions required for a diagnosis of dementia and to detect mild degrees of cognitive impairment [35]. It consists of eight subscales (orientation, language, memory, attention, praxis, calculation, abstract thinking, perception). Its strengths and weaknesses are similar to the MMSE, although it covers a broader range of cognitive functions, is sensitive to milder degrees of cognitive impairment than the MMSE, and does not suffer from ceiling effects to the degree to which the MMSE does.

Alzheimer's Disease Assessment Scale – Cognitive Portion (ADAS-Cog)

The Alzheimer's Disease Assessment Scale (ADAS) [36] has been widely used both as a cognitive screening instrument and as an outcome measure in clinical trials, and has been recognised by the US Food and Drug Administration and the Commission of the European Communities [9,10]. The cognitive portion (ADAS-Cog) includes seven performance-based items and four clinician-rated items assessing memory, language, praxis and orientation, with a total score range of 0 (no impairment) to 70 (maximal impairment). Major strengths of the ADAS-Cog are its broader coverage of the relevant cognitive domains compared with the MMSE, the availability of alternate forms for repeat testing and the availability of extensive longitudinal data. Its main weakness is that it is unsuitable for severely demented patients, and the lack of assessment of attention/concentration. Recently, some additions to the present ADAS-Cog have been proposed to extend the cognitive domains covered to include tests of delayed recall, face recognition, attention, praxis and planning; and to extend the range of symptom severity covered [37].

Mattis Dementia Rating Scale (DRS)

The Mattis Dementia rating Scale (DRS) [38] consists of five subscales measuring attention, initiation and perseveration, conceptualisation, construction, and memory. The items are administered in hierarchical fashion such that a patient unable to complete simple items does not receive more complex ones. The total score ranges from 0 (maximal impairment) to 144 (no impairment), and the test takes up to 45 minutes to administer. The major strengths of the DRS are its broad coverage of the relevant cognitive domains, the inclusion of items designed to assess attention and executive function, and its ability to distinguish different patterns of dementia. Its major weakness is the lack of alternate forms.

Objective Neuropsychological/Psychometric Tests

Syndrome Kurtztest (SKT)

The Syndrome Kurtztest (SKT) consists of nine manually administered, timed subtests, with 60 seconds allowed per subtest [39]. The subtests are designed to assess memory, attention, naming and object arrangement. Its major strengths are its brevity (10–15 minutes to administer) and the inclusion of measures of attention. Furthermore, five equivalent forms are available. Its main weakness is that the SKT is suitable only for patients with mild dementia, and the use of timed tests can lead to difficulties in interpreting the relative effects of cognitive versus motor impairments.

Milan Overall Dementia Assessment (MODA)

The Milan Overall Dementia Assessment (MODA) [40,41] consists of three subtests designed to measure memory, attention, language, praxis, insight, intelligence, perception, orientation and activities of daily living. Its strengths are that it covers broadly the relevant cognitive domains and the availability of longitudinal data. Its main weakness is that no equivalent forms are available.

Neuropsychological Battery of the Consortium to Establish a Registry for Alzheimer's Disease (CERAD)

This battery was designed as part of the CERAD project [42], which was funded by the US National Institute on Ageing with the aim of developing standardised clinical, neuropathological, neuroradiological, and neuropsychological evaluation of patients with AD. The CERAD neuropsychological battery consists of seven subtests including the MMSE and three others which are adapted from the ADAS-Cog. These tests assess orientation, memory, language and praxis. The major strengths of the CERAD battery are its broad coverage of the relevant cognitive domains; its applicability to a broad range of dementia severity, from very early to severe AD; and the availability of extensive longitudinal data. Its main weakness are the lack of alternate forms and the lack of a summary score.

Cambridge Neuropsychological Test Automated Battery (CANTAB)

The Cambridge Neuropsychological Test Automated Battery (CANTAB) [43,44] comprises three batteries, each addressing a specific cognitive domain: (i) visual memory, (ii) attention and (iii) working memory and planning. The visual memory and working memory batteries begin with simple tests, progressing to more complex tests that incorporate the cognitive components of the earlier simple tests. The working memory battery also includes a test of planning that gives a sensitive measure of executive functioning. The attention battery includes tests of selective, divided and sustained attention.

The CANTAB battery has a number of major advantages over other psychometric batteries in use in clinical trials and in fact meets the majority of criteria set out by the International Working Group on Harmonisation of Dementia Drug Guidelines:

1. The CANTAB tests have high construct and content validity, having: (a) strong theoretical underpinnings, with the tests being designed to reflect the latest theoretical developments in the cognitive neuroscience of memory, attention, and executive functions [45,46] and (b) being specifically designed to facilitate cross-species comparisons between rats, primates and humans [47].
2. The tests have been shown to be sensitive to brain pathology in e.g. AD [48] and Huntington's disease [49], as well as to activities of daily living [25].
3. All CANTAB tests have satisfactory levels of test–retest reliability, with some reaching correlations of better than 0.9 [50].
4. The tests are graded in nature, allowing for a wide range of ability while avoiding ceiling effects in young, healthy subjects, and floor effects in the impaired elderly.
5. Longitudinal data are available for both healthy volunteers and patients with AD.
6. The CANTAB battery includes training measures designed to familiarise subjects with the equipment, which reduce subjects' responses to a reasonable baseline level of performance prior to beginning the main battery of tests.
7. There are five equivalent versions available.
8. All the cognitive domains recommended for assessment by the Working Group are assessed, with the exception of language.
9. The CANTAB tests have been used successfully in a number of cross-cultural studies. In fact, tests of language are deliberately not included to make the tests genuinely cross-cultural in nature. Indeed, they can be administered without verbal instruction, and one study with Native Australians revealed no cultural differences in performance [51].
10. The battery is entirely computerised, with detailed automatic recording of response accuracy and speed made via a touch-screen apparatus.
11. The results are instantly available, and standardised scores can be produced from a large pool of normative data.
12. The tests are sensitive to pharmacological challenge models of dementia [52], and also to treatment effects (e.g. tacrine in AD [53], L-dopa in Parkinson's disease [54], idazoxan in dementia of frontal lobe type [55].
13. The tests are sensitive enough to be able to discriminate between different dementia types, such as AD, Parkinson's disease and Huntington's disease, and have been shown to be sensitive enough to detect preclinical cognitive decline in, for example, Huntington's disease [56] and neuroAIDS [57].

Cognitive Drug Research (CDR) Cognitive Test System

The Cognitive Drug Research (CDR) [58] computerised battery consists of 12 subtests designed to measure attention, working memory, episodic and secondary memory. Its major strengths are that it has good construct specificity and efficiency; it has 20 equivalent forms; longitudinal data are available, as are data on practice effects; and is available in several languages [59]. Its main weaknesses are a lack of a summary score, and lack of detailed coverage of important cognitive domains such as executive functions and visuospatial abilities.

New York University Computerised Test Battery (NYU Battery)

The NYU battery is a computerised battery composed of 12 subtests designed to evaluate immediate memory, recent memory, language, concept formation, psychomotor speed and attention [61]. The tests in the NYU battery are adaptations of tests used in cognitive gerontological studies, and thus are suitable for use in mildly demented individuals but are of limited use in assessing severely demented patients. Certain of the tests were designed to simulate ecologically valid processes such as recalling telephone numbers, whereas others were designed to parallel tests used in animals during the preclinical evaluation of putative cognitive enhancing compounds [62]. The major strength of this battery is that it has good construct specificity. There are six equivalent forms available, longitudinal data are available, as are data on practice effects and the effects of cholinergic disruption as a model of dementia. The main weaknesses of the NYU battery are the lack of an overall dementia score, the relatively lengthy time for test administration and the lack of executive tasks such as planning.

Memory Assessment Clinics (MAC) Computerised Test Battery

The Memory Assessment Clinics (MAC) computerised battery consists of 13 memory and attention tests which were selected to mimic real-world activities such as telephone dialling and remembering faces [63]. This battery is best suited to the assessment of non-demented elderly and mildly demented patients, but less suited to moderately or severely demented patients. Its main strengths are the availability of five equivalent forms; availability of longitudinal data; norms for healthy ageing; and its translation into several languages. Its main weaknesses are that it lacks a summary score and that the battery does not cover all the relevant cognitive domains for dementia assessment.

Activities of Daily Living, Global Staging and Behavioural Assessment

In addition to measures of cognitive function, activities of daily living (ADL) assessment, global staging and behavioural ("non-cognitive") assessment are essential components of a complete dementia evaluation.

Activities of Daily Living

Activities of daily living (ADL) refer to basic, physical functions which underlie normal living, such as continence, walking, managing money and shopping [64]. A distinction is usually made between universal, biologically necessary ADLs such as feeding and dressing ("basic" ADL), and higher-level ADLs such as shopping and handling finances ("instrumental ADL") [65]. Deterioration in both basic and instrumental ADL is a component of dementia as reflected in standard definitions such as those of DSM-IV and ICD-10 [66,67].

At present, no ADL instrument has been accepted as a valid measure of clinical significance for antidementia drugs. The instruments assessing ADL that have been published so far have shown little responsiveness to symptomatic antidementia drugs, even in the presence of measurable improvement in cognition.

Current published guidelines for the assessment of dementia stress the importance of assessing "functionality" as by measured by ADL scales [64]. For clinical trial management, ADL should have broad applicability, assess both basic and instrumental ADL, have good test–retest reliability, scaling to cover a broad range of performance, and sensitivity to detect changes with disease progression, and be non-gender-specific [16,64]. Although no specific scale has been recommended, Galasko et al. [68] have recently described the development of an inventory to assess ADL for clinical trials in AD, which meets current guidelines.

Global Change and Staging Instruments

Global change and staging instruments are interview-based instruments which provide a *subjective* assessment of the patient's overall clinical condition. These global, subjective instruments, which are intended to measure "clinical utility", may provide a useful adjunct to objective measures of cognitive function. As yet, however, consensus has not been reached on exactly what constitutes clinical utility. It has been argued that tests of clinical utility could include ADL, quality of life, and caregivers' impressions, as well as clinicians' interview-based global impressions.

The International Working Group on Harmonization of Dementia Drug Guidelines (IWGHDDG) has recently put forward a position paper on clinical global measures of dementia [32]. Readers may consult this document for more detailed discussion of clinical global measures of dementia. The IWGHDDG classified clinical global measures of dementia into two distinct types. Global severity scales such as the Clinical Dementia Rating Scale (CDR) [69] and the Global Deterioration Scale (GDS) [70] evaluate patients according to fixed external standards, whereas global change scales such as the Clinical Global Impression on Change (CGIC) [71] and later modifications such as the ADCS-CGIC [72] and Parke-Davis CIBI [73] rate the patient relative to their own previous condition.

Global Severity Scales

The CDR is based on a work sheet interview, assesses dementia severity, and includes cognitive and functional domains. The GDS assesses the phenomenological global progression of AD, cognitively, functionally and behaviourally. Data exist on the reliability and validity of the CDR and the GDS, and both have been used in clinical trials of the cholinesterase inhibitors tacrine and donepezil [74,75].

Global Change Scales

The original CGIC was based on an unstructured seven-point Likert scale, ranging from "very much improved" to "no change" to "very much worse". More recent adaptations also rate change on a seven-point scale. The ADCS-CGIC uses an organised but somewhat unstructured format in which domains including cognition, behaviour and functioning are assessed. It has been shown to have good reliability and construct validity [76]. Other interview-based change scales have been developed recently including the Parke-Davis Clinical Interview-Based Impression (CIBI), and the New York University Clinician's Interview-Bases Impression of Change-Plus.

Conclusions

Our review has indicated that existing instruments for evaluating cognitive symptoms of dementia are generally adequate to evaluate most drugs proposed for the treatment of cognitive dysfunction in dementia. However, available instruments for evaluating psychiatric symptoms, functional capacity and global clinical utility are less well developed, and considerable work needs to be done before these

aspects of dementia can be evaluated with confidence in clinical trials.

The choice of instrument used in clinical trials should be determined by the questions the investigator wishes to answer. Both phase II and phase III trials require detailed cognitive testing using an objective psychometric test battery, in tandem with a more global subjective measure (e.g. the ADAS). A number of test batteries are available and, in particular, the CANTAB battery meets all the requirements set out by the International Working Group on Harmonization of Dementia Drug Guidelines. When dementia trials wish to compare different types and subtypes of dementia, or to examine an "at-risk" population, then objective psychometric tests are clearly required. For example, the CANTAB battery has been shown to differentiate between AD, Lewy Body dementia and Huntington's disease. In addition, the CANTAB battery has been shown to be sensitive to "preclinical" cognitive impairment in Huntington's disease and neuroAIDS.

Clinicians' global assessments are intended to determine whether a drug can produce a clinically meaningful effect. A number of such scales are available, although in theory change measures might be more sensitive than global staging instruments, because they are, by definition, adjusted for baseline. However, consensus has not been reached on the issue of how best to assess "clinically meaningful change": that is, whether global scales should be required in phase II and phase III trials, or whether other specific assessments such as ADL, cognition and behaviour measures could replace the global as assessments of clinical meaningfulness [32].

ADL assessment and behavioural assessment are useful components of a dementia evaluation [28]. Unfortunately, at present, no ADL instrument has been accepted as a valid measure of clinical significance for antidementia drugs, although there have been recent promising developments [68]. Weiner et al. [76] have recently identified three suitable behavioural scales for clinical trials (see Table 15.1). However, it is too early to specify any single instrument without further studies to confirm the validity and utility of such measures, especially psychometric properties.

Acknowledgements. B.J.S. thanks the Medical Research Council for support. A.D.L. is funded by the British Brain and Spine Foundation, the Royal Society, and the MRC.

References

1. Small GW, Rabins PV, Barry PP, Buckholtz NS, DeKosky ST, Ferris SH, et al. Diagnosis and treatment of Alzheimer disease

and related disorders. Consensus statement of the American Association for Geriatric Psychiatry, the Alzheimer's Association, and the American Geriatrics Society. JAMA 1997;278:1363–1371.

2. Berrios GE. Dementia during the seventeenth and eighteenth centuries: a conceptual history. Psychol Med 1987;17:829–837.

3. Stuss DT, Levine B. The dementias: nosological and clinical factors related to diagnosis. Brain Cogn 1996;31:99–113.

4. Cummings JL, Benson DF. Dementia: a clinical approach. Boston: Butterworth, 1992.

5. Lawrence AD, Sahakian BJ. The neuropsychology of frontostriatal dementias. In: Woods RT, editor. Handbook of the clinical psychology of ageing. Chichester: Wiley, 1996:243–265.

6. Brown RG, Mardsen CD. Subcortical dementia: the neuropsychological evidence. Neuroscience 1988;25:363–387.

7. Antuono P, Doody R, Gilman S, Huff J, Scheltens P, Ueda K, et al. Diagnostic criteria for dementia in clinical trials. Position paper from the International Working Group on Harmonization of Dementia Drug Guidelines. Alzheimer Dis Assoc Disord 1997;11(Suppl 3):22–25.

8. Sahakian BJ. Computerised assessment of neuropsychological function in Alzheimer's disease and Parkinson's disease. Int J Geriatr Psychiatry 1990;5:211–213.

9. Leber P. Guidelines for the clinical evaluation of antidementia drugs, first draft. Rockville, MD: US Food and Drug Administration, 1990.

10. CPMP Working Party on Efficacy of Medicinal Products. Antidementia medicinal products. Brussels: Commission of the European Community, 1992.

11. Charlton BG. Cognitive neuropsychiatry and the future of diagnosis: a "PC" model of the mind. Br J Psychiatry 1995;167:149–153.

12. Morley S, Snaith P. Principles of psychological assessment. In: Freeman C, Tyrer P, editors. Research methods in psychiatry. 2nd ed. London: Gakell, 1992:135–152.

13. Lemke E, Wiersma W. Principles of psychological assessment. Chicago: Rand McNally, 1976.

14. Nunally JC. Psychometric theory. 2nd ed. New York: McGraw-Hill, 1978.

15. Burgess PW. Theory and methodology in executive function research. In: Rabbitt P, editor. Methodology of frontal and executive functions. Hove: Erlbaum, 1997:81–116.

16. Mohs RC. Neuropsychological assessment of patients with Alzheimer's disease. In: Bloom FE, Kupfer DJ, editors. Psychopharmacology: the fourth generation of progress. New York: Raven Press, 1995:1377–1388.

17. Milberg W. Issues in the assessment of cognitive function in dementia. Brain Cogn 1996;31:114–132.

18. Demonet JF, GelyNargeot MC, Bakchine S. Methodological aspects of cognitive assessment. Therapie 1997;52:495–498.

19. Parry CJ, Hodges JR. Spectrum of memory dysfunction in degenerative disease. Curr Opin Neurol 1996;9:281–285.

20. Owen AM, Sahakian BJ, Robbins TW. The role of executive deficits in memory disorders in neurodegenerative disease. In: Troster AI, editor. Memory in neurodegenerative disease: biological, cognitive and clinical perspectives. Cambridge: Cambridge University Press, 1998:157–171.

21. Cipolotti L, Warrington EK. Neuropsychological assessment. J Neurol Neurosurg Psychiatry 1995;58:655–664.

22. Kuhn T. The structure of scientific revolutions. 2nd ed. Chicago: University of Chicago Press, 1970.

23. Farah MJ. Neuropsychological inference with an interactive brain: a critique of the "locality" assumption. Behav Brain Sci 1994;17:43–104.

24. Kosslyn SM. Neural systems and psychiatric disorders. Cogn Neuropsychiatry 1996;1:89–93.

25. Lawrence AD. Executive functions and memory in Huntington's disease. PhD thesis, Department of Experimental Psychology, University of Cambridge, UK, 1997.

26. Weintraub S, Baratz R, Mesulam MM. Daily living activities in the assessment of dementia. In: Corkin S, editor. Alzheimer's disease: a report of progress. New York: Raven Press, 1982:189–192.

27. Plaisted KC, Sahakian BJ. Dementia of frontal lobe type: living in the here and now. Aging Mental Health 1997;1:293–295.

28. Ferris SH. Diagnosis by specialists: psychological testing. Acta Neurol Scand 1992;Suppl 139:32–35.

29. Ferris SH, Lucca U, Mohs R, Dubois B, Wesnes K, Erzigkeit H, et al. Objective psychometric tests in clinical trials of dementia drugs. Alzheimer Dis Assoc Disord 1997;11(Suppl 3):34–38.

30. Cockrell JR, Folstein MF. Mini-Mental State Examination (MMSE). Psychopharmacol Bull 1988;24:689–692.

31. Brandt J, Folstein SE, Folstein MF. Differential cognitive impairment in Alzheimer's disease and Huntington's disease. Ann Neurol 1988;23:555–561.

32. Reisberg B, Schneider L, Doody R, Anand R, Feldman H, Haraguchi H, et al. Clinical global measures of dementia. Position paper from the International Working Group on Harmonization of Dementia Drug Guidelines. Alzheimer Dis Assoc Disord 1997;11:8–18.

33. Blessed G, Tomlinson BE, Roth M. The association between quantitative measures of dementia and of senile change in the cerebral grey matter of elderly subjects. Br J Psychiatry 1968;114:797–811.

34. Roth M, Tym E, Mountjoy CQ, Huppert FA, Hendrie H, Verma S, et al. CAMDEX: a standardised instrument for the diagnosis of mental disorder in the elderly with special reference to the early detection of dementia. Br J Psychiatry 1987;149:698–709.

35. Huppert FA, Brayne C, Gill C, Paykel ES, Beardsall L. CAMCOG: a concise neuropsychological test to assist dementia diagnosis: sociodemographic determinants in an elderly population sample. Br J Clin Psychol 1995;34:529–541.

36. Mohs RC. The Alzheimer's disease assessment scale. Int Psychogeriatr 1996;8:195–203.

37. Mohs RC, Knopman D, Petersen RC, Ferris SH, Ernesto C, Grundman M, et al. Development of cognitive instruments for use in clinical trials of antidementia drugs: additions to the Alzheimer's disease assessment scale that broadens its scope. Alzheimer Dis Assoc Disord 1997;11(Suppl 2):S13–S21.

38. Mattis S. Mental status examination for organic mental syndrome in the elderly patient. In: Bellack R, Karasu B, editors. Geriatric psychiatry. New York: Grune & Stratton, 1976:77–121.

39. Erzigkeit H. The SKT: a short cognitive performance test as an instrument for the assessment of clinical efficacy of cognition enhancers: In: Bergener M, Reisberg B, editors. Diagnosis and treatment of senile dementia. Berlin: Springer, 1989:164–174.

40. Brazzelli M, Capitani E, Della Salla S, Spinnler H, Zuffi M. A neuropsychological instrument adding to the description of patients with suspected cortical dementia: the Milan Overall Dementia Assessment. J Neurol Neurosurg Psychiatry 1994;57:1510–1517.

41. Capitani E, Manzoni L, Spinnler H. Follow-up of 53 Alzheimer patients with the MODA (Milan Overall Dementia Assessment). Eur J Neurol 1997;4:237–239.

42. Morris JC, Heyman A, Mohs RC, Hughes JP, van Belle G, Fillenbaum G, et al. The Consortium to Establish a Registry for Alzheimer's Disease (CERAD). I. Clinical and neuropsychological assessment of Alzheimer's disease. Neurology 1989;39:1159–1165.

43. Fray PJ, Robbins TW. CANTAB battery: proposed utility in neurotoxicology. Neurotoxicol Teratol 1996;18:499–504.

44. Fray PJ, Robbins TW, Sahakian BJ. Neuropsychiatric applications of CANTAB. Int J Geriatr Psychiatry 1996;11:329–336.

45. Robbins TW. Dissociating executive functions of the pre-frontal cortex. Phil Trans R Soc Lond B 1996;351:1463–1471.

46. Owen AM. Cognitive planning in humans: neuropsychological, neuroanatomical and neuropharmacological perspectives. Prog Neurobiol 1997;53:431–450.

47. Roberts AC, Sahakian BJ. Comparable tests of cognitive function in monkey and man. In: Sahgal A, editor. Behavioural neuroscience: a practical approach. Oxford: IRL Press, 1993: 165–184.

48. Forstl H, Sahakian BJ. Thalamic radiodensitiy and cognitive performance in mild and moderate dementia of the Alzheimer type. J Psychiatr Neurosci 1993;18:33–37.

49. Lawrence AD, Weeks RA, Brooks DJ, Andrews TC, Watkins LHA, Harding AE, et al. The relationship between striatal dopamine receptor binding and cognitive performance in Huntington's disease. Brain 1998;121:1343–1355.

50. CENES Cognition. Personal communication, 1998.

51. Maruff P, Tyler P, Burt T, Currie B, Burns C, Currie J. Cognitive deficits in Machado-Joseph disease. Ann Neurol 1996;40:421–427.

52. Robbins TW, Semple J, Kumar R, Truman MI, Shorter J, Ferraro A, et al. Effects of scopolamine on delayed-matching-to-sample and paired associates tests of visual memory and learning in human subjects: comparison with diazepam and implications for dementia. Psychopharmacology 1997;134:95–106.

53. Sahakian BJ, Owen AM, Morant NJ, Eagger SA, Boddington S, Crayton L, et al. Crockford HA, Crooks M, Hill K, Levy R. Further analysis of the cognitive effects of tetrahydroaminoacridine (THA) in Alzheimer's disease: assessment of attentional and mnemonic function using CANTAB. Psychopharmacology 1993;110:395–401.

54. Lange KW, Robbins TW, Marsden CD, James M, Owen AM, Paul GM. L-Dopa withdrawal in Parkinson's disease selectively impairs cognitive performance in tests of frontal lobe function. Psychopharmacology 1992;107:394–404.

55. Coull JT, Sahakian BJ, Hodges JR. The alpha-2 antagonist idazoxan remediates certain attentional and executive dysfunction in patients with dementia of frontal type. Psychopharmacology 1996;123:239–249.

56. Lawrence AD, Hodges JR, Rosser AE, Kershaw A, ffrench-Constant C, Rubinsztein DC, et al. Evidence for specific cognitive deficits in preclinical Huntington's disease. Brain 1998;121:1329–1341.

57. Sahakian BJ, Elliott R, Low N, Mehta M, Clark RT, Pozniak AL. Neuropsychological deficits in tests of executive function in asymptomatic and symptomatic HIV-1 seropositive men. Psychol Med 1995;25:1233–1246.

58. Simpson PM, Surmon DJ, Wesnes KA, Wilcock GR. The cognitive drug research computerised assessment system for demented patients: a validation study. Int J Geriatr Psychiatry 1991;6:95–102.

59. Wesnes K. The pathology of attention of the dementias. J Psychopharm 1996;10(Suppl):A51.

60. Mohr E, Walker D, Randolph C, Sampson M, Mendis T. Utility of clinical trial batteries in the measurement of Alzheimer's and Huntington's dementia. Int Psychogeriatr 1996;8:397–411.

61. Ferris SH, Flicker C, Reisberg B. NYU computerised test battery for assessing cognition in aging and dementia. Psychopharmacol Bull 1988;24:699–702.

62. Flicker C, Dean R, Bartus RT, Ferris SH, Crook T. Animal and human-memory dysfunctions associated with aging, cholinergic lesions, and senile dementia. Ann NY Acad Sci 1985;444:515–517.

63. Larrabee GJ, Crook T. A computerised everyday memory battery for assessing treatment effects. Psychopharmacol Bull 1988;24:695–697.

64. Gauthier S, Bodick N, Erzigkeit E, Feldman H, Geldmacher DS, Huff J, et al. Activities of daily living as an outcome measure in clinical trials of dementia drugs. Alzheimer Dis Assoc Disord 1997;11(Suppl 3):S6–S7.

65. Katz S, Ford AB, Moskowitz RW, Jackson BA, Jaffe MW. Studies of illness in the aged. JAMA 1963;185:914–919.

66. American Psychiatric Association. Diagnostic and statistical manual of mental disorders. 4th ed. Washington, DC: American Psychiatric Association, 1994.

67. World Health Organization. The ICD-10 classification of mental and behavioural disorders. Geneva: World Health Organization, 1992.

68. Galasko D, Bennett D, Sano M, Ernesto C, Thomas R, Grundman M, et al. An inventory to assess activities of daily living for clinical trials in Alzheimer's disease. Alzheimer Dis Assoc Disord 1997;11(Suppl 2):S33–S39.

69. Morris JC. The clinical dementia rating (CDR): current version and scoring rules. Neurology 1993;43:2412–2414.

70. Reisberg B, Ferris SH, de Leon MJ, Crook T. The global deterioration scale for assessment of primary degenerative dementia. Am J Psychiatry 1982;139:1136–1139.

71. Guy W. ECDEU assessment manual. Rockville, MD: US Department of Health Education and Welfare publication no. (ADM) 76-338, 1976.

72. Ferris SH, Mackell JA, Mohs R, et al. A multicenter evaluation of new treatment efficacy instruments for Alzheimer disease clinical trials: overview and general results. Alzheimer Dis Assoc Disord 1997;11(Suppl 1):S1–S2.

73. Knopman DS, Knapp MJ, Gracon SI, Davis CS. The clinician interview based impression (CIBI): a clinician's global change rating scale in Alzheimer's disease. Neurology 1994;44:2315–2321.

74. Knapp MJ, Knopman DS, Solomon PR, et al. A 30-week randomized controlled trial of high-dose tacrine in patients with Alzheimer's disease. JAMA 1994;271:985–991.

75. Rogers S, Doody RS, Mohs R, Friedhoff L. E-2020 produces both clinical global and cognitive test improvement in patients with mild to moderatley severe Alzheimer's disease (AD): results of a 30 week Phase III trial. Neurology 1996;46:A217.

76. Weiner MF, Koss E, Wild KV, Folks DG, Tariot P, Luszczynska H, et al. Measures of psychiatric symptoms in Alzheimer patients: a review. Alzheimer Dis Assoc Disord 1996;10:20–30.

77. Homma A, Brodaty H, Bruno G, Cummings JL, Gilman S, Gracon S, et al. Clinical trials of treatment for noncognitive symptoms of dementia. Position paper from the International Working Group on Harmonization of Dementia Drug Guidelines. Alzheimer Dis Assoc Disord 1997;11(Suppl 3):S54–S55.

78. Ferris SH, Mackell JA. Behavioral outcomes in clinical trials for Alzheimer disease. Alzheimer Dis Assoc Disord 1997;11(Suppl 4):S10–S15.

79. Reisberg B, Auer SR, Monteiro IM. Behavior pathology in Alzheimer's disease (BEHAVE-AD) rating scale. Int Psychogeriatr 1996;8(Suppl 3):301–308.

80. Tariot PN, Mack JL, Patterson MB, et al. The behavior rating scale for dementia of the Consortium to Establish a Registry of Alzheimer's Disease. Am J Psychiatry 1995;152:1349–1357.

81. Koss E, Weiner M, Ernesto C, Cohen-Mansfield J, Ferris SH, Grundman M, Schafer K, Sano M, Thal LJ, Thomas R, Whitehouse PJ. Assessing patterns of agitation in Alzheimer's disease patients with the Cohen-Mansfield agitation inventory. Alzheimer Dis Assoc Disord 1997;11(Suppl 2): 545–550.

16. Dementia: Trial Design and Experience with Large Multicentre Trials

R.J. Harvey and M.N. Rossor

Introduction

Dementia is common, being estimated to affect up to 50% of the population who are aged over 85 years [1]. Rarely, reversible causes, such as a frontal meningioma, normal pressure hydrocephalus or vitamin B_{12} deficiency lead to specific treatments. The majority of cases, however, are due to one of the neurodegenerative diseases, of which Alzheimer's disease (AD) is by far the commonest. The identification of specific cholinergic deficits in the brains of patients with AD in the late 1970s and early 1980s provided considerable impetus to the hope that treatment for the dementias might be possible [2,3]. The development and expansion of world-wide drug development programmes since that time have been dramatic, culminating in the licensing of tacrine in the United States in 1993 [4,5], and more recently, the approval of donezepil [6]. The diseases that cause dementia are defined neuropathologically, yet in life the diagnosis can usually only be made clinically. Moreover, the considerable heterogeneity and broad spectrum of impairment that occurs is difficult to measure in a reliable way. From the earliest clinical trials in AD, drug regulatory authorities, and particularly the US Food and Drug Administration (FDA) have taken a proactive interest in the methodology being used to prove the efficacy of drugs treatments for dementia. This interest has ensured broad standardisation of clinical trial designs, and has promoted the development of standardised guidelines through processes such as the International Working Group on the Harmonization of Dementia Drug Guidelines [7].

The development and licensing of symptomatic treatments for AD represents the first milestone towards effective treatment for all dementias. Drug development programmes are likely to expand into other dementias, and will increasingly focus on other therapeutic targets such as the slowing of disease progression and ultimately disease prevention.

Early Trials in Alzheimer's Disease

It is useful to review the methodology used in early dementia drug trials, and particularly the role tacrine had in defining subsequent guidelines. The first study of tacrine in AD was published in 1981 and was a pilot study of 12 patients, 9 of whom were considered to have improved on treatment [8], a further study appeared to confirm the dramatic benefits of the drug in AD [9]. The magnitude of effect and potential therapeutic importance of the original study [9] led to a FDA audit that revealed methodological flaws in the protocol and performance of the trial. The subsequent enquiry and report [10] resulted in an FDA task force [11] and further report [12] which have influenced the development of current methodologies for therapeutic clinical trials in AD.

The original study by Summers et al. [9] enrolled 23 demented subjects who underwent a variety of laboratory and clinical tests to confirm the diagnosis of AD, as a result of which 17 subjects entered the first phase of the study. In phase I, patients were given open label escalating doses of tacrine. The best dose for each patient was identified by observation of clinical improvement without side effects, or treatment with maximum dose without clinical improvement. In phase II of the study, now as out-patients, subjects were randomised to receive either their optimal dose or placebo in a double-blind manner for 3 weeks, after which they crossed over to the opposite treatment group for a further 3 weeks. In phase III of the study, those who were considered to have responded in phase II were able to continue at their optimal dose for an extended period. In total 17 of 23 subjects entered phase I, 15 of 17 entered phase II, and 12 of 15 entered phase III (Fig. 16.1).

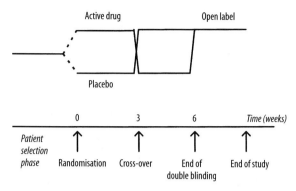

Fig. 16.1. Study design of the earliest study of tacrine [1].

Although the responses reported in the study were dramatic, a number of methodological problems with the study were considered by the FDA audit:

- The randomisation method was not documented, and blinding was not maintained throughout the study.
- Very small numbers of patients took part, which was combined with a high drop-out rate.
- The inclusion and exclusion criteria were poorly defined and lacked clarity. Even after those who were thought not to have AD were excluded, the initial double-blind treatment group included a patient with low vitamin B_{12}, one had Parkinson's disease and clinical depression, and a further patient had multiple cerebral infarcts.
- The crossover design of the trial had short treatment periods and no wash-out between treatments.
- There was no separate analysis of the blinded tacrine versus blinded placebo in the first 3 weeks of phase II, i.e. a parallel-group analysis.
- No allowance was made for the fact that all patients took lecithin throughout the study.
- There was no apparent placebo effect, and this was not commented upon.
- The outcome measures used by the study were a global improvement scale, a name learning test and an orientation test, all of which were considered to be of questionable validity. In particular the global ratings were performed after the trial was completed, in an unsubstantiated manner.

As a result of the audit, the FDA issued guidelines for investigators assessing the effects of drugs in patients with dementia. These recommended a double-blind, randomised, placebo-controlled, parallel group methodology that allows true comparison of a placebo and treatment group and avoids problems with inadequate washout periods between treatments. They also recommended a minimum length of trial of at least 6–12 months. For efficacy to

be demonstrated a statistically significant positive result was required on both a validated cognitive measure and a clinician's global rating. They also stressed the need for careful, standardised patient selection and diagnosis using validated clinical criteria, and well-defined inclusion and exclusion criteria. These recommendations remain the basis upon which most clinical trials in dementia have been designed.

Patient Selection

The selection of carefully defined homogeneous groups of patients is of critical importance, both to ensure validity of the results and to reduce variability in the outcome measures used. However, even within a population of patients with a single disease such as AD there is considerable heterogeneity of clinical, neuropsychological and functional deficits.

The diagnosis of the cause of dementia can only be made with absolute certainty on neuropathological examination of brain tissue; thus patients entering clinical trials are likely to have only a presumptive clinical diagnosis. However, the development of a range of validated clinical diagnostic criteria plays a major role in identifying populations of patients for inclusion in clinical trials.

Diagnostic Instruments: Alzheimer's Disease

AD is a neuropathological diagnosis determined by the presence of neurofibrillary tangles and senile plaques in the brain of a patient with dementia. The disease frequently starts with memory impairment, but is invariably followed by a progressive global cognitive impairment. Neurological examination is often normal early in the disease. Structural neuroimaging may be normal early in the disease, but cerebral atrophy, particularly of the medial temporal lobe structures, is apparent as the disease progresses [13]. Three main sets of diagnostic criteria have become widely accepted: the American Psychiatric Association Diagnostic and Statistical Manual of Mental Disorders version 4 (DSM-IV) [14], the World Health Organization Tenth International Classification of Diseases (ICD-10) and the National Institute of Neurological, Communication Disorders and Stroke/Alzheimer's Disease and Associated Disorders Association (NINCDS/ADRDA) research diagnostic criteria for AD [15].

DSM-IV

A DSM-IV diagnosis of AD requires the patient to have developed deficits in multiple domains of cognitive function which consist of memory impairment, plus one or more impairments in the domains of language (aphasia), motor activities (apraxia), visual perception (agnosia) and executive functioning (frontal lobe function) [14]. Furthermore these deficits should be significant enough to impair social and/or occupational function. The development of these symptoms should have been gradual, progressive and not associated with other central nervous system (CNS) diseases, systemic disorders known to cause cognitive impairment, or substance abuse. The deficits should not occur exclusively during a delirium, and should not be better accounted for by any other DSM-IV diagnosis, for example a major depressive disorder.

ICD-10

The ICD-10 diagnostic guidelines define dementia as a decline in both memory and thinking sufficient to impair personal activities of daily living. In addition to memory impairment there should be impaired thinking and reasoning capacity, and a reduced flow of ideas. Symptoms and impairments should be present for a minimum period of 6 months, and must have been present during periods of clear consciousness. A diagnosis of AD requires the dementia to have had an insidious onset and slow deterioration. The criteria do, however, allow plateaux in the illness. There should be an absence of other systemic or brain diseases that could mimic dementia, excluded by clinical evidence and special investigations. The symptoms should not have a sudden onset, and there should be no neurological signs to suggest focal brain damage.

The ICD-10 criteria are less specific in the definition of the domains of impairment required for a diagnosis of dementia, but like the DSM-IV focus on the course of the disease, and the absence of other signs of systemic or neurological disease.

NINCDS/ADRDA

The NINCDS/ADRDA provide more comprehensive research diagnostic criteria for AD, and permit levels of certainty (definite, probable, possible) to be assigned to the diagnosis [15]:

A diagnosis of *definite* NINCDS/ADRDA AD requires neuropathological confirmation of the disease.

A *probable* or *possible* diagnosis of AD requires that dementia is established clinically with the cognitive impairment documented using a test such as the Mini Mental State Examination [16], and confirmed using formal neuropsychological testing. There must be deficits in two or more areas of cog-

nition with progressive worsening of memory and other cognitive functions. Consciousness should be undisturbed and there should be an absence of systemic or other brain disease that could account for the symptoms. Notably, the criteria require an onset of the disease between the ages of 40 and 90 years.

The criteria then provide several sections to enable probable cases to be differentiated from possible cases. Probable AD is supported by progressive deterioration of specific cognitive functions, impaired activities of daily living and altered behaviour. It also recognises that there may be a family history. Specific investigations such as lumbar puncture should be normal, the electroencephalogram may show slow wave activity, and structural imaging should show progressive cerebral atrophy. Other features are recognised as being consistent with probable AD, including plateaux in the course of the disease, associated psychiatric and behavioural symptoms, neurological abnormalities such as myoclonus and gait disorders, seizures in advanced disease and the occasional finding of a normal CT scan. Features that make a probable diagnosis of AD unlikely include a sudden or apoplectic onset, focal neurological findings, and seizures or gait disorder early in the disease.

Those patients with typical core features but factors making a probable diagnosis unlikely are defined as having possible AD. Reliability and validity studies of the criteria have been carried out and suggest that, when the criteria are diligently applied, 80% specificity is possible [17].

Other Dementias

Although AD accounts for the majority of all dementia, a significant number of demented patients will have other diseases such as vascular dementia, dementia with Lewy bodies and frontotemporal dementia. Improved clinical and neuroimaging investigations, together with neuropathological studies, have resulted in an increasing range of diagnostic criteria, which allow these other dementias to be accurately identified.

Vascular Dementia (VaD)

Diagnostic criteria for VaD are less well developed [18] and there is no firm consensus on the most appropriate criteria to use for clinical trials [19]. DSM-IV criteria [14] are very similar to the criteria for AD, but require the presence of focal neurological symptoms, or neuroimaging signs of multiple infarctions in the cortex. The ICD-10 criteria require a history of transient ischaemic attacks, or a succession of small strokes. The important presence of

Table 16.1. Summary of the NINDS-AIREN criteria for vascular dementia (VaD)

I. For probable VaD
  1. Dementia defined by deficits in multiple domains of cognitive function, confirmed clinically and neuropsychologically, and interfering with everyday life
  2. Cerebrovascular disease confirmed by focal neurological signs and evidence of vascular disease on CT or MRI
  3. A temporal relationship between 2 and 1

II. Features consistent with a probable diagnosis include:
  Early gait disturbance, unsteadiness or falls, urinary symptoms, pseudobulbar palsy, personality and mood changes

III. Features that make the diagnosis unlikely include:
  Early memory deficit and progressive worsening of specific cognitive deficits without evidence of focal brain lesions on neuroimaging, absence of focal neurological signs, the absence of vascular lesions on CT or MRI

IV. Clinical features of possible vascular dementia include:
  1. Features of section I.1, with focal neurological signs, but where neuroimaging has not been performed to confirm the presence of vascular lesions
  2. The absence of a temporal relationship between I.1 and I.2
  3. The presence of a subtle and variable course in the disease

V. Criteria for definite VaD are:
  1. Clinical criteria for probable VaD
  2. Histopathological evidence from biopsy or autopsy
  3. Absence of neuropathological features of Alzheimer's disease
  4. Absence of other clinical or pathological cause for the disease

Adapted from Roman et al. [20].

vascular risk factors is recognised, together with the findings of focal neurological signs and symptoms and neuroimaging confirmation of vascular lesions.

In 1993 a work group of the National Institute of Neurological Disorders and Stroke (NINDS) and the Association Internationale pour la Recherche et l'Enseignement en Neurosciences (AIREN) reported on a workshop held to discuss diagnostic criteria for research in VaD [20]. They recognised the difficulties inherent in the diagnosis, and helpfully classified VaD syndromes as follows:

1. Multi-infarct dementia.
2. Strategic single infarct dementia.
3. Small vessel disease with dementia.
4. Hypoperfusion.
5. Haemorrhagic dementia.
6. Other mechanisms.

This classification shows the difficulty of establishing a single set of diagnostic criteria for a disease with at least six discrete underlying pathological mechanisms. A summary of the criteria that they proposed is presented in Table 16.1. The working group recognised that the criteria were not ideal. Clinical application results in the selection of a "pure" group of vascular dementias, which undoubtedly excludes many patients with a vascular component to their disease.

The International Working Group for Harmonization of Dementia Drug Guidelines (IWG) also dis-

cussed the issue of diagnostic criteria for VaD [20] and recognised that applying the current criteria selected a group of patients who may be of limited clinical comparability to the general population of VaD patients. The recommendation of the IWG was to enrol populations of patients with "pure" VaD, mixed AD/VaD and probable AD. A comparison of efficacy between these three groups would then allow inference of drug efficacy in VaD.

Dementia with Lewy Bodies (DLB)

DLB often presents in a similar way to AD; however, frontal lobe and visuo-spatial impairments occur early in the disease, and there are a number of other features which differentiate DLB from AD: motor features of parkinsonism, prominent visual hallucinations, systematised delusions, marked fluctuation, falls and syncopal episodes are all characteristic of the disease. The consensus criteria for DLB reflect these features (Table 16.2) [21]. Patients with DLB have a marked cholinergic deficit [22], and have been identified as possible preferential responders in AD clinical trials [23].

Frontotemporal Dementia (FTD)

FTD describes a clinical syndrome of behavioural disorder associated with fronto-temporal cerebral atrophy [24,25], usually beginning before the age of 65 years. The syndrome has three main pathological

Table 16.2. Consensus criteria for diagnosis of probable dementia with Lewy bodies (DLB)

1. Progressive cognitive decline of sufficient magnitude to interfere with normal social or occupational function. Prominent memory impairment may not occur in the early stages but is evident with progression of the disease. Deficits on tests of attention and of frontal subcortical skills and visuospatial ability may be especially prominent

2. Two of the following core features are essential for a diagnosis of probable DLB:
    (a) fluctuating cognition with pronounced variations in attention and alertness
    (b) visual hallucinations which are typically well formed and detailed
    (c) motor features of parkinsonism

3. Features supportive of the diagnosis include:
    (a) repeated falls
    (b) syncope
    (c) transient disturbances of consciousness
    (d) neuroleptic sensitivity
    (e) systematised delusions
    (f) hallucinations in other modalities

4. A diagnosis of DLB is less likely in the presence of:
    (a) stroke disease, evident as local neurological signs or on brain imaging
    (b) evidence on physical examination and investigation of any physical illness, or other brain disorder, sufficient to account for the clinical picture

Adapted from McKeith et al. [21].

substrates: In the frontal lobe degeneration type nerve cell loss and spongiform change is seen; in the Pick's disease type, swollen or "ballooned" neurones (Pick cells) and intraneuronal inclusion bodies (Pick bodies) are present; and in the third variant of the disease, spinal motor neurone degeneration is seen, usually associated with the frontal lobe degeneration type pathology [26].

The core clinical features of these patients are the insidious onset of a selective loss of cognitive abilities, namely language and/or frontal executive function, with the relative preservation in other domains such as memory, orientation and visuoperceptual function. Personal and social awareness is lost early, and the disease is associated with disinhibition, mental rigidity and inflexibility in association with maintained general independence.

The diagnostic criteria are useful for identifying groups of patients with this syndrome; however, the disparate pathology underlying the disease suggests a variety of possibly aetiologies that may require different treatment strategies. The development of more specific criteria capable of accurately identifying the subgroups of FTD will be needed once potential treatments for these diseases appear.

The Application of Diagnostic Criteria in Clinical Trials

The lack of objective diagnostic markers, and the clinical subjectivity of the available diagnostic criteria, raise a number of methodological problems in multicentre clinical trials. Investigator training is the most important factor in ensuring consistency of diagnosis across a number of centres. The training should cover the rationale of the criteria being applied and the group assessment of clinical material to identify areas of disagreement in diagnosis between investigators. Particularly in multi-national studies cultural biases will be inherent in the diagnostic process and a consensus on application of the diagnostic criteria must be agreed between all centres before recruitment commences.

The IWG has suggested a filtered approach to diagnosis that leads the investigator through a structured diagnostic route, commencing with the history and examination, and progressively adding clinical investigations such as neuroimaging, and possibly other diagnostic markers, until the diagnosis is either confirmed or refuted [19]. This structured approach, if carefully documented, permits sponsors and regulators to review the individual process of diagnosis for each patient.

Clinical Trial Design

The design of clinical trial protocols for anti-dementia drugs is influenced by a number of factors. First, as discussed in the section on diagnosis, the patient population is heterogeneous. Secondly, the lack of objective outcome measures results in significant variability in the data that are collected. Finally, the likely effects of the drug need to be considered in the design of a trial. For example, a trial to demonstrate symptomatic efficacy of the drug will require a different design from one to demonstrate the effects of the drug on disease progression.

Early Phase Development of Anti-dementia Drugs

Phase I: Early Pharmacology and Pharmacokinetic Studies

Initial studies with potential anti-dementia drugs are carried out with the recognition that the target population for the drug will be elderly people. The expected pharmacological principles on which the effectiveness of the drug is anticipated are established and early side effects or markers of effectiveness in normal volunteers are used to plan the dose ranges for phase II studies.

Phase II: Initial Therapeutic Studies

Phase II studies aim to document efficacy and identify dose ranges and administration regimes in small groups of carefully selected patients with the target dementia. Patients are generally more mildly affected and free of concomitant medical conditions and medications. Patients may be selected on the basis of a positive response to the drug in pre-randomisation challenge, as in the early tacrine studies – a methodology that would not be acceptable beyond this phase of development.

Late Phase II and Phase III Pivotal Efficacy Studies

The aim of phase III studies is to establish the efficacy of the drug in a population of patients representative of those who are likely to be receiving it after licensing. The population should include patients from various subgroups of the disease: varying severity, other illnesses and medications, younger and older patients, and those with renal and hepatic impairment. However, there are often inadequate safety and tolerability data to justify such studies, and therefore pivotal studies, i.e. those designed to demonstrate conclusive efficacy for licensing purposes, are often performed in late phase II. In late phase II studies, large groups of relatively selected patients are assessed for safety, tolerability and efficacy.

Trials to Demonstrate Symptomatic Efficacy

The demonstration of symptomatic efficacy has been the primary aim of clinical trials carried out in the field of dementia to date. Although improving the patient's symptoms may appear to delay the pro-

gression of the disease, the clear distinction between symptomatic and biological progression of the disease is critical in determining whether the drug has had any permanent biological effect on the disease process. For a purely symptomatic treatment, patients taking the drug will have a significant benefit in terms of symptoms when compared with untreated patients or those receiving a placebo, but if the drug is withdrawn they return to the same state as the control group. If a drug has a biological effect on the disease process then the patients who have taken the drug will maintain a symptomatic advantage over those who have not been exposed to the drug, even when the drug is withdrawn.

Two main clinical trial designs have been used to demonstrate symptomatic efficacy of anti-dementia drugs: the crossover study and the parallel group study:

The Crossover Trial. In a crossover design (Fig. 16.1), once included in the trial, patients are randomised to receive either active drug or placebo. Following a period of treatment and assessment the groups cross over. The advantage of this design is its ability to reduce inter-group and inter-subject variability as all subjects are part of both the control and treatment groups. However, this type of design is only suitable for relatively short treatment periods and where persistent effects of the drug, withdrawal effects and half-life are so insignificant that they will not confound the results of the study [12,27]. In a dementia treatment for chronic use, these requirements are unlikely to be fulfilled and this is rarely a suitable design. In studies where it has been used, analysis of the first section of the study, prior to crossover, can be analysed as a separate parallel group study, and it has been possible to show efficacy for anti-dementia drugs at this stage [28,29].

The Parallel Group Trial. In a parallel group study, patients are randomised to receive either active treatment or placebo, and remain in these groups throughout the trial. Larger group sizes, combined with randomisation, reduce variability and there are no issues of drug wash-out or symptomatic carry-over. The limiting issue in trials of this design is the willingness of patients to take a placebo for 6–12 months. Prior to the licensing of treatments for AD this has been a relatively minor issue; however, in the future placebo-controlled studies will inevitably disappear with the appearance of studies involving comparator drugs of proven efficacy. Group sizes are based on power calculations made according to the magnitude of effect expected from the compound. To compensate for measurement variability, however,

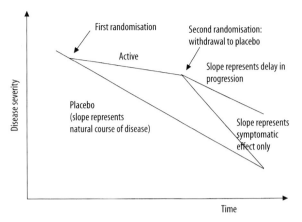

Fig. 16.2. Randomised withdrawal design.

a minimum of 100–150 patients per arm is usually required.

Fixed Dose Versus Variable Dose Studies

Phase II studies classically aim to establish, dose, dosing regimen, adverse effect and efficacy relationships. Having established this at phase II, phase III studies can be based upon two or more fixed dose levels compared with placebo. However, with a more rapid move to pivotal studies, and the involvement of a more heterogeneous and frail population, a fixed high dose may lead to unacceptable levels of drop-out due to adverse effects. Two strategies are available to improve tolerability and compliance.

First, maintaining the fixed dose design, patients begin on a low dose and gradually titrate to the fixed dose for their group. To ensure valid results patients must reach the full dose level to which they were randomised and an adequate period should be allowed at the maximum dose for a steady state to be established prior to efficacy measures.

A second strategy is the maximum tolerated dose design. Patients are randomised to placebo or one of two or more dose ranges. A titration period follows, but patients may stop titration at a dose level that is below the maximum. Blinding is maintained throughout the titration by moving all patients, including those in the placebo group, through a series of "dosing levels". The benefits of this strategy are improved tolerability, reduced drop-out from the study and potentially improved efficacy by ensuring the patients are taking their optimal dose. However, the data may be more difficult to analyse, particularly if the majority of patients remain on lower doses. Logistically this design is difficult to administer and requires at least one unblinded pharmacist to dispense the specific dose for each patient at each visit,

as it is impossible to provide pre-packaged drug supplies that cover all eventualities. The FDA has recommended the adoption of parallel group studies with three widely spaced, fixed doses (with titration) versus placebo as a method for documenting efficacy, optimum dosing regimen and tolerability [12].

Length of Trial

Most dementias are chronically progressive conditions, with a duration of disease measured in years. An effective treatment for dementia therefore has to have efficacy measured over a realistic duration. Guidelines on anti-dementia drug development from the United States, Canada, Europe and Japan encourage a minimum duration of 3 months, with a more realistic target of at least 6 months treatment, and ideally 1 year or more [12,27,30,31].

Trials to Demonstrate Disease Modifying Efficacy

Within the protocols designed to demonstrate symptomatic efficacy, the end of study analysis will prove or refute a difference between the treatment and control groups on cognitive, functional and global measures. However, this analysis cannot determine whether the underlying disease has been biologically altered. Two possible trial designs that theoretically may be able to demonstrate the effect of a drug of biological disease progression have been proposed [32]: withdrawal design and randomised start design.

Withdrawal Design. Fig. 16.2 represents a withdrawal design. This is a modification of the standard parallel group study, where, at intervals during the trial, patients in the active group are randomly reassigned either to continue active treatment or switch to placebo (withdrawal). At the end of the study all patients are on placebo. If those patients who have received the active treatment for longest have a symptomatic advantage over those who have received less treatment then this would be evidence that exposure to the drug has altered the course of their disease. The major disadvantages of this design are the practical and ethical issues of having patients on placebo for long periods.

Randomised Start Design. In the randomised start design [33], all patients commence on placebo and at intervals during the study are re-randomised to either remain on placebo or switch to active treatment. At the end of the trial all patients are taking active treatment (Fig. 16.3). If the results show greatest benefit for those patients who have been exposed to the drug for the longest period, and particularly if

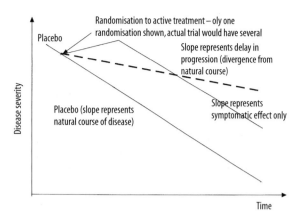

Fig. 16.3.   Randomised start design.

the slope of their continuing decline is not convergent with the control group then this suggests that the drug has modified the progression of the disease.

Primary Prevention Trials

Primary prevention trials aim to prevent or treat a disease before it expresses itself. The primary prevention of dementia would have major economic and public health benefits were it possible. The IWG has considered primary prevention trials and suggested possible methodology [34]. Given the projected incidence of AD and an effect size of a 50% reduction in the incidence, studies with 2500 individuals per arm would be required with follow-up over 5 years. Subjects selected on the basis of significantly increased risk of dementia may be able to reduce group sizes. This type of study would be expensive, estimated at $25–$50 million, and difficult to replicate. To justify such a study there would need to be very strong evidence for efficacy, adequate information on dosing and excellent safety data. Nevertheless, prevention is probably the ultimate aim in dementia.

Outcome Measures

The choice of outcome measure is guided by the regulatory guidelines. The FDA guidelines have been the most explicit and require that the major outcome variables are clearly defined before the study commences. Moreover, the outcome measure chosen must be able to show that the drug has a clinically meaningful effect, and that it is exerting its effects on the "core" manifestations of dementia [12]. It is suggested that this is achieved by demonstrating effectiveness on a global assessment performed by a skilled clinician, and on a performance-based, objective measure which provides a comprehensive as-

sessment of cognitive function. More recently, other domains of function such as activities of daily living (ADL) and quality of life (QOL) have been proposed as additional primary outcome measures. A range of secondary outcome measures encompassing the cognitive, functional, behavioural and clinical domains are usually also included. The use of a wide range of outcome measures with post-hoc selection of the "best" measure is strongly discouraged.

Clinical Global Rating Scales

Clinical global rating scales are commonly used in psychopharmacological research. This reflects the fact that for a drug to be of benefit, those benefits should be recognisable by a clinician familiar with the manifestations of the disease. A range of global assessments have been developed and used. The assessments fall into two categories: those that assess global severity and those that measure global change relative to baseline. They have been classified as follows [35]:

Global Interview-Based Severity Scales

Assessments using global interview-based severity scales are primarily aimed at placing the patient on the spectrum of disease in a cross-sectional way. The assessment may be unanchored, anchored to fixed descriptive points, or made on the basis of guidelines for severity. The anchored measures can be used as absolute severity outcomes, while the unanchored and guideline-based assessments usually have a corresponding change scale associated with them.

Anchored Assessments

CDR (Clinical Dementia Rating) [36].   The CDR is assessed using a structured interview completed with both the patient and a caregiver independently. Performance in six domains of function (memory; orientation; judgement and problem solving; community affairs; home and hobbies; and personal care) are rated using a 5-point scale (0 = normal, 0.5 = questionable, 1 = mild, 2 = moderate, 3 = severe). A global CDR rating is then generated either using a weighted rubric to combine the six individual domain scores, or simply by summing the domains. The weighted scoring system gives a CDR rating of 0–5, with points as above plus 4 representing profound dementia and 5 representing terminal.

GDS (Global Deterioration Scale) [37].   As for the CDR, the GDS scale provides a single-figure rating of dementia severity, on a 7-point scale from 1 (normal) to 7 (very severe cognitive decline). The rating is made by a clinician who has access to all available sources of information about the patient. It is easy to use and incorporates evaluations of cognition, function and behaviour.

Unanchored Assessments

Clinical Global Impression of Severity (CGIS) [38]. The CGIS is an assessment made by a skilled clinician. There is no specified assessment and the assessor is asked to place the patients on a 7-point scale representing severity of disease based upon their clinical experience (1 = amongst the most mildly affected; to 7 = amongst the most severely affected patients).

Sandoz Clinical Assessment Scale Geriatric (SCAG) [39]. For the SCAG a semi-structured interview is used to assess 18 cardinal signs and symptoms of dementia. A final item requires an unanchored rating of severity to be made on a 7-point scale.

Guideline-Based Assessments

Clinical Interview-Based Impression of Severity (CIBIS) [12]. The CIBIS represents the first part of the global rating recommended in the FDA guidelines and requires an absolute global severity rating to be made on an unanchored 7-point scale from very mild to very severe judged in relation to the full range of symptomatology in dementia.

Global Interview-Based Change Scales

Clinical Global Impression of Change (CGIC) [38]. There are minimal instructions or guidelines for the CGIC and it primarily requires a skilled clinician to make a judgement of change on a 7-point scale (1 = very much improved through 4 = no change to 7 = very much worse). The physician is instructed to rate only change relative to base line (CGIS), whether or not they attribute it to drug treatment.

Clinicians Interview-Based Impression of Change (CIBIC) [12]. The CIBIC is the second part of the FDA-recommended global assessment. It requires an experienced clinician to rate change in the patient on an unanchored 7-point scale based upon their own personal interview with the patient and no other sources of information. In particular the rater should not have access to psychometric tests, investigation results, or reports from nurses or caregivers.

CIBI (Parke-Davis) [40]. Used in many of the tacrine studies, the CIBI recognised the difficulty and discrepancy from clinical practice of assessing a demented person in isolation. At the baseline assessment a thorough interview is carried out with both the patient and caregiver, addressing eight specific areas including the mental state. The follow-up assessments are performed solely with the patient and the rating of change is made on the 7-point scale as for the CIBIC.

CIBIC+. The CIBIC+ is a variation on the CIBIC using the same 7-point unanchored scale; however, the rater has access to the caregiver at each assessment.

Alzheimer's Disease Collaborative Study – CGIC (ADCS-CGIC) [41]. The ADCS-CGIC uses a semi-structured interview to assess 15 domains of function with both the patient and the caregiver, it includes sample probes in each domain. The rating is made on the standard CGIC 7-point scale.

New York University CIBIC/CIBIC+ (NYU-CIBIC/ CIBIC+). The NYU-CIBIC/CIBIC+ is a more structured assessment that requires separate interviews with the patient and caregiver assessing multiple domains of function. Elements of other validated assessments are incorporated and anchors are provided on the 7-point scale.

Overview of Global Measures

Global measures are an important part of many regulatory guidelines and there has been an extensive debate on the best methodology. A gradual shift has occurred from unstructured, unanchored assessments to more structured assessments on anchored scales, primarily in an attempt to increase sensitivity without compromising reliability.

Objective Cognitive Measures

A core manifestation of dementia is impairment of cognitive function, and thus an objective cognitive measure is always likely to be a primary outcome measure. Guidelines from both the United States [12] and Europe [27] require the objective cognitive measure used to be validated, sensitive enough to detect even modest changes in symptoms, reliable, practical, calibrated with various populations, free of cultural bias and available in equivalent forms for repeated administration (see also Chapter 15). Other requirements include acceptance of the measure by experts in the field of dementia and its documented ability to measure change in clinical trials. Very few instruments are capable of fulfilling all these requirements and thus of being used in multicentre international trials.

Mini Mental State Examination (MMSE) [16]

The MMSE was developed to be a simple method of grading a patient's cognitive state. It consists of 30 items that are administered to the patient by an assessor. Despite fulfilling few of the criteria for objective cognitive tests it has been included almost universally in dementia clinical trials. It is primarily used as staging instrument within the inclusion criteria and lacks sensitivity for use as a primary outcome measure.

Alzheimer's Disease Assessment Scale (ADAS-Cog) [42]

The ADAS is a battery of brief tests that divides into two main parts: cognitive (ADAS-Cog) and non-cognitive (ADAS-Noncog). It is probably the only objective cognitive measure that comes close to fulfilling the regulatory guidelines and thus it has been widely employed in anti-dementia trials, where it now has the documented ability to demonstrate the effects of drugs on AD.

The ADAS-Cog has 12 sections and is scored by the number of errors made. A score of 0 therefore represents perfect performance. The graded difficulty of the assessment, however, means that even normal individuals are unlikely to achieve a perfect score. A maximum error score of 70 would indicate failure on every section. The demanding nature of some sections means that only mildly to moderately affected patients can complete the whole assessment. It is divided into eight sections:

- *Word recall.* The patients ability to recall 10 words is tested over three trials.
- *Naming objects and fingers.* The patient is asked to name 12 objects selected to have names of high, medium and low frequency, and then to name the fingers on their dominant hand.
- *Commands.* Five sequences of commands are given to the patient in turn. The first sequence is a single command, increasing each time until a sequence of five actions is given.
- *Constructional praxis.* A sequence of four drawings is presented that the patient is asked to copy.
- *Ideational praxis.* The patient is asked to fold and place a piece of paper in an envelope, seal the envelope, and address it to themselves, including placing the stamp.
- *Orientation.* A set of eight standard orientation questions are asked.
- *Word recognition.* The patients reads out 12 words. They are then asked to identify the 12 "target" words which have been mixed with 12 "distracter" words. This is repeated for three trials with fresh distracters for each trial.

- *Observer-rated sections.* The test administrator then scores the patients on the five remaining sections: remembering test instructions; spoken language ability; word finding difficulty in spontaneous speech; comprehension; and concentration/distractibility.

The test requires 30–60 minutes to administer. For international clinical trials there are now Euro-ADAS versions in French, German, Italian and Spanish.

Other Objective Cognitive Tests

The ADAS is widely accepted as the de facto cognitive test in AD trials [43], and the restrictions imposed by the current guidelines effectively stifle the development of other assessments for AD. However, the ADAS has a strong bias towards memory function and is much less suitable for use in other dementias, such as VaD and DLB. In DLB in particular, attention deficits may predominate, and there are no attentional components in the ADAS. Computerised cognitive assessments such as the Computerised Dementia Rating (CDR) [44] and Cambridge Neuropsychological Test Automated Battery (CANTAB) [45] are able to fulfil many of the guideline requirements, and in addition include timed components and other tests that assess attention. It is likely that the ADAS will remain the test of choice for AD but that alternative batteries will be needed for other dementias.

Magnetic Resonance Imaging

There have been significant advances in the methodology available to monitor disease progression in dementia in the last three years. Serial volumetric MRI is now the technique of choice and is being applied in the majority of new clinical trials, particularly of more recent agents that are intended to interact with the disease process. A detailed description of the technique is beyond the scope of this chapter and the reader is referred to the key publications in this area (70–74).

Measuring Functional Ability and Activities of Daily Living

A wide range of assessment scales has been developed for measuring impairment in functional ability in activities of daily living (ADL). ADL assessments have been proposed as an additional primary outcome measure for anti-dementia trials, and are discussed in the European and US regulatory guidelines. However, the majority of available instruments

Table 16.3. Functional (ADL) scales for dementia

Instrumental Activities of Daily Living (IADL) [53]	Developed for the assessment of functional ability in elderly people, this scale is rated by the carer in eight domains of IADL
Physical Self Maintenance Scale (PSMS) [53]	A companion to the IADL, this assesses basic ADLs including toileting, feeding, dressing, bathing, grooming and ambulation and is rated from an informant
Functional Assessment Staging (FAST) [54]	A combined basic and IAL scale assessed in 16 areas in an interview with the caregiver
Blessed Dementia Scale [55]	An early ADL assessment used for assessing functional impairment in dementia
Nurses Observational Scale for Geriatric Patients (NOSGER) [56]	Although this scale also incorporates some behavioural, memory and mental state measures it primarily covers ADL function in 30 areas. It is intended to be completed by a nurse observing the patient in a residential or hospital setting, though has also been used by caregivers in the home environment
Disability Assessment in Dementia (DAD) [57]	A relatively new assessment scale based upon either a questionnaire or a structured interview administered to the caregiver. Assesses the patient's initiative and ability to carry out a range of basic and IADL tasks
Interview for Deterioration in Daily Living in Dementia (IDDD) [58]	Widely used in more recent Alzheimer's disease clinical trials this scale consist of 33 items covering basic and IADL activities. For each item initiative and ability are assessed on a 3-point scale with scale points relative to previous ability
Cleveland Scale for ADL [59]	
Progressive Deterioration Scale (PDS) [60]	Assesses changes in quality of life and ADLs on 29 items
Rapid Disability Rating Scale-2 [61]	This scale incorporates ADL abilities, rated by a carer, and also includes some items on mental state, orientation and behavioural change

have shown little responsiveness to treatment effects, even when efficacy is seen in cognitive and global domains. ADL can be divided into basic ADL abilities such as feeding, washing, dressing and continence, and instrumental ADL (IADL) which include driving, cooking, using the telephone and making tea or coffee. The major scales used in anti-dementia clinical trials are summarised in Table 16.3.

Assessing Behavioural Disturbance

Behavioural disturbance in dementia includes mood disturbance, delusions, hallucinations, aggression, agitation, wandering and more general behaviour that is "troublesome" to the caregiver. Behavioural disturbance is common in dementia; however, such patients are likely to be difficult to maintain in a clinical trial, often requiring protocol-prohibited psychoactive medication, and are thus often excluded. Nevertheless, the assessment of behavioural changes during a trial is an important secondary outcome measure, but when choosing a particular assessment scale it should be recognised that it is likely that only patients with milder degrees of behavioural change will be recruited.

More recently there has been increasing interest in developing effective treatment strategies specifically for behavioural disturbance in patients with dementia. In trials of medication primarily to control problem behaviour, the behavioural scale will form the primary outcome measure. As with ADL measures the majority of the published assessments were not developed to measure subtle changes behaviour

in response to medication. Table 16.4 summarises the major behavioural scales that are available.

Quality of Life

Quality Of Life (QOL) has been defined by the World Health Organization (WHO) as "the individual's perceptions of their position in life in the context of the culture and value system in which they live, and the relationship to their goals, expectations, standards and concerns" [46]. Attempting to measure such a concept is both a difficult and an essential topic in the evaluation of anti-dementia drugs. None of the current guidelines for the evaluation of anti-dementia drugs refer to the measurement of QOL. In the assessment of patients with dementia, the QOL for the caregiver is probably as significant as the patient's QOL, and doubles the problems inherent in assessment.

Health economic research has developed single-figure QOL scales such as the Euro-QOL [47]; however, these are biased towards physical disability and are difficult to use with demented patients. A further issue is whether the patient's QOL should be measured directly from the patient or as the caregiver's view of the patient's QOL.

Health Economics

The development of anti-dementia drugs raises many economic issues. AD is a major cost burden, in terms of both health and social costs, in all developed countries [48]. The introduction of drug treatments

Table 16.4. Behavioural assessments for anti-dementia trials

Alzheimer's Disease Assessment Scale – Non-Cognitive Part (ADAS-nonCog) [42]	The non-cognitive sections of the ADAS assess tearfulness, depression, concentration, uncooperativeness, hallucinations, delusions, pacing, motor activity, tremors and appetite. It is usually rated by the psychometrician following the ADAS-Cog and may only be based upon the period of contact with the patient
Brief Psychiatric Rating Scale (BPRS) [62]	A general psychopathology scale that is not specific for dementia. It focuses on the mental state assessment and is performed by an experienced clinician in an interview with the patient
Present Behavioural Examination (PBE) [63]	This assessment is based on in-depth interviews with the patient and caregiver. It provides detailed and reliable data but is too long for routine use in clinical trials. Other scales such as the NPI and MOUSEPAD have good concurrent validity with the PBE
Neuropsychiatric Inventory (NPI) [64]	Widely used in clinical trials this 13-item structured assessment uses a series of probes to identify areas of disturbed behaviour. It can be rapidly completed in the absence of behavioural problems, but can assess problems in depth when they are present. Includes ratings of both frequency of behaviour and distress to the caregiver
Manchester and Oxford Universities Scale for the Psychopathological Assessment of Dementia (MOUSEPAD) [65]	A newly published assessment that has been validated against the PBE and NPI. It is simple to apply and covers the behavioural disturbances seen in a range of dementias. Untested in published clinical trials
Behaviour Rating Scale for Dementia of the Consortium to Establish a Registry for AD (CERAD BRSD) [66]	Based on a semi-structured interview with the caregiver and rates frequency of behaviour in eight domains relevant to Alzheimer's disease. The frequency rating is helpful in clinical trials and may be more sensitive to treatment effects than a simpler present/absent assessment
Behavioural Pathology in AD Scale (BEHAVE-AD) [67]	Seven areas of behaviour disturbance are assessed on 25 items. The scale is specific for AD symptoms. It does not cover many behavioural disturbances seen in other dementias
Cohen-Mansfield Agitation Inventory (CMAI) [68]	Twenty-nine items relating to agitation are rated by an observer on a 7-point scale. The items render down to four factors: aggressive behaviour, physically non-aggressive behaviour, verbally agitated behaviour and hiding/hoarding behaviour. Primarily useful in more severely demented, institutionalised patients
Cornell Scale for Depression in Dementia [69]	The only depression rating scale developed specifically for patients with dementia. Rated by separate interviews with the patient and caregiver covering the same domains of mood. A consensus rating is made and an overall depression score is generated

for dementia inevitably raises questions about the economic impact of the treatment. There is little consensus on the methods or data to be collected in the economic evaluation of patients with dementia. Direct costs, including health and social service usage, can be recorded, yet for patients early in the disease the majority of the cost is likely to be indirect, relating to loss of employment for both patient and caregiver, and in informal caregiver time.

Economic evaluations of anti-dementia drugs are also problematic in phase III studies. Patients are selected for these studies by their relative lack of behavioural or functional impairment, and then both they and the caregiver receive intensive investigation and supportive contact – all of which will significantly bias the economic outcome.

Economic evaluation is likely to be ideally placed in phase IV studies, yet for a drug to become licensed, and thus reach phase IV, some regulators now require evidence of economic efficacy. Furthermore it is likely to be the long-term economic outcome for patients treated with the drug that is more important than short-term benefits seen during the 6–12 month duration of most clinical trials.

Ethics

The major principles of ethical research enshrined in the Nuremberg Code and the Declaration of Helsinki are:

- The minimisation of harm;
- The maximisation of benefit (beneficence);
- Truth telling;
- Autonomy and self-determination through the process of informed consent.

Dementia is a devastating disease of significant humanitarian importance and thus potentially more than minimal risk can be accepted if significant benefits are anticipated. Truth telling and disclosure can present considerable problems in patients with dementia. In particular, caregivers are often unwilling to allow the patient to be told their diagnosis, and even when told the diagnosis, patients with significant anosognosia may deny their disabilities. Thus during the process of informed consent these four principles need to be constantly balanced depending upon the patient's reactions and responses to the information they are being given. In general the principles of beneficence are probably the strongest in making ethical decisions about entering demented patients into clinical trials. The importance of involving the caregiver and patient's family in the decision to enter a clinical trial cannot be overemphasised.

A significant ethical issue does arise in patients with more severe dementia who are unable to give consent. A drug that prolongs the life of a severely demented patient may not be in the best interest of the patient. Similarly, a drug that controls behavioural disturbance and thus reduces the need for nursing home care, yet has significant side effects is also not being given primarily for the benefit of the patient and thus may not be ethically justified [49,50].

Ethics Committee Review of Protocol

Ethics committees are charged with a responsibility to review clinical trial protocols, and to take particular care when "vulnerable" subjects, such as demented patients, are to be included. In particular, the information sheet must be clearly drafted in simple language that could be understood by someone of reduced intelligence. The process of consent, and those to be involved in the process, should be clearly documented. The involvement of both a caregiver and an independent witness to the process is vital to ensure that no coercion is involved.

Ethics committees will also need to assure themselves that the principles of ethical research are being adhered to and in particular that the potential risks to the patient are mitigated by the likely beneficence [51].

The International Working Group on Harmonisation of Dementia Drug Guidelines

Dementia represents a major public health problem in all countries, and particularly those with a high proportion of elderly citizens. The development and licensing of anti-dementia drugs has prompted the issuing of regulatory guidelines on the demonstration of efficacy for these drugs from a number of countries including the United States, Canada, Europe and Japan. However, the guidelines vary in their requirements, and for global licensing trials often having to be repeated with different designs in order to satisfy different regulators. The IWG was formed in 1994 as a collaborative working group of representatives from academia, clinical practice, industry and governmental regulatory agencies. The

intention of the process has been to develop worldwide harmonised guidelines for the development of anti-dementia drugs.

The IWG has 13 working groups covering: length of trials; objective cognitive measures; clinical global measures; ADL; non-cognitive symptoms; health economics; ethics; translation issues; cultural issues; QOL; diagnostic criteria; primary prevention protocols; and trials to demonstrate delay in progression. The IWG process is likely to continue for some time until harmonised guidelines are agreed upon; however, the process stimulates and guides developments in this area and, it is hoped, will eventually lead to significant benefits.

The Organisation of Dementia Trials

Clinical trials of anti-dementia drugs are intensive and time-consuming studies. The subjects are cognitively impaired and require special care and attention, combined with time and an unpressured environment if a reliable assessment is to be performed. The assessments themselves are complex and include physical, neuropsychological and functional assessment of the patient, together with caregiver assessments to monitor adverse events, functional changes and quality of life. It is unlikely that clinical trials in dementia can be successfully performed without dedicated research staff to support the investigator.

Staffing

Dementia drug trials require staff from a number of different disciplines. The minimum staffing is the principal investigator with a research nurse or psychometrician. However, if independent global ratings are required then this number increases. With trials lasting from first recruitment to last patient completion there is a significant risk of staff changes occurring during the study. In subjective longitudinal global assessments it is unlikely that a valid rating could be made by someone who has not performed the baseline assessment. Therefore, to ensure consistency and validity it is helpful to have back-up raters available for the primary outcome measures who also completed a baseline assessment.

The staff needed for dementia trials broadly fall into the following categories:

Principal Investigator

The principal investigator (PI) will usually be a neurologist, psychiatrist or geriatrician as they are likely to have suitable patient populations. The PI is usually of consultant/senior lecturer grade – a requirement of most ethics committees and licensing authorities. General practitioners may also act as PIs, although a large practice size, or group of practices, would be needed to ensure an adequate recruitment rate. The PI will usually have an interest in the field of dementia and should be able to demonstrate an adequate source of patients from which to recruit subjects. Good Clinical Research Practice (GCRP) [51,52] requires the sponsor to obtain documentation of the PI's qualifications for participation in the study, and to assess the PI's centre for suitability for performing the study.

The PI may be directly involved with the day-to-day running of the trial, but these responsibilities may also be delegated to other members of the research team.

Co-investigators

Co-investigators are other consultant or sub-consultant grade doctors who participate in the study. A medically qualified person is always required to carry out physical examinations, review the results of blood tests and other investigations, make the initial diagnostic assessment and prescribe study medication.

Research Nurses

Research nurses bring valuable skills in clinical trials unit. Their practical abilities make them ideal as study co-ordinators, ensuring the successful recruitment and smooth running of the study. Their clinical abilities allow them to record patient observations, carry out psychological testing, take blood samples and arrange tests and investigations. Administrative skills are vital to deal effectively with paperwork and correspondence, and to liaise with the monitors and sponsoring company involved.

Psychometrician

At larger trial centres a dedicated psychometrician may be employed to carry out the psychological testing. This is usually a psychologist or assistant psychologist, although research nurses often assume this role. Psychologists also have good skills in patient care and administration, but their lack of clinical training usually means that they cannot record patients observations or take blood samples.

Clinical Global Rater

An independent person who has no access to other study data makes the clinical global rating. This effectively means that they must not be involved in the study, or with any of the patients except for their own focused assessment. The definition of what constitutes a "clinician" is often an issue during the development of clinical trial protocols. A generally accepted requirement is that this is someone who has experience in the assessment and care of patients with dementia but is not necessarily medically qualified. The global rater may thus be a physician, a nurse or a psychologist, the defining factor being their ability to justify their experience of assessing patients with dementia.

The Caregiver

Although not a member of staff, the involvement of a caregiver is vital in dementia drug trials, and a factor that differentiates these from other trials. The caregiver is in effect a "proxy" for the subject, and as such should give his or her own informed consent to participate in the study. The primary responsibilities of the caregiver are:

- To act as the patient's advocate during the informed consent process.
- To provide verification of the history during the initial diagnostic assessment.
- To provide baseline and follow-up observer data for the outcome assessments.
- To supervise the patient's compliance with study medication.
- To monitor and report adverse events that the patient may have forgotten or be unaware of.

The caregiver should have contact with the patient on at least a daily basis and the same caregiver should accompany the patient for each visit.

Conclusions

Clinical trials of anti-dementia drugs incorporate many practical, methodological and ethical issues. Many large multicentre national and international trials in AD are currently under way involving substantial investment from the pharmaceutical industry, with the effort and interest, such as through the IWG, gradually solving the methodological issues involved. The development of proven objective measures of disease progression, by means of MRI or other imaging modalities, represent a major methodological advance in dementia trials, and this will supplement the sensitive cognitive and global measures that are now in use.

The ethical issues involved require constant consideration with every patient who is enrolled to maintain the balance of minimisation of harm, beneficence and autonomy – inevitably the primary goal of developing effective treatments for dementia.

References

1. Jorm AF, Korten AE, Henderson AS. The prevalence of dementia: a quantitative integration of the literature. Acta Psychiatr Scand 1987;76:465–479.
2. Rossor MN, Garrett NJ, Johnson AL, Mountjoy CQ, Roth M, Iversen LL. A post-mortem study of the cholinergic and GABA systems in senile dementia. Brain 1982;105:313–330.
3. Perry EK, Tomlinson BE, Blessed G, Bergmann K, Gibson PH, Perry RH. Correlation of cholinergic abnormalities with senile plaques and mental test scores in senile dementia. BMJ 1978;ii:1457–1459.
4. Charatan FB. New tacrine hopes for Alzheimer patients in US. BMJ 1994;308:999–1000.
5. Knapp MJ, Gracon SI, Davis CS, Solomon PR, Pendlebury WW, Knopman DS. Efficacy and safety of high-dose tacrine – a 30-week evaluation. Alzheimer Dis Assoc Disord 1994;8:S22–S31.
6. Kelly CA, Harvey RJ, Cayton H. Treatement for Alzheimer's disease raises clinical and ethical issues. BMJ 1997;314:693–694.
7. Ferris SH, Hasegawa K, Homma A, Khachaturian ZS, Post S, Rossor M, Whitehouse PJ. International efforts to improve Alzheimer disease treatment. Alzheimer Dis Assoc Disord 1995;9:181.
8. Summers WK, Viesselman JO, Marsh GM, Candelora K. Use of THA in treatment of Alzheimer-like dementia: pilot study in twelve patients. Biol Psychiatry 1981;16:145–153.
9. Summers WK, Majovski LV, Marsh GM, Tachiki K, Kling A. Oral tetrahydroaminoacridine in long-term treatment of senile dementia, Alzheimer type. New Engl J Med 1986;315:1241–1245.
10. Division of Neuropharmacological Drug Produces Office of New Drug Evaluation (I) Center for Drug Evaluation and Review. An Interim Report from the FDA. New Engl J Med 1991;324:349–352.
11. Ad Hoc Dementia Assessment Task Force. Meeting Report. Anti-dementia drug assessment symposium. Neurobiol Aging 1991;12:379–382.
12. Leber P. Guidelines for the clinical evaluation of antidementia drugs. Rockville MD: US Food and Drug Administration, 1990.
13. Rossor MN. Alzheimer's disease. BMJ 1993;307:779–782.
14. American Psychiatric Association. Diagnostic and statistical manual of mental disorders, 4th ed. (DSM-IV). Washington, DC: APA, 1994.
15. McKhann G, Drachman D, Folstein M, Katzman R, Price D, Stadlan EM. Clinical diagnosis of Alzheimer's disease: report of the NINCDS-ADRDA work group under the auspices of Department of Health and Human Services Task Force on Alzheimer's Disease. Neurology 1984;34:939–944.
16. Folstein M, Folstein S, McHughs P. The "Mini Mental State": a practical method for grading the cognitive state of patients for the clinician. J Psychiatr Res 1975;12:189–198.
17. Blacker D, Albert MS, Bassett SS, Go RCP, Harrell LE, Folstein MF. Reliability and validity of NINCDS-ADRDA criteria for Alzheimer's disease. Arch Neurol 1994;51:1198–1204.
18. Verhey FR, Lodder J, Rozendaal N, Jolles J. Comparison of seven sets of criteria used for the diagnosis of vascular dementia. Neuroepidemiology 1996;15:166–172.
19. Antonuono P, Doody R, Gilman S, Huff J, Scheltens P, Ueda K, Khachaturian ZS. Diagnostic criteria for dementia in clinical trials. Position paper from the International Working Group on Harmonization of Dementia Drug Guidelines. Alzheimer Dis Assoc Disord 1997;11(S3):22–25.
20. Roman GC, Tatemichi TK, Erkinjuntti T, Cummings JL, Masdeu JC, Garcia JH, et al. Vascular Dementia: Diagnostic criteria for research studies. Report of the NINDS-AIREN International Workshop. Neurology 1993;43:250–260.
21. McKeith IG, Perry RH, Fairbairn AF, Jabeen S, Perry EK. Operational criteria for senile dementia of Lewy body type (SDLT). Psychol Med 1992;22:911–922.
22. Perry EK, Haroutunian V, Davis KL, Levy R, Lantos P, Eagger S, et al. Neocortical cholinergic activities differentiate Lewy body dementia from classical Alzheimer's disease. Neuroreport 1994;5:747–749.
23. Levy R, Eagger S, Griffiths M, Perry E, Honavar M, Dean A, Lantos P. Lewy bodies and response to tacrine in Alzheimer's disease. Lancet 1994;343:176.
24. The Lund and Manchester Groups. Clinical and neuropathological criteria for frontotemporal dementia. J Neurol Neurosurg Psychiatry 1994;57:416–418.
25. Gustafson L. Frontal lobe degeneration of non-Alzheimer type II. Clinical picture and differential diagnosis. Arch Gerontol Geriatr 1987;6:209–223.
26. Neary D, Snowden JS, Mann DM. The clinical pathological correlates of lobar atrophy. Dementia 1993;4:154–159.
27. CPMP Working Party on Efficacy of Medicinal Products. Anti-dementia Medicinal Products. Commission of the European Communities, 111/3705-91-EN, 1992.
28. Eagger SA, Morant NJ, Levy R. Parallel group analysis of the effects of tacrine versus placebo in Alzheimer's disease. Dementia 1991;2:207–211.
29. Eagger SA, Levy R, Sahakian BJ. Tacrine in Alzheimer's disease. Lancet 1991;338:50–51.
30. Mohr E, Feldman H, Gauthier S. Canadian guidelines for the development of antidementia therapies: a conceptual summary. Can J Neurol Sci 1995;22:62–71.
31. Kameyama M, Ito E, Otomo E, Kogure K, Goto H, Sawada T, et al. Guideline on clinical evaluation of cerebral circulation and metabolism improvers. Kyoto, Japan: Kyoto University, 1994.
32. Bodick N, Forette F, Hadler D, Harvey RJ, McKeith I, Riekkinen P, et al. Protocols to demonstrate slowing of disease progression. Position paper from the International Working Group on Harmonization of Dementia Guidelines. Alzheimer Dis Assoc Disord 1997;11(S3):50–53.
33. Leber P. Observations and suggestions on antidementia drug development. Alzheimer Dis Assoc Disord 1996;10.
34. Thal L, Carta A, Doody R, Leber P, Mohs R, Schneider L, et al. Report of the working group on prevention protocols for Alzheimer's disease. Position paper from the International Working Group on Harmonization of Dementia Drug Guidelines. Alzheimer Dis Assoc Disord 1997;11(S3):46–49.
35. Ferris S. Report of the working group on clinical global measures. Position paper from the International Working Group on Harmonization of Dementia Drug Guidelines. Alzheimer Dis Assoc Disord 1997;11(S3):8–18.
36. Hughes CP, Berg L, Danziger WL, et al. A new clinical scale for the staging of dementia. Br J Psychiatry 1982;140:566–572.
37. Reisberg B, Ferris SH, de Leon MJ, Crook T. The Global Deterioration Scale for assessment of primary degenerative dementia. Am J Psychiatry 1982;139:1136–1139.
38. Guy W. Clinical Global Impressions (CGI). In: Anonymous ECDEU assessment manual for psychopharmacology. Rockville, MD: US Department of Health and Human Services, 1976:218–222.
39. Shader RI, Harmatz JS, Salzman C. A new scale for clinical assessment in geriatric populations: Sandoz Clinical Assessment–Geriatric (SCAG). J Am Geriatr Soc 1974;22:107–113.
40. Schneider LS, Olin JT. Clinical global impressions in clinical trials. Int Psychogeriatrics 1996;8:277–288.

41. Schneider LS. Validity and reliability of the Alzheimer's Disease Study–Clinical Global Impression of Change (ADCS-CGIC). Alzheimer Dis Assoc Disord 1997;11(S2):S22–S32.

42. Rosen WG, Mohs RC, Davis K. A new rating scale for Alzheimer's disease. Am J Psychiatry 1984;141:1356–1364.

43. Ferris S, Lucca U, Mohs R, Dubois B, Allain H, Erzkeit H, et al. Workgroup report: objective psychometric tests. Position paper from the International Working Group on Harmonization of Dementia Drug Guidelines. Alzheimer Dis Assoc Disord 1997;11(S3):34–38.

44. Simpson PM, Surmon DM, Wesnes KA, Wilcock GK. The Cognitive Drug Research Computerised Assessment System for demented patients: a validation study. Int J Geriatr Psychiatry 1991;6:95–102.

45. Robbins TW, James M, Owen AM, Sahakian BJ, McInnes L, Rabbitt P. Cambridge Neuropsychological Test Automated Battery (CANTAB): a factor analytic study of a large sample of normal elderly volunteers. Dementia 1994;5:266–281.

46. The World Health Organization Quality of Life – 100. Geneva: Division of Mental Health, WHO, 1995.

47. EuroQol Group. A new facility for the measurement of health-related quality of life. Health Policy 1990;18:25–36.

48. Gray A, Fenn P. Alzheimer's Disease: the burden of the illness in England. Health Trends 1993;25:31–37.

49. Post SG, Ripich DN, Whitehouse PJ. Discourse ethics: research, dementia, and communication. Alzheimer Dis Assoc Disord 1994;8(Suppl 4):58–65.

50. Post SG, Whitehouse PJ. Dementia and the life-prolonging technologies used: an ethical question. Alzheimer Dis Assoc Disord 1992;6:3–6.

51. Good clinical practice for trials on medicinal products in the European Community. Committee for Proprietary Medicinal Products (CPMP), EEC 111/3976/88-EN, 1990.

52. Guidelines on good clinical research practice. London: Association of the British Pharmaceutical Industry, 1988.

53. Lawton M, Brody E. Assessment of older people: Self-maintaining and instrumental activities of daily living. Gerontologist 1969;9:179–186.

54. Reisberg B. Functional assessment staging. Psychopharmacol Bull 1988;24:653–659.

55. Blessed G, Tomlinson BE, Roth M. Blessed-Roth Dementia Scale (DS). Psychopharmacol Bull 1988;24:705–708.

56. Spiegel R, Brunner C, Ermini Funfschilling D, Monsch A, Notter M, Puxty J, Tremmel L. A new behavioral assessment scale for geriatric out- and in-patients: the NOSGER (Nurses' Observation Scale for Geriatric Patients). J Am Geriatr Soc 1991;39:339–347.

57. Gauthier L, Gauthier S, Gelinas I, McIntyre M, Wood-Dauphinee S. Assessment of functioning and ADL. Abstract BOOK of the 6th congress of the International Psychogeriatric Association 5–10 September, 1993:9.

58. Teunisse S, Mayke M, Van Creval H. Assessing the severity of dementia. Arch Neurol 1991;48:274–277.

59. Patterson MB, Mack JL, Neundorfer MM, Martin RJ, Smyth KA, Whitehouse PJ. Assessment of functional ability in Alzheimer disease: a review and a preliminary report on the Cleveland Scale for Activities of Daily Living. Alzheimer Dis Assoc Disord 1992;6:145–163.

60. Dejong R, Osterlund OW, Roy GW. Measurement of quality-of-life changes in patients with Alzheimer's disease. Clin Ther 1989;11:545–555.

61. Linn MW, Linn BS. The rapid disability rating scale: 2. J Am Geriatr Soc 1982;30:378–382.

62. Overall JE, Gorham DR. The Brief Psychiatric Rating Scale. Psychol Rep 1962;10:799–812.

63. Hope T, Fairburn CG. The Present Behavioural Examination (PBE): the development of an interview to measure current behavioural abnormalities. Psychol Med 1992;22:223–230.

64. Cummings JL, Mega M, Gray K, Rosenberg Thompson S, Carusi DA, Gornbein J. The Neuropsychiatric Inventory: comprehensive assessment of psychopathology in dementia. Neurology 1994;44:2308–2314.

65. Allen NHP, Gordon S, Hope T, Burns A. Manchester and Oxford Universities Scale for the Psychopathological Assessment of Dementia (MOUSEPAD). Br J Psychiatry 1996;169:293–307.

66. Tariot PN, Mack JL, Patterson MB, Edland SD, Weiner MF, Fillenbaum G, et al. The behavior rating-scale for dementia of the consortium to establish a registry for Alzheimer's disease. Am J Psychiatry 1995;152:1349–1357.

67. Reisberg B, Borenstein J, Salob SP, Ferris SH, Franssen E, Georgotas A. Behavioral symptoms in Alzheimer's disease: phenomenology and treatment. J Clin Psychiatry 1987;48(Suppl):9–15.

68. Cohen Mansfield J. Reflections on the assessment of behavior in nursing home residents. Alzheimer Dis Assoc Disord 1994;8(Suppl 1):S217–22.

69. Alexopoulous GS, Abrams RC, Young RC, Shamoian CA. Cornell scale for depression in dementia. Biol Psychiatry 1988;23:271–284.

70. Fox NC, Cousens S, Scahill R, Harvey RJ, Rossor MN. Using serial registered brain magnetic resonance imaging to measure disease progression in Alzheimer disease: power calculations and estimates of sample size to detect treatment effects. Archives of Neurology 2000;57(3):339–344.

71. Fox NC, Jenkins R, Leary SM, Stevenson VL, Losseff NA, Crum WR, Harvey RJ, Rossor MN, Miller DH, Thompson AJ. Progressive cerebral atrophy in MS: a serial study using registered, volumetric MRI. Neurology 2000;54(4):807–812.

72. Harvey RJ. Modifying the Alzheimer's disease process: establishing criteria for demonstrating a delay in disease progression. International Journal of Geriatric Psychopharmacology 2000;2:55–59.

73. Fox NC, Scahill RI, Crum WR, Rossor MN. Correlation between rates of brain atrophy and cognitive decline in AD. Neurology 1999;52(8):1687–1689.

74. Fox NC, Warrington EK, Rossor MN. Serial magnetic resonance imaging of cerebral atrophy in preclinical Alzheimer's disease. Lancet 1999;353:2125.

17. Cerebrovascular Disease: Basic Designs, Sample Sizes and Pitfalls

P.M. Rothwell

Introduction

Cerebrovascular disease is a major public health problem; over the next 10 years approximately 15 million people will suffer an acute stroke in Europe and the United States [1]. There is a clear need for more effective treatments both to prevent stroke and to treat the acute event. There has, in response to this, been a substantial increase in interest in the design, methodology and analysis of randomised controlled trials in cerebrovascular disease in recent years [2,3]. Indeed, trials have changed clinical practice in the primary prevention of stroke, e.g. treatment of hypertension [4]; the secondary prevention of stroke, e.g. antiplatelet treatment [5], anticoagulation [6], and carotid endarterectomy [7,8]; rehabilitation following stroke, e.g. stroke units [8]; and in the treatment of acute stroke, e.g. Nimodipine in subarachnoid haemorrhage [9] and more recently aspirin [10,11] and thrombolytic therapy [12] in cerebral infarction. There are trials in progress of many other potentially promising treatments such as angioplasty for symptomatic carotid stenosis [13] and neuroprotective treatments for acute ischaemic stroke [3].

This chapter deals with current issues relating to the design, performance and interpretation of clinical trials in cerebrovascular disease. Although general methodology and statistical considerations have been dealt with in earlier chapters (see Part I), the way in which a trial is performed is dependent to a very great extent on the type of patients included and the nature of the disease under study. The majority of patients with cerebrovascular disease are elderly, many are relatively frail, and some may already have a degree of physical disability. Each of these considerations affects the design and analysis of trials in cerebrovascular disease. For example, patients with cerebrovascular disease frequently have coexisting systemic vascular pathology, and are more likely to suffer a myocardial infarction or die of ischaemic heart disease during follow-up than they are to have a further stroke or die as a consequence of their cerebrovascular disease. Trials of secondary prevention of stroke should, therefore, assess the effect of the intervention on the overall risk of stroke, myocardial infarction and vascular death rather than on the neurological outcome alone.

However, there are many ways in which cerebrovascular disease lends itself to clinical trials. Vascular disease is common, and so there is no shortage of patients. Treatments usually aim to prevent acute events or improve outcome following an acute event, and so trial design is usually relatively simple. Measurement of outcome can require little more than the counting of specific follow-up events. In contrast, trials in other areas of neurology, in which a poor outcome is not manifest by an easily appreciated acute event, require measurement of disease progression in all patients. Indeed, the choice of outcome measure is the main issue in trial design in many neurological diseases. The use of objective outcome measures such as death or disabling stroke also means that blinded outcome assessment is often unnecessary in trials in cerebrovascular disease. By contrast, the subjective nature of the outcome measures necessary in trials in other more variable and slowly progressive diseases means that blinding of those assessing outcome is of great importance. This can, of course, be very difficult to achieve, and many trials are undermined by ineffective blinding. It is probably for these reasons that cerebrovascular disease has produced more than its fair share of large, methodologically sound, and consequently influential clinical trials.

Ethics, Uncertainty, and Recognising the Need for a Trial

The ethics of randomisation in clinical trials are dealt with in detail elsewhere [14] (Chapter 1), but some points are worth emphasising here. It is often argued that when a clinician is uncertain about the efficacy of a treatment in a particular patient, the only scientifically valid response, in theory at least, is to randomise the patient in a well-organised clinical trial. The patient may not receive the best treatment but at least the trial result will help improve the management of future patients. The present patient loses nothing because the clinician does not know how best to treat him or her anyway. However, this may not be the case. In order to be entered into the trial patients must give informed consent. They must understand that their doctors do not know how best to treat them and that they may well be randomised to no treatment. This uncertainty, although scientifically valid, may well undermine the confidence of the patient in the doctor, and thereby diminish the therapeutic effect of the doctor–patient relationship. However, if the detrimental effect of uncertainty on trial patients was clinically important, then one might expect the outcome of patients randomised into the control group of clinical trials to be worse than those treated similarly outwith the trial. In fact, the opposite is usually found to be the case. Patients within clinical trials do better than those without [15]. Although one can never exclude the possibility that this may be due to differences in case-mix or subtle differences in treatment, we can at least conclude that there is no clear evidence that participation in a clinical trial has a detrimental effect on patients.

Clinical trials are set up to establish the efficacy of treatments, new or established, about which there is still some uncertainty, at least in the minds of the trialists. However, simply because there is no clear evidence from clinical trials as to whether a treatment is beneficial, ineffective or harmful, does not mean that there is necessarily widespread uncertainty about the use of the treatment in clinical practice. Individual clinicians may have formed a definite opinion about a treatment on the basis of their own clinical experience or following recommendations by a respected authority. In fact, somewhat paradoxically, the consistency with which individual clinicians use a treatment is often inversely proportional to the amount of clinical trial evidence about the treatment. Treatments for which efficacy has been defined accurately for various indications tend to be used by most clinicians to a similar extent in similar patients. However, there is often great variation in the use of unproven treatments, with many clinicians using the treatment in all their patients and many others never using the treatment. For example, there is very little evidence as to whether or not the use of a carotid arterial shunt to bypass the clamped

portion of the internal carotid artery during carotid endarterectomy is beneficial [16]. However, of those surgeons participating in the European Carotid Surgery Trial [7], 60% used a shunt in fewer than 20% of their patients whereas 25% used a shunt in 80% or more (Fig. 17.1). Thus for both groups of surgeons a clinical trial in which they used a shunt in only half their patients would be a significant departure from their normal practice. The situation was even more polarised for intra-operative electroencephalograph monitoring (Fig. 17.1). If large numbers of patients are required and a multicentre trial is envisaged, it will, therefore, be necessary, prior to setting up the trial, to persuade colleagues that the treatment is of uncertain value and that a trial is necessary.

The first step in demonstrating the need for a clinical trial is to highlight the lack of definitive evidence about the efficacy of the treatment. This will usually require a systematic review of previous randomised controlled trials (RCTs) and possibly also any non-randomised comparisons with other treatments. Having demonstrated a lack of definitive evidence, the second step is to illustrate the extent of variation in the use of the treatment in everyday clinical practice. For example, with reference to Fig. 17.1, the two groups of surgeons cannot both be right. The lack of consistency between surgeons is strong evidence in support of the need for a trial. The argument is particularly strong if the treatment in question is expensive or has a significant associated morbidity or mortality. A similar lack of consistency is also frequently evident in studies of the variation in use of treatments between different countries (Table 17.1). There is no definite evidence for or against the use of

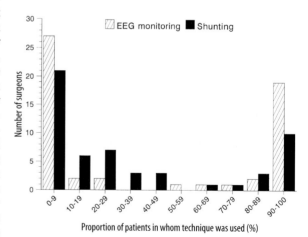

Fig. 17.1. The frequency (proportion of operations) with which surgeons taking part in the European Carotid Surgery Trial [7] used arterial shunts and intra-operative electroencephalographic (EEG) monitoring. Analysis was limited to surgeons who included at least 20 patients in the trial.

Table 17.1. Variations between 36 different countries in the use of ancillary treatments for acute ischaemic stroke

Treatment	Countries in which treatment was used most frequently (% of patients treated)	Average usage in remaining countries (% of patients treated)
Glycerol	Italy (50% of 1473 patients)	3% of 14 647 patients in 35 countries
Steroids	Turkey (32% of 225 patients)	4% of 15 895 patients in 35 countries
Haemodilution	Austria (54% of 206 patients)	3% of 15 523 patients in 34 countries
	Czech Republic (38% of 391 patients)	

Data derived from the International Stroke Trial [51].

steroids, glycerol or haemodilution in acute stroke, yet there is great variability between countries in the use of these drugs.

In practice, one of the most useful arguments to use in order to encourage colleagues to enter patients into a trial is the "uncertainty principle". If the clinician is certain that a particular treatment is indicated for a particular patient, then the patient should not be entered into a trial. If the clinician is certain that the patient will not benefit from the treatment, then the patient should not be entered into the trial. However, if the clinician is uncertain about the likely efficacy of the treatment in a particular patient then the patient should be randomised in the trial. Clinicians will differ in the type of patients about which they feel uncertain, their "grey area" of uncertainty. As a consequence, if a sufficiently large number of clinicians enter patients into the trial a broad spectrum of patients is likely to be included. The uncertainty principle is, therefore, a solid ethical and practical basis for a trial.

Trial Design

One of the most frequent and damning criticisms of clinical trials is that the results cannot be applied to everyday clinical practice. This section will concentrate on the design considerations in trials in cerebrovascular disease which influence the generalisability of the eventual results to clinical practice. The details of different trial designs have been discussed in previous chapters. The majority of trials in cerebrovascular disease are performed in three areas: primary or secondary prevention of stroke in particular patient groups; treatment of acute stroke; and rehabilitation following stroke. Cross-over design trials or n-of-1 trials cannot be used in the first two areas and are rarely used in the last. Thus the vast majority of trials in cerebrovascular disease use the parallel group design.

Pragmatic Versus Explanatory Trials

The *effectiveness* of a treatment is not the same as the *usefulness* of a treatment. For example, a treatment for acute ischaemic stroke may be *effective* in that it reduces infarct size, but may not be *useful* because it is too poorly tolerated by patients, too expensive or too complex to administer. An ineffective drug is, on the other hand, always useless (excluding the placebo response). It is frequently argued, therefore, that a pragmatic trial to establish usefulness should always be preceded by an *explanatory* trial to establish efficacy. An explanatory trial seeks to measure the specific effect of the treatment on the pathophysiology of the disease. Such trials are often small, include only a tightly defined group of patients, ensure that all patients receive their allotted treatment, and frequently have non-clinical measures of outcome. Pragmatic trials seek to measure the usefulness of treatments in conditions which, as far as possible, mimic normal clinical practice. Ideally they should include a broad spectrum of patients with the disease in question, they should be analysed on an intention-to-treat basis and they should have a clinically important measure of outcome. As a consequence pragmatic trials usually need to be much larger than explanatory trials in order to confirm or exclude a useful treatment effect. They are, however, much more likely than explanatory trials to change clinical practice. For the most part, this chapter will be concerned with pragmatic trials.

Selection of Patients

Patient entry criteria determine whether the results of the trial will be highly *applicable* to a very tightly defined, and probably small, group of patients, or whether they will be widely *generalisable* to a less stringently defined, and probably much larger, population of patients with the condition. For example, a trial of carotid endarterectomy for asymptomatic stenosis might include all patients with a certain degree of stenosis or it might be limited to the small proportion of patients with an ulcerated carotid plaque and an asymptomatic cerebral infarction in the territory of the stenosed artery. The advantage of a highly *applicable* result is that it can be applied with a degree of confidence to an individual patient, assuming that he or she fits the trial criteria. The disadvantage is that the result may not inform management of the majority of patients with the condition who would not fit the trial criteria. The disadvantage of a widely *generalisable* result is that it cannot be used with any confidence to predict the likely response to treatment of an individual patient. All that can be said is that if the treatment is given to a sufficiently large number of patients, on average it will have a given effect. However, large trials with broad entry criteria do have a number of important advantages. Firstly, generally speaking the broader the entry criteria, the more likely it is that the trial will recruit sufficient patients to produce a definitive result. This is partly because more patients will be eligible, but also because the entry criteria will overlap with the grey area of uncertainty of a higher proportion of clinicians resulting in a larger number of collaborators. Secondly, even if the trialists are mainly interested in a specific group of patients, it often makes more sense in practice to adopt broad entry criteria as this will probably result in the randomisation of a greater number of patients with the specific characteristics of interest than if entry is specifically limited to such patients. The main reasons for this are that the trial will have access to the patients of a larger number of collaborators and, of particular importance, clinicians will be randomising patients regularly and will, therefore, be familiar with the randomisation procedure and trial protocol. By contrast, if only a small proportion of patients are eligible, clinicians will tend to forget about the trial and miss the rare patient who does actually fit the criteria. A large trial with broad entry criteria may well have sufficient power to allow analysis of the efficacy of treatment in predefined groups of patients who are of particular interest. For example, the International Stroke Trial [10], which examined the effect of antithrombotic treatment in acute ischaemic stroke, had a time window of up to 48 hours between stroke onset and randomisation. It recruited 19 436 patients, 3165 (16%) of whom were randomised within 6 hours. It is therefore the largest trial of very early intervention after acute stroke and has sufficient power to examine the effect of treatment given within 6 hours of onset.

Entry Requirements

Trials often require certain investigations to be performed or protocols followed prior to entry. Similar arguments to those regarding patient selection apply to trial entry requirements. Again a balance has to be achieved between what might be possible in an ideal world and what can be achieved in practice. For example, a trial of carotid endarterectomy for asymptomatic carotid stenosis that insisted on four vessel selective carotid arterial angiography in all patients prior to randomisation would not only accrue patients very slowly but, since the degree of carotid stenosis is now increasingly measured by non-invasive methods, any recommendations made in the results which were based on the findings at angiography would rapidly become redundant. Moreover, if the trial is to have a chance of being completed in the first place one cannot exclude too many patients. One hospital taking part in one particular multicentre acute stroke trial screened 192 patients over a 2-year period but was able to enter only one patient into the trial [17]. This is an extreme example, but trial entry rates following screening of 10–20% are very common, particularly in explanatory trials [18,19]. Lasaga's Law states that "As soon as a clinical trial begins, the supply of patients becomes one tenth of that which it was thought to be before the trial started" [19]. This is particularly problematic for trials of treatments for acute stroke which are likely to have a narrow time window, such as thrombolysis or neuroprotection. In order to minimise the delay between hospital admission and treatment, pre-randomisation investigations should be limited only to those which are absolutely essential. For example, there is no good reason why brain imaging should be performed before rather than after randomisation in trials of neuroprotective agents [3].

Ensuring Comparability with Other Trials

It is often difficult for a single trial to recruit sufficient patients to confirm or exclude moderate treatment effects on relatively low-risk outcomes, such as are found in trials of primary prevention and secondary prevention of stroke. In this situation the only practical way of determining the efficacy of treatment with sufficiently narrow confidence limits is to perform a meta-analysis of trials as part of a systematic review. However, attempts to combine the results of independent trials are frequently hampered by major differences in the design of trials, particularly in the measurement of outcome. It is important, therefore, if it seems likely that a meta-analysis of all trials may be necessary in future, that some consideration be given to maximising the comparability of the trial design with those of previous or current trials.

Sample Size

Statistical issues relating to sample size have been discussed elsewhere. There are, however, a number of issues relating specifically to cerebrovascular disease. Firstly, and most importantly, the treatment effects involved in the treatment or prevention of stroke are often relatively small. For example, one would probably not expect a neuroprotective agent to yield much more than a 20% relative reduction in mortality following acute stroke. A similar relative risk reduction might be expected in the risk of recurrent stroke with an antiplatelet drug in a secondary prevention trial. Given that in neither these examples would the absolute risk of the trial outcome in the control group be much more than 10%, the expected reduction in the absolute risk of the trial outcome with treatment would only be about 2%. Table 17.2 gives details of the power to demonstrate such a treatment effect which different sample sizes would have. To be reasonably sure of documenting the true efficacy of treatment the trial would require at least 12 000 patients and ideally 20 000 patients. Although large simple trials do have some limitations [20,21], the case in favour of them is very strong [22]. The fact that it is possible to recruit such numbers is illustrated by the recent success of the International Stroke Trial [10] and the Chinese Acute Stroke Trial [11].

Secondly, the lack of power inherent in small trials is compounded by the tendency for the outcome in patients entered into clinical trials to be better, irrespective of treatment, than that in those who are not entered. It is important not to over-estimate the expected untreated risk of a poor outcome in the control group when calculating the sample size. Simply extrapolating from the risks reported in observational studies is likely to be inappropriate. For example, the risk of stroke in patients randomised in the UK-TIA Aspirin trial [23] was lower than a comparable hospital-referred series of patients with apparently similar disease and very much lower than in a comparable community-based series [24] (Fig. 17.2). As a consequence of this the trial was not able to demonstrate a significant reduction in the risk of stroke with aspirin treatment.

Thirdly, trials in patients with cerebrovascular disease not infrequently have a sizable number of drop-outs and cross-overs from treatment to no treatment or vice versa. This is at least partly because they involve an elderly population of patients who tend to be more liable to develop side-effects of treatment. Since the trial will be analysed on an intention-to-treat basis, significant numbers of cross-overs and drop-outs will undermine the power of the trial to demonstrate a given treatment effect. This should be taken into account in the initial sample size calculation. Fourthly, if long follow-up is required, as is the case in primary or secondary prevention trials, sample size calculations must also take

Table 17.2. Effect of sample size on the reliability of the result of a trial of a hypothetical treatment for acute stroke The treatment is assumed to reduce case-fatality from 10% to 8%, i.e. a 20% relative risk reduction

Total Patients	p value[a]	Trial power (%)	Comments on trial size
200	0.99	1	Completely inadequate
400	0.98	2	Completely inadequate
800	0.96	4	Completely inadequate
1 600	0.90	10	Completely inadequate
3 200	0.75	25	Inadequate
6 400	0.43	57	Barely adequate
12 800	0.09	91	Probably adequate
20 000	0.01	99	Definitely adequate

Adapted from Dorman and Sandercock [3].
[a] Approximate probability of failing to achieve $p < 0.01$ significance if true relative risk reduction is 20%.

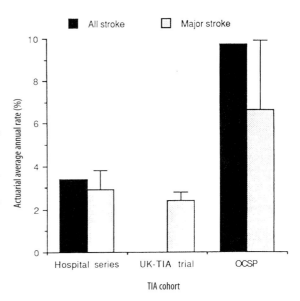

Fig. 17.2. The annual risk of stroke in three different cohorts of patients with transient ischaemic attacks: a series of hospital-referred patients (Hospital Series), patients randomised in a large clinical trial (UK-TIA Trial), and patients identified in a community-based incidence study (OCSP). For further information see [24].

Table 17.3. Baseline clinical characteristics of patients randomised to treatment intervention versus control in a hypothetical trial of an intervention to reduce the risk of stroke and death due to carotid endarterectomy. The likely effect of each characteristic on the difference in operative risk between the intervention group and the control group is calculated from the respective hazard ratios derived from a previous study [50]

	Randomised allocation		Significance[a]	Effect of characteristic on predicted operative risk (hazard ratio and 95% CI)[b]	Difference between operative risk in the intervention group versus control group (change in expected relative risk)
	Intervention ($n = 20$)	Control ($n = 20$)			
Baseline characteristic					
Female sex	6	12	$p = 0.11$	1.41 (1.16–1.70)	+12%
Ocular symptoms only	12	6	$p = 0.11$	0.46 (0.24–0.91)	+35%
Peripheral vascular disease	1	4	$p = 0.34$	1.44 (1.17–1.79)	+7%
Systolic blood pressure BP >180 mmHg	3	8	$p = 0.16$	1.93 (1.22–3.04)	+23%
Overall increase in expected operative risk in the intervenion group versus the control group (% increase in expected relative risk) = 77%					

[a] Chi squared test.
[b] Derived from Rothwell et al. [50].

account of a relatively high mortality from vascular incidents other than stroke and causes other than vascular disease. Finally, the trial entry criteria can, of course, be defined in such a way as to minimise the sample size required. For example, it has been argued that both minor strokes and very severe strokes should be excluded from a trial of a treatment for acute ischaemic stroke. Those who suffer minor strokes are likely to recover completely with or without treatment and those who have had very severe strokes will probably die irrespective of treatment. If one accepts these assumptions, both groups could be excluded from the trial without loss of power since only the outcome in patients with strokes of intermediate severity is likely to be influenced by the treatment.

Treatment Allocation

The purpose of randomisation in a clinical trial is to ensure that neither the patients nor the clinician can predict in advance which treatment the patient will receive. Randomisation does not necessarily ensure that the prognosis in the treatment and control groups will be equal at baseline. Indeed, in a small trial this is very unlikely to be the case. There is an argument, therefore, that randomisation should be stratified according to important prognostic variables or that a balance should be achieved using minimisation. However, these methods are best suited to large, preferably multicentre trials in which there is central computer randomisation.

There are a number of outcomes in cerebrovascular disease for which there are important prognostic variables. For example, there are established models for predicting recovery after acute stroke [25] or the risk of stroke following a transient ischaemic attack [26]. Trials should consider balancing treatment allocation for these variables. The effect of imbalance is illustrated in Table 17.3 which details a hypothetical trial of an intervention intended to reduce the risk of stroke and death due to carotid endarterectomy. There is a non-significant imbalance in five important prognostic variables in favour of the intervention group. Using the hazard ratios obtained in a recent systematic review of risk factors for stroke and death due to endarterectomy [27], the predicted risk of a poor outcome in the control group is more than twice that in the intervention group independently of any effect of the intervention itself. This degree of prognostic imbalance will, not infrequently, result from simple randomisation in small and medium-sized trials.

Trials should, of course, detail the balance of prognostic variables across the treatment groups when reporting results. It is important to bear in mind, however, that if a prognostic variable is particularly important, a relatively minor imbalance between the treatment groups may have a major effect on the trial result, irrespective of whether or not the imbalance is of statistical significance. Reports of trials which do not give any information on the characteristics of the different treatment groups should be interpreted with caution. For example, a recent small randomised trial of gastrostomy feeding versus nasogastric feeding following acute stroke reported a significant reduction in mortality in the gastrostomy group [12% (2/16) vs 57% (8/14)] [28]. The result was impressive, albeit somewhat implausible, but would have been more convincing had the baseline data also been reported.

Blinding

As stated in the introduction, the necessity for blinding depends to a certain extent on the design of the trial, particularly the outcome measures used. There are two main reasons for blinding the trial clinicians. The first is in order that the use of non-trial treatments and interventions is not influenced by a knowledge of whether or not the patient received the trial treatment. The second is in order that clinicians are not biased in their assessment of clinical outcomes. However, there is less potential for bias in assessment of outcome in trials in which the outcomes are objective, such as death or major stroke. Thus trials of carotid endarterectomy have not gone to elaborate lengths to blind assessors to whether or not the patient had had the operation [7,8]. Such trials do, however, usually have a blinded audit committee which studies a report by the trial clinician of any potential trial outcome event and decides how the event should be classified. Non-blinded trials cannot, of course, exclude the possibility that knowledge of the treatment which the patient received did influence non-trial management in a way which might have led to a bias. They should, therefore, document all potentially important non-trial treatments given to patients during follow-up and report these data with the trial results (Fig. 17.3).

In contrast, blinded outcome assessment is vital in trials in which the outcome measure is subjective. The subjectivity of an outcome measure is best judged by measuring its inter-observer reproducibility. For example, inter-observer agreement in the diagnosis of transient ischaemic attacks or in the detection of abnormal neurological signs is relatively poor [29,30]. Thus a non-blind trial in which a transient ischaemic attack was an outcome event or in which outcome was measured using some sort of neurological impairment scale would be susceptible to bias. In the case of measurement of neurological impairment and disability, the potential for biased assessment was clearly demonstrated in a recent multiple sclerosis trial in which blinded and non-blinded outcome assessment produced very different results [31].

The term "double-blind" is frequently misused. Simply because the patients and clinicians were not actually told the treatment allocation does not mean that they were not able to work it out for themselves! If it is decided that clinicians should be blinded to the treatment allocation, then some effort should be made during and at the end of the trial to test whether or not blinding was effective. Trials in cerebrovascular disease are no exception. For example,

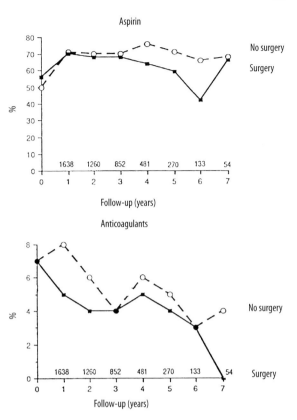

Fig. 17.3. The proportion of patients (%) receiving aspirin or anticoagulants following randomisation to surgery or no-surgery in the European Carotid Surgery Trial [7].

treatments such as steroids or heparin are difficult to blind, and if subjective outcome measures are used then it is quite possible that outcome assessment may be biased.

Length of Follow-up

One of the major potential shortcomings of clinical trials in cerebrovascular disease is insufficient follow-up. Long follow-up is likely to increase the cost of the trial and make complete follow-up more difficult to achieve. However, it is quite possible for the effectiveness of treatments to change with time. Recovery following acute stroke may continue for 6 months to 2 years [32,33], and so measurement of functional outcome at hospital discharge in an acute stroke trial will give a very incomplete picture of the effect of treatment and may well be less sensitive than assessment of outcome at 6 months.

Similar considerations apply to secondary prevention trials. The result of a trial with 2 years follow-up may be very different from the result that would be obtained after 5 years follow-up. For example, although endarterectomy for asymptomatic carotid stenosis does reduce the risk of ipsilateral ischaemic stroke [34,35], the benefit is small and the procedure is regarded by many as being of little value [36]. The benefit derived from the operation is determined to a great extent by the risk of stroke without treatment. This is relatively low after 2 or 3 years of follow-up, and only just offsets the risk of the operation itself. However, a 50-year-old man with a severe asymptomatic carotid stenosis may survive for 20 or more years. The cumulative risk of stroke due to the carotid stenosis is likely to be considerable over that length of time. The results of a trial performed in an elderly population with only a few years follow-up may well underestimate the likely benefit of surgery in a patient such as this. Clearly, 20-year follow-up is impractical, but trialists should consider the potential problems which may result from too short a period of follow-up.

Outcome Measures

The choice of outcome measure can be a difficult issue in trial design in cerebrovascular disease. It has implications for the cost of the trial, the sample size required to obtain a clear result, and the likelihood that the trial will influence clinical practice. Important considerations in choosing an outcome measure include validity, reproducibility, sensitivity to change, clinical meaning, and the burden it places on patients and clinicians taking part in the trial. Outcome measures which have been used in trials in cerebrovascular disease include event rates, neurological impairment, disability or handicap, quality of life, and various other indicators such as length of hospital stay, proportion of patients returning home, and health-economic assessments of the cost of illness. The most commonly used outcomes are discussed below.

Single Events or "Endpoints"

Assessment of the relative frequency of particular events across the treatment groups is probably the simplest method of measuring the efficacy of treatment. The event could be death in a trial of a treatment for acute stroke or stroke in a trial of a preventive treatment. In acute treatment trials with short follow-up it may be reasonable simply to compare the proportion of events in each group. In trials of treatments aiming to prevent stroke, in which long follow-up is required, the comparison of event rates should be based on an actuarial analysis.

The use of single events as outcome measures has several advantages over the use of more complex scales or surrogate outcome measures. Firstly, in the majority of cases the occurrence of the event in question will be fairly obvious (e.g. death or disabling stroke). In other words, the outcome assessment will have good inter-observer agreement. The true efficacy of the treatment will not, therefore, be blurred by variation between different observers in the measurement of outcome. This does, of course, depend on the choice of event. For example, the diagnosis of transient ischaemic attacks has relatively poor inter-observer agreement [29]. Secondly, if an objective measure of outcome is used, such as death or disabling stroke, then there is much less potential for bias in non-blind or poorly blinded trials than if a more subjective measure, such as an impairment score or stroke scale were used. Thirdly, assessment of the frequency of specific events will usually be cheaper and will place less of a burden on the patient and clinician than measurement of more complex scores. Finally, the actual value of the treatment can be more easily appreciated by future patients and clinicians if it is analysed as an event rate than if it is expressed as a change in the mean value of a particular stroke scale.

Measurement of event rates does, however, have certain disadvantages. It takes no account of the consequences of the event on the impairment, disability or handicap of the patient. A stroke, for example, can range in severity from slight numbness in one hand to a complete hemiplegia with dysphasia or neglect. It seems wrong that these two events should be given the same weight in any analysis of the effectiveness of a treatment. In certain trials even stroke and transient ischaemic attack have been lumped together as a single composite outcome event [35]. Not only does this make it difficult for clinicians to assess the utility of the treatment (Does it prevent major strokes or just transient ischaemic attacks?), but it assumes that the relative proportion of strokes and transient events will be the same in each treatment group. This is, however, by no means always likely to be the case. For example, in trials of carotid endarterectomy the majority of outcome events in patients randomised to surgery occur during or shortly after the operation. Since the procedure is usually carried out under general anaesthetic, it is likely that many transient ischaemic attacks and minor strokes will be missed. By contrast, outcome events in patients randomised to medical treatment occur gradually over the next few years and a significant proportion of reported events are transient or minor. A direct comparison of event rate in such trials is likely, therefore, to be biased in favour of surgery. However, there are circumstances where different outcomes should be combined. For example, in acute stroke trials death and non-fatal outcomes such as disabled survival should probably be combined as a single outcome:

otherwise non-fatal adverse outcomes could be "prevented" completely by using a suitably poisonous treatment.

A further disadvantage of using the number of patients experiencing a particular event as an outcome measure is the difficulty in dealing with multiple events in single patients. This can be difficult to accommodate in standard survival analyses. However, it is quite possible for a single patient to have several disabling strokes during follow-up. This is also a problem when composite outcomes, such as stroke, myocardial infarction or vascular death, are used. A single patient may suffer all these events during follow-up. It is possible to look at the cumulative event rate in each treatment group rather than simply the number of patients suffering an event, but further research is required in order to produce a consensus about the most appropriate techniques to use.

Surrogate Outcomes

Non-clinical surrogate outcomes can be used to measure the effect of treatment, such as infarct size on CT brain scan in an acute stroke trial, or cerebrovascular reactivity in trials of treatment for carotid stenosis. They are looking for a biological effect. Is the treatment doing anything at all? Surrogate outcome measures are important in explanatory trials in order to determine whether or not a treatment is worth investigating further in large pragmatic clinical trials. They do not, however, tell us anything about the clinical usefulness of the treatment. However, one major advantage of surrogate outcome measures, such as infarct size, is that the measurement which is used for the trial analysis can be made by a radiologist who has not seen the patient and who is, therefore, more likely to be blinded to treatment allocation than a clinician who has to examine the patient in order to derive a score on a stroke scale. Ideally, of course, measurements such as infarct size should be automated, thereby precluding assessor bias altogether.

Impairment

Several stroke scales have been used as outcome measures in trials in cerebrovascular disease. These are usually impairment scales which allot scores to various neurological signs and then sum them to produce an overall score. It is, of course, very difficult for either patients or doctors to know exactly what a particular score represents or, more importantly, whether a treatment which results in a given change in mean score is worthwhile. It has been argued that a patient is more than the sum of their signs, and that

adding up arbitrary scores for speech, power, level of consciousness, eye signs and reflex changes is as meaningless as adding up the concentrations of blood urea, sodium, potassium and glucose to make up an overall "metabolic score" [37]. This argument is difficult to oppose.

One important disadvantage of many of the impairment scores used in stroke trials is their tendency to concentrate mainly on motor signs. Subtle difficulties with speech or visuospatial functioning may not contribute much to the stroke severity score even though they can be extremely disabling for the patient. The true impact of such impairments is much more likely to be registered by measurements of handicap or health-related quality of life. Moreover, the assumption made by many that a detailed neurological score will necessarily be more sensitive to any effect of treatment than a simple disability or handicap scale is by no means self-evident. Complex scores tend to have greater inter-observer variability, which will introduce background noise into the analysis and reduce the power of the trial. More research is required into the sensitivity to change of different types of outcome measure.

Disability, Handicap and Simple Questions

There are several generic disability scales, such as the Barthel scale [38], which have been used in stroke trials. These are based on the ability of the patient to perform specific tasks and, as such, have more obvious meaning to doctors and patients. Although the Barthel scale is similar to an impairment score in that it simply sums scores for different activities of daily living, the total score (ranging from 0 to 100) has been shown to have a degree of validity in that it predicts the level of autonomy following stroke rehabilitation. For example, a score of 20 or more immediately after a stroke or a score of 40 or more at the time of transfer to a rehabilitation centre are highly predictive of a return to home following rehabilitation [39]. Moreover, the absolute score at a given time can be roughly equated with a level of independence. A score of 60 corresponds to the level of function required to live at home with moderate assistance, and a score of 85 corresponds to independence with minimal assistance [40].

However, even with scales such as the Barthel it is still difficult to know exactly what a change of a given number of points actually means. Simple handicap scores overcome this difficulty to some extent. The most widely used of these is the Rankin scale, which has five levels of disability from no significant disability to totally bedridden [41]. The score is analysed as a categorical variable and the meaning of both absolute scores and changes in score are rela-

Table 17.4. The reduction in variance (i.e. "the statistical power") of a measurement according to the number of subdivisions of the measurement. The example assumes that the quantity being measured has true integer values of 0 to 100

No. of possible values	Approximate variance of measurement	Reduction in variance achieved by measurement
1 (0–100, i.e. not measured)	900 (i.e. SD = 30)	0
2 (0–50, 50–100)	225 (i.e. SD = 15)	75%
3 (0–33, etc.)	100	89%
5 (0–20, etc.)	36	96%
10 (0–10, etc.)	9	99%
100 (0–1, etc.)	0	100%

tively easily understood by clinicians and patients. It has also been shown to have good inter-observer reproducibility [41].

One common misconception regarding outcome scales is that the more complex a scale is, i.e. the greater the number of possible scores, the more discriminating it will be. In other words, a scale which divides patients into a large number of groups has much greater statistical power to detect a difference between treatment groups than a scale which divides patient into just a few groups. In fact the increase in "statistical power" with increasing number of subdivisions is very much a case of diminishing returns (Table 17.4). The logical extension of this observation is to limit outcome assessment to a series of simple questions, such as "Have you made a complete recovery from your stroke?" This approach was used in the International Stroke Trial [10,42].

One of the main advantages of disability scales, handicap scales and simple questions is that they can often be completed by the patient themselves or administered by non-clinical assistants. Both options are cheaper than medical assessment and are often particularly appropriate in large multicentre trials. Self-assessment by patients has the advantage that it eliminates the potential for external assessor bias, although it does not avoid bias due to placebo effects experienced by patients. Postal or telephone follow-up using very simple scales is easily standardised and relatively inexpensive.

Quality of Life and the Importance of the Patient's Point of View

It can be argued that the most important overall measure of the effect which a treatment has on a patient is the effect on overall health-related quality of life. Let us consider a hypothetical new antiplatelet drug intended for use in the secondary prevention of ischaemic stroke. The drug produces a modest, but worthwhile, 25% relative reduction in the risk of recurrent stroke over the next few years, and appears to be marginally more effective than aspirin. However, it causes significant malaise, nausea or diarrhoea in 15% of patients, and milder symptoms in over 30%. How should the benefit of a reduced risk of stroke be balanced against the distress caused by the side-effects of the drug? Side-effects are rarely incorporated into the overall trial result, and are usually simply listed separately. The decision as to whether the benefits of treatment justify the side-effects is therefore left for doctors reading the paper to decide for themselves. However, since the concerns of doctors and patients may not coincide this may be inappropriate. Measuring outcome using an overall measure of health-related quality of life would at least record the patients' perspective as to whether or not the treatment was worse than the disease itself. Measures of health-related quality of life which have been studied in stroke patients include the Short Form-36 [43,44] and the EuroQol [44,45].

Assessment of Serious Complications of Treatment

Treatments used in cerebrovascular disease often have an associated risk of serious complications e.g. thrombolysis in acute ischaemic stroke and carotid endarterectomy or anticoagulation in the prevention of stroke. Whilst it is always desirable to reduce this risk as much as possible, clinical trials often go to such lengths that the eventual result may no longer be generalisable to normal clinical practice. For example, trials of carotid endarterectomy sometimes allow only surgeons who can demonstrate very low operative complication rates to participate in the trial and have mechanisms in place to prevent a surgeon entering further patients if his complication rate in the patients operated on in the trial exceeds a certain figure. The risk of stroke or death due to endarterectomy in one such trial was remarkably low [34], and significantly lower than that obtained from a systematic review of the published literature [27], which is itself likely to be an underestimate due to publication bias. The benefit derived from endarterectomy in this particular trial might well exceed that which would be obtained in everyday clinical practice. Similarly, trials of anticoagulants, such as warfarin, often insist on very frequent INR testing and probably partly as a consequence of this have relatively few haemorrhagic complications [46]. The risks of treatment with warfarin may be much greater in clinical practice when such tight control is not always possible. The underlying issue is, of course, whether a trial should attempt to determine the efficacy of a treatment when used in the context of best possible practice or in the context of everyday clinical practice. Trialists may not agree about which option is more valid, but the issue should certainly be borne in mind when designing a trial protocol.

Multicentre Trials

Multicentre trials are often required to determine the efficacy of treatments in cerebrovascular disease. In fact, the vast majority of trials which have had a major impact on clinical practice in cerebrovascular disease over the last 10 years have been multicentre trials. This is simply a reflection of the fact that very large numbers of patients are required in order to demonstrate moderate but important treatment effects, particularly if the absolute risk of a poor outcome is low [22]. Multicentre trials allow large numbers of patients to be randomised over a relatively short period of time. This produces a quick result before people lose interest in the treatment. As has been discussed elsewhere [47], multicentre trials also have other advantages:

1. They lead to wide dissemination of results and have the credibility to change clinical practice.
2. They allow inclusion of a broader range of patients than would be likely from a single centre.
3. They benefit from a pooling of skills and expertise from different centres in many countries.

In addition, they foster national and international collaboration and often lead to further collaborative studies and trials.

The nuts and bolts of performing a multicentre trial in cerebrovascular disease have been discussed in detail by experienced trialists [47,48]. Briefly, the most important advice is to keep the trial as simple as is possible. This includes basic design, randomisation procedure, collection of baseline data, and follow-up. Entry criteria should be broad and simple. Few if any extra investigations should be required prior to randomisation. Randomisation should be performed by telephone to a central office, and as much baseline information as is required should be collected over the 'phone at the time of randomisation. Care must be taken to collect only data which will be required to answer the main trial questions and to perform planned subgroup analyses. Forms should be kept to a minimum and should rarely be longer than a single page. Baseline data and clinical assessments should be simple to obtain. Simple data

are usually the most reproducible, and reproducibility of assessments across different centres and different countries is vital in a multicentre trial. Ideally, entering the patient into the trial and following them up should involve no more work than would be done as part of normal clinical practice outwith the trial. Follow-up should, therefore, be performed when patients would usually be seen anyway or, if possible, by telephone or questionnaire from the trial centre. Collaborating clinicians are inevitably busy and the trial will not be their highest priority. "Randomise and forget" trials are most likely to recruit patients. Finally, and of great importance in obtaining funding, the simpler the trial is, the less expensive it is likely to be.

Reporting of Trial Results

There are several issues relating to the analysis of trial data and reporting of results which are particularly important in trials in cerebrovascular disease.

Intention-to-Treat Analysis

The primary analysis in any randomised controlled trial is usually an intention-to-treat analysis. This is important in cerebrovascular disease, in which there is often a high rate of non-compliance with the randomised treatment allocation. It may be reasonable to perform an efficacy analysis, but the results should be interpreted with caution and a bias cannot be excluded. The potential for bias is illustrated by examining the outcome in patients who were randomised to surgical treatment in the European Carotid Surgery Trial, but who were not operated on and "crossed-over" to medical treatment (Fig. 17.4). The risk of stroke was considerably greater in this group than in those patients who were randomised to medical treatment alone. In other words, the cross-over patients were a particularly poor prognostic group. This is perhaps to be expected when one considers the main reasons why the patients were not operated on: the anaesthetist considered them to be too high an operative risk; the patient declined the operation; the patient suffered a stroke or myocardial infarction before the operation could be performed. In an efficacy analysis this group would be removed from the surgery group and added to the medical treatment group. In other words, a group of patients with a high risk of a poor outcome would be removed from the treatment group and added to the control group, leading to a considerable bias.

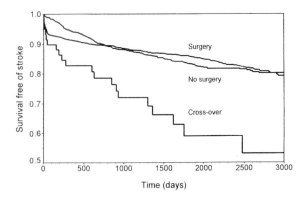

Fig. 17.4. Survival free of stroke during follow-up in patients randomised in the European Carotid Surgery Trial [7] for patients randomised to medical treatment (no-surgery), patients randomised to surgical treatment who underwent surgery (surgery) and patients who were randomised to surgery but were not operated on (cross-over).

Subgroup Analysis

Subgroup analysis is not intrinsically bad. Although it is frequently criticised, it can be essential to the proper understanding of a trial result. Problems arise with subgroup analysis when trial data are stratified according to several different baseline characteristics without any clear pre-hoc hypothesis. If enough analyses are performed, one will almost invariably find a subgroup of patients in whom the treatment effect is significantly different from the remainder. It is not usually difficult then to produce a seemingly plausible hypothesis to explain why the finding was, in fact, exactly what might have been expected. If it is stated how many other analyses were done in order to produce the one significant result, then it is possible to adjust the level of significance for multiple comparisons. However, this information may not always be given. Likewise, one suspects that subgroup analyses which were genuinely post-hoc may sometimes be presented as if they had been pre-hoc hypotheses. It is for these reasons that subgroup analyses are generally viewed with caution.

There are several instances of subgroup analyses producing misleading results in trials in cerebrovascular disease. For example, the results of one influential trial of aspirin and sulfinpyrazone in threatened stroke suggested that aspirin was effective in the secondary prevention of stroke in men but not in women [49]. Many theories were produced to explain why this was exactly what would be expected, and for a period of time women were not given aspirin. However, subsequent trials and a definitive meta-analysis have demonstrated that the benefit of aspirin in women is equal to that in men [5].

Generalising the Trial Result to Individual Patients

It is often difficult, given the very heterogeneous population of individuals who tend to be included in large trials in cerebrovascular disease, to know to what extent an overall trial result can be applied with confidence to the decision whether or not to treat an individual patient. The absolute benefit a patient will derive from a treatment will, of course, vary depending on the absolute risk of a poor outcome without treatment, but the relative treatment effect is generally assumed to be qualitatively, if not quantitatively, constant. Thus the overall relative risk reduction is assumed to be generalisable to all future patients who fit the trial entry criteria. However, this may not always be the case. Heterogeneity of relative treatment effect is especially likely when, as is often the case in cerebrovascular disease, a treatment has an appreciable risk of serious harm. It is quite conceivable that a treatment might be beneficial in some patients and harmful in others, the overall trial result merely reflecting the balance between these two groups. For example, carotid endarterectomy reduces the overall risk of ischaemic stroke in patients with a recently symptomatic stenosis of the internal carotid artery, but has a 5–7% operative risk of stroke or death [7,8,27]. Although it now widely recommended that all such patients be considered for surgery, in neither of the major trials did more than 25% of patients randomised to medical treatment actually have a stroke on follow-up. In other words, the remaining 75% of patients who remained stroke-free could not possibly have benefited from surgery had they been randomised to endarterectomy. Indeed, given the risk of stroke or death due to the operation, they would, as a group, undoubtedly have been harmed.

Application of the overall results of clinical trials to all patients is predicated on the assumption that we cannot identify in advance those patients who will do badly without treatment, and who should therefore be treated, and those patients who will do well without treatment, and who therefore should not be subjected to the risks of treatment. However, this negative approach may not be justified. Whilst we can seldom predict outcome with 100% accuracy, there are validated prognostic models in several branches of medicine which can reliably stratify patients according to their likely level of risk of various clinical outcomes. Stratification of the results of clinical trials using such models can provide an insight into the potential unreliability of overall trial results. For example, when patients with severe carotid stenosis in the European Carotid

Surgery Trial were stratified into "low", "medium" and "high" risk groups according to their predicted baseline absolute risk of stroke on medical treatment, using an independently derived and validated prognostic model, the effectiveness of endarterectomy was found to differ. Despite significant overall benefit in patients with severe carotid stenosis as a whole, patients with a "low" predicted stroke risk on medical treatment appeared to have possibly been harmed by endarterectomy (relative risk of stroke or surgical death with endarterectomy = 1.16, 95% CI = 0.6–2.4), whereas patients at "moderate" or "high" risk of stroke showed clear benefit (0.53, 0.3–0.9, and 0.34, 0.1–0.7, respectively) – a significant trend in relative treatment effect [21]. The overall trial result was not telling the whole story. Endarterectomy was of no obvious value in one group of patients but was highly beneficial in another and, most importantly, these groups could be defined.

The approach suggested is most applicable to treatments which are associated with a risk of serious harm, but should also be considered for low-risk but expensive treatments. If clinicians were able to treat only those patients who actually needed treatment and avoid unnecessary treatment of patients who were destined to do well without treatment, the financial savings could be considerable. In general, the relative efficacy of a safe treatment would seem less likely to vary qualitatively than that of a risky treatment. However, the efficacy of treatment might, for example, depend on the extent to which a disease has already progressed or the specific pathophysiology of the disease in a particular patient. While multiple subgroup analyses are undesirable and potentially misleading, we should be cautious about assuming that overall trial results can necessarily be applied to all patients.

References

1. Sandercock PAG, Celani MG, Ricci S. The likely public health impact in Europe of simple treatments for acute ischaemic stroke. Cerebrovasc Dis 1992;2:236.
2. Bogousslavsky J. () Acute stroke trials: from morass to nirvana? Cerebrovasc Dis 1995;5:3–6.
3. Dorman PJ, Sandercock PAG. Considerations in the design of clinical trials of neuroprotective therapy in acute stroke. Stroke 1996;27:1507–1515.
4. Collins R, Peto R, MacMahon S, et al. Blood pressure, stroke and coronary heart disease. Part 2, short term reductions in blood pressure: overview of randomised drug trials in their epidemiological context. Lancet 1990;335:827–838.
5. Antiplatelet Trialists' Collaboration. Collaborative overview of randomised trials of antiplatelet therapy. I. Prevention of death, myocardial infarction and stroke by prolonged antiplatelet therapy in various categories of patients. BMJ 1994; 308:81–106.
6. European Atrial Fibrillation Trial Study Group. Secondary prevention in nonrheumatic atrial fibrillation transient ischaemic attack or minor stroke. Lancet 1993;342:213–220.
7. European Carotid Surgery Trialists' Collaborative Group. MRC European Carotid Surgery Trial: interim results for symptomatic patients with severe (70–99%) or with mild (0–29%) carotid stenosis. Lancet 1991;337:1235–1243.
8. North American Symptomatic Carotid Endarterectomy Trial Collaborators. Beneficial effect of carotid endarterectomy in symptomatic patients with high-grade carotid stenosis. N Engl J Med 1991;325:445–453.
9. Pickard JD, Murray GD, Illingworth R, et al. Effect of oral nimodipine on cerebral infarction and outcome following subarachnoid haemorrhage: British aneurysm nimodipine trial. BMJ 1989;298:636–642.
10. International Stroke Trial Collaborative Group. The International Stroke Trial (IST): a randomised trial of aspirin, subcutaneous heparin, both or neither among 19 435 patients with acute ischaemic stroke. Lancet 1997;349:1569–1581.
11. Chinese Acute Stroke Trial Collaborative Group. CAST: a randomised placebo controlled trial of early aspirin use in 20 000 patients with acute ischaemic stroke. Lancet 1997;349:1641–1649.
12. National Institute of Neurological Disorders and Stroke rt-PA Stroke Study Group. Tissue plasminogen activator for acute ischaemic stroke. N Engl J Med 1995;333:1581–1587.
13. Major ongoing stroke trials. Carotid and Vertebral Artery Transluminal Angioplasty Study (CAVATAS). Stroke 1996; 27:358.
14. Harrison MJG. Ethics of stroke trials. In: Amery WK, Bousser M-G, Clifford-Rose F, editors. Clinical trial methodology in stroke. London: Baillière Tindall, 1989:267–281.
15. Stiller CA. Centralised treatment, entry to trials and survival. Br J Cancer 1994;70:352–362.
16. Counsell C, Salinas R, Naylor R, Warlow C. The role of routine or selective carotid artery shunting during carotid endarterectomy and the different methods of monitoring in selective shunting. The Cochrane Library. London: BMJ Publishing, 1997.
17. LaRue LJ, Alter M, Traven ND, et al. Acute stroke therapy trials: problems in patient accrual. Stroke 1988;19:950–954.
18. Steiner TJ, Clifford Rose F. Towards a model stroke trial. The single centre naftidrofuryl study. Neuroepidemiology 1986;5: 121–147.
19. Gorringe JAL. Initial preparartion for clinical trials. In: Harris EL, Fitzgerald JD, editors. The principles and practice of clinical trials. Edinburgh: Churchill Livingstone, 1970: 41–46.
20. Woods KL. Megatrials and management of acute myocardial infarction. Lancet 1995;346:611–614.
21. Rothwell PM. Can overall results of clinical trials be applied to all patients? Lancet 1995;345:1616–1619.
22. Yusef S, Collins R, Peto R. Why do we need some large, simple randomized trials? Stat Med 1984;3:409–420.
23. UK-TIA study group. The United Kingdom transient ischaemic attack (UK-TIA) aspirin trial: final results. J Neurol Neurosurg Psychiatry 1991;54:1044–1054.
24. Hankey GJ, Dennis MS, Slattery J, Warlow CP. Why is the outcome of transient ischaemic attacks different in different groups of patients? BMJ 1993;I:1107–1111.
25. Hier DB, Edelstein G. Deriving clinical prediction rules from stroke outcome research. Stroke 1991;22:1431–1436.
26. Hankey GJ, Slattery JM, Warlow CP. Transient ischaemic attacks: which patients are at high (and low) risk of serious vascular events? J Neurol Neurosurg Psychiatry 1992;55:640–652.

27. Rothwell PM, Slattery J, Warlow CP. A systematic review of the risks of stroke and death due to endarterectomy for symptomatic carotid stenosis. Stroke 1996;27:260–265.

28. Norton B, Homer-Ward M, Donnelly MT, Long RG, Holmes GKT. A randomised prospective comparison of percutaneous endoscopic gastrostomy and nasogastric tube feeding after acute dysphagic stroke. BMJ 1996;312:13–16.

29. Kraaijeveld CL, van Gijn J, Schouten HJA, Staal A. Interobserver agreement for the diagnosis of transient ischaemic attacks. Stroke 1984;15:723–725.

30. Hansen M, Sindrup SH, Christensen PB, Olsen NK, Kristensen O, Friis ML. Interobserver variation in the evaluation of neurological signs: observer dependent factors. Acta Neurol Scand 1994;90:145–149.

31. Noseworthy JH, Ebers GC, Vandervoort MK, Farquhar RE, Yetisir E, Roberts R. The impact of blinding on the results of a randomized, placebo-controlled multiple sclerosis clinical trial. Neurology 1994;44:16–20.

32. Kotila M, Waltimo O, Niemi ML, et al. The profile of recovery from stroke and factors influencing outcome. Stroke 1984;15:1039–1044.

33. Skilbeck CE, Wade DT, Langton-Hewer R, Wood VA. Recovery after stroke. J Neurol Neurosurg Psychiatry 1983;46:5–8.

34. Executive Committee for the Asymptomatic Carotid Atherosclerosis Study. Endarterectomy for asymptomatic carotid artery stenosis. JAMA 1995;273:1421–1428.

35. Hobson RW, Weiss DG, et al. and the Veterans Affairs Cooperative study group. Efficacy of carotid endarterectomy for asymptomatic carotid stenosis. N Engl J Med 1993;328:221–227.

36. Warlow CP. Endarterectomy for asymptomatic carotid stenosis? Lancet 1995;345:1254–1255.

37. van Gijn J, Warlow C. Down with stroke scales. Cerebrovasc Dis 1992;2:244–246.

38. Mahoney FI, Barthel DW. Functional evaluation. The Barthel Index. Md State Med 1965;14:61–65.

39. Granger CV, Sherwood CC, Greer DS. Functional status measures in comprehensive stroke care program. Arch Phys Med Rehabil 1977;58:555–561.

40. Granger CV, Dewis LS, Peters MC, et al. Stroke rehabilitation: analysis of repeated Barthel index measures. Arch Phys Med Rehabil 1979;60:14–17.

41. Van Swieten JC, Koudstaal PJ, Schouten HJA, van Gijn J. Interobserver agreement for the assessment of handicap in stroke patients. Stroke 1988;19:604–607.

42. Lindley RI, Waddell F, Livingstone M, Warlow C, Dennis M, Sandercock P, Smith B. Can simple questions assess outcome after stroke? Cerebrovasc Dis 1994;4:314–324.

43. Brazier JE, Harper R, Jones NMB, O'Cathain A, Thomas KJ, Usherwood T, et al. Validating the SF-36 health survey questionnaire: new outcome measure for primary care. BMJ 1992;305:160–164.

44. Dorman PJ, Slattery J, Farrell B, Dennis MS. A randomised comparison of the EuroQol and Short-Form 36 after stroke. BMJ 1997;315:461.

45. The EuroQol Group. Euroqol: a new facility for the measurement of health-related quality of life. Health Policy 1990;16:199–208.

46. Koudstaal PJ. Stroke prevention in non-valvular atrial fibrillation. Some methodological aspects. In: Amery WK, Bousser M-G, Clifford Rose F, editors. Clinical trial methodology in stroke. London: Baillière Tindall, 1989.

47. Warlow C. How to do it: Organise a multicentre trial. BMJ 1990;300:180–183.

48. Candelise L. Clinical trial methodology in stroke multicentre studies: keep the protocol simple. In: Amery WK, Bousser M-G, Clifford Rose F, editors. Clinical trial methodology in stroke. London: Baillière Tindall, 1989.

49. Canadian Cooperative Study Group. A randomised trial of aspirin and sulfinpyrazone in threatened stroke. N Engl J Med 1978;299:53–59.

50. Rothwell PM, Slattery J, Warlow CP. A systematic review of clinical and angiographic predictors of stroke and death due to carotid endarterectomy. BMJ 1997;315:1571–1577.

51. Ricci S, Celani MG, Righetti E, Cantisani AT for the International Stroke Trial Collaborative Group. Between country variations in the use of medical treatments for acute stroke: An update. Cerebrovasc Dis 1996;6(Suppl 2):133.

18. Clinical Trials in Stroke Prevention in North America

H.J.M. Barnett, H. Meldrum and M. Eliasziw

Introduction

The randomized clinical trial has been applied in cerebral vascular disorders for nearly 30 years. The amount of research coming from Canada and the United States in the field of stroke prevention by biological agents and drugs is appropriate because of historical events. For example, heparin emerged from the laboratories of Dr. Charles Best at the University of Toronto [1], and Dr. Hugh Smythe working in Dr. Fraser Mustard's laboratory at the same institution was the first to detect the platelet-inhibiting properties of any potentially therapeutic compound, sulfinpyrazone [2]. Within a year, Dr. Harvey Weiss in New York described the platelet-inhibiting action of aspirin [3]. It is somewhat artificial to divide the work of North Americans from that of Europeans in any field because of the cross-fertilization of ideas and collaborative studies. The first platelet-inhibiting drug to be put to the test of a clinical trial was dipyridamole. Its mode of action as a platelet antagonist was defined by a Canadian, Dr. Patricia Emmons, working in the Department of Hematology in Oxford [4].

This chapter will consider only the randomized clinical trials which have been conducted from North America. Trials evaluating platelet inhibitors, anticoagulants and surgical measures to prevent stroke will be reviewed.

Platelet Inhibitors

In the mid-1960s it was becoming clear that the passage of platelet fibrin material into the cerebral and retinal arteries was an important component of the phenomenon of transient hemisphere and retinal ischemic symptoms. These transient ischemic events (TIA) were identified as a warning symptom to many impending ischemic strokes. Mustard's observations

[5] on the alteration of platelet survival by sulfinpyrazone and Weiss' observation [3] on the alteration in platelet aggregation by aspirin were the sparks which led to this era of collaboration between clinicians, statisticians and pharmacologists to execute trials evaluating the potential usefulness of platelet inhibitors in stroke prevention.

The Canadian Cooperative Study

The seminal Canadian Cooperative Study was launched in 1971 [6]. In a factorial design patients with TIA or nondisabling stroke, judged to be related to noncardiac sources, received either aspirin 1300 mg daily with placebo, or sulfinpyrazone 800 mg daily with placebo, or both active treatment drugs, or only placebo. After an average treatment period of 26 months, the results in 585 patients from 16 Canadian centers indicated a benefit in stroke and death significant at a p value of <0.05. For all patients there was a 30% relative risk reduction arrived at by combining the two arms containing aspirin and comparing them with the two non-aspirin groups. Subgroup analysis did not detect a benefit in the 200 women in the trial. Analyzing the subgroup which was confined to men, the benefit for stroke and death reached a 48% relative risk reduction, ($p < 0.005$) (Fig. 18.1).

Criticisms arose soon after this trial was published. It was declared that synergism between sulfinpyrazone and aspirin could not be denied absolutely and that it was improper to make a comparison between the two arms with aspirin and the two arms without aspirin. Had the trial been much larger by modern design, this question might have been settled. There was concern expressed about looking at the gender subgroups without prior plan to do so in the design of the trial. Observations which followed upon this startling absence of demonstrated benefit for women disclosed that in women the outlook is more favorable than for men after they ex-

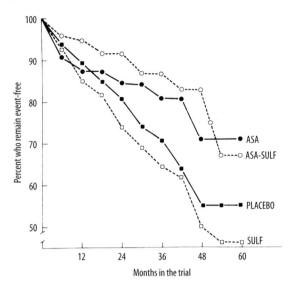

Fig. 18.1. Lack of benefit of sulfinpyrazone (SULF), benefit of aspirin (ASA) (<0.005) and lack of synergism or antagonism of a combination of the two in male patients. Reproduced with permission from the *Canadian Medical Association Journal*, 1980;122:295.

perience TIA or non-disabling stroke [7]. The appropriate sample size, had this fact been known, would have included more women than men. Instead, there was a ratio of 2 men to every 1 woman. The final problem in this first trial was the use of a single dose of aspirin. The dose was decided empirically, based on perceived levels of tolerance for aspirin and in ignorance of the mode of enzymatic action of aspirin upon the platelet – and, of course, in ignorance of the concept that the endothelial cell played a role in preventing thrombogenesis. This knowledge was to come later and to spark a major dose controversy based on hypotheses favoring the lowest possible dose.

Although there were faults in this first randomized trial of aspirin as an antithrombotic the stage was set for three decades of new studies involving aspirin and subsequent platelet inhibitors.

The Aspirin in Transient Ischemic Attacks Trial (AITIA)

The AITIA was launched in 1972 and terminated because of administrative problems in 1975. The investigators were able to report a trend toward benefit from aspirin in TIA and nondisabling stroke [8]. A total of 88 patients received aspirin and 90 received placebo. Eleven strokes occurred in the treatment arm and 14 in the placebo arm. For the combined outcome events of stroke or vascular death

there were 13 in the treatment arm and 18 in the placebo arm.

The American-Canadian Aspirin and Persantine Trial

The American-Canadian Aspirin and Persantine Trial addressed the question of benefit from a combination of 975 mg of aspirin and 400 mg of dipyridamole daily compared with 975 mg of aspirin alone [9]. This trial, in common with two French studies addressing the same question and using a similar dosage of the two preparations, concluded, in a total of 1589 patients, that dipyridamole added to aspirin was no more efficacious than was aspirin alone in these doses [10,11].

Skepticism lingers in the minds of some, including the authors, about the value of dipyridamole in stroke prevention. A very large trial reported in 1996 on 6602 patients, one quarter of whom were denied any platelet inhibitor, one quarter of whom each received either 50 mg of aspirin or 400 mg of dipyridamole and one quarter of whom received a combination of both of these active drugs. The investigators did not explain why they did not include a group with the dose of aspirin used in the previous studies with dipyridamole. They chose an aspirin dose that had never been shown against placebo to be effective in stroke prevention [12]. They utilized a placebo despite existing proof of the efficacy of aspirin. The data center was not at arms length from the manufacturer. Serious fraudulent practice on the part of one investigator was detected only after he had accumulated hundreds of nonexistent patients [13]. Data from this center were not entered in the analyses but a shadow lingers over the conduct of the trial.

Wilterdink and Easton recommend that another trial of similar size to ESPS-2 (about 3000 patients with TIA or stroke, comparing dipyridamole combined with 325 mg aspirin with 325 mg of aspirin alone) may be required to confirm these findings and dramatically alter clinical practice. "If dipyridamole plus aspirin truly reduces the risk of stroke by 23% (and nonfatal stroke by 27%) over aspirin alone, it will be difficult for new antiplatelet agents to do substantially better" [14]. Regulatory agencies have approved the combination of aspirin and dipyridamole so that, despite concerns about the conflicting trials, the drugs much higher cost and the exceptionally low dose of aspirin used in the trial, the use of the combination has been commonly accepted by practitioners. The authors recommend its use if aspirin fails.

The Ticlopidine Aspirin Stroke Study (TASS)

The TASS introduced the second platelet inhibitor which has proven to be effective in stroke prevention [15]. Its action on the platelet is not the same as aspirin. It interferes with the platelet-fibrinogen binding mechanisms. The end result is a decrease in platelet aggregation and fibrinogen binding to inhibit the formation of a thrombus. Unlike aspirin, which has maximal effect in 20 min, ticlopidine requires 24–48 h for maximal benefit.

The TASS trial involved 3069 patients with TIA or minor stroke randomized to receive 500 mg of ticlopidine or 1300 mg of aspirin daily. A relative risk reduction of 12% favoring ticlopidine for nonfatal stroke or death was observed at 3 years. These events occurred in 19% of the aspirin and 17% of the ticlopidine group, for a 2% absolute risk reduction favoring ticlopidine. Stroke alone, either fatal or nonfatal, was observed in 10% of the ticlopidine and 13% of the aspirin group, a relative risk reduction of 21% and an absolute risk reduction of 3% in favor of ticlopidine. Subgroup analyses have claimed superiority of ticlopidine over aspirin on a gender basis, and in posterior circulation ischemia, but this data-generated information is based on unconvincing numbers [16,17].

The Canadian-American Ticlopidine Study (CATS)

The CATS was different from the TASS in that patients with TIA were not randomized [18]. Ticlopidine in the CATS was tested against placebo. The disability of the stroke in the randomized patients varied but it could not be severe enough to preclude follow-up visits. A relative risk reduction of 30% was observed in the combined outcomes of stroke, myocardial infarction, and deaths from vascular causes.

As a consequence of these two trials, ticlopidine has been accepted as a treatment to be used after cerebral ischemic events. It has been touted by some as the only drug proven to be of value after a developed stroke [19]. This is misleading because all the aspirin trials included a large proportion of patients with ischemia ranging from TIA to moderately disabling stroke. The inclusion of patients with strokes in these trials has been ignored and has not deterred enthusiasts from recommending ticlopidine as the drug of first choice over aspirin after infarction has occurred.

Ticlopidine should be regarded as another alternative to aspirin and used as the platelet inhibitor of later choice for the following reasons. First, the use of ticlopidine rests on only two trials: one with and one without TIA patients. Experience proving the usefulness of aspirin is 10-fold greater. Second, the difference between aspirin and ticlopidine in the one direct comparison study (TASS) is modest. The absolute risk reduction of 2–3% is unimpressive. Third, the drug is more expensive. If the absolute difference between the drugs had proven to be considerable, the expense would have to be accepted because stroke itself is an expensive and distressing phenomenon. Fourth, at least 20% of those given ticlopidine suffer diarrhea. In a quarter of these, the drug must be discontinued permanently.

Finally, and most disturbingly, there is evidence of bone marrow suppression. Fortunately, it was uncommon in the trials (no more than 2%) and it was reversible. Subsequent evidence has emerged that fatalities have occurred because of irreversible bone marrow suppression [20,21]. Of the 645 patients known to the manufacturers of ticlopidine to have suffered bone marrow suppression, 16% died [22]. In some of these patients, it is known that appropriate steps had been taken to monitor blood counts and yet this precaution did not prevent the disastrous results. In others, the amount of monitoring has not been reported. Subsequently serious and fatal instances of thrombotic thrombocytopenia purpura have been reported in patients receiving short-term therapy with ticlopidine as an anti-thrombotic protection during coronary artery angioplasty and stenting and in the weeks following the procedure [22,23]. Careful supervision of bone marrow function is essential to the use of ticlopidine.

In conclusion, ticlopidine is to be recommended when aspirin cannot be tolerated or when ischemic events continue despite its use. Ticlopidine must only be administered to patients in whom there is no doubt about the diagnosis of cerebral or retinal ischemic events.

The Clopidogrel Versus Aspirin in Patients at Risk of Ischemic Events (CAPRIE) Trial

A trial tested a drug closely related to ticlopidine. [24] This very large trial randomized 19 185 patients to receive either 75 mg of clopidogrel or 325 mg of aspirin daily. It is not known why the investigators of this drug, who had already evaluated ticlopidine against 1300 mg daily of aspirin, elected to utilize only 325 mg in this subsequent trial. It is unfortunate that clopidogrel was not tested against a second, larger dose of aspirin. In any event, only a modest

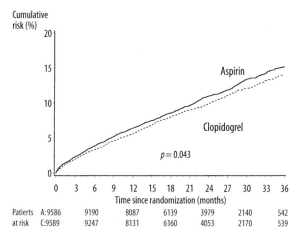

Fig. 18.2. Cumulative risk of ischaemic stroke, myocardial infarction or vascular death. *A*, aspirin; *C*, clopidogrel. Reproduced with permission from *The Lancet* 1996;348:1333.

benefit was shown for clopidogrel compared with this dose of aspirin. (Fig. 18.2) The absolute difference in benefit between clopidogrel and aspirin was 0.5%. It has been calculated that 200 patients need be switched to clopidogrel from aspirin to prevent one ischemic event within 2 years in the cerebral, coronary or peripheral arterial circulations. The study was able to show a mildly favorable result for the aggregation of outcomes in favor of clopidogrel, (Plavix®). Definite benefit was observed in patients who entered the trial with peripheral vascular disease. They experienced significantly reduced numbers of peripheral vascular outcomes. A significant reduction in strokes was not reported for those entering the trial with stroke as the entry event. Negative benefit in terms of myocardial infarction was reported in patients who entered the trial because of recent coronary artery symptoms. Neurologists confronted with patients who have had repeat cerebral ischemic symptoms will find it difficult to be enthusiastic about the use of this drug if the goal of therapy is stroke prevention. The investigators reported that the incidence of side effects in the gastro-intestinal tract was lower than with ticlopidine and that the incidence of bone marrow suppression was only one tenth as frequent as with ticlopidine. The drug has been accepted by the regulatory agencies, but in the opinion of the authors it is uncertain that it should replace ticlopidine as the alternate drug of choice when aspirin or aspirin with dipyridamole is not tolerated or fails. Since clopidogrel came on the market one disturbing report of 13 patients who developed thrombotic thrombocytopenia purpura in association with the use of Plavix has been published [25–29]. If these

reports continue, serious reservations will arise about its widespread use. Clearly these post-marketing monitoring for both ticlopidine and clopidogrel point to the need for scrupulous post-marketing observations and immediate frank disclosures about the alarming complications.

The Physician's Health Study

The Physician's Health Study was a primary prevention trial in which 22 071 middle-aged male American physicians, free of heart disease and stroke history, were randomized to take 325 mg of aspirin every other day or to take a placebo [30]. At the conclusion of the trial, and an average follow-up of 5 years, it was declared by the investigators that there was a 44% reduction in nonfatal myocardial infarction in those taking aspirin but that there was no reduction in the occurrence of stroke. When the preliminary report was published on the basis of 13 hemorrhagic strokes out of 80 strokes in the aspirin arm and 6 hemorrhagic strokes out of 70 in the placebo arm, it was postulated that aspirin might be the cause of this phenomenon [31]. Despite the small numbers, significance in this subgroup was reported. After one further year of follow-up, the risk of hemorrhagic stroke, now a total of 23 of 119 total strokes in the aspirin arm and 12 of 98 strokes in the placebo arm, was not significant. In a nonrandomized study of 87 678 women who took aspirin in variable doses as compared with no aspirin, a lack of stroke benefit was reported. Once again, myocardial infarction reduction was observed, with 32% fewer in the aspirin compared with the non-aspirin group [32]. No trial has specifically addressed the question of primary prevention of stroke by aspirin nor addressed the optimum dose of aspirin to be used for this purpose.

The Asymptomatic Cervical Bruit Study

The Asymptomatic Cervical Bruit Study involved 372 patients who were known to have asymptomatic carotid artery stenosis of ≥50% [33]. The individuals in the trial received either placebo or 325 mg daily of aspirin. After a median of 2.3 years of therapy, the trial did not detect any reduction in stroke or myocardial infarction. There were 11 strokes in the aspirin and 10 in the placebo group, and 7 and 4 myocardial infarctions in the aspirin and placebo groups respectively. The possibility cannot be dismissed that the failure to observe a benefit was due to a combination of factors, including the fact that the number of individuals in the trial was too small, the outcome events too few, and the dose of aspirin not optimal for the prevention of stroke.

Anticoagulants

Introduced to medical practice nearly 30 years before platelet inhibition was feasible, anticoagulants lagged behind in terms of critical evaluation. The science of methodology and biostatistics was not mature. There were a few randomized trials attempted by the pioneering trialist, Dr. Robert Baker, in the Veterans Administration hospitals [34]. A British group under Dr. J.M.S. Pearce also made early contributions [35]. Their combined efforts yielded a mere 185 patients with TIA or stroke were who randomized to receive warfarin or anticoagulants. There were too few patients and outcomes for any conclusions. Ten strokes occurred in the placebo group and 8 in the warfarin group. The hazards of administration of warfarin yielded an excess of cerebral hemorrhage in the treated ($n = 15$) compared with the placebo group ($n = 10$).

Warfarin for Patients with Noncardiac Cerebral Ischemic Symptoms

Modern clinical evaluation is more precise and the type of stroke can be identified and hemorrhage excluded. Furthermore methodologists and biostatisticians can estimate the number of patients with threatened stroke needed to prove the efficacy of therapy [36]. Thus the stage has been set to rectify previous failure to carry out the definitive trials. A trial currently in progress, the Warfarin-Aspirin Recurrent Stroke Study (WARSS) [37], is looking at TIA patients provided they have a CT lesion supporting the diagnosis; they and recent stroke patients are being given either aspirin or warfarin in a randomized study. Results are expected within the next year. Another trial is in progress evaluating aspirin and warfarin in patients experiencing TIA or stroke in the carotid territory who have intracranial stenosis [38]. The reader will be aware from other chapters about large trials in Europe and China comparing anticoagulants and heparin in patients with recent cerebral infarction.

Heparin in Progressing Stroke

Patients with ischemic stroke who are worsening, either progressively or in a step-like fashion, commonly have been given heparin therapy. The question of efficacy remains unclear. One small randomized trial found that among 225 patients who appeared to have progressing deficit, the patients given heparin progressed as often as those given placebo [39]. A smaller observational series ($n = 36$) noted worsening in half the patients given heparin.

The introduction of tissue plasminogen activator (tPA) for ischemic stroke and its efficacy for selected patients with a lesion of less than 3 h duration, will probably diminish interest in testing heparin in these patients. Patients with stroke symptoms for longer than 3 h will continue to raise the unanswered question of the value of heparin. Further studies are required and the problem is far from settled. Many of these patients will be worsening because of deleterious changes in the neurons due to the accumulation of toxic excitatory neurotransmittors and will be unresponsive to an anticoagulant.

Heparin and Warfarin To Prevent Stroke After Myocardial Infarction

The Cerebral Embolism Task Force [40] was a multicenter trial planned to evaluate heparin in patients who had evidenced a cerebral ischemic event after myocardial infarction. The trial was terminated when 45 patients had been randomized, because there were already 8 events in the placebo and none in the treatment group. More convincingly, two other North American controlled studies and one from Italy have studied large numbers of patients with anterior myocardial infarction. The study by Turpie et al. [41] indicated that a high dose (12 500 units) of subcutaneous heparin twice daily was comparable to a low dose (5000 units) twice daily. The investigators reported a reduction in left ventricular thrombus at day 10 of 11% in the high-dose compared with 32% in the low-dose group. Non-hemorrhagic infarction occurred in 1% of the high-dose and 4% of the low-dose group.

Warfarin was tested in 1214 patients following a myocardial infarction. The patients entered the study at a mean of 27 days after the myocardial infarction and were followed for an average of 37 months [42]. For those assigned to warfarin, the target INR was 2.8–4.8. A reduction in the relative risk of stroke of 55% was observed in the treated group compared with placebo, and there was a relative risk reduction of 24% and 34% respectively for death and risk of reinfarction.

Warfarin in Prevention of Stroke in Patients with Non-valvular Atrial Fibrillation (NVAF)

Six North American [43,44,45,46,47,48] and two European randomized trials [49,50] have found conclusively that the risk of stroke from non-valvular atrial fibrillation is reduced significantly with the use

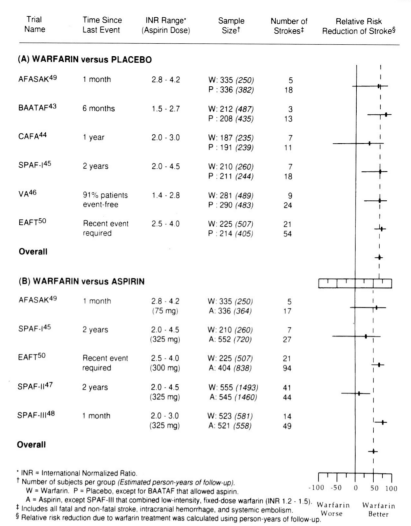

Trial Name	Time Since Last Event	INR Range* (Aspirin Dose)	Sample Size†	Number of Strokes‡	Relative Risk Reduction of Stroke§
(A) WARFARIN versus PLACEBO					
AFASAK[49]	1 month	2.8 - 4.2	W: 335 *(250)* P: 336 *(382)*	5 18	
BAATAF[43]	6 months	1.5 - 2.7	W: 212 *(487)* P: 208 *(435)*	3 13	
CAFA[44]	1 year	2.0 - 3.0	W: 187 *(235)* P: 191 *(239)*	7 11	
SPAF-I[45]	2 years	2.0 - 4.5	W: 210 *(260)* P: 211 *(244)*	7 18	
VA[46]	91% patients event-free	1.4 - 2.8	W: 281 *(489)* P: 290 *(483)*	9 24	
EAFT[50]	Recent event required	2.5 - 4.0	W: 225 *(507)* P: 214 *(405)*	21 54	
Overall					
(B) WARFARIN versus ASPIRIN					
AFASAK[49]	1 month	2.8 - 4.2 (75 mg)	W: 335 *(250)* A: 336 *(364)*	5 17	
SPAF-I[45]	2 years	2.0 - 4.5 (325 mg)	W: 210 *(260)* A: 552 *(720)*	7 27	
EAFT[50]	Recent event required	2.5 - 4.0 (300 mg)	W: 225 *(507)* A: 404 *(838)*	21 94	
SPAF-II[47]	2 years	2.0 - 4.5 (325 mg)	W: 555 *(1493)* A: 545 *(1460)*	41 44	
SPAF-III[48]	1 month	2.0 - 3.0 (325 mg)	W: 523 *(581)* A: 521 *(558)*	14 49	
Overall					

* INR = International Normalized Ratio.
† Number of subjects per group *(Estimated person-years of follow-up)*.
  W = Warfarin. P = Placebo, except for BAATAF that allowed aspirin.
  A = Aspirin, except SPAF-III that combined low-intensity, fixed-dose warfarin (INR 1.2 - 1.5).
‡ Includes all fatal and non-fatal stroke, intracranial hemorrhage, and systemic embolism.
§ Relative risk reduction due to warfarin treatment was calculated using person-years of follow-up.

Fig. 18.3.   Meta-analyses showing the relative risk reduction of stroke among patients with nonvalvular atrial fibrillation receiving *A* warfarin as compared with placebo, and *B* warfarin as compared with aspirin. The relative risk reduction is indicated by a *black rectangle*, with its corresponding 95% confidence interval as a *horizontal line*. The overall relative risk reduction is represented by the *broken vertical line*: *A* 64%, 95% confidence interval 51–74%, $p < 0.001$; and *B* 48%, 95% confidence interval 33–60%, $p < 0.001$. All *p* values are two-tailed. Test for heterogeneity among relative risk reductions in each analysis was statistically nonsignificant. Adapted from the *New England Journal of Medicine*;332:239.

of warfarin. As seen in Fig. 18.3, this benefit is translated into a reduction in the relative risk of stroke of 64% ($p < 0.001$) for warfarin compared with placebo and of 48% ($p < 0.001$) for warfarin compared with aspirin.

The INR range now recommended is 2.0–3.0. The evidence that has accumulated during these trials points clearly to the fact that the individuals under the age of 60 years have a sufficiently low risk of stroke that they should not be considered for warfarin therapy unless they have a high-risk vascular profile consisting of: (a) evidence of systemic embolism, (b) congestive heart failure, (c) hypertension with left ventricular hypertrophy. Patients with paroxysmal fibrillation are not considered candidates for long-term therapy. This recommendation will change if the condition reverts to a chronic dysrhythmia. For patients older than 75 years, the risk of hemorrhage increases. The trialists are recommending extra precautions in assuring a compliant patient, an excellent laboratory, and an INR not exceeding 3.0. Aspirin can be recommended for those patients with NVAF who do not need anticoagulants, such as young patients with low risk profile or patients considered at high risk of complication from anticoagulants.

Surgical Therapy in Stroke Prevention: Patients with Symptomatic Carotid Artery Arteriosclerosis

The Joint Study of Extracranial Carotid Occlusion

The Joint Study of Extracranial Carotid Occlusion was a trial to evaluate the benefit of carotid endarterectomy against best contemporary medical care [51]. It was initiated within a decade of the introduction of carotid artery surgery. It proved to be a negative trial. There were a number of reasons for this, most related to the study design and execution. Fortunately, negative results of the Joint Study were ignored by many clinicians, and the procedure was not prematurely nor erroneously abandoned. The Joint Study was too small, with only 316 patients entered into the trial. The entry characteristics were not properly identified and 42% of the patients were not affected with appropriate focal carotid hemisphere or retinal symptoms. There was a large number of patients lost to follow-up and many crossed over from the medical to the surgical arm. The report optimistically expressed positive benefit and achieved this claim by comparing the medical and surgical outcomes beginning at the point when the patients left hospital. This flawed method overlooked the fact that 11% of the patients had a stroke or died in the postoperative, pre-discharge period.

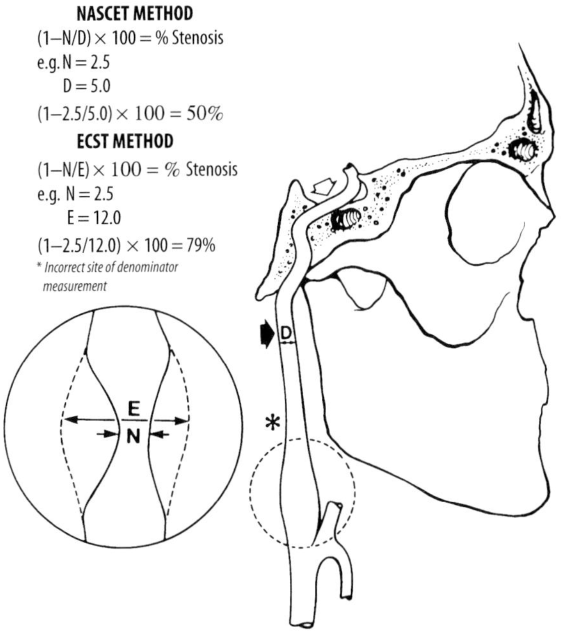

The North American Symptomatic Carotid Endarterectomy Trial (NASCET)

Primary Observations

The NASCET was the second North American trial evaluating carotid endarterectomy and was conducted in two phases [52]. The first phase was for those with symptoms appropriate to severe (70–99% stenosis) atherosclerotic lesions and the second phase was confined to those with less than 70% stenosis. Both phases of the NASCET were launched in 1987 and ran in parallel to each other and to the European Carotid Surgery Trial (ECST), launched in 1981 [45].

NASCET METHOD

$(1-N/D) \times 100 = \%$ Stenosis

e.g. $N = 2.5$

$D = 5.0$

$(1-2.5/5.0) \times 100 = 50\%$

ECST METHOD

$(1-N/E) \times 100 = \%$ Stenosis

e.g. $N = 2.5$

$E = 12.0$

$(1-2.5/12.0) \times 100 = 79\%$

* Incorrect site of denominator measurement

Fig. 18.4. The NASCET calculates the percentage of stenosis by using the narrowest linear diameter in two (or three planes) as the numerator, and the artery well beyond the carotid bulb (*circled*) and any post-stenotic dilatation as the denominator (*filled arrow*). Measurement of the artery too close to the bulb produces a misleading denominator (*asterisk*). The NASCET measures were conducted at a site well beyond the usual post-stenotic or arteriosclerotic dilatation. The ECST used the same numerator but used the imagined site of the wall of the carotid bulb as the denominator. The ECST calculations yielded 46% more patients in the "severe" category than the NASCET. The *open arrow* points to the common site of stenosing atheroma in the intracranial portion of the internal carotid artery. Reproduced with permission of Quality Medical Publishing from *Current Critical Problems in Vascular Surgery* 1994:291.

The NASCET randomized patients to receive either best medical care alone or best medical care plus carotid endarterectomy. The study required a history within 180 days of focal hemisphere or retinal symptoms with an angiographically proven lesion in the ipsilateral carotid artery. The degree of stenosis was calculated by determining the percentage of luminal diameter using the narrowest part of the stenosed segment of the artery as the numerator, and the diameter of the artery below the base of the skull where the walls become parallel beyond the bulb and any post-stenotic dilatation as the denominator (Fig. 18.4). Patients were excluded at entry if they had a probable cardiac source of embolism, serious disease likely to cause death within 5 years, or intracranial disease that was more significant than the carotid lesion. Neurologists followed the patients and the underlying cause of all deaths, and the territory, type, severity, and cause of all strokes were assessed.

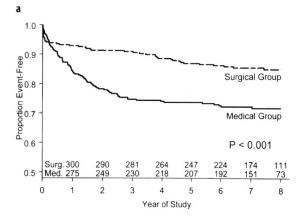

a

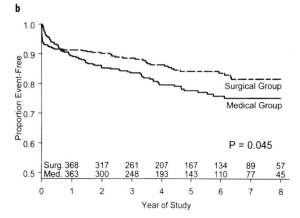

b

Fig. 18.5. **a** Kaplan-Meier Curves for Event-free Survival among Patients with 70–99% Carotid Stenosis. The curves show the probability of avoiding an ipsilateral stroke of any degree of severity for each treatment group. Also shown is the p-value from the Mantel-Haenszel chi-square test used to compare the event-free survival curves. The numbers along the horizontal axis are the numbers of patients in each group who were still at risk during each year of follow-up. *Reproduced with permission from New England Journal of Medicine 1998;339:1415–1425.* **b** Kaplan-Meier Curves for Event-free Survival among Patients with 50–69% Carotid Stenosis. The curves show the probability of avoiding an ipsilateral stroke of any degree of severity for each treatment group. Also shown is the p-value from the Mantel-Haenszel chi-square test used to compare the event-free survival curves. The numbers along the horizontal axis are the numbers of patients in each group who were still at risk during each year of follow-up. *Reproduced with permission from New England Journal of Medicine 1998;339:1415–1425.*

Stopping rules were defined at the beginning of the NASCET to ensure that neither benefit would be denied nor harm would be done to patients. Confidential analyses of the outcome events began after 1 year of randomization and were repeated at regular intervals. The first patient was admitted in December 1987, and by February 1991 the Monitoring Committee advised that the severe phase of the trial must be terminated. An unequivocal benefit was found in

Table 18.1. NASCET: Risk of ipsilateral stroke or any perioperative stroke or perioperative death

Month of study	Risk (%)			RRR (%)	NNT
	Medical	Surgical	Difference		
30 days	3.3	5.8	−2.5	–	–
1 year	17.3	7.5	9.8	57	10
2 years	26.0	9.0	17.0	65	6

Reproduced with permission from *Neurology* 1996;46:603–608.
From the North American Symptomatic Carotid Endarterectomy Trial (NASCET), the risk of stroke for 331 medically treated and 328 surgically treated patients with symptoms appropriate to severe stenosis are given at 30 days, 1 and 2 years. To prevent one stroke in 2 years, 6 patients need to have endarterectomy. RRR, relative risk reduction; NNT, number needed to treat.

favor of endarterectomy in the patients with 70–99% stenosis (Fig. 18.5). These results were obtained from only 659 patients admitted from 50 participating centers. The 30-day (perioperative) risk of any stroke or death from endarterectomy was 5.8%. In terms of disabling stroke and death, the perioperative risk was 2.1%. The risk for medically treated patients, of any ipsilateral stroke at 2 years was 26.0% in comparison to 9.0% for patients treated surgically. The relative risk reduction favoring surgery was 65%, and the absolute risk reduction was 17.0%. The number needed to treat (NNT) to prevent one stroke in 2 years was calculated at 6 patients. Although randomization of patients with 70–99% stenosis was stopped in 1991, patients continued to be followed to the end of the study in December 1997. The benefit of endarterectomy persisted out to 8 years.

For the 858 patients with 50–69% stenosis, the benefit was muted (Fig. 18.5). The 5-year risk of ipsilateral stroke was 22.2% among patients treated medically and 15.7% among those treated surgically. The absolute reduction in risk was only 6.5% and the NNT to prevent one stroke in two years was 15. For this group, benefit was greater in patients presenting with hemisphere not retinal symptoms, with stroke rather than TIA, and male sex. Among the 1368 patients who had <50% stenosis, no benefit from endarterectomy was observed.

Two important considerations must be borne in mind when interpreting these results and generalizing them to other patients with symptoms related to carotid lesions. First, the surgical skill must be equivalent or nearly equivalent to that of the surgeons who participated in NASCET. If the skill is less or is not known, it is unacceptable. Endarterectomy is a dangerous procedure and the referring physicians and patients must know that a perioperative

Table 18.2. NASCET: Failure of ultrasound to prove the need for Crossover

Center's opinion	Moderate on angiography (n = 30)	Severe on angiography (n = 38)
Moderate on ultrasound	10 (33%)	4 (11%)
Severe on ultrasound	19 (63%)	32 (84%)
Occluded on ultrasound	1 (3%)	2 (5%)

NASCET centers investigated 68 patients initially exhibiting moderate stenosis (<70%) suspected of advancement of disease to severe (70–99%) stenosis. Thirty remained "moderate" on conventional angiography; the ultrasound findings agreed in only 33% and judged 63% to be "severe" and 3% to be occluded. Thirty-eight were confirmed by angiography to have severe stenosis (70–99%). Of these, ultrasound judged 11% to remain "moderate"; agreed with the angiogram in 84% and erroneously categorized 5% as an occlusion.

rate of stroke or death of 6% or less can be achieved and that this complication rate confers on them a real benefit compared with medical care. At complication rates of 8–10%, the risk of the procedure approaches the point where benefit is negated.

Second, these results relate to an accurate measurement of the degree of stenosis seen in a conventional angiogram. Ultrasound is used in an increasing number of institutions as a substitute for this stringent and demanding method [54]. This is not recommended. Despite claims to the contrary, there are still difficulties encountered in attempts to correlate ultrasound findings, even of the most sophisticated variety, with the measurements from arteriography [55]. Mistakes are commonly made even with modern equipment in sophisticated centers. A lesion may be labelled moderate or totally occluding when in fact it is neither but is a near-occlusion. Patients with symptoms due to near-occlusion benefit from endarterectomy. It is undesirable that the degree of stenosis from a lesion be either underestimated or overestimated. If a lesion is not severe but is called severe, the patient is subjected to a procedure for which data may not exist to justify it. Conversely, patients are denied a beneficial surgical procedure if lesions are called moderate on ultrasound when they in fact are ≥70% by arteriography (Table 18.2).

There are several other reasons for not substituting non-invasive imaging for conventional angiography. First, magnetic resonance angiography has not overcome the tendency to overread the degree of stenosis due to turbulence. This may come. Second, the degree of intracranial stenosis in the carotid siphon cannot be measured accurately by ultrasound, including transcranial Doppler. Finally, the NASCET and some small case-series have pointed to the fact that a soft intraluminal arterial thrombus pushes the risk of endarterectomy to triple or quadruple (18–25%) what is expected when this

thrombus is not present [56,57]. Ultrasound and MRI are less reliable than conventional angiography in detecting this dangerous lesion.

Some clinicians claim that angiography is too risky. A literature review determined that, in published series, the average complication rate was 1% [51]. There are institutions that have reported unusually high levels of complications. If this is the case, patients may receive their therapeutic advice on the basis of ultrasound studies alone and know that there is a reasonable chance they are facing a significant surgical risk (5–6% at best) in circumstances where the indications are not certain. Alternatively, and preferably in high-risk angiogram institutions, patients should be sent for these studies to institutions where reasonable levels of complication have been demonstrated by institutional audit.

The risk of conventional angiography in 2885 patients with moderate or severe arteriosclerosis submitted to the procedure in 100 NASCET centers was 0.6% for mild to moderate non-disabling stroke and an estimated 0.1% for disabling stroke. This is an acceptable level because it is only a small fraction of the 2.0% risk of disabling stroke from endarterectomy.

Secondary Observations

From the follow-up of 659 patients symptomatic with severe disease and 2226 patients symptomatic with moderate disease over an average of 5 and 4 years respectively, a number of observations relating to patients with these lesions have been possible:

1. The surgical procedure to which 1409 moderate and severe patients were randomized proved to be of durable benefit up to 8 years of follow-up (Fig. 18.6).
2. Among the 1039 strokes that occurred in all patients over NASCET's follow-up period, 112 were of cardioembolic, 211 were of lacunar, and

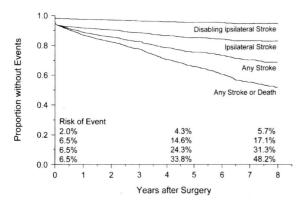

Fig. 18.6. Kaplan-Meier Curves for Event-free Survival after Carotid Endarterectomy in 1409 Patients with Severe and Moderate Stenosis. The curves show the probability of avoiding an event, according to 4 different definitions of outcome. Point estimates (at the bottom as percentages) are shown for the risk of each event at 30 days, 5 years, and 8 years after the surgery and include all perioperative outcome events. *Reproduced with permission from Stroke 1999;30:1751–1758.*

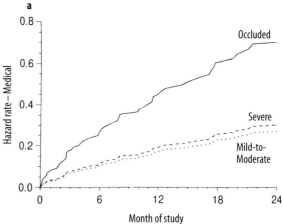

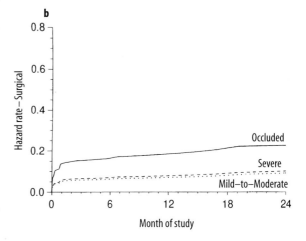

Fig. 18.7. **a** Cumulative hazard curves showing risk (hazard rate) of ipsilateral stroke for medically treated patients at three degrees of contralateral carotid artery disease. **b** Cumulative hazard curves showing risk (hazard rate) of ipsilateral stroke for surgically treated NASCET patients with ≥70% stenosis at three levels of contralateral carotid artery disease. Severe contralateral stenosis carried the same prognosis as did a mild to moderate stenosis. By contrast, a contralateral occlusion added greatly to the risk in medically treated patients. The surgical risk was double that of patients without contralateral occlusion but substantially less than in those treated medically. Reproduced with permission from *Journal of Neurosurgery* 1995;83:781.

698 were of large-artery origin. There were 17 due to primary intracerebral hemorrhage and 1 patient had subarachnoid hemorrhage [59]. The 5-year risk for a cardioembolic stroke in any territory was 2.6%, for lacunar stroke it was 6.9%, and for large-artery stroke it was 19.7%. Approximately 20% of the strokes in the territory of a symptomatic artery with 70–99% stenosis were unrelated to carotid stenosis. By contrast 40% of the strokes in patients with 60–69% stenosis were of lacunar or cardioembolic origin.

3. When an occlusion is present in the artery contralateral to the severe stenosis which is causing the symptoms, with medical treatment alone the risk of stroke in the symptomatic territory is increased three-fold compared with patients whose contralateral asymptomatic artery is the site of stenosis but not occlusion. Endarterectomy on the symptomatic artery carries a two-fold risk compared with the risk for patients who do not have an occlusion but is decidedly beneficial compared with medical therapy (Fig. 18.7).

4. The presence of an increasingly high vascular risk profile adds progressively to the poor outlook and risk of stroke in medical patients with severe (70–99%) stenosis (Fig. 18.8). Endarterectomy is equally effective at all risk levels.

5. In patients with severe stenosis, the presentation with hemisphere events carries a risk that is triple that for patients who present exclusively with retinal ischemic symptoms. The risk increases with increasing degrees of severity of stenosis (Fig. 18.9).

6. In patients with severe stenosis (70–99%) in whom an ulcer is obviously visible on angiography, the prognosis in those treated medically is worse than when the lesion is not present and the negative impact of ulceration on the prognosis increases with increasing degree of severity of the stenosis. Surgical therapy once again confers benefit equally in all levels of stenosis and regardless of the presence of ulceration (Fig. 18.10).

7. In the severe phase of NASCET, 25 patients were observed with an intraluminal thrombus

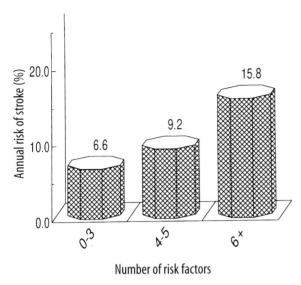

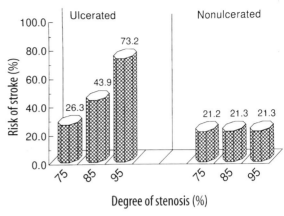

Fig. 18.8. Kaplan–Meier estimates of the average annual risk of ipsilateral stroke related to the number of risk factors present in the medically treated patients of NASCET symptomatic with 70–99% stenosis of the carotid artery. The list of 16 risk factors that comprise the risk profile has been previously published [42]. The risk of stroke rises with an increasing number of risk factors. Reproduced with permission from *Neurology* 1996;46:606.

Fig. 18.10. Two-year estimates of ipsilateral stroke risk by presence (and absence) of definite plaque ulceration and degree of stenosis for medically treated NASCET patients with 70–99% stenosis, calculated from a Cox proportional hazards regression model. The presence of definite carotid plaque ulceration on an angiogram is a marker for poor prognosis, which is exacerbated by increasing degrees of stenosis. In the absence of plaque ulceration, the risk of stroke remains relatively constant. Reproduced with permission of Med-Orion Publishing from *Cerebrovascular Ischaemia: Investigation and Management* 1996:386.

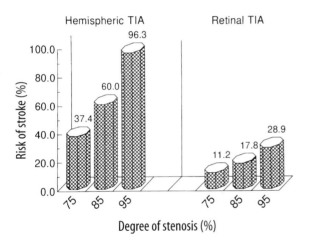

Fig. 18.9. Two-year estimates of ipsilateral stroke by type of transient ischemic attack (TIA) and degree of stenosis for medically treated NASCET patients with ≥70% stenosis, calculated from a Cox proportional hazards regression model. The overall prognosis for patients presenting with a first-ever hemispheric TIA is worse than for patients presenting with a first-ever retinal TIA. In both cases, the outlook is affected by the degree of carotid artery stenosis. Reproduced with permission of Med-Orion Publishing from *Cerebrovascular Ischaemia: Investigation and Management* 1996:386.

beyond the severely stenosing lesion. The 30-day outlook in terms of ipsilateral stroke for those randomized to the surgical arm was poor, with 22% postoperative strokes. Likewise, the 30-day outlook in the medical patients was poor, with 25% suffering ipsilateral strokes. Accordingly the accepted empirical management for these patients has been to recommend a 4- to 6-week period on warfarin, followed by repeat imaging to ensure clearing of the thrombus and continued patency of the artery. When these studies have been completed and the thrombus is no longer seen, endarterectomy should proceed.

8. The risk of stroke is directly related to the degree of stenosis in the patients treated medically. The worst outlook was encountered in patients whose stenosis was 90–94% (Fig. 18.11). Additionally, in the 95–99% range, patients exhibited features of collateral intracranial anastomoses, delayed flow up the internal carotid artery, narrowing of the artery beyond the lesion and in some, a narrowing sufficiently extreme as to be designated a "string sign" [60]. For patients within this extreme range of stenosis, the outlook with medical care is better than for those in the 90–94% range.

9. The severity of ischemic stroke which occurs in the long-term follow-up of patients who have been subjected to endarterectomy is less than for those patients with severe disease who have an ischemic stroke while still on medical therapy alone (unpublished NASCET data; P.H. Lyrer, personal communication 1996).

10. Prospective observations were made upon the asymptomatic carotid artery, on the side

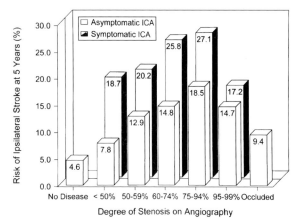

Fig. 18.11. The Risk of an Ipsilateral Stroke at 5 Years after Study Entry in the Territories of Asymptomatic and Symptomatic Carotid Arteries, According to the Degree of Stenosis. Stenosis of 95–99% represents near-occlusion. *Reproduced with permission from New England Journal of Medicine 2000;342: 1693–1700.*

contralateral to the symptoms which preceded randomization (N = 1820). The risk of stroke increased with the degree of stenosis but was substantially less than it was for the same degree of stenosis in a symptomatic artery (Fig. 18.11). Moreover, 45% of the strokes that occurred in the territory of an asymptomatic artery with 60–99% stenosis were attributable to cardioembolism or lacunar disease [61].

The VA Symptomatic Carotid Trial

A second North American trial evaluating carotid artery surgery was conducted in VA hospitals [62]. A total of 189 patients with stenosis measuring 50–99% were randomly assigned to best medical care or to endarterectomy. When the trial was stopped short of its goal because of the compelling results from the NASCET and the ECST, a trend towards benefit in favor of endarterectomy was observed.

Surgical Therapy in Stroke Prevention: Patients with Asymptomatic Carotid Artery Stenosis

Between North America and Europe, four randomized trials have concluded and one is in progress to determine the benefit of endarterectomy in asymptomatic individuals. The three trials conducted in North America will be reviewed.

The Mayo Clinic Asymptomatic Carotid Endarterectomy Study (MACE)

The MACE was designed to determine whether endarterectomy without aspirin therapy was superior to aspirin therapy in the management of this lesion [63]. After 71 patients had been randomized and there were 8 instances of myocardial infarction and 3 instances of cerebral ischemic events in the surgical arm and none of either in the medical arm, the trial was stopped. The trial was inappropriately designed because the medical and surgical arms received dissimilar therapy.

The Veterans Administration Asymptomatic Trial

The Veterans Administration Asymptomatic Trial was larger than the MACE study. Nevertheless, it was smaller than calculations had predicted would be required because of the paucity of outcome events in asymptomatic patients [64]. A total of 444 patients followed for an average of 47.9 months reported a perioperative stroke and death risk of 4.4% [65]. The patients had angiographic evidence of 50–99% stenosis. Significant benefit was claimed for surgical therapy but was evident only if the outcome event of TIA was added to that of stroke and perioperative death. Confining the analyses to stroke and death, the survival curves for the medical and surgical arms were superimposed throughout the entire length of surveillance of the patients out to 96 months. A nonsignificant trend for benefit in the reduction of stroke, omitting perioperative death, has been identified but its value as an isolated observation is questionable.

The Asymptomatic Carotid Atherosclerosis Study (ACAS)

The ACAS multicenter study, randomized 1662 patients with asymptomatic carotid disease to receive either best medical care alone or best medical care plus endarterectomy [57]. The study found a benefit for endarterectomy and a relative risk reduction for ipsilateral stroke of 53%, an absolute risk reduction of 5.9% (11% medical versus 5.1% surgical). Patients with 60–99% stenosis, as measured by a conversion from Doppler ultrasound, were randomized. A demanding evaluation of the participating surgeons' record of perioperative complications was required prior to their acceptance into the study. The perioperative complication rate during the trial was reported at 2.3%. This rate included the risk of angiography mandated only for the patients randomized to endarterectomy. There are a number of disappointing aspects to this trial which must be studied carefully before applying the results to the large numbers of individuals who are harboring a silent carotid artery lesion:

1. The sample-size represented a reasonably small number of patients and there were a small number of outcome events. Patients were followed for an average of only 2.7 years.
2. The investigators did not identify any reduction in the numbers of disabling strokes in the surgical as compared with the medical group. It is possible to speculate that this was due to the small number of events.
3. The perioperative risk was calculated on the basis of the 825 patients randomized to the surgical arm including 101 patients who never had the operation. The actual perioperative stroke and death complication rate including angiography calculated from only those patients who underwent endarterectomy rose to 2.6%.
4. The absolute difference in risk of ipsilateral stroke or perioperative stroke or perioperative death in the surgical group compared with the medical group was 5.9% at 5 years (Table 18.3). This converts to slightly more than 1% benefit per year between the treatment groups. If the perioperative rate is adjusted to reflect the actual level of the complication rate of 2.6%, this absolute difference is reduced to 5.6%.
5. At 2 years, the number needed to be treated with endarterectomy to prevent one stroke is 67 patients (Table 18.3). Adjusting the perioperative rate to the actual achieved, this procedure must be extended to 83 patients. This is in sharp contrast to the 6 patients who must have endarterectomy to prevent one stroke in 2 years in symptomatic patients with 70–99% stenosis. Only 4 symptomatic patients need to receive endarterectomy to prevent one stroke in 2 years if the stenosis is 90% or more.
6. Women were not shown to benefit from endarterectomy in the ACAS. The perioperative complication rate was 3.6% compared with 1.7% in men and this probably explains the lack of demonstrated benefit for women. This lack of demonstrated benefit is further evidence of the fine line separating benefit from lack of benefit achieved by this procedure and the fact that only the most expert surgeons with a proven record of a low complication rate should attempt to operate on asymptomatic carotid artery lesions. Several reports from multi-institutional studies and from administrative databases (notably Medicare) report complication rates of 4–5%. Many patients

Table 18.3. ACAS: Risk of ipsilateral stroke or any perioperative stroke or perioperative death

Month of study	Risk (%)			RRR (%)	NNT
	Medical	Surgical	Difference		
30 days	0.4	2.3	−1.9	–	–
1 year	2.4	3.0	−0.6	–	–
2 years	5.0	3.5	1.5	30	67
5 years	11.0	5.1	5.9	53	17

Reproduced with permission from *Neurology* 1996;46:603–608.
From the Asymptomatic Carotid Atherosclerosis Study (ACAS), the risk of stroke is compared between the medically and surgically treated patients. To prevent one stroke in 2 years, 67 patients need to have endarterectomy. Adjusting the surgical group to include only the patients who had endarterectomy, the 30 day surgical risk becomes 2.6%, and the 1, 2 and 5 year risks rise to 3.3%, 3.8%, and 5.4% respectively. The number of endarterectomies needed to treat to prevent one stroke in 2 years becomes 83.
RRR, relative risk reduction; NNT, number needed to treat.

receiving endarterectomy would be better treated by medical management [67].

7. The ACAS was unable to determine whether there was a difference in surgical benefit for patients with the lower (60–79%) or the higher (80–99%) degrees of stenosis. This is disappointing. The symptomatic studies and the observational case-series have all found a compelling difference in outlook, with the worst outlook in the highest deciles of stenosis [68,69].

All efforts to date have failed to answer satisfactorily the vexed question of benefit or lack thereof from endarterectomy in patients with asymptomatic disease. Estimates place the number of individuals in the United States over 50 years of age who have 50% or greater stenosis at 2 million [70]. It would be rewarding to have guidelines allowing a selection from these individuals of the ones most likely to remain stroke-free after endarterectomy. There will not be many and it is predicted that they will be in the upper two deciles of stenosis and probably have, in addition, a high vascular risk profile. A worsening of the prognosis accompanying a high vascular risk profile was observed in the patients with asymptomatic lesions in the NASCET population [61].

The Aspirin in Carotid Endarterectomy Trial (ACE)

The ACE trial was designed and conducted in the NASCET centers between July 1994 and April 1998. All patients not eligible for the NASCET, who were scheduled for endarterectomy in these centers, were randomly assigned one of four doses of aspirin between 81 mg and 1300 mg daily, and then followed by neurologists for 3 months. Among the 2804 patients who underwent surgery, the combined rate of stroke, myocardial infarction, and death was lower in the low-dose groups (81 or 325 mg) than in the high-dose groups (650 or 1300 mg) at 30 days (5.4% versus 7.0%) [71].

In the 74 ACE centers, with experienced surgeons in academic and large practice institutions, 46% of the endarterectomies were done for symptomatic and 54% for asymptomatic lesions. The overall perioperative stroke and death rate was 5.4%, with 4.6% in the patients who were asymptomatic and 6.4% in those with appropriate symptoms. The ACAS perioperative complication rate of 2.6% was not reproduced in ACE. This illustrates the difficulty of reproducing in practice the results reported in ACAS.

Extracranial Intracranial Bypass Study

Microvascular surgery perfected the technique of anastomosing small arteries under the microscope using hair-like sutures. It was learned that the superficial temporal artery could be joined to the largest available cortical branch of the middle cerebral artery. The possibility was attractive that this bypassing procedure might be of use in stroke prevention in patients who had occluded arteries or intracranially stenosed major arteries and were continuing to have ischemic events. The anecdotal experiences were encouraging. A multicenter randomized trial entered 1377 patients who had occluded internal carotid or middle cerebral arteries or surgically inaccessible stenosis of the internal carotid and stenosis of the main stem of the middle cerebral artery [72]. Symptoms had to have occurred within 90 days. In the patients randomized to surgery, the perioperative morbidity and mortality was low at a rate of 3.1%, the success of the anastamosis was excellent with a patency rate of 96%. Nevertheless, the medically treated patients fared slightly better than did those who received the bypass. Fewer strokes occurred and the long-term stroke-free survival rates favored the medically treated patients. This was true of all patients in the medical group. Furthermore no benefit was noted in separate analyses of the radiological subgroups, some of whom might have had hemodynamic cause for their ischemic attacks and for which this compromise nowadays would be sought by newer technological advances. In the subgroup of 74 patients most likely to be suspected of hemodynamic insufficiency because they had bilateral occlusion of the carotid arteries, the medical patients survived free

of stroke more often than did the surgical patients. No subsequent studies, utilizing sophisticated techniques, have been able to confirm that a small hemodynamically impaired group will improve or survive more free of stroke with the procedure.

A randomized trial done early in the history of this procedure, being decidedly negative, was able to prevent the spread of a procedure which, by anecdote and uncontrolled case series, looked promising.

Summary

North American trials of stroke prevention have been able to make important contributions by a number of disciplined studies:

1. The Canadian Collaborative Study launched the era of aspirin therapy as an antithrombotic preparation to be used in patients presenting with TIA or minor stroke.
2. The Cerebral Embolism Task Force, the first randomized study of patients with cerebral ischemic complications following myocardial infarction, established that heparin was effective in reducing the risk of stroke.
3. In conjunction with European studies, major trials have established that warfarin is a powerful tool to be employed in patients with non-valvular atrial fibrillation. Anticoagulants are preferred over platelet inhibitors in patients threatening with cardioembolic stroke.
4. Ticlopidine became available as an alternative platelet inhibitor and was recommended for patients unable to take aspirin, or who continue to experience events despite the use of aspirin. More recently hematological complications from the use of ticlopidine have diminished enthusiasm for it.
5. Clopidogrel was introduced as an alternative to ticlopidine. Its effectiveness on reducing the occurrence of stroke in stroke-threatened patients has not been convincing.
6. In agreement with the ECST results, NASCET has produced convincing evidence that patients with focal symptoms due to 70–99% carotid stenosis will benefit from carotid endarterectomy done by expert surgeons. In NASCET the benefit is less for patients with 50–69% stenosis. Below 50% stenosis there was no benefit.
7. Progress has been made in clarifying the role, if any, of endarterectomy in asymptomatic carotid stenosis. Major uncertainties persist.
8. Superficial-temporal to middle cerebral artery bypass surgery is not an effective procedure in stroke prevention.

References

1. Best CH. Preparation of Heparin its use in the first Clinical Case. Circulation 1959; Vol. 19:79–86.
2. Smythe HA, Orygzlo MA, Murphy EA, et al. The effect of sulfinpyrazone (Anturan) on platelet economy and blood coagulation in man. Can Med Assoc J 1965;92:818–821.
3. Weiss HJ, Aledort LM. Impaired platelet/connective-tissue reaction in man after aspirin ingestion. Lancet 1967;II: 495–497.
4. Emmons PR, Harrison MJ, Honour AJ, Mitchell JR. Effect of a pyrimido pyrimidine derivative on thrombus formation in the rabbit. Nature 1965;208:255.
5. Mustard JF, Rowsell HC, Smythe HA, Senyi A, Murphy EA. The effect of sulfinpyrazone on platelet economy and thrombus formation in rabbits. Blood 1967;29:859–866.
6. The Canadian Cooperative Study Group. A randomized trial of aspirin and sulfinpyrazone in threatened stroke. New Engl J Med 1978;299:53–59.
7. Dyken ML. Antiplatelet aggregating agents in transient ischemic attacks and the relationship of risk factors. In: Breddin K, Loew D, Uberla K, et al., editors. Prophylaxis of venous, peripheral, cardiac and cerebral vascular diseases with acetylsalicylic acid. Stuttgart: Schattauer Verlag, 1981: 141–148.
8. Fields WS, Lemak NA, Frankowski RF, et al. Controlled trial of aspirin in cerebral ischemia. Stroke 1977;8:301–316.
9. The American-Canadian Co-operative Study Group. Persantine Aspirin Trial in cerebral ischemia: endpoint results. Stroke 1985;16:406–415.
10. Bousser MG, Eschwege E, Haguenau M, et al. "AICLA" controlled trial of aspirin and dipyridamole in the secondary prevention of athero-thrombotic cerebral ischemia. Stroke 1983;14:5–14.
11. Guiraud-Chaumeil B, Rascol A, David JL, Boneu B, Clanet M, Bierme R. Prévention des récidives des accidents vasculaires cérébraux ischémiques par les anti-agrégants plaquettaires: résultats d'un essai thérapeutique contrôlé de 3 ans. Rev Neurol (Paris) 1982;138:367–385.
12. Diener HC, Cunha L, Forbes C, Sivenius J, Smets P, Lowenthal A. European Stroke Prevention Study 2. Dipyridamole and acetylsalicylic acid in the secondary prevention of stroke. J Neurol Sci 1996;143:1–13.
13. Enserink M. Fraud and ethics charges hit stroke drug trial. Science 1996;274:2004–2005.
14. Wilterdink JL, Easton JD. Dipyridamole Plus Aspirin in Cerebrovascular Disease. Arch Neurol 1999;56:1087–1092.
15. Hass WK, Easton JD, Adams HP Jr, et al. A randomized trial comparing ticlopidine hydrochloride with aspirin for the prevention of stroke in high-risk patients. New Engl J Med 1989;321:501–507.
16. Hershey LA. Stroke prevention in women: role of aspirin versus ticlopidine. Am J Med 1991;91:288–292.
17. Grotta JC, Norris JW, Kamm B, TASS Baseline and Angiographic Data Subgroup. Prevention of stroke with ticlopidine: who benefits most? Neurology 1992;42:111–115.
18. Gent M, Blakely JA, Easton JD, et al. The Canadian American Ticlopidine Study (CATS) in thromboembolic stroke. Lancet 1989;I:1215–1220.
19. Harbison JW. Ticlopidine versus aspirin for the prevention of recurrent stroke: analysis of patients with minor stroke from the Ticlopidine Aspirin Stroke Study. Stroke 1992;23:1723–1727.
20. Oh PI, Lanctôt KL, Naranjo CA, Shear NH. Fatal aplastic anemia associated with ticlopidine therapy – approaches to an adverse drug reaction. Can J Clin Pharmacol 1995;2:19–22.
21. Shear NH. Prevention of ischemic stroke [letter]. New Engl J Med 1995;333:460.
22. Barnett HJM, Eliasziw M, Meldrum HE. Prevention of ischemic stroke [reply]. New Engl J Med 1995(August 17); 333:460.
23. Bennett CL, Weinberg PF, Rozenberg-Ben-Dror K, Yarnold PR, Kwaan HC, Green D. Thrombotic thrombocytopenic purpura associated with ticlopidine: a review of 60 cases. Ann Intern Med 1998;128:541–544.
24. CAPRIE Steering Committee. A randomised, blinded, trial of cloppidogrel versus aspirin in patients at risk of ischaemic events (CAPRIE). Lancet 1996;348:1329–1339.
25. Tholl U, Anlauf M, Helmchen U. Clopidogrel and membranous nephropathy. Lancet 1999;354:1443–1444.
26. Chinnakotla S, Leone JP, Fidler ME, Hammeke MD, Tarantolo S. Clopidogrel-Associated Thrombotic Thrombocytopenic Purpura/Hemolytic Uremic Syndrome in a Kidney/Pancreas Transplant Recipient. Transplantation 2000;70:550–552.
27. Moy B, Wang JC, Raffel GD, Marcoux II JP. Hemolytic Uremic Syndrome Associated with Clopidogrel. Arch Intern Med 2000;160:1370–1372.
28. Bennett CL, Connors JM, Carwile JM, Moake JL, Bell WR, Tarantolo SR, McCarthy LJ, Sarode R, Hatfield AJ, Feldman MD, Davidson CJ, Tsai HM. Thrombotic Thrombocytopenic Purpura Associated with Clopidogrel. N Engl J Med 2000;342:1773–1777.
29. Wood AJJ. Thrombotic Thrombocytopenic Purpura and Clopidogrel – A Need for New Approaches to Drug Safety. N Engl J Med 2000;342:1824–1826.
30. Steering Committee of the Physicians' Health Study Research Group. Final report on the aspirin component of the ongoing Physicians' Health Study. New Engl J Med 1989;321:129–135.
31. Steering Committee of the Physician's Health Study Research Group. Special report: preliminary report: findings from the aspirin component of the ongoing Physicians' Health Study. New Engl J Med 1988;318:262.
32. Manson JE, Stampfer MJ, Colditz GA, et al. A prospective study of aspirin use and primary prevention of cardiovascular disease in women. JAMA 1991;266:521–527.
33. Côté R, Battista RN, Abrahamowicz M, et al. Lack of effect of aspirin in asymptomatic patients with carotid bruits and substantial carotid narrowing. Ann Intern Med 1995;123:649–655.
34. Baker RN, Schwartz WS, Rose AS. Transient ischemic strokes: a report of a study of anticoagulant therapy. Neurology 1966; 16:841.
35. Pearce JMS, Gubbay SS, Walton JN. Long-term anticoagulant therapy in transient cerebral ischaemic attacks. Lancet 1965; I:6.
36. Taylor DW, Sackett DL, Haynes RB. Sample size for randomized trials in stroke prevention: how many patients do we need? Stroke 1984;15:968.
37. WARSS, APASS, PICSS, HAS and GENESIS Study Groups. The feasibility of a collaborative double-blind study using an anticoagulant. Cerebrovasc Dis 1997;7:100–112.
38. Major ongoing clinical trials. Warfarin vs. aspirin for symptomatic intracranial disease (WASID). Stroke 2000;31:1479–1480.
39. Duke RJ, Block RF, Turpie AGG, et al. Intravenous heparin for the prevention of stroke progression in acute partial stable stroke: a randomized controlled trial. Ann Intern Med 1986; 105:825.
40. Cerebral Embolism Task Force. Cardiogenic brain embolism: the second report of the cerebral embolism task force. Arch Neurol 1989;86:727.
41. Turpie AGG, Robinson JG, Doyle DJ, et al. Comparison of high-dose with low-dose subcutaneous heparin to prevent left ventricular mural thrombosis in patients with acute transmural

anterior myocardial infarction. New Engl J Med 1989;320: 352.

42. Smith P, Arnesen H, Holme I. The effect of warfarin on mortality and reinfarction after myocardial infarction. New Engl J Med 1990;323:147.

43. The Boston Area Anticoagulation Trial for Atrial Fibrillation Investigators. The effect of low-dose warfarin on the risk of stroke in patients with nonrheumatic atrial fibrillation. New Engl J Med 1990;323:1505.

44. Connolly SJ, Laupacis A, Gent M, et al. Canadian atrial fibrillation anticoagulation (CAFA) study. J Am Coll Cardiol 1991; 18:349–355.

45. Stroke Prevention in Atrial Fibrillation Investigators. Stroke Prevention in Atrial Fibrillation Study: final results. Circulation 1991;84:527–539.

46. Ezekowitz MD, Bridgers SL, James KE, et al. Warfarin in the prevention of stroke associated with nonrheumatic atrial fibrillation. New Engl J Med 1992;327:1406–1412. (Erratum, New Engl J Med 1993;343:687–691.)

47. Stroke Prevention in Atrial Fibrillation Investigators. Warfarin versus aspirin for prevention of thromboembolism in atrial fibrillation: Stroke Prevention in Atrial Fibrillation II Study. Lancet 1994;343:687–691.

48. Stroke Prevention in Atrial Fibrillation Investigators. Adjusted-dose warfarin versus low-intensity, fixed-dose warfarin plus aspirin for high-risk patients with atrial fibrillation: Stroke Prevention in Atrial Fibrillation III randomised clinical trial. Lancet 1992;348:633–638.

49. Petersen P, Godtfredsen J, Boysen G. Placebo-controlled, randomized trial of warfarin and aspirin for prevention of thromboembolic complications in chronic atrial fibrillation: The Copenhagen AFASAK study. Lancet 1989;I:175.

50. EAFT (European Atrial Fibrillation Trial) Study Group. Secondary prevention in non-rheumatic atrial fibrillation after transient ischaemic attack or minor stroke. Lancet 1993;342:1255–1262.

51. Fields WS, Maslenikov V, Meyer JS, Hass WK, Remington RD, Macdonald M. Joint study of extracranial arterial occlusion. V. Progress report of prognosis following surgery or nonsurgical treatment for transient cerebral ischemic attacks and cervical carotid artery lesions. JAMA 1970;211:1993–2003.

52. North American Symptomatic Carotid Endarterectomy Trial Collaborators. Beneficial effect of carotid endarterectomy in symptomatic patients with high-grade carotid stenosis. New Engl J Med 1991;325:445–453.

53. European Carotid Surgery Trialists' collaborative Group. MRC European Carotid Surgery Trial: interim results for symptomatic patients with severe (70–99%) or with mild (0–29%) carotid stenosis. Lancet 1991;337:1235–1243.

54. Chervu A, Moore WS. Carotid endarterectomy without arteriography. Ann Vasc Surg 1994;8:296–302.

55. Eliasziw M, Rankin RN, Fox AJ, Haynes RB, Barnett HJM, for the North American Symptomatic Carotid Endarterectomy Trial (NASCET) Group. Accuracy and prognostic consequences of ultrasonography in identifying severe carotid artery stenosis. Stroke 1995;26:1747–1752.

56. Buchan A, Gates P, Pelz D, Barnett HJM. Intraluminal thrombus in the cerebral circulation. Stroke 1988;19:681–687.

57. Barnett HJM. Prospective randomized trial of symptomatic patients: results from the NASCET Study. In: Moore WS, editor.

Surgery for cerebrovascular disease, 2nd ed. Philadelphia: Saunders, 1996:537–539.

58. Hankey GJ, Warlow CP, Molyneuz AJ. Complications of cerebral angiography for patients with mild carotid territory ischaemia being considered for carotid endarterectomy. J Neurol Neurosurg Psychiatry 1990;53:542–548.

59. Barnett HJM, Gunton RW, Eliasziw M, Fleming L, Sharpe B, Gates P, Meldrum H, for the North American Symptomatic Carotid Endarterectomy Trial (NASCET) Group. The Causes and Severity of Ischemic Stroke in Patients with Internal Carotid Artery Stenosis. JAMA 2000;283(11):1429–1436.

60. Morgenstern LB, Fox AJ, Sharpe BL, Eliasziw M, Barnett HJM, Grotta JC for the North American Symptomatic Carotid Endarterectomy Trial (NASCET) Group: The risks and benefits of carotid endarterectomy in patients with near occlusion of the carotid artery. Neurology 1997;48:911–915.

61. Inzitari D, Eliasziw M, Gates P, Sharpe B, Chan RKT, Meldrum HE, Barnett HJM, for the North American Symptomatic Carotid Endarterectomy Trial (NASCET) Group. The Causes and Risk of Stroke in Subjects with an Asymptomatic Internal Carotid Artery. N Engl J Med 2000 Jun 8;342(23):1693–1700.

62. Mayberg MR, Wilson SE, Yatsu F, et al. Carotid endarterectomy and prevention of cerebral ischemia in symptomatic carotid stenosis. JAMA 1991;266:3289–3294.

63. Mayo Asymptomatic Carotid Endarterectomy Study Group. Results of a randomized controlled trial of carotid endarterectomy for asymptomatic carotid stenosis. Mayo Clin Proc 1992;67:513–518.

64. Chambers BR, Norris JW. The case against surgery for asymptomatic carotid stenosis. Stroke 1984;15:964–967.

65. Hobson RW II, Weiss DG, Fields WS, et al. Efficacy of carotid endarterectomy for asymptomatic carotid stenosis. New Engl J Med 1993;328:221–227.

66. Executive Committee for the Asymptomatic Carotid Atherosclerosis Study. Endarterectomy for asymptomatic carotid artery stenosis. JAMA 1995;273:1421–1428.

67. Barnett HJM, Broderick JP. Carotid endarterectomy: Another wake-up call. Neurology 2000 (in press).

68. Hennerici M, Hulsbomer HB, Hefter H, Lemmerts D, Rautenberg W. Natural history of asymptomatic extracranial arterial disease: results of a long-term prospective study. Brain 1987;110:777–791.

69. Norris JW, Zhu CZ, Bornstein NM, Chambers BR. Vascular risks of asymptomatic carotid stenosis. Stroke 1991;22:1485–1490.

70. Barnett HJM, Eliasziw M, Meldrum HE, Taylor DW. Do the facts and figures warrant a 10-fold increase in the performance of carotid endarterectomy on asymptomatic patients? Neurology 1996;46:603–608.

71. Taylor DW, Barnett HJM, Haynes RB, Ferguson GG, Sackett DL, Thorpe KE, Simard D, Silver FL, Hachinski V, Clagett GP, Barnes RW, Spence JD for the ASA and Carotid Endarterectomy (ACE) Trial Collaborators. Low Dose and High Dose acetylsalicylic acid for Patients Undergoing Carotid Endarterectomy: a randomised controlled trial. Lancet 1999;353:2179–2184.

72. The EC/IC Bypass Study Group. Failure of extracranial-intracranial arterial bypass to reduce the risk of ischemic stroke: results of an international randomized trial. New Engl J Med 1985;313:1191–1200.

19. Cerebrovascular Disease: Experience Within Large Multicentre Trials

M.M. Brown and A.C. Pereira

Introduction

Stroke is defined as rapidly developing clinical signs of focal (or global) disturbance of cerebral function, with symptoms lasting 24 h or longer or leading to earlier death, with no apparent cause other than of vascular origin. Transient ischaemic attack (TIA) is defined identically except that the symptoms and signs resolve within 24 h [1]. There is no fundamental difference between a TIA and a stroke except for the duration. Stroke is therefore a syndrome with numerous symptoms and signs; it has different aetiologies and the prognosis can vary enormously. Disability may be considered by some to be a worse outcome than death since stroke can affect every aspect of normal life, from higher mental functions such as intelligence, personality and expression to more mundane tasks such as toileting, dressing and feeding. The extremely wide definition of stroke and the enormous variety of outcomes has made the conduct of clinical trials in stroke and the choice of outcome measures problematic. In spite of this, there is more information available from clinical trials to facilitate evidence-based practice in stroke than in any other neurological discipline. In this chapter, we discuss the major issues, problems and solutions derived from the most important multicentre trials of cerebrovascular disease.

Stroke is a very common condition. It is the third commonest cause of death in Britain, causing 10–12% of all deaths, and the commonest cause of adult disability. The annual incidence in industrialised countries is about 2/1000 population [2]. The incidence of TIA is about 25% that of stroke, but following a TIA there is a 5–10% risk of stroke each year. Until recently, clinical management has been largely conservative. However, prevention of stroke has been improved by the recent clinical trials which have demonstrated the benefits of treating carotid stenosis [3,4] and atrial fibrillation [5–9], while acute stroke treatment is likely to be revolutionised by trials examining the role of thrombolysis [10–12] and anticoagulation [13,14].

The Need for Clinical Trials in Stroke

Clinical practice is based on a complex combination of common sense, intuition and science. As evidence-based practice evolved, it has been realised that treatment should be based on the results of well-conducted clinical trials and many entrenched attitudes have had to be dislodged. Until recently, evidence-based medicine had little influence on the management of cerebrovascular disease, particularly in Britain, where nihilist attitudes prevailed. Elsewhere in the world, numerous treatments were advocated because they seemed to make sense on haemodynamic grounds, and not because there was any clinical evidence of benefit. Because the outcome of stroke is so variable, anecdotal reports and even case series have little value in assessing the value of potential treatments in cerebrovascular disease. Thus, in stroke, randomised clinical trials are the only acceptable way of proving a therapy is beneficial. Several popular treatments have been shown to be inadequate when subjected to the rigour of a randomised controlled trial. Haemodilution, a practice widely used in Europe and supported by small studies, was the subject of two large trials in Scandinavia and Italy. Both failed to show any benefit of haemodilution, and suggested it might even be harmful [15]. Another popular treatment in acute stroke is anticoagulation with heparin. However, the recent final analysis of the International Stroke Trial (IST) [16] suggests high-dose subcutaneous heparin significantly worsens the outcome after a stroke because of an increased risk of intracranial haemorrhage.

Design of Clinical Trials in Cerebrovascular Disease

Recruitment

Entrenched views about the benefits of treatment frequently affect recruitment to clinical trials. Recruitment to the early trials of surgical therapy was adversely influenced by preconceived views about efficacy. Some surgeons refused to take part in the European Carotid Surgery Trial (ECST) [3] because they "knew" that surgery worked, while other clinicians did not join because their experience was that surgery caused stroke rather than prevented it. Recruitment may also be influenced by financial or personal considerations.

In surgical trials, an active, participating surgeon will "lose" randomised patients from surgery to medical care. Recruitment to surgical trials is therefore much more successful in countries such as the UK where reimbursement is salaried and not on a fee-for-service basis. In the ECST, which started in 1981, an attempt was made to encourage surgical recruitment by randomising more patients (60%) to surgery than to medical care (40%). This caused considerable confusion when the results were first presented because the numbers in each group were not equal, and this approach has not been repeated in any other large-scale trials.

Attempts to accommodate preconceived ideas about efficacy may lead to complex trial protocols and frequent crossovers, diminishing the value of any results. For example, the Carotid Surgery Versus Medical Therapy in Asymptomatic Carotid Stenosis (CASANOVA) Trial [17] was particularly affected by preconceived views. The trial tested the utility of carotid endarterectomy in patients with asymptomatic carotid stenosis. However, at that time it was considered unethical to withhold an operation from patients with a greater than 90% stenosis. In addition, patients randomised in the trial in whom the stenosis progressed or became bilateral were also operated on. As a consequence, the final results were degraded by the large number of crossovers and the most important question of how to treat patients with a severe but asymptomatic stenosis could not be answered.

To incorporate the wide range of clinical opinions and maximise recruitment within a wide range of potential indications, the ECST developed the concept of the "grey area". This allows individual investigators to randomise patients who lie in the investigator's grey area, where the investigator is uncertain which treatment is best for the patient. This grey area, so-called clinical equipoise, is different for different investigators and may change with time. As new treatment becomes available with a modest benefit to patients, it becomes necessary for trials to incorporate the advance. For this reason, surgical trials usually compare surgery plus best medical treatment with best medical treatment alone. This leaves open the question of what is "best medical treatment". Whether the results of a trial are accepted and translated into clinical practice depends on the power of the trial, and the degree of benefit.

Randomisation

The most useful trials are prospective, randomised, controlled trials which may or not be blinded. A control group is essential. Because the causes and risk factors for stroke are so variable, it is essential that any stroke trial includes similar numbers of men and women in each group with similar aetiology of stroke and risk factor profiles, such as hypertension, diabetes and smoking. In general, the randomisation process will result in the two groups being very similar. In some multicentre trials such as the ECST [3], randomisation was stratified by centre, i.e. each centre was treated as its own small trial. This ensures that randomisation equalises different types of patients in each group within each centre and adjusts for differences between centres in the characteristics of patients caused by variation in referral patterns (i.e. case mix), patient selection or treatment procedures (e.g. surgical skill or use of other non-trial treatment).

Sample Size

The simpler the trial design, the more likely a trial is to reach a definite answer. This is because recruitment will be facilitated if the minimum amount of data is collected. Stroke is a complex disorder with numerous causes and very variable outcome. Clear and simple definitions of inclusion and exclusion criteria and of outcomes to be measured are essential. The main question asked is the "primary question", and the trial is designed to answer it, but in such a way that additional data may provide answers to other, "secondary" questions. For example, the primary question might be whether carotid endarterectomy in a recently symptomatic patient would prevent that patient having a stroke. However, the trial may provide enough data to determine whether the degree of stenosis matters: a secondary question. However, since trials are powered only to answer primary questions, there may not be enough information generated to answer secondary questions with statistical significance, and considerable caution needs to be used in interpreting such sub-group analyses.

The sample size and the power of the trial needed to answer the primary question are estimated from the size of the expected difference between the test and control groups. If the expected difference is small, a very large sample is required to demonstrate the difference and be confident that it is truly significant. In general, in prevention trials, the expected outcome event occurs infrequently (e.g. the incidence of recurrent stroke after TIA is only about 5% per annum) [18]. In this case, very large samples sizes are required to stand a good chance of showing a difference. For example, in the UK TIA Trial [19] 2435 patients were randomised but the benefit of aspirin in preventing stroke still did not reach significance. It required a meta-analysis pooling results from 145 trials totalling 70000 patients for the benefits of aspirin in preventing stroke to reach statistical significance [20]. Similar problems of sample size affect the analysis of trials of treatment for acute stroke. There are considerable difficulties assessing the outcome of stroke in terms of disability (see below) and therefore mortality is often chosen as an important "hard" end-point. However, the mortality from stroke in general is only about 10% [21], which again means that very large sample sizes are required to show a reduction in mortality with a new treatment. Some trials have attempted to get round this problem by selecting only patients with large cortical middle cerebral artery territory infarcts (who have a much higher mortality (30%) or risk of permanent disablity) [22]. However, in patients who already have large infarcts there may be little to be gained by reducing the size of the infarct by a small amount and hence a possible benefit of the same treatment in milder strokes may be missed by being too selective. It is important that the results of any trial should be applicable to as many patients with stroke as possible. Sample size calculations are often made on the assumption that only a considerable benefit, e.g. 25% reduction in risk, is going to be clinically worthwhile. However, in a common disease such as stroke, even a 1% absolute risk reduction in mortality would save 1000 lives per annum in the UK.

Most stroke treatment trials have therefore been far too small to exclude even a large benefit of the treatment examined. One partial solution to the problem of small trials missing important benefits is to carry out a meta-analysis in an attempt to combine results from different trials. However, this technique relies on there being more than one trial of a particular treatment available to analyse. There is also the danger that negative trials will not be published or only appear in obscure journals. The Cochrane stroke Review Group has therefore set up a database of clinical stroke trials, which at present lists over 100. This facilitates systematic reviews and meta-analyses, which are published in the Cochrane database of systematic reviews [23]. An example of the value of meta-analysis is the overview of stroke unit care published by Langhorne et al. [24] Only 1 in 10 trials of stroke units demonstrated a significant benefit of stroke unit care against general medical ward but the largest recruited only 311 patients. When a meta-analysis was carried out, a highly significant benefit of stroke unit care on mortality emerged, with a 28% reduction in mortality at 6 months [24]. Hence, because of small numbers, a benefit sufficient to save 2 lives per month in the average District General Hospital was missed before the meta-analysis was published. Many trials sponsored by the drug industry have been abandoned on commercial grounds too early to be certain that a potential benefit was not present.

The importance of a very large sample size in stroke trials is only now beginning to be appreciated. Three very large trials published their results at the end of 1996 and beginning of 1997. For example, the CAPRIE trial (see below) was powered to detect a difference of 10% between aspirin and a new antiplatelet agent, clopidogrel; this required 19185 patients to be randomised. Despite these very large numbers, the difference only just reached significance. The International Stroke Trial (IST) [16] was also powered to detect a 15% difference in the outcome between aspirin, heparin and either drug and randomised 19435 patients. The IST required considerable international co-operation throughout the world to achieve such numbers, but despite such efforts, failed to demonstrate any significant benefit. The Chinese Acute Stroke Trial (CAST) [13] recruited a similar number of patients, examining aspirin versus placebo in the acute treatment of stroke, and, although demonstrating a significant but very small benefit of aspirin on stroke recurrence, failed to show any benefit of aspirin on the combined outcome of stroke and death. It was only when the IST and CAST were combined in a meta-analysis to give a total of about 40000 patients that a significant benefit of aspirin emerged. The figures make sobering reading for anyone contemplating organising a trial of acute stroke treatment. Only treatments with dramatic effects are likely to show significant benefit with smaller numbers of patients. Such dramatic effects are rather unlikely given the very variable nature of human stroke and the known vulnerability of neurones to even brief periods of cerebral ischaemia. Further, if the effect of treatment is less than expected then the chosen sample size may not allow the results to be significant. It should be borne in mind that even a small absolute benefit in a trial may translate into a large benefit in the population as a whole. For example, the 1% reduction in death and disability shown for aspirin in acute stroke, would benefit over 1000 patients per annum in the UK if every stroke patient was treated.

Trials are normally designed so that a single treatment group is compared with a control group, such as in the ECST and NASCET [3,4]. Another approach uses a 2 × 2 factorial design as employed by the IST and the Multicentre Acute Stroke Trial–Italy (MAST-I) [10,16]. Patients were recruited in MAST-I into four groups: no treatment, streptokinase only, aspirin only and both. This allowed the outcomes of all the patients receiving streptokinase to be compared with those of all the patients not receiving that drug. A proportion of each group received aspirin which, if it interacted with streptokinase, would ruin the primary comparison. Factorial trials are useful as they provide answers to several questions using a smaller group of patients than would be required for two separate trials because the placebo group can be compared with both drug treatments. However, clinicians tend to be confused by the results of factorial trials and simpler trials often appear more convincing. Simple trials produce less ambiguous results.

Choice of Outcome Variables in Stroke Prevention Trials

Although ultimately the aim is to prevent death and disability, it has been usual to use recurrent stroke as one of the major outcome measures in stroke prevention trials. Some of the earlier carotid surgery trials such as the Veterans Affairs Asymptomatic Trial (VAAT) [25] included TIA as an outcome measure and stopped the trial when the number of TIAs and strokes together reached significance. Although the authors interpreted the result as positive, in fact there was no benefit of surgery on the outcomes of stroke and sudden death alone, and most observers concluded that the trial actually showed no useful benefit of surgery. TIAs are not of great importance because, by definition, the patient makes a complete and rapid recovery. In addition, it is not easy to be certain that transient neurological symptoms have been the result of cerebral ischaemia, and the patient is rarely examined during an attack. The reliability of a diagnosis of TIA is poor because considerable interpretation is required by the observer subject to bias if the treatment is not blinded. Even between neurologists, inter-observer

agreement concerning the diagnosis of TIA is only about 85% [26]. Stroke is therefore preferred as the outcome measure. Even if stroke is chosen there may be arguments about whether symptoms lasting only a few days are relevant. The ECST therefore only counted strokes lasting more than 7 days. However, this definition has not been generally accepted and almost all other trials have counted any stroke using the standard definition of symptoms or signs lasting more than 24 h. Nevertheless, a stroke from which the patient has made a full recovery is less important than a disabling stroke. Most trials therefore analyse disabling strokes separately, but the definition of disabling stroke varies from trial to trial.

It may also be important to consider the side or territory in which the stroke occurs. In trials of an antiplatelet agent this will be irrelevant, but becomes important in trials of treatment of carotid stenosis. Carotid surgery can only be expected to reduce the incidence of stroke in the territory of the operated artery, but might cause stroke in any territory at the time of operation. It has therefore been usual in the carotid surgery trials to analyse stroke in any territory when considering operative risks but to analyse ipsilateral carotid territory stroke separately during follow-up. Analysing ipsilateral stroke rates will tell us about the efficacy of carotid surgery, but when assessing the utility or benefit to the patient, it is important to assess the overall stroke rate, since it does not matter much to the patient whether their stroke occurs on the ipsilateral or contralateral side. For example, in the Asymptomatic Carotid Atherosclerosis Study (ACAS) [27], carotid surgery reduced the relative risk of ipsilateral stroke over 10 years by 51%, which was statistically significant, but had no effect on contralateral stroke, which was about as likely to occur as ipsilateral stroke in medically treated patients. The benefit of surgery on overall stroke was therefore a reduction of 26%, which did not reach significance.

Death must always be an important outcome, especially in prevention trials. All deaths are important, not just deaths due to stroke, because the cause of death is irrelevant to the patient. Deaths need to be analysed together with stroke as an outcome because otherwise an individual patient might not have survived long enough to have a stroke or other primary outcome event. Furthermore, there is little point in reducing the risk of stroke if the patient is going to die anyway. There is a very strong association between stroke and ischaemic heart disease and a patient with a TIA, for example, has the same chance of dying from myocardial infarction as of suffering a stroke over the next 5 years [28]. Death from myocardial infarction has a far more important influence on outcome than stroke. For example, in the VAAT, although the incidence of TIA and stroke was halved by carotid surgery (from 9.4% to 4.7%), this was of little importance to the subjects in the trial because 33% had died (mainly from myocardial infarction) by the end of 5 years follow-up. The relevant combined end-point of stroke or death was therefore only reduced from 44.2% to 41.2%, which was not significant [25].

Most of the drugs used to prevent stroke, such as antiplatelet agents, are expected to prevent other vascular events, such as myocardial infarction, as well as stroke. It has therefore become customary to use the combined cluster of stroke, myocardial infarction or vascular death as the primary end-point for statistical analysis [20,29]. This has the advantage that a smaller sample size is needed, as there will be more combined outcome events than there will be strokes or myocardial infarcts alone. However, this will mean that any benefit is unlikely to reach statistical significance in any subgroup analysis of stroke alone. This type of analysis assumes that the drug, e.g. antiplatelet agent, has a similar benefit in each type of vascular disease. There is some evidence that this is the case for aspirin from the Antiplatelet Trialists Collaboration [20] but it may be not true for other agents. For example, in CAPRIE [29], subgroup analysis suggested that clopidogrel might be better at preventing vascular events in patients with peripheral vascular disease and stroke than in patients with recent myocardial infarction. However, because the trial was only powered to show a difference in the combined outcome cluster in the combined groups of subjects with all three types of vascular disease, any subgroup analysis must be treated with great caution and no firm conclusion can be drawn. This highlights the need to choose a clinically relevant end-point for the conduct and interpretation of clinical trials in stroke.

Choice of Outcome Variables in Acute Stroke Trials

Unlike trials of stroke prevention, where it is relatively easy to choose outcomes such as non-disabling, disabling or fatal stroke, trials of acute stroke treatment face much greater difficulty when choosing an appropriate outcome relevant to the patient. The only outcome which is undisputed is death, but even here it is not certain that death is a worse outcome than very severe disability. There are a great many shades of recovery from stroke: from complete recovery with no residual symptoms or signs to a requirement for complete nursing care. It is not easy to decide whether the treatment saves lives and improves the quality of life in the survivors or whether patients who would have succumbed to their stroke are now surviving very disabled.

One problem of choosing death as a primary outcome is that risk of early death in unselected groups of patients with acute ischaemic stroke is low. The Oxford Community Stroke Project showed a mortality of 10% after 30 days and the TRUST study showed a 12% mortality after 3 weeks in untreated controls [28,30]. If a treatment reduced mortality from 10% to 8%, this decline would save 20 deaths per 1000 patients treated, which would be worthwhile. To demonstrate such a small benefit from treatment, a large number of patients would have to be studied. It is only recently that a trial (the IST) of sufficient size to show such benefits has been organised [16]. To achieve such numbers without major sponsorship from a pharmaceutical company it was essential to use simple, widely available treatments such as aspirin and heparin and to make entry and follow-up in the trial extremely simple. These principles allowed the IST to randomise almost 20 000 patients. However, such simple trials sacrifice collection of detailed information which may be essential to assessing the value or risks of a new drug. For example, CT scanning was not mandatory in the IST. In the case of most treatments, more complicated assessment and access to emergency CT scanning facilities are required. Such trials can only recruit relatively small numbers of patients and if the true benefit is small the results of the trials will not reach significance. A recent review of all medical treatments of acute stroke concluded that almost all trials were not large enough to exclude a definite benefit of the treatment [31]. The only trials large enough to stand a good chance of showing any benefit were those of haemodilution, but interestingly they demonstrated no benefit from what had hitherto been a widely used treatment [15]. This conclusion reinforces the need for clinical trials to be large enough and for them to be carried out before any hopeful treatment become widely practised.

Fundamental to the design of the trial is the choice of the primary and secondary outcome measures. These are clearly dictated by the primary question. Often the desired outcome is obvious, but trying to define an accurate and clinically relevant outcome measure is far more difficult. For example, one might want to know whether patients do better if given thrombolysis soon after having a stroke. The problem lies in deciding how to define "do better". Although death is an obvious outcome measure, in stroke care one is often more concerned about the quality of, rather than just the fact of, survival. This has led to the use of various rating scales to provide soft outcome measures in the evaluation and description of the degree of residual handicap following a stroke. The spectrum of these scales in predictably wide. Some (e.g. the National Institute of Health Stroke Scale, NIHSS) [32] concentrate mainly on the neurological outcome, such as the return of power to a limb, but they then do not address the question of whether the improvement is useful (Table 19.1). Some, such as the Barthel Index [33], use a brief account of the activities of daily living to assess how useful the return of function has been, but often there is an overemphasis on limb function, ignoring the problems of communication or other cognitive impairments (Table 19.2). Such scales tend to be useful for following an individual patient and so have clinical utility, but patients with the same score might have very different clinical deficits or infarct sizes, so such scales have little scientific utility. Others, such as the Rankin Scale [34], rely on the patient, family or doctor to decide on the degree of handicap (whether mild, moderate or severe) that the patient is suffering without defining exactly how these categories should be distinguished (Table 19.3).

On the principle that simple is best, the IST outcome score has much merit [16]. Patients were telephoned at home and asked whether they had made a full recovery after their stroke or whether they were dependent on others. The problem with such a scale is that it is not very sensitive. The patient may be dependent on others for reasons other than the stroke. A minor degree of dependence is very different from major dependence. Thus significant effects of treatment may be missed by the simple scales, but the data can be collected quickly by

Table 19.1. National Institutes of Health Stroke Scale[32]

Item	Name	Response
1A	Level of consciousness	0 = Alert
		1 = Not alert, obtunded
		2 = Unresponsive
1B	Questions	0 = Answers both correctly
		1 = Answers one correctly
		2 = Answers neither correctly
1C	Commands	0 = Performs both tasks correctly
		1 = Performs one task correctly
		2 = Performs neither task
2	Gaze	0 = Normal
		1 = Partial gaze palsy
		2 = Total gaze palsy
3	Visual fields	0 = No visual loss
		1 = Partial hemianopia
		2 = Complete hemianopia
		3 = Bilateral hemianopia
4	Facial palsy	0 = Normal
		1 = Minor paralysis
		2 = Complete paralysis
5	Motor arm	0 = No drift
	a. Left	1 = Drift before 10 seconds
	b. Right	2 = Falls before 10 seconds
		3 = No effort against gravity
		4 = No movement
6	Motor leg	0 = No drift
	a. Left	1 = Drift before 5 seconds
	b. Right	2 = Falls before 5 seconds
		3 = No effort against gravity
		4 = No movement
7	Ataxia	0 = Absent
		1 = One limb
		2 = Two limbs
8	Sensory	0 = Normal
		1 = Mild loss
		2 = Severe loss
9	Language	0 = Normal
		1 = Mild aphasia
		2 = Severe aphasia
		3 = Mute or global aphasia
10	Dysarthria	0 = Normal
		1 = Mild
		2 = Severe
11	Extinction/inattention	0 = Normal
		1 = Mild
		2 = Severe

Table 19.2. Barthel Index[33]

Item	Score	Categories
Bowels	0	Incontinent or needs enemas
	1	Occasional incontinence (less than once a week)
	2	Continent
Bladder	0	Incontinent/unable to manage catheter
	1	Occasional accident (less than once a day)
	2	Continent
Grooming	0	Needs help with shaving, washing, hair or teeth
	1	Independent
Toilet use	0	Dependent
	1	Needs some help
	2	Independent on, off, dressing and cleaning
Feeding	0	Dependent
	1	Needs some help (e.g. with cutting, spreading)
	2	Independent if food provided within reach
Transfer	0	Unable and no sitting balance
(e.g. bed	1	Needs major help
to chair)	2	Needs minor help
	3	Independent
Mobility	0	Unable
	1	Wheelchair independent indoors
	2	Walks with help or supervision
	3	Independent (but may use aid)
Dressing	0	Dependent
	1	Needs some help
	2	Independent including fasteners
Stairs	0	Unable
	1	Needs some help or supervision
	2	Independent up or down
Bathing	0	Dependent
	1	Independent in bath or shower
Total	20	

Table 19.3. Modified Rankin Scale[34]

Grade	Description
0	No symptoms
1	Minor symptoms which do not interfere with lifestyle
2	Minor handicap. Symptoms which lead to some restriction in lifestyle but do not interfere with the patient's ability to look after themselves
3	Moderate handicap. Symptoms which significantly restrict lifestyle and prevent totally independent existence
4	Moderately severe handicap. Symptoms which clearly prevent independent existence although not needing constant care and attention
5	Severe handicap. Totally dependent, requiring constant attention day and night

relatively untrained observers, which may be essential in very large unsponsored trials. There is also likely to be greater inter- and intra-observer reliability. Blinding the observer, recording the outcome after treatment, can be a problem in stroke trials, particularly if a surgical procedure is involved; scales such as the IST which can be completed by telephone interview are much easier to blind. In conclusion, in a large multicentre trial with many different clinicians assessing patients, it is probably better to have a very simple scale and sacrifice some sensitivity.

Duration of Follow-up

In acute stroke trials there has been no accepted time period at which to conduct the outcome assessment. For example, in IST analyses were carried out at 14 days (or earlier discharge) and 6 months, in CAST at 1 month or earlier discharge only, in the National Institute of Neurological Diseases and Stroke (NINDS) tissue plasminogen activator (tPA) trial at 3 months [12], and in FISS at 3 and 6 months [14]. These variations may lead to difficulties in interpreting the results. For example in FISS there was no benefit of fraxiparine evident at 3 months but a significant benefit was seen at 6 months, which is difficult to explain. However, the disability from stroke does continue to improve in most patients for a year or more and even 6 months might be too early to assess eventual outcome. Moreover, a drug that shows a benefit at an early stage might simply be speeding up recovery (e.g. reducing oedema) but have no worthwhile long-term benefit, particularly if it saved lives but did not reduce final disability. Trials with long-term follow-up for at least 6 months are therefore to be preferred.

In stroke prevention trials the follow-up period is determined by the expected outcome event rate,

which usually requires a minimum of 2 years follow-up. Some trials, e.g. ACAS [27], have required as long as 5 years to reach significant differences between the two groups, while the ECST continued follow-up for 15 years before concluding that there was no worthwhile benefit of operating on moderate carotid stenosis. By convention, operative complications are usually assessed at 1 month after surgery. Any strokes or death occurring within 30 days are counted against surgery on the basis that some events caused by surgery (such as pulmonary embolism, cerebral haemorrhage caused by hyperperfusion or death from infection) may not occur for some weeks after the operation.

Stopping Rules

Another important question is at what stage a trial should be terminated for ethical reasons. This requires that the treatment tested is either significantly beneficial or significantly harmful. For example, the arm of the North American Symptomatic Carotid Endarterectomy Trial (NASCET) [4] recruiting patients with greater than 70% stenosis was terminated early by the Data Monitoring Committee when they found that symptomatic patients denied a carotid endarterectomy had a substantial risk of suffering a stroke. Predefined stopping rules, which required the statistical difference between the two arms to be substantial, were applied and it was therefore unethical to allow these patients to remain untreated. This action was supported by the publication of the ECST results for the same group of patients [3]. As soon as the NASCET and ECST results were known, the Veterans Affairs Symptomatic Trial [35], a similar study, was terminated early before any significant result was reached, demonstrating the extent to which the ECST and NASCET findings were rapidly accepted by the research community. This rapid acceptance highlights the perceived value of large, well-conducted, multicentre trials run by well-respected principal investigators. The fact that the trials were not stopped until a substantial, highly significant difference was reached between the two treatments, and the fact that there were two trials, both contributed to the rapid acceptance of the results.

Interpretation of the Results

One particular problem which has yet to be fully addressed is how to interpret the results of a trial in which treatment may have an immediate hazard but then a large long-term benefit. For example, the European Co-operative Acute Stroke Study (ECASS), a randomised, multicentre, double-blind, placebo-controlled trial comparing the outcome at 3 months in patients treated within 6h of the onset of stroke with tPA or placebo showed a considerable excess of intracranial haemorrhage caused by tPA, but in those who survived treatment there was a better long-term outcome [36]. Overall, there was no benefit on an intention-to-treat analysis but if those patients with a visible infarct on CT who had a much greater hazard of intracranial haemorrhage were removed from the analysis, tPA appeared to be effective. Research is needed on patient preferences to see how much initial hazard of death they would accept to stand a better chance of less disability if they survived.

In stroke prevention trials, it is usual to express benefit in terms of an odds ratio or reduction in relative risk. Calculation of these two statistics usually results in very similar values in stroke prevention trials since the incidence of outcome events is low. In interpreting the clinical utility of the treatment studied, it is very important to convert this as far as possible into measures of absolute benefit. For example, an impressive-sounding 50% reduction in the relative risk of ipsilateral stroke resulting from carotid surgery in ACAS was actually only a reduction in absolute risk of about 1% per annum, meaning that nearly 100 patients had to be operated on to prevent one stroke per year. To give another example, in CAPRIE, the relative benefit of clopidogrel over aspirin was an 8% reduction in vascular events. However, in absolute terms this translates to a saving of 5 vascular events per 1000 patients treated with clopidogrel rather than aspirin.

The final decision as to whether to choose a particular treatment according to the results of a clinical stroke trial will often depend on a cost-benefit analysis. To date very few such economic analyses have been done. In general, stroke is a very expensive disorder consuming approximately 5% of National Health Service expenditure in the UK. In one study in America, the average cost of a stroke patient admitted to hospital was $90981 [37]. There is an urgent need for more accurate health economic data to allow the cost-benefit ratios of different treatment for stroke to be assessed.

Description of the Major Stroke Trials

Prevention of Stroke: Symptomatic Carotid Stenosis (Table 19.4)

Carotid artery disease accounts for about 10% of stroke, but only recently has there been evidence that carotid endarterectomy is beneficial in preventing stroke. This has been established by two major trials: the European Carotid Surgery Trial (ECST) and the North American Symptomatic Carotid Endarterectomy Trial (NASCET) [3,4]. It should be noted that both trials examined the policy of adding surgery to 'best medical treatment'. The latter was not defined, but most cases were treated with aspirin. Very few patients were anticoagulated and it is impossible to know if the results would have been different if anticoagulation had been stipulated as best medical treatment. The ECST began in 1981 and was completed in 1996. An interim analysis was published in l991. Three thousand and twenty-six patients were randomised in the ECST; the interim analysis was based on 2518 patients. Following a clinical alert based on the NASCET results, the ECST published the results in patients who had either mild (0–29%) or severe (70–99%) carotid artery stenosis. Of those patients who had severe carotid artery stenosis and were assigned to surgery, 7.5% had a stroke or died within 30 days of surgery. Over the following 3 years this group's risk of an ipsilateral ischaemic stroke was an extra 2.8%, making a total risk of stroke follow-ing surgery of 10.3%. The risk for patients treated medically was 16.8%. The Kaplan–Meier curve of survival without stroke showed that the main excess of disabling or fatal ipsilateral ischaemic strokes occurred within the first year. In contrast, patients with a mild stenosis treated medically only had a 1.3% risk of an ipsilateral ischaemic stroke lasting more than 7 days over the 3 year follow-up period compared with 16.8% for those who had severe stenosis. The equivalent figures for the surgical groups were 3.3% and 2.8% respectively. There was no significant difference apparent in patients with a moderate stenosis.

The risks of surgery in the mild and severe stenosis groups were similar to each other. The preoperative rate of stroke or death was 4.6%, and of disabling stroke or death was 2.6% in the mild stenosis group compared with 3.7% and 7.5% respectively in the severe stenosis group. Thus one can conclude that surgery is beneficial in recently symptomatic patients with more than 70% stenosis but harmful in those with lesser degrees of stenosis.

NASCET began in 1988 and randomised patients with 30–99% carotid artery stenosis and recent symptoms (within 120 days) to receive either best medical therapy (modification of risk factors and 300 mg aspirin per day) or best medical therapy and endarterectomy [4]. The interim results were published in 1991 after the Safety and Monitoring Committee had invoked the stopping rule and ended recruitment of patients with greater than 70–99% stenosis. This group contained 659 patients. The

Table 19.4. Results of the major symptomatic and asymptomatic trials of surgery for carotid stenosis (values are percentages unless otherwise stated)

Trial	No. of patients entered	Length of actuarial follow-up (years)	Rate of stroke or death		Perioperative stroke and death rate at 1 month	Disabling and fatal stroke rate	
			Medical group	Surgical group		Medical group	Surgical group
Symptomatic trials							
NASCET[4] – severe stenosis > 82%[a]	659	2	32.3	15.8***	5.8	13.1	3.7***
ECST[3] – severe stenosis > 70%	778	3	21.9	12.3**	7.5	11.0	6.0*
ECST – moderate stenosis 50–69%	942	8	19.1	24.0	7.9	NA	NA
ECST – moderate stenosis 30–49%	648	8	16.1	20.4	8.0	NA	NA
ECST – mild stenosis < 30%	374	3	6.2	11.8	4.6	1.2	5.6
Asymptomatic trials							
VAAT[25] – 70–99% stenosis[a]	444	4	44.2	41.2	5.7	NA	NA
ACAS[27] – 60–99% stenosis[b]	1662	5	31.9	25.6	2.3	25.5	20.7

The stroke rates are those determined over the full length of the trials, which differ in each trial. Only stroke lasting more than 7 days and surgical death are included in the figures from ECST.
NA, not recorded in report.
[a] Angiographic measurements of stenosis adjusted to be equivalent to the CC and ECST methods.
[b] Measured using the ultrasound criteria specified in ACAS.[27]
* $p < 0.05$, ** $p < 0.01$, *** $p < 0.001$ respectively for comparison of the surgical group with the medical group. Any other difference in event rates did not reach statistical significance.

cumulative risk of any ipsilateral stroke at 2 years was 26% in the medical group compared with 9% in the surgical group, an absolute risk reduction of 17% and a 65% relative risk reduction in favour of surgery. For major or fatal ipsilateral stroke the risks were 13.1% and 2.5% respectively.

The combined perioperative stroke and death rate in the surgical group (defined as being from the day of randomisation to 30 days after surgery) was 5.5% compared with 3.3% in the medical group during the same time period. This gives an excess surgical event rate of 2.2%. Kaplan–Meier curves of survival and any stroke showed that the initial disadvantage to surgical patients was rapidly overcome by 3 months after randomisation and, as the curves did not converge after surgery, the benefit of surgery was long lived.

A secondary analysis of the deciles of carotid artery stenosis (70–79%, 80–89%, 90–99%) showed that an increase in stenosis correlated with an increased risk reduction after surgery [38]. The overall risk reduction for all ipsilateral stroke at 2 years in patients with a 70–79% stenosis was 12%, in those with 80–89% stenosis it was 18% and in those with 90–99% stenosis it was 26%. NASCET also

looked at how risk factors affected the risk of stroke in the medically treated group. Thirty-nine per cent of patients with more than six risk factors experienced an ipsilateral stroke within 2 years compared with 7% of patients with fewer than six risk factors. Those with six risk factors exactly had an intermediate risk of 23%. NASCET did not include patients with mild stenosis. The final published results of ECST [39] and NASCET [40] confirmed that clinically significant benefit was only confirmed by surgery in patients with severe stenosis.

The ECST and NASCET also provided evidence that severe carotid stenosis was the likely cause of an ipsilateral stroke, rather than it being an epiphenomenon of widespread atherosclerosis. Ninety-five per cent of first strokes in the medical group in NASCET were ipsilateral to the tight stenosis, whereas in ECST 76% of strokes occurred in the ipsilateral carotid territory of patients with severe stenosis. However, in patients with mild stenosis only 22% of the strokes occurred ipsilaterally.

The Veterans Affairs (VA) Symptomatic Trial ran at the same time and also examined the efficacy of carotid artery surgery in symptomatic carotid artery stenosis [35]. It was terminated early once the results of NASCET and the ECST were known. It sought to compare men with at least 50% carotid artery stenosis who had suffered cerebral or retinal ischaemia within the previous 120 days (like NASCET). They were randomised to receive either best medical treatment or carotid endarterectomy. At the time of trial termination, 197 men had been randomised and the results were similar to NASCET and the ECST. Only 7.7% of the surgical group suffered TIAs or stroke compared with 19.4% of the medically treated group. The benefit was more pronounced (7.9% vs 25.6%) in patients with carotid artery stenosis greater than 70%. There were fewer individuals in the range of 50–69%; 1% of surgical patients suffered a stroke or TIA compared with 6.7% of medically treated patients; this was not significant. The perioperative stroke mortality/morbidity was 5.5%, similar to that of NASCET and the ECST.

NASCET and the ECST are probably the most influential trials in cerebrovascular disease of the last decade. Quality of data and uniformity of the results are quite striking in spite of minor methodological differences (e.g. method of measuring stenosis: see below). They provide the benchmark with which further surgical trials will be compared. The importance of patients receiving their treatment as soon after randomisation as possible is highlighted by the presence of so many strokes occurring between randomisation and the day of surgery. The choice of end-points is also critical. For example, are we interested in any stroke or TIA, or in events that are disabling or fatal? Even large well organised trials do not answer more than one or two questions clearly. For example, the relative benefits of anticoagulation or aspirin as best medical treatment for carotid stenosis remains uncentain.

It is laudable that once the benefit of surgery was known, this was communicated to participating and other physicians promptly. Up to this point, it was necessary to maintain data confidentiality in order not to affect referral to the trial. Recruitment for the trial was based on the uncertainty principle and information leaking about the results might have affected the referring physicians' referral policy.

The ECST and NASCET used different methods to measure the degree of stenosis. The ECST used the diameter of the carotid artery at the point of maximum visible stenosis as the numerator and the estimated original diameter of the carotid artery at the same site (usually the carotid bulb) as the denominator. NASCET compared the same numerator with the diameter of the disease-free distal portion of the carotid artery. The ECST denominator is greater than the NASCET denominator and hence produces an apparently more severe stenosis. This begs the question as to which clinical trial one should base one's practice on. Does one give medical treatment to 60% NASCET stenosis or offer surgery to the same stenosis which is now 70% by the ECST method? The most reproducible method for measuring the degree of carotid artery stenosis is the common carotid method which compares the diameter of the stenosis with the diameter of the common carotid artery below the bifurcation [41]. If the ECST and NASCET data are reanalysed using such a method, the trial results are similar. Analysis of future studies would be eased if the Common Carotid method were generally adopted (see also Chapter 18).

Prevention of Stroke: Asymptomatic Carotid Stenosis

In contrast to symptomatic stenosis, asymptomatic carotid stenosis is a more benign disease. Hennerici et al. [42] prospectively followed up 339 patients with either unilateral or bilateral asymptomatic carotid stenosis. These patients were recruited from other clinics specialising in coronary or peripheral vascular disease, or were noted to have neck bruits. They form a reasonable cohort of hospital-based patients with carotid disease and other vascular risk factors. The annual mortality was high at 7%, the majority of deaths being cardiac, but the combined annual stroke rate was 0.97%. The annual stroke mortality was low at 0.6% and the annual morbidity was 0.4%. The risk of suffering a stroke without a premonitory TIA was similarly low at 0.4%. This is an extremely important point because it suggests that carotid surgery would have to be extremely safe to warrant being undertaken prophylactically. It also demonstrates that it is normally safe to wait for the patient to become symptomatic before treating them, because a patient's first symptoms are more likely to be TIAs than a devastating stroke.

Doppler ultrasound showed that the disease progressed in 36% of patients, while 59% remained the same. Only in 5% did the disease remit. Progression occurred more frequently in symptomatic than asymptomatic patients. The mean annual rate of progression in asymptomatic patients was 12.7% compared with that in symptomatic patients of 22.5%. Of the people alive at end of the study, 87% were asymptomatic, 10% had had TIAs and 3% had had a stroke without a warning TIA.

The above study described the natural history of the disease, but several trials have now examined the policy of operating on asymptomatic carotid stenoses. The first was the romantically named CASANOVA (Carotid Artery Stenosis and Asymptomatic Narrowing: Operation Versus Aspirin) Trial

[17]. This prospective, multicentre, controlled trial randomised patients with an asymptomatic carotid stenosis of 50–90% to either surgery with best medical treatment or to best medical treatment alone. The primary outcome events were surgical death or any stroke. At the time little was known about the natural history of the disease, and as conventional practice then favoured treating all carotid artery disease, there were clear ethical difficulties in setting up the trial and these affected the quality and interpretation of the results. Patients in the surgical group received either a bilateral (11%) or a unilateral (72%) endarterectomy operation, but 17% never had their operation. In the medical group, 80% had only medical care but 20% had an endarterectomy at entry. A further 26% of the medical group went on to have an endarterectomy because of progression of the disease. Criteria for endarterectomy were development of a stenosis greater than 90% (with or without symptoms), development of bilateral 50% stenoses, symptomatic stenosis greater than 50%, and development of a stenosis greater than 50% on the contralateral side. Further problems with the study were that only 69% of patients took aspirin, mainly because of side effects from the high dose prescribed, and 76 patients who had previously had a carotid endarterectomy and later developed contralateral stenosis were retrospectively enrolled in the study. The large number of confounding variables and protocol violations made interpretation of the study difficult.

The result of the primary outcome analysis, the intended method of analysing the data when the trial was planned, showed that 10.7% of patients in the surgical group had a stroke or died compared with 11.3% in the medically treated group. This gives an odds ratio of 0.94 in favour of surgery, which is not significant and has very wide confidence limits from 0.57 to 1.98. That means that the possibility of a relative risk reduction by surgery of up to 43% cannot be excluded by this study. The CASANOVA trial therefore suggested that there was little benefit to be gained from operating on asymptomatic carotid artery stenoses but was insufficiently powerful or well controlled to be convincing. It also suffered by excluding those with a 90% stenosis – the group most likely to benefit from or be harmed by surgery.

The next trial to address this problem was the Mayo Asymptomatic Carotid Endarterectomy Study, a randomised study designed to compare the outcomes of patients with an asymptomatic stenosis treated surgically or medically [43]. Here again there were great methodological problems. Only the medical patients were given aspirin. The trial was stopped early after only 71 patients had been entered.

The reason was the high incidence (22%) of myocardial infarctions in the surgical group. Fifty per cent of the infarcts occurred before surgery, and were attributed to the withholding of aspirin. This highlights the importance of comparing the effect of surgery in addition to best medical treatment, with medical treatment alone.

A much more informative trial was the Veteran Affairs Asymptomatic Trial (VAAT) [25]. This recruited men only, randomly assigning 444 patients with greater than 50% asymptomatic carotid stenosis to either best medical treatment plus endarterectomy or best medical treatment. The primary outcome events were TIA, amaurosis fugax and stroke. Of the patients in the surgical group 12.8% suffered these events compared with 24.5% in the medical group. This was significant but included contralateral events too. If one considers ipsilateral events only, 8% occurred in the surgical group compared with 20.6% in the medical group. This difference was significant but included transient symptoms. From the previous trials mentioned, we know that when an asymptomatic stenosis becomes symptomatic, it is usually first manifested as a TIA [42]. These can then be investigated and treated by surgery, so the important question is whether there is any difference between the groups when those patients with transient symptoms are removed. The frequency of all strokes was 8.6% and of all stroke plus all deaths was 41.2% in the surgical group compared with 12.7% and 44.2% respectively in the medical group. These differences are not significant. The rate of permanent stroke and death within 30 days of randomisation was 4.7% in the surgical group compared with 1.3% in the medical group.

The trial therefore does not support taking the risk of early operation in an asymptomatic patient, but suggests that it is a better to wait until that patient becomes symptomatic. The cohort of patients studied in the VAAT was atypical in that the patients were mostly elderly men who often had significant heart disease. The mortality rate during the course of the trial was very high (33%), emphasising the importance of analysing all outcomes.

The most recent trial, ACAS [27], randomised over 1600 subjects with more than 60% stenosis determined by ultrasound. This reported a significant benefit in the combined end-point of ipsilateral stroke (or death) during follow-up and any ipsilateral stroke (or death) in the perioperative period, favouring surgery. The calculated 5 year risk of these end-points was significantly reduced by surgery from 11.0% in the medical group to 5.1% in the surgical group. The results of ACAS have not been generally accepted as supporting the general policy of surgery in asymptomatic patients and the policy varies from centre to centre. Enthusiasts use the ACAS results to justify the policy of operating on all patients known to have asymptomatic carotid stenosis and even of setting up ultrasound screening in clinics for the general population. Many neurologists do not believe that the results justify promoting carotid surgery for asymptomatic patients, for several reasons [44,45]. Firstly, ACAS did not show a significant benefit of surgery for the end-point of most interest to the patient of any stroke or death, which was only reduced from 31.9% at 5 years in the medical group to 25.6% in the surgical group. This demonstrates that the reduction of ipsilateral risk by surgery is not of much benefit to the patient because they have still have significant risk of contralateral stroke and death from myocardial infarction. Secondly, the surgeons collaborating in the trial were very highly selected and had to show a very low rate of morbidity, which was reflected in a low perioperative stroke rate, which implied above-average expertise or a case mix favouring low-risk patients. The results are therefore not generalisable to the average vascular centre. Finally, ACAS was not able to show a greater medical risk in patients with increasing severity of stenosis, which does not accord with the symptomatic trial data. On balance, taking all the asymptomatic trials into account, it is difficult to advocate a general policy of surgery for asymptomatic stenosis.

Prevention of Stroke: EC-IC Bypass

Occlusion of the internal carotid artery would normally be expected to reduce cerebral perfusion pressure. An attractive a priori hypothesis is that improving perfusion by diverting blood from the extracranial to the intracranial circulation would improve cerebral perfusion and lessen the risk of recurrent cerebral ischaemia in patients with atherosclerotic disease in the carotid or middle cerebral arteries. Extracranial to intracranial bypass surgery (EC-IC bypass) was first performed in 1967 and in the ensuing decade became widely applied. However, patients with carotid occlusion but only minor symptoms or a non-disabling infarct must have a good collateral blood supply to compensate for the loss of perfusion through one carotid artery. Bypass surgery might therefore have little to offer and in 1977 an international multi-centre randomised trial, the EC-IC bypass study, was started to test the hypothesis that the rate of subsequent stroke among patients was indeed reduced [46]. A total of 1377 patients with hemispheric stroke, retinal infarction or transient ischaemic attack and atherosclerotic narrowing of the distal internal carotid artery or middle cerebral arteries or carotid occlusion were randomised to best

medical care or best medical care plus EC-IC bypass surgery. The trial failed to show any benefit in the operation. In fact, the average effect of surgery over the entire trial showed a 14% increase in the relative risk of fatal and non-fatal strokes. The bulk of this risk occurred soon after surgery. Defining the perioperative period as the time from randomisation to 30 days after the actual operation, 12.2% of surgical patients had cerebral or retinal ischaemic events and 4.5% had major strokes. In a comparable time period, 3.4% of the medically treated patients had some sort of cerebral or retinal ischaemic event and 1.3% had major strokes, i.e. there was an excess of 3.2% fatal or non-fatal strokes in the surgical group. This trial highlighted the fact that a randomised control trial may demonstrate that a treatment which was expected to have been beneficial is actually harmful. It also highlights the need for all new treatments to be assessed by a randomised trial before they gain wide clinical acceptance. Publication of the results of the trial led to a rapid decline in EC-IC bypass operations, which are now rarely performed.

Prevention of Stroke: Atrial Fibrillation

Atrial fibrillation is an important risk factor for stroke, being present in about 15% of all stroke patients. Non-rheumatic valvular atrial fibrillation without a previous history of embolism is associated with a risk of stroke of 4% per year [47] but only recently have there been good trial data regarding the benefits of anticoagulation. The results of six major primary prevention clinical trials – the Copenhagen Atrial Fibrillation Aspirin and Anticoagulation (AFASAK) Study [5], the Boston Area Anticoagulation Trial for Atrial Fibrillation (BAATAF) [48], the Veterans Affairs Stroke Prevention in Atrial Fibrillation Study (SPINAF) [49], Stroke Prevention in Atrial Fibrillation Study (SPAF 1) [47], Stroke Prevention in Atrial Fibrillation Study (SPAF II) [7] and Canadian Atrial Fibrillation Anticoagulation Study (CAFA) [50] – have clearly shown a reduction in the incidence of stroke with antithrombotic therapy, with a relative risk reduction of about two-thirds [51].

The first trial published was the Copenhagen Atrial Fibrillation Aspirin and Anticoagulation Study (AFASAK), which randomised patients to receive warfarin, 75 mg of aspirin daily or placebo [5]. Warfarin was given open labelled. Primary end-points were thromboembolic events or major haemorrhage. There was a reduction from 5.5% to 1.6% of reaching the primary end-point on warfarin. There was no significant reduction with aspirin.

Blinding is a very important principle in treatment trials. However, in AFASAK, warfarin administration

Table 19.5. Atrial fibrillation trials

	No. in trial	Mean age (years)	Effect of warfarin			Effect of aspirin	
			Stroke rate in controls (% per annum)	Stroke rate on warfarin (% per annum)	Major haemorrhage rate on warfarin (% per annum)	Stroke rate on placebo (% per annum)	Stroke rate on aspirin (% per annum)
Primary prevention trials							
AFASAK[5]	1007	74	4.6	1.9	0.8	4.6	3.9
SPAF[7]	1330	67	7.0	2.3	1.5	5.8	3.2
BAATAF[9]	420	68	3.0	0.4	1.8		
CAFA[48]	378	68	4.3	3.0	2.5		
SPINAF[8]	525	67	4.3	0.9***	1.5		
Overall analysis	3660	69	4.4	1.4***	1.6	5.3	3.4*
Risk reduction (%)				68***			36*
Secondary prevention trial							
EAFT[52]	1007	73	12.3	3.9***	2.8	12.6	10.5[NS]
Risk reduction (%)				68			16[NS]

NS, not significant.

*$p < 0.05$, **$p < 0.001$, ***$p < 0.001$ compared with placebo.

was unblind. The need for warfarin therapy to be monitored by regular blood tests would inevitably lead to unblinding unless a complex system of issuing dummy results for control patients was instituted. Knowing that a patient was being treated with warfarin from the start could introduce bias so the threshold for drug withdrawal might be lowered. Thus in AFASAK, 38% of patients in the warfarin group stopped treatment compared with 13% and 15% in the aspirin and placebo groups respectively. In contrast, in CAFA (Canadian Atrial Fibrillation Anticoagulation Study), a double-blind trial, only 26% of warfarin-treated patients permanently discontinued treatment compared with 23% of controls [50]. The high rate of drop-out from treatment in these drug trials is important when stroke trials are analysed by intention-to-treat, because it means that the efficacy of warfarin may be much higher than initially appears.

The Boston Area Anticoagulation Trial for Atrial Fibrillation (BAATAF) was an unblind study in which 420 patients were randomised to low-dose warfarin (prothrombin time prolonged to 1.2–1.5 normal) or placebo [48]. The control group could choose to take aspirin, which confused interpretation of the results. The trial was stopped early because of the favourable results in the warfarin-treated group. The incidence of stroke in the warfarin group was 0.4% per year compared with 3% in the controls, an 86% risk reduction. The death rate in the two groups was 2.3% and 6% respectively. There was one fatal haemorrhage in each group.

The Veterans Affairs Stroke Prevention in Atrial Fibrillation Study (SPINAF) was a randomised, double-blind, placebo-controlled men-only trial of low-dose warfarin (prothrombin time prolonged to 1.2–1.5 normal) [49]. Two samples of patients were studied: 525 who had never previously had a stroke, and 46 who had. Therefore the trial combined primary and secondary prevention. The incidence of stroke in warfarin-treated patients was 0.9% per year compared with 4.3% per year in the placebo group, a relative risk reduction of 79% and sufficient to result in the trial being stopped early. The rate of haemorrhage in the warfarin group was 1.3% per year and 0.9% per year in the placebo group. The secondary prevention arm of the trial showed a reduction in the rate of recurrent infarction from 9.3% to 6.1%.

The Stroke Prevention in Atrial Fibrillation Study (SPAF I) was stopped early having randomised 1330 patients to receive 325 mg aspirin (double-blind) or warfarin (prothrombin time prolonged to 1.3–1.8 normal) or placebo [47]. The trial looked at primary end-points of stroke or systemic embolism. Warfarin reduced the incidence of primary endpoints from 7.4% to 2.3%, a 67% relative risk reduction. Aspirin reduced the incidence of primary events from 6.3% to 3.6%, a 42% relative risk reduction. There were too few events in the warfarin-eligible group to be able to differentiate the effects of aspirin from warfarin directly. The risk of significant bleeding was 1.5%, 1.4% and 1.6% per year in patients assigned to warfarin, aspirin and placebo respectively.

The Canadian Atrial Fibrillation Anticoagulation Study (CAFA) randomised 378 patients between double-blind warfarin and placebo [50]. The target INR was 2–3. Primary outcome events were systemic thromboembolism and haemorrhage. The trial addressed the problem of patients discontinuing medication by using an analysis of efficacy for primary outcome events that occurred within 28 days of treatment discontinuation, and excluding those that occurred beyond then. The rate of occurrence of primary outcome events was 3.5% per year in the warfarin-treated group compared with 5.2% in the placebo group. The results agree with those in the other warfarin trials but did not reach statistical significance because the trial was stopped early when the results of AFASAK and SPAF were published.

The preceding trials compared aspirin or warfarin with placebo in patients with non-rheumatic valvular atrial fibrillation, but none had compared aspirin directly with warfarin. The Stroke Prevention in Atrial Fibrillation Study II (SPAF II) was the first trial to make this important comparison, and also examined the benefit of anticoagulation in different age groups [7]. In two parallel trials, patients above and below the age of 75 years were randomised to receive warfarin (target prothrombin time 1.3–1.8 times normal) or 325 mg aspirin daily. In younger patients, the primary event rate was 1.3% on warfarin and 1.9% on aspirin. Haemorrhage rates were 1.7% and 0.9% respectively. In older patients, the primary event rate was 3.6% on warfarin and 4.8% on aspirin. Haemorrhage rates were 4.2% and 1.6% respectively. The trial showed that warfarin was superior to aspirin in either age group, but that in the older age group much of the beneficial effect was negated by the increased incidence of haemorrhage.

Taken together, the trials show a very large relative risk reduction for patients below the age of 75 years with non-rheumatic valvular atrial fibrillation taking warfarin, and it is undoubtedly important to anticoagulate patients at risk. The risks of anticoagulation were less than expected. Despite moderate levels of anticoagulation, major haemorrhage requiring hospital admission or blood transfusion occurred in 1.6% per year of patients on warfarin compared with 1.0% per year on placebo. This implies that haemorrhage would need to be 6 times worse than thromboembolism to justify withholding warfarin [50]. However results must be tempered by clinical realism. The actual event rates were quite low. SPAF II suggested that the event rate in patients with lone atrial fibrillation without hypertension, heart failure or previous thromboembolic events was 0.5% per year on aspirin. This implies that, in young patients at least, atrial fibrillation without other attendant risk factors is not a sufficient reason to start anticoagulation.

Perhaps one of the surprising lessons from these primary atrial fibrillation trials is the relative lack of benefit of aspirin. There was no significant benefit of 75 mg aspirin in the AFASAK study. The SPAF I trial also used a randomised, blinded comparison of 325 mg of aspirin against placebo and demonstrated a 42% relative risk reduction. SPAF II, which compared the same dose of aspirin with warfarin, showed there was about a 30% benefit of warfarin over aspirin.

The fact that five or six separate trials of warfarin for atrial fibrillation were required before the benefits of warfarin over aspirin were accepted, demonstrates how difficult it is to overcome pre-existing prejudices about the value of particular treatments in stroke medicine. There was undoubtedly a widely held view that warfarin was dangerous and aspirin very effective, which led to the results of the earlier trials being doubted or ignored. There is also the problem that the results of trials, however good the treatment, may be ignored if the new treatment requires considerable extra work for the doctor and perceived inconvenience for the patient, such as the requirement for regular monitoring of warfarin therapy. The messages of primary prevention also need to be taught to family practitioners and, because warfarin is not a major source of income for drug companies, this relies on haphazard educational opportunities rather than wholesale promotion. Even in hospitals, the uptake of warfarin treatment for patients with known atrial fibrillation has been extremely low [53].

The results of the primary prevention trials of anticoagulating patients with atrial fibrillation were not necessarily generalisable to secondary prevention, i.e. to those patients presenting after the onset of symptoms of cerebrovascular disease. It was argued that the common association of atrial fibrillation with stroke might be coincidence because the patients often have possible causes of stroke, such as hypertension, which would not necessarily benefit from anticoagulation. The European Atrial Fibrillation Trial addressed this problem [54]. In this study 1007 patients with a recent TIA or minor ischaemic stroke were randomised to open anticoagulation or double-blind treatment with aspirin (300 mg) or placebo. Patients with a contraindication to anticoagulation were randomised between aspirin and placebo. The primary end-points were stroke, vascular death or systemic embolism. The annual rate of outcome events in patients assigned to anticoagulants was 8% compared with 17% in the placebo group. The risk of stroke alone was reduced from 12% to 4%, which was highly significant. The annual incidence of outcome events on aspirin was 15% compared with 19% in the placebo group, which was not statistically significant. The relative reduction in embolism rate at about 60% was almost identical to the primary prevention effect of warfarin, but since the event rate was so much higher the absolute benefit was even greater. Again, aspirin proved much less effective for secondary prevention in patients with atrial fibrillation than expected.

The problem of translating the results of clinical trials to everyday clinical practice is well illustrated by the atrial fibrillation trials. The results of clinical trials apply only to the type of patients included in the trials. In the case of the atrial fibrillation trials, because of the requirement for frequent follow-up, the majority of patients included in the trials were under 75 years of age and most were otherwise fit and well. In clinical practice, most patients with atrial fibrillation are over 75 years old and many have other medical problems or reduced mobility. There has been considerable concern that the control of the level of anticoagulation was better in the clinical trials than is achieved in routine practice and it is noteworthy that any significant increase in the incidence of cerebral haemorrhage over about 3% per annum will quickly negate any benefit [52]. The conclusion is that patients need to be carefully selected for anticoagulation and their treatment carefully monitored. These considerations emphasise the important principle that clinical trials should include as wide a range of patients with the potential to benefit from treatment as possible and should mimic real life as closely as possible. Hence, the intention-to-treat analysis should be paid attention but there are also lessons to be learnt for clinical practice from an efficacy analysis. For example, in AFASAK there were 5 strokes on warfarin, of which 4 were ischaemic. One occurred on the day of randomisation, two after treatment had been discontinued and only one in an "adequately" anticoagulated patient. If one could ensure precise anticoagulation, then the benefit of warfarin would be even more marked. However, it is important to know how efficacious and acceptable a treatment is likely to be in daily practice. The strength of the trials is that they show such a significant benefit in spite of the fluctuations in the level of warfarinisation.

Prevention of Stroke: Aspirin

Aspirin is accepted as an effective agent in the prevention of stroke, but the evidence of its benefit in this context is less impressive than many imagine. The UK-TIA Aspirin Trial [55], the largest trial of aspirin after TIAs in which 2435 patients were randomised between aspirin (600 mg twice daily),

aspirin (300 mg once daily) and placebo, failed to show a statistically significant effect of aspirin in preventing stroke, although there was a significant reduction in the combined end-point of major stroke, myocardial infarction or vascular death. There was an non-significant reduction in stroke risk of 15%, but even with this large number of patients the trial was not powerful enough to show that the reduction was significant. Confirmation of aspirin's benefit has therefore relied on the meta-analysis of all the aspirin trials together, which was performed by the Antiplatelet Trialist's Collaboration [20]. This produced an overview of 145 randomised trials of antiplatelet agents including 70 000 patients and confirmed the utility of aspirin in reducing vascular events in patients with a variety of vascular diseases. The vascular events were defined as the cluster of myocardial infarction, stroke and vascular death. The Collaboration analysed four subgroups of patients: those with cerebrovascular disease who had suffered a previous stroke or TIA, those who had had a previous myocardial infarct, those who had suffered an acute myocardial infarction, and those who were at high risk of suffering adverse vascular events (e.g. those with peripheral vascular disease or angina). The data pertinent to patients with cerebrovascular disease was taken from 18 trials studying the use of an antiplatelet agent for secondary prevention. A highly significant 22% relative risk reduction of suffering a myocardial infarction, stroke or vascular death was demonstrated in these patients. Similarly, the risk of suffering a non-fatal stroke was reduced by 23% in this group of patients, and again this was highly significant when the trials were combined. The risk reduction of vascular death or death from any cause was 14% and 16% respectively, but neither was significant. The benefit of antiplatelet treatment in the cerebrovascular disease group appeared to be less than in the other subgroups.

The overview confirms the definite benefit of aspirin in symptomatic patients, but interestingly the group of patients that benefit least are those who have cerebrovascular disease. Although vascular diseases are atherosclerotic in nature, there is no doubt that the behaviour of the atherosclerotic plaque is different in the carotid, coronary and peripheral arteries, and this might be reflected by the different responses to antiplatelet therapy. Further, many strokes occur secondary to hypertensive small vessel disease or cardioembolic mechanisms, neither of which may benefit in the same way from antiplatelet therapy. With the exception of atrial fibrillation, no trials have been large enough to examine the benefit of aspirin in these subgroups of stroke.

There is clearly a need for antiplatelet agents better than aspirin, and recently the results of the CAPRIE trial, a randomised, blinded, trial of clopidogrel (75 mg once daily) and aspirin (325 mg once daily), have been published. The population studied comprised three cohorts of patients with vascular disease. The groups were those with a recent ischaemic stroke, a recent myocardial infarction or symptomatic peripheral arterial disease. Primary outcome events were any stroke, any myocardial infarction and other vascular death. When all the groups were combined, there was an overall benefit of clopidogrel compared with aspirin, with a reduction in the combined event outcome cluster of 8%, which was just conventionally significant at $p = 0.043$. The event rate reduction for the subgroup of stroke patients was from 7.71% on aspirin to 7.15% on clopidogrel, a 7.3% relative risk reduction which was not significant. However, the sample size of the stroke subgroup was not large enough for a difference of this size to be expected to reach significance and so the lack of significance does not exclude benefit. The corresponding figures for the myocardial infarction group were 4.84% and 5.03% respectively, which again was not significant. Interestingly, the group suffering from peripheral vascular disease enjoyed a highly significant reduction in the risk of further vascular events from 4.86% to 3.71%, a reduction of 23.8%. A test of heterogeneity was significant suggesting that the true benefit may not be identical across all the groups, implying that clopidogrel might be equivalent to aspirin in patients presenting with stroke or myocardial infarction, but greatly beneficial in those patients presenting with peripheral vascular disease. On the other hand, the confidence limits of the estimates of benefit of clopidogrel overlapped in all these groups, so there may be no true difference between the effectiveness of clopidogrel in the different disorders. Combining different diseases in one trial therefore led to difficulty interpreting the results, although it is clear that clopidogrel is an effective antiplatelet agent with an excellent safety profile. Future trials may need to take account of the possibility that different antiplatelet agents might have roles to play in different thromboembolic disorders.

Acute Stroke Treatment: Heparin and Aspirin

There have been exciting developments recently in the treatment of acute cerebral infarction. The similarity between the mechanisms of myocardial and brain infarction suggest that treatment that works in one might succeed in the other. In cardiology the ISIS-2 trial showed that aspirin given as soon after the onset of major symptoms as possible significantly reduced mortality from myocardial infarction [56]. Several trials have looked at the role of aspirin given acutely in stroke. One of the most important

recent trials has been the International Stroke Trial (IST) [16]. The trial employed a 2×2 factorial design. Patients were randomised to receive aspirin or no aspirin and subcutaneous heparin or no heparin. Two doses of subcutaneous heparin were used. The design allowed two conditions to be studied using a smaller group of patients than would otherwise have been necessary. It was possible to compare all the patients taking aspirin with all the patients avoiding that drug, bearing in mind that half the patients in each group were receiving heparin. This is valid, provided there is no strong effect of any one drug, and the test drugs do not interact. The greatest achievement of the trial was to succeed in recruiting almost 20 000 patients from centres around the world within 48 h of the onset of symptoms, making the IST the largest acute stroke trial in the world, and, as 2322 patients were randomised within 6 h of onset, it was the largest trial of very early stroke treatment. The trial reported that a 9 per thousand reduction in early death was offset by a 7 per thousand excess in intracranial haemorrhages in patients treated with heparin, making any overall benefit from heparin non-significant. Haemorrhage was more frequent and more serious in the patients receiving the higher dose of heparin.

An equally large trial, the Chinese Acute Stroke Trial (CAST) [13], examining the effect of aspirin in acute stroke, was published soon after the IST and included a meta-analysis of the data from both trials. Patients were recruited to CAST from within 48 h of onset of stroke and were treated with either 160 mg of aspirin daily or placebo for up to 4 weeks. The primary outcomes were death during the 4 weeks of treatment and death or dependency at discharge. CAST showed a small but significant reduction in mortality from 3.9% in the placebo group to 3.3% in the aspirin-treated group. There was no significant benefit in terms of reduction in incidence of recurrent ischaemic stroke, reduction in frequency of death or non-fatal stroke or death or dependency at discharge. However, the meta-analysis of the data together with data from the IST and MAST-I showed a small but definite benefit. There were about 9 fewer deaths or non-fatal strokes per 1000 in the first few weeks and 13 fewer dead or dependent patients per 1000 after 3 months of follow-up.

The aspirin story was more promising. The Antiplatelet Trialists' Collaboration [20] found that aspirin therapy reduced the risk of non-fatal stroke by 23% in secondary prevention of stroke. Less benefit was found in the IST but there was still an 11 per 1000 reduction in death and recurrent ischaemic stroke, offset by an increase in intracranial haemorrhage of 1 per 1000. This is a small benefit, but when one considers that 120 000 people suffer a stroke each year in the UK and the simplicity of the treatment, this amounts to a substantial saving in recurrent stroke in the UK and worldwide. Also, patients started on aspirin in hospital are probably more likely to be discharged on it. Thus the benefit is likely to be sustained. The results from the IST showed that 13 per 1000 more patients treated with aspirin were independent at 6 months compared with controls [16].

Only a trial as large as the IST could demonstrate these small benefits convincingly, but a smaller trial using a low-molecular-weight heparin, nadroparin, has produced some startling results [14]. This simple randomised, double-blind, placebo-controlled trial of two doses of nadroparin versus control showed that there were fewer poor outcomes in the groups treated with the low-molecular-weight heparin and this effect was dose dependent. There were two particularly fascinating observations from this study. The first was that the positive effects were not significant at 3 months and only became conventionally significant after 6 months. This highlights the importance of the outcome measures chosen and the timing of assessment. The second was that most of the benefit appeared to be in those patients who had suffered a lacunar infarct. The most likely explanation for findings such as these, which are difficult to explain, is that they are the result of chance. The results emphasise the importance of stratifying patients in terms of infarct subtype. A further trial of nadroparin was therefore carried out with larger numbers of patients. This second trial of nadroparin failed to confirm the initial trial, but has never been published in full, illustrating the potential dangers of basing treatment decisions on a single small trial.

Acute Stroke Treatment: Thrombolysis

Thrombolysis is another treatment that has been shown to improve the management of acute myocardial infarction and is now being assessed in the treatment of stroke. Myocardial infarction and stroke are not entirely comparable; the therapeutic time window may be different and the risk of haemorrhage is greater after cerebral infarction. To date, four major trials of thrombolytic therapy in stroke have been published. Most have been stopped early because of adverse safety findings. Three trials – MAST-I (Multicentre Acute Streptokinase Trial–Italy) [10] and MAST-E (Multicentre Acute Streptokinase Trial–Europe) [11] and the Australian Streptokinase Trial [57] – used streptokinase whereas ECASS (European Co-operative Acute Stroke Study) [36] and NINDS (National Institute for Neurological Disorders and Stroke) [12] used tissue plasminogen activator (tPA). Only the NINDS trial showed a definite benefit of early thrombolysis.

MAST-I employed a 2×2 factorial design investigating the use of streptokinase and aspirin administered within 6 h of the onset of symptoms. [10] The 10 day case fatality was higher in treatment groups including streptokinase (26.5% vs 11.7%) and was even greater when streptokinase was combined with aspirin (34% vs 10%). However, after 6 months there was no difference in the outcome in terms of death and disability. In fact, treated patients seemed to be less disabled after 6 months. This suggested that treatment with thrombolysis may have improved the long-term outcome at the expense of an excess of early deaths.

In contrast, MAST-E was a simple comparison of streptokinase against placebo administered within 6 h of the onset of symptoms [11]. Again, the 10 day mortality was much higher (34% vs 18.2%) in the thrombolysis group compared with placebo. However the 6 month outcome, like that in MAST-I, was not significantly different.

The ASK trial examining the use of streptokinase administered within 6 h of the onset of stroke was also stopped early because of significantly adverse outcomes in the treated group [57].

There has been a suggestion from the cardiological trials that tPA has slightly better efficacy and fewer adverse bleeding events than streptokinase; ECASS and NINDS therefore examined the benefit of tPA in acute stroke. ECASS randomised 620 patients within 6 h of the onset of symptoms in a double-blind, placebo-controlled design [36]. Unlike the other streptokinase trials, ECASS had strict inclusion criteria to reduce the risks of the treatment and maximise benefit. The target population was defined as patients between the ages of 18 and 80 years with a stable moderate to severe hemispheric stroke with no or only minor early infarct signs on the initial CT scan who could be treated within 6 h. A large number of patients who did not fit these criteria were included in the trial. The authors therefore carried out a retrospective analysis of the target population after completion of the trial. Thus out of 620 patients recruited, 109 were excluded from the target population for major protocol violations, mainly because a large infarct was visible on the original CT scan when reviewed by the experienced principal neuroradiologists. The overall results analysed on an intention-to-treat basis were similar to those of the MAST trials. The outcome in terms of disability at 3 months was better in those patients receiving tPA but was outweighed by an excess of earlier death from intracerebral haemorrhage. However, in the selected target population, the benefit appeared to be highly significant. The penalty of increased early mortality was much lower.

The results emphasise the importance of selecting appropriate centres and investigators when conducting clinical trials. It appears that in ECASS, many of the investigators did not have the experience or skill to recognise the early signs of infarction on CT. There were also considerable difficulties in recruiting patients within 6 h of onset of stroke, which may have led investigators to ignore the CT findings so as to include at least some patients in the trial. Clearly decisions about using treatments have to be made on the intention-to-treat results. A further European trial of tPA in acute stroke was therefore started in which the centres were carefully instructed about entry criteria and the interpretation of the CT scan in stroke before entering the study. Disappointingly, this trial also failed to demonstrate a benefit of thrombolysis within 6 h of onset in the primary analysis of patients making an almost complete recovery (Rankin grade 0 or 1). However, a post-hoc analysis examining recovery to Rankin grade 0, 1 or 2 (the more usual dichotomy) showed a significant benefit for tPA [58].

In contrast to all the other trials, the NINDS trial unequivocally showed a benefit of thrombolysis [12]. Six hundred and twenty-four patients were randomised to receive either placebo or tPA. Unlike the other trials, patients were entered within 3 h of onset of symptoms. No matter which outcome scale was used – Barthel Index, Modified Rankin Score, Glasgow Outcome Score or NIH Stroke Scale – patients treated with tPA fared better than the controls. Twenty per cent more patients treated within 90 min of the onset of their symptoms improved with an increase of at least 4 points on the NIH Stroke Scale over the ensuing 24 h, compared with controls. The 30 day mortality was similar between the groups (12.8% vs 15.7%), and the incidence of symptomatic intracranial haemorrhage was not significantly different. Patients randomised in NINDS were highly selected and closely monitored by experienced stroke neurologists. Although tPA has received a licence in North America for the treatment of acute stroke under these conditions, the results are clearly not generalisable to the average stroke patient or the average hospital. Furthermore, it was difficult to recommend thrombolysis on the basis of one positive trial when there have been negative trials and meta-analysis does not reveal any definite benefit when the results are combined. [59] However, more recent meta-analysis concentrating on patients treated with tPA within 3 h only suggest a significant benefit to thrombolysis within this narrow time window [60]. The cohorts of patients enrolled in the thrombolysis trials are clearly different in terms of their propensity to intracranial haemorrhage. MAST-E and ECASS had the highest incidence of intracranial haemorrhage (39.6% and 36.8% respectively) whereas MAST-I had 10.9% and NINDS only 3.5%.

This cannot be explained simply in terms of the agent used or the dose. However, the NINDS trial used the smallest dose and the narrowest treatment window. Clearly, the results emphasise the difficulty of forming conclusions from a single trial of treatment in stroke.

These studies highlight the complexity involved in carrying out treatment trials in acute stroke. There was clearly no consensus as to the correct thrombolytic agent to administer, and the time window was not known. The NINDS trial suggests that this therapeutic window is very narrow and ECASS suggests that it might be too late to give a patient thrombolysis once the infarct is visible on the CT scan. Careful selection of patients will clearly be essential in the future. It will no longer be enough to scan patients simply to exclude haemorrhage; the size and extent of ischaemic changes will need to be assessed. Newer imaging techniques, such as diffusion-weighted MRI, will make it easier to categorise an infarct within minutes of onset in terms of size and location (for example, lacunar or cortical) and then enrol patients with more comparable diseases into subsequent trials.

Acute Stroke Treatment: Stroke Units

Enthusiasts for treating stroke have always favoured stroke units, but until recently have not been able to prove their benefit. The difficulties that have already been encountered in drug trials of stroke discussed earlier are even greater when considering the impact of stroke units. Not only is the disease, the outcomes measured and the patients included in the trials heterogeneous, but even the management is heterogeneous on stroke units. There is even no consensus regarding what constitutes a stroke unit. The definition varies from a specialist team on a dedicated ward to a specialist team that visits stroke patients all over the hospital.

Almost all the published trials of stroke unit care failed individually to show a significant benefit of stroke unit care (Table 19.6). However, each trial included very small numbers of patients: the largest included only 311. Most of the trials of stroke units showed better outcome in the stroke unit group but only Indredavik et al.'s study showed a benefit that was significant [61]. In this study, 220 patients were randomised between the stroke unit and general wards. The mortality after 6 weeks was 7.3% for the stroke unit group and 17.3% for the general medical wards group, rising to 24.6% and 32.7% respectively after 1 year. Furthermore, at 1 year, 62.7% of the stroke unit group and 44.6% of the general medical wards group were at home. An overview of these 10 trials which was published in 1993 [24] and updated

Table 19.6. Overview of stroke unit care[57]

Trail	Treatment observed/total	Control observad/total	Observed minus expected	Variance	Odds ratio (95% CI) (Treatment: control)	Odds reduction (SD)
Dedicated stroke unit versus general medical ward						
Dover	54/98	60/89	−5.74	11.16		
Edinburgh	93/155	94/156	−0.20	18.70		
Kuopio	31/50	31/45	−1.63	5.43		
Montreal	58/65	60/65	−1.00	2.74		
Nottingham	63/98	52/76	−1.77	9.65		
Orpington (1995)	34/34	37/37	0.00	0.00		
Orpington (1993)	38/53	39/48	−2.41	4.61		
Perth	10/29	14/30	−1.80	3.62		
Trondherm	54/110	81/110	−13.50	13.10		
Umea	52/110	102/183	−5.82	17.19		
Subtotal	487/802	570/839	−33.86	86.20		32 (8)
Mixed assessment/rehabilitation unit versus general medical ward						
Birmingham	8/29	9/23	−1.48	2.88		
Helsinki	47/121	65/122	−8.77	15.13		
Illinois	20/56	17/35	−2.77	5.25		
New York	23/42	23/40	−0.56	5.11		
Newcastle	26/34	28/33	−1.40	2.66		
Uppsala	45/60	41/52	−1.07	5.01		
Subtotal	169/342	183/305	−16.05	36.07		36 (12)
Dedicated stroke unit versus mixed assessment/rehabilitation unit						
Dover	11/18	19/28	−0.74	2.54		
Nottingham	60/78	48/63	−0.26	6.29		
Orpington (1993)	63/71	69/73	−2.08	2.77		
Tampere	53/98	55/113	2.84	13.18		
Subtotal	187/165	191/177	−0.27	24.78		1 (25)
Total	843/1409	944/1421	−49.65	147.04		29 (7)

0.1   0.3 0.5   1   2   4

Odds of death or dependency at the end of scheduled follow-up, with stroke unit compared with conventional care. Points to the left of the pecked line suggest that stroke unit care is better; those to the right suggest it is worse. Confidence lines that cross unity suggest the result is not significant.

in 1997 [62] showed a highly significant benefit in favour of stroke unit care when the results of each trial were combined, and is therefore extremely important in demonstrating the value of meta-analysis. All the trials compared an intervention group (stroke unit or rehabilitation) with routine non-specialist care on a general medical or neurology ward [24]. To allow the data from several trials to be pooled, the main outcome used was usually mortality rather than degree of disability, although in the subsequent publication individual data were pooled to allow an estimate of dependency [59]. Patients who did not require physical assistance for transfers, mobility, dressing, feeding or toileting were considered to be independent. Any who failed any of those criteria were considered dependent. Thus it was possible to compare disability between one trial and another only by going back to the original data and constructing a new, simpler scale applicable to all trials. Langhorne et al. [24] originally showed that patients treated in a stroke unit had a 28% reduction in mortality compared with controls. The later overview included 19 trials and confirmed this finding. It further demonstrated an increase of about 15% in the number of patients who regained their independence after being managed in a stroke unit [62].

Langhorne et al.'s overviews highlight the importance of having sufficient patients in a clinical trial to be able to answer the primary question. If one took the results of the trials alone, one might be misled into thinking that as nine trials had shown no significant benefit from being managed in a specialist unit, there was no justification in conducting further trials. The results of the overviews show that a very striking benefit of treatment had been overlooked.

Conclusion

The studies reviewed in this chapter illustrate the wide variety of treatments available for stroke and the value of subjecting them to assessment by a randomised clinical trial. Despite the difficulties of defining the disease of interest, choosing appropriate outcome assessments and recruiting sufficient numbers of patients, major advances have been made which allow rational decisions to be made about the treatment of stroke based on solid scientific evidence.

References

1. Who Monica Project principal investigators. The World Health Organisation Monica Project (Monitoring Trends and Determinants in Cardiovascular Disease): a major international collaboration. J Clin Epidemiol 1988;41:105–114.
2. Bonita R, Stewart AW, Beaglehole R. International trends in stroke mortality 1970–1985. Stroke 1990;21:989–992.
3. European Carotid Surgery Trialists Collaboration Group. MRC European carotid surgery trial: interim results for symptomatic patients with severe (70–99%) or with mild (0–29%) carotid stenosis. Lancet 1991;337:1235–1243.
4. North American Symptomatic Carotid Endartectomy Trial Collaborators. Beneficial effect of carotid endarterectomy in symptomatic patients with high-grade carotid stenosis. N Engl J Med 1991;325:445–453.
5. Petersen P, Boysen G, Godtfredsen J, Andersen ED, Andersen B. Placebo-controlled, randomised trial of warfarin and aspirin for prevention of thromboembolic complication in chronic atrial fibrillation. Lancet 1989;I:175–178.
6. Wade JP, Wong W, Barnett HJ, Vandervoort P. Bilateral occlusion of the internal carotid arteries: presenting symptoms in 74 patients and a prospective study of 34 medically treated patients. Brain 1987;110:667–682.
7. Stroke Prevention in Atrial Fibrillation Investigators. Warfarin versus aspirin for prevention of thromboembolism in atrial fibrillation: Stroke Prevention in Atrial Fibrillation II Study. Lancet 1994;343:687–691.
8. Ezekowitz MD, Bridgers SL, James KE, et al. Warfarin in the prevention of stroke associated with nonrheumatic atrial fibrillation. N Engl J Med 1992;327:1406–1412.
9. Boston Area Anticoagulation Trial for Atrial Fibrillation Investigators. The effect of low-dose warfarin on the risk of stroke in patients with non-rheumatic atrial fibrillation. N Engl J Med 1990;323:1505–1511.
10. Multi-centre Acute Stroke Trial–Italy (MAST-I) Group. Randomised controlled trial of streptokinase, aspirin and combi-

nation of both in treatment of acute ischaemic stroke. Lancet 1995;346:1509–1514.
11. The Multicenter Acute Stroke Trial–Europe Study Group. Thrombolytic therapy with streptokinase in acute ischemic stroke. N Engl J Med 1996;335:145–150.
12. The National Institute of Neurological Disorders and Stroke rt-PA Stroke Study Group. Tissue plasminogen activator for acute ischemic stroke. N Engl J Med 1995;333:1581–1587.
13. CAST (Chinese Acute Stroke Trial) Collaborative Group. CAST: randomised placebo-controlled trial of early aspirin use in 20 000 patients with acute ischaemic stroke. Lancet 1997;349:1641–1649.
14. Kay R, Wong KS, Yu YL, et al. Low-molecular-weight heparin for the treatment of acute ischemic stroke. N Engl J Med 1995;333:1588–1593.
15. Asplund K. Hemodilution in acute stroke. Cerebrovasc Dis 1991;1(Suppl 1):129–138.
16. International Stroke Trial Collaborative Group. The International Stroke Trial (IST): a randomised trial of aspirin, subcutaneous heparin, both, or neither among 19 435 patients with acute ischaemic stroke. Lancet 1997;349:1569–1581.
17. The CASANOVA Study Group. Carotid surgery versus medical therapy in asymptomatic carotid stenosis. Stroke 1991;22:1229–1235.
18. Dennis MS, Bamford JM, Sandercock PA, Warlow CP. Incidence of transient ischemic attacks in Oxfordshire, England. Stroke 1989;20:333–339.
19. UK-TIA Study Group. The United Kingdom transient ischaemic attack (UK-TIA) aspirin trial: final results. J Neurol Neurosurg Psychiatry 1991;54:1044–1054.
20. Antiplatelet Trialists' Collaboration. Collaborative overview of randomised trials of antiplatelet therapy. I. Prevention of death, myocardial infarction, and stroke by prolonged antiplatelet therapy in various categories of patients. BMJ 1994;308:81–106.
21. Bamford J, Sandercock P, Dennis M, et al. A prospective study of acute cerebrovascular disease in the community: the Oxfordshire Community Stroke Project 1981–86 1. Methodology, demography and incident cases of first-ever stroke. J Neurol Neurosurg Psychiatry 1988;51:1373–1380.
22. Bamford JM, Sandercock PAG, Dennis MS, Warlow CP. Classification and natural history of clinically identifiable subtypes of cerebral infarction. Lancet 1997;337:1521–1526.
23. Cochrane Stroke Review Group. A systematic overview of specialist multidisciplinary team (stroke unit) care of stroke inpatients. Cochrane Database of Systematic Reviews, 2000.
24. Langhorne P, Williams BO, Gilchrist W, Howie K. Do stroke units save lives? Lancet 1993;342:395–398.
25. Hobson RW, Weiss DG, Fields WS, et al. Efficacy of carotid endarterectomy for asymptomatic carotid stenosis. N Engl J Med 1993;328:221–227.
26. Kraaijeveld CL, Van Gijn J, Schouten HJA, Staal A. Interobserver agreement for the diagnosis of transient ischaemic attacks. Stroke 1984;15:723–725.
27. Executive Committee for the Asymptomatic Carotid Atherosclerosis Study. Endarterectomy for asymptomatic carotid artery stenosis. JAMA 1995;273:1421–1428.
28. Bamford J, Sandercock P, Dennis M, Burn J, Warlow C. A prospective study of acute cerebrovascular disease in the community: the Oxfordshire Community Stroke Project – 1981–86. 2. Incidence, case fatality rates and overall outcome at one year of cerebral infarction, primary intracerebral and subarachnoid haemorrhage. J Neurol Neurosurg Psychiatry 1990;53:16–22.

29. CAPRIE Steering Committee. A randomised, blinded, trial of clopidogrel versus aspirin in patients at risk of ischaemic events. Lancet 1996;348:1329–1339.

30. TRUST Study Group. Randomised double-blind placebo controlled trial of nimodipine in acute stroke. Lancet 1990;336:1205–1209.

31. Sandercock PAG, van den Belt AGM, Lindley RI, Slattery J. Antithrombotic therapy in acute ischaemic stroke: an overview of the completed randomised trials. J Neurol Neurosurg Psychiatry 1993;56:17–25.

32. Brott T, Adams HP, Olinger CP, et al. Meaurements of acute cerebral infarction: a clinical examination scale. Stroke 1989;20:864–890.

33. Mahoney F, Barthel D. Functional evaluation the Barthel Index. Ma State Med J 1965;14:61–65.

34. Van Swieten JC, Koudstaal PJ, Visser MC, Schouten HJA, Van Gijn J. Interobserver agreement for the assessment of handicap in stroke patients. Stroke 1988;19:604–607.

35. Mayberg MR, Wilson SE, Yatsu F, et al. Carotid endarterectomy and prevention of cerebral ischaemia in symptomatic carotid stenosis. JAMA 1991;266:3289–3294.

36. Hacke W, Kaste M, Fieschi C, et al. Intravenous thrombolysis with recombinant tissue plasminogen activator for acute hemispheric stroke. JAMA 1995;274:1017–1025.

37. Taylor TN, Davis PH, Torner JC, Holmes J, Meyer JW, Jacobsen MK. The lifetime cost of stroke in the United States: summary of findings. Stroke 1996;27:1459–1466.

38. Easton JD, Wilterdink JL. Carotid endarterectomy: trials and tribulations. Ann Neurol 1994;35:5–17.

39. European Carotid Surgery Trialists Collaborative Group. Randomised trial of endarterectomy for recently symptomatic carotid stenosis: final results of the MRC European Carotid Surgery Trial. Lancet 1998;351:1379–1387.

40. Barnet HJ, Taylor DW, Eliasziw M, et al. Benefit of carotid endarterectomy in patients with symptomatic moderate or severe stenosis. New Engl J Med 1998;339:1415–1425.

41. Williams MA, Nicolaides AN. Predicting the normal dimensions of the internal and external carotid arteries from the diameter of the common carotid. Eur J Vasc Surg 1987;1:91–96.

42. Hennerici M, Hulsbomer HB, Hefter H, Lammerts D, Rautenberg W. Natural history of asymptomatic extracranial arterial disease: results of a long-term prospective study. Brain 1987;110:777–779.

43. Mayo Asymptomatic Carotid Endarterectomy Study. Results of a randomised controlled trial of carotid endarterectomy for asymptomatic carotid stenosis. Mayo Clin Proc 1992;67:513–518.

44. Brown MM. Balloon angioplasty for cerebrovascular disease. Neurol Res 1992;14(Suppl):159–173.

45. Brown MM. Surgery, angioplasty, and interventional neuroradiology. Curr Opin Neurol Neurosurg 1993;6:66–73.

46. EC-IC Bypass Study Group. Failure of extracranial-intracranial arterial bypass to reduce the risk of ischemic stroke: results of an international randomised trial. N Engl J Med 1985;313:1191–1200.

47. Stroke Prevention in Atrial Fibrillation Investigators. Stroke Prevention in Atrial Fibrillation Study: final results. Circulation 1991;84:527–539.

48. The Boston Area Anticoagulation Trial for Atrial Fibrillation Investigators. The effect of low-dose warfarin on the risk of stroke in patients with non-rheumatic atrial fibrillation. N Engl J Med 1990;323:1505–1511.

49. Ezekowitz MD, Bridgers SL, James KE, SPINAF Investigators. Interim analysis of VA co-operative study, Stroke Prevention in Non-rheumatic Atrial Fibrillation. Circulation 1991;84:SII–450.

50. Conolly SJ, Laupacis A, Gent M, Roberts RS, Cairns JA, Joyner C. Canadian Atrial Fibrillation Anticoagulation (CAFA) study. J Am Coll Cardiol 1991;18:349–355.

51. Morley J, Marinchak R, Rials SJ, Kowey P. Atrial fibrillation, anticoagulation and stroke. Am J Cardiol 1996;77:38A–44A.

52. Jaime Caro J, Groome PA, Flegel KM. Atrial fibrillation and anticoagulation: from randomised trials to practice. Lancet 1993;341:1381–1384.

53. Bath PMW, Prasad A, Brown MM, MacGregor GA. Survey of use of anticoagulation in patients with atrial fibrillation. BMJ 1993;307:1045.

54. The European Atrial Fibrillation Trial Study Group. Optimal oral anticoagulant therapy in patients with nonrheumatic atrial fibrillation and recent cerebral ischemia. N Engl J Med 1995;333:5–10.

55. Wardlaw JM, Warlow CP. Thrombolysis in acute ischemic stroke: does it work? Stroke 1992;23:1826–1839.

56. ISIS-2 Collaborative Group. Randomised trial of intravenous streptokinase, oral aspirin, both or neither among 17187 of acute myocardial infarction. Lancet 1988;91:311–322.

57. Donnan GA, Hommel M, Davis SM, McNeil JJ, for the steering committees of the ASK and MAST-E trials. Streptokinase in acute ischaemic stroke. Lancet 1995;346:56.

58. Hacke W, Kaste M, Fieschi C, et al. Randomised double-blind placebo-controlled trial of thrombolytic therapy with intravenous alteplase in acute ischaemic stroke (ECASS-II). Lancet 1998;352:1245–1251.

59. Wardlaw JM, Yamaguchi T, del Zoppo G. Thrombolytic therapy versus control in acute ischaemic stroke. In: Warlow CP, van Gijn J, Sandercock P, Candelise L, Langhorne P, editors. Stroke module of the Cochrane Database of Systematic Reviews. Oxford, 1997.

60. Ford G, Freemantle N. ECASSII Intravenous alteplase in ischemic stroke. Lancet 1999;353:365.

61. Indredavik BO, Bakke F, Solberg K, Rosketh R, Haahein LL, Holme IO. Benefit of stroke unit: a randomised controlled trial. Stroke 1991;22:1026–1031.

62. Stroke Unit Trialists' Collaboration. Collaborative systematic review of the randomised trials of organised inpatient (stroke unit) care after stroke. BMJ 1997;314:1151–1159.

20. Epilepsy: Ethics, Outcome Variables and Clinical Scales

M.C. Walker, J.W. Sander and S.D. Shorvon

Introduction

The Need for New Antiepileptic Drugs (AEDs) and Antiepileptic Drug Trials

Approximately 70–80% of patients with epilepsy will become seizure free with presently available AEDs, and over half of these will be able to stop treatment successfully [1]. The remainder have epilepsy that is resistant to present antiepileptic medication, and less than 5% of such patients are suitable for curative epilepsy surgery. Recently launched AEDs, which are initially licensed for use in this refractory group, have had little impact, rendering fewer than 5% of this group seizure free [2,3]. Thus effective novel AEDs are still required for treatment of those with refractory epilepsy. Most of these patients have partial epilepsy, as the generalised epilepsies respond better to current AED treatment.

Even in those in whom established AEDs are effective, side-effects often restrict their use. In comparative drug studies in newly diagnosed patients, treatment failure is more often due to drug side-effects than to lack of efficacy. Indeed, in a large trial of 421 newly diagnosed patients comparing the efficacy of carbamazepine, phenobarbital, phenytoin and primidone, 212 withdrew because of toxicity. Of these, 85 had good seizure control [4]. Only 11 patients withdrew because of lack of efficacy alone. There were no differences between the four drugs in treatment failure due to lack of efficacy (with or without side-effects), yet there were marked differences in treatment failure due to side-effects alone. AED tolerability thus plays a pivotal role in the choice of AEDs. In those AEDs in which side-effects are predominantly dose-related, the maximum dose is often restricted by tolerability and in some instances this can reduce the potential efficacy of the AED [5]. Thus improving the tolerability of AEDs is a second and important aim.

A third aspect is that of pharmacokinetics and ease of use. Phenytoin, for example, has difficult pharmacokinetics which can result in difficulty in adjusting the dose. The ideal pharmacokinetics for an AED are: rapid and complete oral absorption; once or twice daily administration, which for most drugs means a half-life of 12–24h, as this improves compliance; little interpatient variability, and linear kinetics (both of which aid dose predictions for patients); no metabolism, and no drug interactions [6]. Unfortunately no such drug exists, but realisation of the importance of these pharmacokinetic parameters has halted the development of some AEDs (e.g. loreclezole, which has an active metabolite with an unacceptably long half-life) and has slowed the development of others (e.g. stiripentol).

Ideally, an AED should improve the prognosis of epilepsy. There have been previous suggestions that early AED treatment favourably alters the prognosis of epilepsy, yet there is a growing body of evidence, mainly from untreated populations in developing countries, to suggest that present AED treatment has little or no influence on the prognosis [1]. Indeed, the prognosis of a patient with epilepsy is likely to relate to the underlying cause of the epilepsy and a number of other factors that have yet to be identified. There is, also, substantial evidence that established AEDs have no effect when used as prophylaxis to prevent the occurrence of epilepsy following head injury, neurosurgery or tumour [5]. There thus remains a place for new AEDs that alter the course of the condition.

Clinical trials should thus determine: (1) the efficacy of a novel AED in refractory epilepsy; (2) the tolerability and side effect profile of the novel AED; (3) the pharmacokinetic suitability of the novel AED and (4) the effect of the novel AED on the prognosis of epilepsy. Lastly, if it is to be considered for use in specific populations (e.g. children, newly diagnosed patients, patients with Lennox-Gastaut syndrome), a

Table 20.1. Potential prognostic factors

Aetiology of epilepsy
Seizure type
Seizure frequency
Age of onset
Duration of seizures
Age of patient
Sex of patient
Additional handicaps

Adapted from Shorvon et al. [7].

Table 20.2. Summary of ILAE classification of seizures

I. *Partial seizures*
A. Simple partial seizures
B. Complex partial seizures
C. Secondary generalised seizures
II. *Generalised seizures*
A. 1. Absence seizures ("petit mal")
2. Atypical absence seizures
B. Myoclonic seizures
C. Clonic seizures
D. Tonic seizures
E. Tonic-clonic seizures ("grand mal")
F. Atonic seizures
III. *Unclassified epileptic seizures*

From [8].

novel AED's efficacy and side-effect profile should be specifically determined in these populations.

Finally, it should be clearly recognised that there are two disparate reasons for carrying out clinical trials: (1) regulatory, i.e. a drug company wishes to get their drug licensed and marketed, and (2) clinical, i.e. physicians wish to have clinically useful information about the drug. Although these aims are not wholly divergent, they are not always addressed by the same type of trial. It is important to realise that drug companies' main aim is the licensing and marketing of a drug. Drug companies are also the sponsors of almost all new AED trials. Thus care should be taken not to over-interpret AED trials, and not to retrieve clinically useful information that is not there. This dichotomy will be met on numerous occasions in the discussion that follows.

Advances in the Methodology of AED Trials

In an analysis of 155 studies of the efficacy of either phenytoin or carbamazepine taking place between 1938 and 1980, a number of important, neglected methodological considerations have been identified [7], and, to a large extent, these have now been rectified. It is mandatory to define those factors that are of prognostic significance in a trial, yet many of the 155 trials failed to do this. Even when prognostic factors were identified, they were often poorly defined so that, for example, seizure type was often recorded in an imprecise fashion [7]. It is now commonplace to define trial populations in terms of potential prognostic factors (Table 20.1), and seizure type has been defined by the International League against Epilepsy (Table 20.2) [8]. It is salutary, however, to note that a factor that is likely to be of major prognostic influence, aetiology of seizures, is still largely ignored.

It was also noted that in the trials analysed too few patients were studied, and duration of follow-up was not stated or was too short to permit useful statistical analysis [7]. It was thus not surprising that in only 16% of the 155 studies were statistical methods used (other than calculating percentages), and these were often of doubtful validity [7]. It is now customary to use statistical tests in comparative trials, and indeed statisticians often help in the analysis and design of new AED trials.

Lastly, compliance has always been a problem in the treatment of epilepsy, yet few of the 155 trials even considered this subject [7]. AED trials now include tablet counts and serum monitoring as methods of assessing compliance. In addition, in adjunctive trials, serum monitoring of all the AEDs is performed in order to identify pharmacokinetic interactions that could influence the results of the trial.

Ethics

Monotherapy Versus Adjunctive Therapy

There are two distinct populations that may be helped by new AEDs: newly diagnosed patients and refractory patients. Ideally, the efficacy of a new AED would best be shown in newly diagnosed patients with the AED as monotherapy, as refractory patients by their nature are likely to be more resistant to treatment [7]. Initial assessment of new AEDs in newly diagnosed patients is, however, unethical as it involves denying patients known effective therapy – up to 80% may expect to become seizure free on monotherapy with established AEDs [9]. Assessment in this group is therefore reserved for new AEDs that have been established as effective add-on therapy in refractory patients. In newly diagnosed patients, new AEDs cannot be compared with placebo, as this would deny those patients effective therapy. Thus, a comparison has to be made with established drugs. This comparison is confounded by suggestions that there is a spontaneous remission rate of at least 30% for this group regardless of AED therapy [1], and large numbers of patients will be needed to demonstrate a difference in efficacy.

Comparative trials can compare the side-effects of a new AED and to an established AED. A well-designed study of carbamazepine against lamotrigine in newly diagnosed patients showed no difference in efficacy but fewer side-effects and fewer drop-outs in those taking lamotrigine [10]. Although the difference was statistically significant, its clinical importance has yet to be established especially considering the vast difference in cost between the two drugs (lamotrigine is approximately 10 times the price of carbamazepine) [11]. Most of the side-effects of carbamazepine occurred during titration, and it has been claimed that they were due to too rapid a titration rate. Finally, a problem for all monotherapy studies in epilepsy is the question of dose used, and comparisons of different drugs at different doses will produce different results.

New AED trials are usually carried out in patients with refractory epilepsy. Since it is, apart from exceptional circumstances (see below), unethical to take these patients off medication, the new AED or placebo has to be added to a patient's medication. The drug trial can then be complicated by the effects of the concomitant medication. Although new AEDs should be chosen and developed on the basis of their good pharmacokinetic profiles, some do have pharmacokinetic interactions that can confound the interpretation of such trials. Stiripentol, for example, increases the serum levels of phenytoin and carbamazepine, and felbamate increases the serum levels of phenytoin and decreases the serum levels of carbamazepine [6]. These interactions are not always obvious; the spectrum and concentration of bioactive metabolites can change in the face of unvarying serum concentrations of the parent drug. Such interactions are seen with lamotrigine, which possibly increases the serum concentration of an active metabolite of carbamazepine, carbamazepine epoxide, and with topiramate that possibly changes the pattern of metabolism of sodium valproate [6]. In both these cases the serum concentrations of the parent compound remain unchanged. As well as pharmacokinetic interactions, there are pharmacodynamic interactions, which are often poorly characterised. These can increase the observed efficacy and adverse events of the drug under investigation. It has certainly been noted that AEDs have a better side-effect profile when used as monotherapy compared with their use as adjunctive therapy [12].

Choice of Patients

For the ethical reasons outlined above, initial trials of new AEDs are restricted to patients with refractory epilepsy. In order to define refractory epilepsy, it is usual to determine a criterion of a minimum number of seizures that a patient should have per month prior to the trial (commonly 4 per month). Determining a subpopulation that has at least a certain number of seizures in the baseline month and excluding those with fewer seizures inevitably results in regression to the mean. This phenomenon is due to the population included in a clinical trial having a greater than mean seizure frequency in the baseline period (because there is a minimum inclusion seizure frequency), and thus by chance alone having fewer seizures in the trial periods.

Further ethical restrictions are applied to the patients chosen for initial drug trials. Age restrictions are common. Children are usually excluded from initial trials because of problems with consent, and the ethical consideration of first trying a drug in an adult prior to testing it in a child. This leads to difficulties in extrapolating early data to children, as they have a different spectrum of aetiologies for their epilepsy, and often in later trials it is found that they have different adverse events. Thus, separate trials for children are usually carried out much later in a drug's development. Trials often exclude the elderly, who may have different pharmacokinetic and pharmacodynamic responses to drugs, and whose epilepsy has a different aetiological spectrum from younger adults. This exclusion is rarely addressed in later trials, as drug licences are restricted to adults but give no upper age limit. Even when AED trials have no upper age limit, the presence of concomitant disease and medication usually excludes the majority of the elderly; thus although the clinical trials of gabapentin in partial epilepsy had no age limit, out of a total of 1160 patients recruited, only 10 were over 65 years old [13].

Pregnant women are excluded from AED trials, and there is thus a paucity of data on teratogenicity of new AEDs. Also, in order to prevent pregnancy occurring in a member of the trial population, women of child-bearing age have to be on adequate contraception (often defined as the contraceptive pill). Many female patients object to this, and there is thus often a male bias in the selection of patients for new AED trials.

Exclusions can be indirect. In double-blind studies exclusion criteria often include chronic alcohol or drug abuse, and only patients reasonably expected to complete the study are enrolled. These are criteria necessary for the proper running of a drug trial, but they nevertheless exclude many people with psychiatric disease, learning difficulties or behavioural problems. Indeed, many AED trials explicitly exclude patients with psychiatric disease or with a history of psychiatric illness. Thus, AED trials are carried out in a population that has a lower incidence of psychiatric disease than the general population of people with epilepsy, and this population is likely to be less sensitive to the adverse psychiatric effects of AEDs. Trials also exclude patients whose seizures are not accurately quantifiable, and may thus exclude patients with minor seizures or those who are amnesic for their seizures. Care must be taken in extrapolating the results of a trial to groups indirectly or directly excluded from the trial. From our experience this represents over three quarters of the patients in tertiary referal clinics.

Structure of Trials

Uncontrolled, Placebo-Controlled, and Comparative Studies

Because trials in epilepsy lack an objective measure and because seizure frequency and adverse events are particularly sensitive to patient expectations, patient stresses and, indeed, the more regular consultations that patients have with their treating physician during a trial period, there is a large and significant placebo or "honeymoon" effect in AED trials. Uncontrolled studies are useful for hypothesis generation and for long-term safety data, but a comparison with placebo in double-blind fashion is necessary for hypothesis testing. There are, however, problems with using a placebo in AED trials, as patients can often recognise the difference between taking a powerful drug with associated side-effects and taking a dummy pill. This problem is usually apparent in crossover studies in which patients are exposed to both placebo and drug, and thus these studies are to some extent unblind.

The alternative to using a placebo is to use an active control (i.e. an established AED); this is in effect a comparative trial. In this situation one drug is compared with another in blinded fashion. The immediate problem with this type of trial is that if no difference is shown between the two treatments, then rather than considering them equally effective, it is equally justifiable to consider them equally ineffective; thus, no antiepileptic effect is shown. This type of evidence is often not admissible to regulatory authorities that issue drug licences. In order to show an antiepileptic effect, the drug under investigation has to be compared against a low dose of an established AED [14,15]. This is not a true (or fair) comparative trial, but should be considered an active

placebo trial – in this instance, no useful comparative information is available for the physician, but the trial may show that the drug under investigation is efficacious. Also by using a low dose of an established AED as the control, it is possible to overcome some of the ethical problems in carrying out monotherapy trials in patients with refractory epilepsy. An alternative approach has been to demonstrate a dose in response to a drug, thus avoiding the problem of equal efficacy. This has been successful in a monotherapy trial of different doses of gabapentin against carbamazepine [16].

Designs of Controlled, Double-Blind Studies

Crossover Versus Parallel Designs

Crossover AED studies have two main problems: wash-over effect and withdrawal from study. The wash-over effect is due to the influence or presence of a drug from the first arm carrying over, when a patient crosses from one arm of the study to the next. There are two chief mechanisms. If not enough time is left between one stage and the next, the first drug could still be present in the serum and thus could still be influencing seizure frequency. This would result in a loss of power of the study in distinguishing between the two treatments. Vigabatrin, for example, increases brain gamma-aminobutyric acid (GABA) by irreversibly inhibiting the enzyme GABA transaminase, and even after the drug is eliminated from the serum, its effect is still present until new enzyme is produced (approximately 10 days) [17]. The second wash-over effect is due to too rapid withdrawal of the drug. Rapid drug withdrawal in some instances can result in an increase in seizure frequency. Thus too rapid tapering off one drug before entering the next stage of the trial could result in an increase in seizures which could be interpreted as a treatment difference. There has to be an adequately long wash-out period between the two arms of a crossover study during which there has to be a sufficiently slow tapering of the drug.

Withdrawal from study can also confound the results. Patients may withdraw on transfer from one arm to another because of the differences between the treatments. Thus, for example, if a patient transfers from the drug to placebo, and this results in an increase in seizure frequency, then the patient may withdraw from the study. The efficacy analysis for this patient cannot be included as the patient has not completed both arms of the study, even though the drug was probably effective.

Because of these particular difficulties and the interpretational problems that they cause, parallel studies are preferred. In these there are separate control and treatment groups. The main disadvantage is that larger numbers of patients have to be used in order to eliminate the effects of inter-patient variability.

Enrichment Studies

Enrichment studies are also known as response-dependent studies and are divided into two phases: an open label screening phase and a double-blind crossover phase. This was used for the assessment of the new AED, tiagabine [18]. Patients are initially given the active drug in an open-label study, and only those that respond to the drug (response being defined, in the case of tiagabine, as a 25% or greater reduction in seizures) can enter the double-blind phase. This type of study is designed to reject before the double-blind stage patients who do not respond to the drug; this maximises the chance of showing a difference between the drug and placebo. This sort of trial gives no useful information on a population response and thus little information for the treating physician in normal practice: when faced with a patient it is not possible to determine the probability of response or tolerability of the drug. The sole purpose of these studies is to demonstrate whether a drug has any antiepileptic activity compared with placebo (i.e. a regulatory not a clinical purpose). A problem in these studies is that, during the open-label phase, patients could learn to distinguish the drug from placebo. This would effectively unblind the study, and could result in a greater difference being observed between the effects of placebo compared with drug. These biases can be present in many phase III studies. Most centres have a pool of suitable patients for refractory epilepsy drug trials. Many of these patients are entered into phase I and II trials. Recruitment for phase III trials is from the same pool of patients, some of whom may have already experienced the drug: thus those who have previously tolerated the drug poorly will not wish to enter the trial and those who have had a previous beneficial effect from the drug will be keen to participate.

Monotherapy Designs in Refractory Epilepsy

If a new AED affects the serum levels of other AEDs, then add-on studies can become uninterpretable. To overcome this problem and also the problem of pharmacodynamic interactions, monotherapy trials in refractory epilepsy have been developed. As alluded to earlier, the major problem is ethical, and relates to taking patients with refractory epilepsy off their medication in order to compare in a blinded fashion a new AED with unknown efficacy and placebo or active control. These problems have been overcome to a certain extent by two new trial designs used in the assessment of felbamate. An active control trial of felbamate as monotherapy compared felbamate with low-dose valproate in a double-blind parallel group trial in partial epilepsy [14]. In this study patients were randomised to receive either valproate or felbamate, and were then tapered from their previous AEDs. Escape criteria were then used such as a twofold increase in monthly seizure frequency, a twofold increase in the highest 2-day seizure frequency or the occurrence of a generalised tonicclonic seizure, and efficacy determined by the number of patients meeting these criteria over the trial period. This study suffers in that the outcome measures are not those generally thought to be clinically relevant. Also the dose of valproate was lower than that used in clinical practice, thus not offering a fair comparison. A similar protocol has been used in patients whose AEDs have been reduced or discontinued as part of a presurgical evaluation [19]. A surrogate measure of efficacy was used such as time to fourth seizure. In this study, however, not all patients are on monotherapy, because some have had their AEDs reduced rather than halted. Thus the outcome could be the result of a pharmacokinetic effect (i.e. the levels of concomitant AEDs could have risen in the felbamate group as compared with the control group). Furthermore, rapid withdrawal effects could not be accounted for, especially in a trial that was so short (29 days) The results of these trials are impossible to apply clinically.

Outcome Measures

Efficacy

The main aim of AED trials is to prevent seizures with minimal side-effects. In addition there are wider considerations such as changes in quality of life and cost analysis. Most AED trials have as their primary aim seizure reduction, but the analysis of this is far from simple.

Seizure Counts

An effect of AEDs on seizure reduction can be measured in different ways. Seizure frequency is the simplest measure, and can be analysed as a continuous variable comparing the effect of drug against placebo. It is not, however, a normally distributed variable and the analysis requires non-parametric tests (e.g. Mann–Whitney U-test). Medians rather than means give a fairer reflection of the data. The range is often large. Attempts have been made to back-transform the data in order to get a normal distribution which is easier to analyse and which increases the statistical power of the analysis. The most successful has been the response ratio, which was used in the analysis of some of the gabapentin trials [20]. This was the ratio of change in seizure frequency from baseline to trial period as a proportion of the seizure frequency at baseline. This artificial measure may demonstrate an antiepileptic effect, but the results are difficult to interpret clinically.

Seizure frequency is determined usually by patient or carers. It is generally accepted that minor seizures are occasionally missed, but the size of this problem has been emphasised by a study that has shown that over 60% of all seizures are unrecognised by patients with partial epilepsy being monitored in an epilepsy unit [21]. Tonic-clonic seizures were missed more often than complex partial seizures. The environment of an epilepsy monitoring unit may not be conducive to seizure recognition, as in real-life situations there are external clues such as the gathering of a crowd and injury. Nevertheless the results of this study bring into question the validity of patient seizure counts, and indeed following a successful treatment which reduces seizure severity from tonic-clonic to simple partial, there may be an increase in reported seizure frequency simply due to the increased recognition of seizures. In epilepsy syndromes in which there are very frequent seizures, such as absence epilepsy or Lennox-Gastaut syndrome, the seizure counts are completely unreliable. Attempts to overcome this have been the use of a video-seizure count over a fixed period of time [22], but this is costly and difficult to interpret.

In order to simplify the statistical analysis, and also to give a more clinically applicable measure, seizure reduction is often categorised according to the percentage seizure reduction, e.g. 0–25%, 26–50%, 51%–75%, 76%–100%. This can then be analysed by a chi-squared method. A simpler measure that is commonly used is based on the assumption that a clinically significant decrease in seizure frequency is 50% or greater, and patients are then divided into those that experience a 50% or greater reduction in seizure frequency and those that do not, i.e. the data are reduced to a binary response that can easily be analysed using chi-squared tests. A 50% or greater reduction in seizure frequency is easy to analyse but it is not necessarily clinically significant. If seizure frequency is reduced from 2 per week to 1 per week, the patient is still unable to drive, still has difficulty getting a job and still has problems maintaining a relationship.

In the measurement of epilepsy surgery outcome, seizure freedom is generally taken as the outcome measure of success. This is based on the assumption that patients only have a significantly improved quality of life with complete freedom from seizures

(and thus freedom from the social stigmatisation of epilepsy). Indeed, even the presence of auras has a significant effect on quality of life [23]. Interestingly, in the same study the number of seizures after surgery had a greater correlation with quality of life than percentage reduction of seizures. These stringent criteria have become necessary for judging the success of epilepsy surgery due to its inherent morbidity and cost.

Seizure freedom is rarely used as the primary measure of efficacy in new AED trials. As discussed, for ethical reasons new AEDs are initially tried as add-on medication in populations with refractory epilepsy resistant to previous AEDs (i.e. those patients with easily controlled seizures are by definition excluded from the trials). Disappointingly, the number of these patients who become seizure free even with "successful" new AEDs is small, and consequently the impact of these drugs on the prognosis of epilepsy is modest. In reviewing double-blind, placebo-controlled studies from which an estimate of seizure freedom could be made, out of a total of 10 trials involving over 300 patients taking a new AED (vigabatrin, lamotrigine or zonisamide as this data could not be obtained from gabapentin and felbamate trials) only 6 (less than 2%) became seizure free [3]. Thus, in order to show a statistically significant effect for seizure freedom very large trials would have to be done. We should recognise that the standard of what we consider a clinically significant effect has been reduced simply to get a statistically significant effect with fewer patients.

Of 16 double-blind, placebo-controlled trials of new AEDs, 13 do not mention the number of patients who became seizure free and in 6 of these trials it was not possible to retrieve this information from the data given; thus seizure freedom has become a secondary measure of efficacy [3].

For an AED that is undergoing monotherapy trials in newly diagnosed patients, there are different considerations. The difficulty is the generally good prognosis for newly diagnosed epilepsy, with similar numbers of patients becoming seizure free regardless of the AED chosen; indeed over time approximately 40% of this group may become seizure free without any drug treatment [1]. Seizure freedom is not an absolute measure and is time dependent. Thus the analysis is carried out as a survival analysis (usually Mantel–Cox) in which percentages of patients who are recurrence free are plotted against time. This is a time to first recurrence analysis. A separate analysis that has more clinical relevance is the elimination of seizures for a fixed period of time, and this is analysed and presented as the percentage achieving a 1 year seizure remission at selected times. This again is a survival analysis, and the endpoint is arbitrary; analyses for 3 and 5 year remissions are used in epidemiological studies. Interestingly, this analysis consistently fails to find a difference between AEDs; it is thus burdened by the equal efficacy/inefficacy dilemma. Furthermore, since AEDs are found to be equally efficacious, other criteria for determining clinical practice have to be used. This has led to the growing importance of analysing the number of patients who continue to take a drug despite the opportunity to change. Using this analysis (again as a survival analysis), it is possible to differentiate between AEDs in newly diagnosed patients. This measure is determined by a combination of the drug's efficacy and tolerability.

Measures of Tolerability and Adverse Events

Adverse events are usually patient-reported in AED trials, with consequent under-reporting of side-effects not recognised to be associated with the drug. To overcome this, many trials use questionnaires. These questionnaires may miss adverse events that were not considered, and they over-report adverse events unconnected with the trial drug. In addition to patient reporting, monitoring of vital signs, weight, neurological and general medical examination and blood tests are used to further detect adverse events. In order that different descriptions of the same adverse event are included together in the analysis, the adverse events are categorised by the investigator using generally accepted terms (e.g. the WHO inventory). The 95% confidence intervals should be calculated for the difference between rates of occurrence of each event between placebo and trial drug.

Drug trials give a good overview of short-term adverse events, but for longer-term side-effect profiles, continuation and open-label studies are performed. Four main problems exist. The first is that some long-term side-effects will not be evident because of the time limit imposed on AED trials, and will thus only be detected in post-marketing surveys. The second is that the total number of patients included in these trials is relatively small, and thus rare but clinically important side-effects such as, for example, aplastic anaemia will be missed (as with the new AED felbamate). Thirty thousand patient-years are required in order to have 95% confidence in detecting an adverse event that occurs once in every 10 000 patient-years (most AEDs are exposed to approximately 2000 patient-years before being licensed). Thirdly, new AED trials exclude pregnant patients or those on inadequate contraception, and thus there are scarce data on the safety of new AEDs during pregnancy and on the developing fetus.

Lastly, drug trials are performed in selected populations. The drug could have a different side-effect and tolerability profile in different populations, not only because of physiological differences but also because of environmental and perceptual differences.

There are further considerations when assessing tolerability. Tolerability is not an absolute quality of an AED, but depends upon rate of drug titration and final dose. Thus in the comparison between lamotrigine and carbamazepine as monotherapy in newly diagnosed patients, lamotrigine appeared to be better tolerated as fewer patients taking lamotrigine withdrew [10]. However, most of the withdrawals on carbamazepine took place in the titration period, and were probably related to the rapid titration of carbamazepine in this trial (more rapid than is used in clinical practice). Similarly, adverse events that were reported in topiramate trials may have been due to the rapid (3–6 week) titration that occurred during these trials [24].

Scales and scores have been used that take into account the presence and severity of adverse events, and result in an overall adverse event score for the drug [25]. These have been used to great effect in the large comparative Veterans Administration studies comparing AEDs as monotherapy in newly diagnosed patients. These scores are, however, supplementary to the more traditional methods, and still have not been fully validated.

Seizure Severity

Seizure counts are not the only possible efficacy endpoint in AED trials; AEDs can also reduce the severity of seizures (perhaps via decreasing the spread of the epileptic discharge) without necessarily changing the frequency. Some AED trials attempt to investigate this by breaking up seizure counts by seizure type (simple partial, complex partial or secondary generalised). Often there are too few patients in one or all of these groups to permit meaningful statistical analysis, and so arbitrary weighting has been used: for example, a tonic-clonic seizure scores 50 points, a complex partial seizure 10 points and a simple partial seizure 1 point [26]. These scoring systems have not been validated, and are unable fully to determine seizure severity as it relates to the impact that a seizure has on a patient's life; this depends not only on seizure type but also on the length of the seizure, injuries that occur during the seizure and other such considerations. A number of more sophisticated scales have been devised to be used in AED trials. Two such scales are the Liverpool Seizure Severity Scale [27] and the National Hospital Seizure Severity Scale (Table 20.3) [28]. The former is a 16-item scale, containing two subscales; 6 items

Table 20.3. Items in the National Hospital Seizure Severity Scale

Each seizure type for a patient is scored by the physician according to: Presence of generalised convulsion Frequency of associated falls Injuries caused by the seizure Incontinence of urine Presence of warning long enough for patient to protect him/herself Time for full recovery following seizure Severity of automatisms

From [28].

refer to perception of control and 10 items refer to ictal/post-ictal effects. The latter is an easily used 7-item scale, which concentrates on only objectively determinable events (Table 20. 3). Such scales have been shown to be reliable, to correlate with a patient's subjective impression of seizure severity and to relate to other psychosocial measures, but no comparison of the scales has been undertaken.

Quality of Life Measurements

Although the aim of AED treatment is to reduce seizure frequency and/or severity, the overall objective of any treatment must be to improve the life of the patient. Thus a very effective AED that had unacceptable side-effects would not be chosen as a treatment despite its efficacy. A combination of a seizure rating score and an adverse event score would give a better idea of a drug's usefulness. Although such scores exist [25], they have yet to be validated. An alternative is to look at measures of quality of life as an indicator of medical outcome. These may be sensitive not only to the antiepileptic and adverse effects of an AED, but also to such qualities as the mood-enhancing properties of the AED. Quality of life scales have been developed and validated for use in assessing the outcomes of neurosurgery for epilepsy [29]. Quality of life measures have recently been applied to AED trials. A health-related quality of life (HRQL) model was developed which contained previously validated measures of anxiety, depression, happiness, overall mood, self-esteem, and mastery [30]. This HRQL model was used in a randomised, placebo-controlled, double-blind, crossover study of lamotrigine. Interestingly in this study, only 14% of the patients had a 50% or greater reduction in seizure frequency, yet over 50% of the patients wished to continue on lamotrigine; this suggest that factors other than seizure frequency determine patient satisfaction with an AED [30]. There was, however, no change in the social and physical scores of the HRQL, but both perceived internal control and mood improved on lamotrigine. The inability of the scale

to detect a difference in certain of the HRQL scores was possibly due to the short time period of the trial (18 weeks). Herein lies a major disadvantage, as it is naive to think that important changes in quality of life can be detected in the short term. Neurosurgical trials have assessed these issues over years, and this is far more appropriate. Non-randomised, unblind longitudinal studies are difficult to interpret, but large, blinded, randomised studies would be unethical over long time scales.

Sample Size, Duration of Follow-up and Meta-analysis

There are a number of confounding factors in determining the sample size and duration of follow-up needed to achieve a statistically significant result in an AED trial [7]. (1) In direct comparisons of AEDs (especially in newly diagnosed patients, who have a high spontaneous remission rate) there is likely to be only a small difference in efficacy of the two drugs. (2) Seizure frequency in most populations is extremely variable. (3) The seizure frequency in an individual patient can also vary considerably over time. Indeed, the need to use non-parametric statistical tests in order to analyse seizure frequency can result in a more than 50% increase in the number of patients needed to achieve a certain statistical power compared with calculations based on a normal distribution of seizure frequency [7].

The duration of follow-up is determined not only by the intra-patient and inter-patient variability in seizure frequency but also by the generally held rule that 5 attacks are necessary before seizure frequency estimates can be considered accurate [7]. In trials in refractory patients this limitation is largely overcome by defining refractory as a seizure frequency of 4 or more seizures per month. In newly diagnosed patients, however, this limitation can have a profound effect. For example, if a population has a mean of 1 seizure per month (normally distributed) with a standard deviation of 0.4 seizures per month, then in order for 5 attacks to occur in more than 75% of that population (to a power of 80%), the patients would have to be followed up for 11 months. In a similar population with a mean seizure frequency of 1 seizure per 3 months, follow-up would be 51 months.

In recent double-blind trials of new AEDs as add-on in refractory epilepsy, the phase III studies have been carried out over a period of usually 3 months and have required more than 20 patients for crossover studies and more than 120 patients for parallel-group studies in order to achieve a statistical difference between placebo and active drug, using 50% or greater reduction in seizure severity as the outcome measure [31].

In order to increase the statistical power of studies, they can be amalgamated as a meta-analysis – this increases the number of patients in each treatment group. This is a more sensitive method of detecting significant but rare adverse events. Using it as a method of determining the efficacy of an AED compared with placebo, and then using this as a method of comparing different AEDs, is, however, fundamentally flawed. By amalgamating trials, prognostic factors (e.g. age, seizure frequency, seizure type) cannot be controlled for. Even AED doses can vary from trial to trial. Drug comparisons thus become difficult to interpret. Indeed, in one extensive meta-analysis [31], differences between the efficacy or adverse events for new AEDs could not be determined with any statistical certainty due to the large confidence intervals for each drug.

Conclusion and the Effect of New AEDs on Prognosis

Randomised trials of new AEDs in newly diagnosed patients do not determine the effect that a new AED has on the prognosis in this group. This is because clinical trials just compare one drug against another, and this is not sufficient. In order to establish the effect of a new AED on prognosis, very large trials need to be carried out comparing present management of newly diagnosed patients (i.e. the substitution of one first-line AED by another if initial therapy is not successful) against present management with the new AED included amongst the first-line therapies.

This extrapolation of clinical trials to clinical practice is even more troublesome in refractory epilepsy. The failure of new AED trials in refractory patients to use seizure freedom as the primary outcome measure, and the short time-span of these trials have meant that they have failed to give a good indication of the effect of new AEDs on the prognosis in this group. Two recently marketed new AEDs, vigabatrin and lamotrigine, appear not to have significantly changed the long-term prognosis in terms of mortality or seizure freedom of patients with severe refractory epilepsy, despite "good results" in short-term studies in this same group [32]. Furthermore, very few patients (far fewer than had a 50% or greater reduction in seizure frequency) continued these drugs in the long term [32].

Perhaps, however, the greatest failing of present AED trials is not recognising aetiology as a major prognostic factor. Epilepsy should be considered as analogous to anaemia in so far that it is a state that is the result of distinct underlying conditions each with its own prognosis and treatment. Most AED trials, however, only classify patients in terms of seizure type. What are required are large multicentre studies in well-defined populations with well-defined epilepsy syndromes and with seizure freedom as the primary measure of efficacy.

References

1. Sander JW. Some aspects of prognosis in the epilepsies: a review. Epilepsia 1993;34:1007–1016.
2. Wong IC, Chadwick DW, Fenwick PB, Mawer GE, Sander JW. The long-term use of gabapentin, lamotrigine and vigabatrin in patients with chronic epilepsy. Epilepsia 1999;40:1439–1445.
3. Walker MC, Sander JWAS. The impact of new antiepileptic drugs on the prognosis of epilepsy: seizure freedom should be the ultimate goal. Neurology 1996;46:912–914.
4. Mattson RH, Cramer JA, Collins JF, et al. Comparison of carbamazepine, phenobarbital, phenytoin and primidone in partial and secondary generalised tonic-clonic seizures. N Engl J Med 1985;313:145–151.
5. Walker MC, Sander JWAS. Overtreatment with antiepileptic drugs: how extensive is the problem? CNS Drugs 1994;2:335–340.
6. Walker MC, Patsalos PN. Clinical pharmacokinetics of new antiepileptic drugs. Pharmacol Ther 1995;67:351–384.
7. Shorvon SD, Johnson AL, Reynolds EH. Statistical and theoretical considerations in the design of anticonvulsant trials. In: Dam L, Gram L, Penry JK, editors. Advances in epileptology XIIth Epilepsy International Symposium. New York: Raven Press, 123–128.
8. Commission on Classification and Terminology of the International League Against Epilepsy. Proposal for revised clinical and electroencephalographic classification of epileptic seizures. Epilepsia 1981;22:289–501.
9. Elwes RDL, Johnson AL, Shorvon SD, Reynolds EH. The prognosis for seizure control in newly diagnosed epilepsy. N Engl J Med 1984;311:944–947.
10. Brodie MJ, Richens A, Yuen AWC. Double-blind comparison of lamotrigine and carbamazepine in newly diagnosed epilepsy. Lancet 1995;345:476–479.
11. Cockerell OC, Hart YM, Sander JWAS, Shorvon SD. The cost of epilepsy in the United Kingdom: an estimation based on the result of two population-based studies. Epilepsy Res 1994;18:244–260.
12. Reynolds EH, Shorvon SD. Monotherapy or polytherapy for epilepsy? Epilepsia 1981;22:1–10.
13. Chadwick D. Gabapentin: clinical use. In: Levy RH, Mattson RH, Meldrum BS, editors. Antiepileptic drugs, 4th edition. New York: Raven Press, 1995:851–856.
14. Sachdeo R, Kramer LD, Rosenberg A, Sachdeo S. Felbamate monotherapy: controlled trial in patients with partial onset seizures. Ann Neurol 1992;32:386–392.
15. Faught E, Sachdeo RC, Remler MP, et al. Felbamate monotherapy for partial-onset seizures: an active-control trial. Neurology 1993;43:688–692.
16. Chadwick DW, Anhut H, Greiner MJ et al. A double-blind trial of gabapentin monotherapy for new diagnosed partial seizures. Neurology 1998;51:1282–1288.
17. Grant SM, Heel RC. Vigabatrin: a review of its pharmacodynamic and pharmacokinetic properties, and therapeutic

potential in epilepsy and disorders of motor control. Drugs 1991;41:889–926.

18. Richens A, Chadwick DW, Duncan JS, et al. Adjunctive treatment of partial seizures with tiagabine: a placebo-controlled trial. Epilepsy Res 1995;21:37–42.

19. Bourgeois B, Leppik IE, Sackellares JC, et al. Felbamate: a double-blind controlled trial in patients undergoing presurgical evaluation of partial seizures. Neurology 1993;43:693–696.

20. Anonymous. Gabapentin in partial epilepsy. UK Gabapentin Study Group. Lancet 1990;335:1114–1117.

21. Blum DE, Eskola J, Bortz JJ, Fisher RS. Patient awareness of seizures. Neurology 1996;47:260–264.

22. Anonymous. Efficacy of felbamate in childhood epileptic encephalopathy (Lennox–Gastaut syndrome). The Felbamate Study Group in Lennox–Gastaut Syndrome [see comments]. N Engl J Med 1993;328:29–33.

23. Vickrey BG, Hays RD, Engel J, et al. Outcome assessment for epilepsy surgery: the impact of measuring health-related quality of life. Ann Neurol 1995;37:158–166.

24. Walker MC, Sander JWAS. Topiramate: a new antiepileptic drug for refractory epilepsy. Seizure 1996;5:199–203.

25. Cramer JA. A clinimetric approach to assessing quality of life in epilepsy. Epilepsia 1993;34(Suppl 4):S8–S13.

26. Ojemann LM, Wilensky AJ, Temkin NR, Chmelir T, Ricker BA, Wallace J. Long-term treatment with gabapentin for partial epilepsy. Epilepsy Res 1992;13:159–165.

27. Baker GA, Smith DF, Dewey M, Morrow J, Crawford PM, Chadwick DW. The development of a seizure severity scale as an outcome measure in epilepsy. Epilepsy Res 1991;8:245–251.

28. O'Donoghue MF, Duncan JS, Sander JW. The National Hospital Seizure Severity Scale: a further development of the Chalfont Seizure Severity Scale. Epilepsia 1996;37:563–571.

29. Vickrey BG, Hays RD, Rausch R, et al. Outcomes in 248 patients who had diagnostic evaluations for epilepsy surgery. Lancet 1995;346:1445–1449.

30. Smith D, Baker G, Davies G, Dewey M, Chadwick DW. Outcomes of add-on treatment with lamotrigine in partial epilepsy. Epilepsia 1993;34:312–322.

31. Marson AG, Kadir ZA, Chadwick DW. New antiepileptic drugs: a systematic review of their efficacy and tolerability. BMJ 1996;313:1169–1174.

32. Walker MC, Li LM, Sander JW. Long term use of lamotrigine and vigabatrin in severe refractory epilepsy: audit of outcome. BMJ 1996;313:1184–1185.

21. Epilepsy: Basic Designs, Sample Sizes and Experience with Large Multicentre Trials

D. Chadwick and A. Marson

Introduction

There have been hundreds, perhaps thousands, of studies assessing the efficacy of antiepileptic drugs (AEDs). Coatsworth [1] produced what could claim to be one of the first systematic reviews in medicine. Penry wrote in the foreword that "in keeping with the general philosophy of thorough documentation for better evaluation, a bibliography of publications judged unworthy of profile has been included, in addition to the bibliography of profiled articles". Coatsworth identified articles from 64 different journals published between 1920 and 1970. Of 120 articles, 43% were based on fewer than 50 patients, 27% on more than 100 and nearly half did not report the duration of the study. Three were multiple crossover studies which employed randomisation, two of which were double-blind and one of which was single-blind. One hundred and six were single group studies with no information about patient evaluation in 74. He concluded "the average reported clinical trial may be characterised as a study of one drug given over a variable period to a group of 20–29 outpatients of differing seizure types. No controls are used, and the drug is varied in dosage by the needs of the patient. Seizure counts, types of seizure and side-effects are the data collected by an unreported evaluator using the clinical examination and laboratory data as his observational methods. The patients were evaluated before the trial and irregularly during the trial. The results of treatment are reported by the percentage of patients improved. In those studies with fair to good results, the investigator's opinion is that the drug is a valuable addition to the present regimen of antiepileptics."

There can be no doubt that the quality of studies has improved considerably over the last three decades. In spite of this, the number of high-quality randomised controlled trials (RCTs) in epilepsy remains small, the quality of many questionable, and the size of most inadequate. By 1982 Gram et al. [2] were able to identify over 50 published RCTs, almost all of which were related to AEDs. Marson and Chadwick [3] were able to identify 355 studies by a mixture of electronic and hand searching techniques in 1996. The interventions investigated are listed in Table 21.1. Currently, the Cochrane database of RCTs in epilepsy identifies over 600 studies. The great majority of such studies examine AEDs and have been sponsored by the pharmaceutical industry. Inevitably, they tend to address limited regulatory issues rather than matters of clinical importance.

Clinical Factors Affecting the Design of Clinical Trials

Clinical trials in epilepsy present a wide range of challenges. Perhaps the most important is the considerable heterogeneity of the disorder and our relative lack of understanding of the basic mechanisms of many human epilepsies. It must be remembered that seizures, most commonly used as an outcome measure in studies, are simply common and relatively easily defined events that result from a wide variety of disturbances within the central nervous system. Because of our limited abilities to define specific epilepsy syndromes with identified aetiologies and mechanisms, most clinical trials in epilepsy select more or less heterogeneous populations of patients. This inevitably means that there may be considerable variation in the size of treatment effects between patients and samples of patients, and that sample sizes will as a consequence need to be large. A striking example of this has been the difficulty of even the largest of comparative drug studies [4,5] to

Table 21.1. The first 357 RCTs

Intervention	No. of RCT reports
AED	292
Vitamins	20
Drug withdrawal	11
Stimulation (Cerebellar, vagus, thalamic)	10
Hormones (steroids/oestrogens)	9
Psychosocial interventions	8
Giving information	2
Intravenous immunoglobulins	2
Treated or not treated after the first seizure(s)	2
Therapeutic drug monitoring	1

detect differences in efficacy between commonly used AEDs, when patients with broad classifications of epilepsy are recruited. In contrast, a study of 22 patients with infantile spasm syndrome due to tuberous sclerosis was able to show a large difference between hydrocortisone and vigabatrin [6]. This emphasises the need for adequate clinical information about patients entering studies in order that judgements can be made about whether the results of a study can be applied to an individual patient. The later can be aided if studies are large enough to allow the development of predictive models or subgroup analyses.

The problems of the classification of epilepsy can produce even more complications. Some AEDs are not broad-spectrum agents. Drugs such as vigabatrin and carbamazepine may not only be ineffective against some seizure types, but can, in the case of absence and myoclonus, cause an increase in seizure frequency [7]. If patients with generalised epilepsies are randomised in error into studies of partial epilepsy, the interpretation of results may become difficult. This could be responsible for some of the different results in studies that compare valproate and carbamazepine.

Outcomes in Epilepsy

There has been difficulty in arriving at a consensus on the outcome measures that are most appropriate in clinical trials. Most trials focus on some measure of seizure frequency and there is an inevitable temptation to investigate continuous variables such as changes in seizure frequency rather than clinically meaningful event (binary) rates such as the proportion of patients becoming seizure-free. Inevitably seizure counts are a somewhat blunt instrument, particularly when total counts of all seizures are used. Giving a simple partial seizure the same

weight as a secondary generalised seizure is a clinical nonsense!

Seizures and Seizure Frequency

A large number of methods exist for measuring and comparing seizure frequency. These include the change in seizure frequency between different periods of time, the change in seizure or seizure-free days, or rates at which patients achieve a given seizure-free state. The most statistically powerful measures compare changes in mean or median seizure frequency as they study a continuous variable. The use of seizure frequency is, however, by no means simple. In particular, expressing changes in terms of percentages can be hazardous. The distribution is unlikely to be normal as there is no limit to the percentage increase in seizures whereas percentage decreases will be smaller and finite. For this reason some form of transformation of the data may be used (log transformation or the use of a response ratio). The latter has been used in studies of gabapentin [8]. It is a ratio of the difference between treatment and baseline seizure frequency over the sum of treatment and baseline seizure frequency. It will vary between +1 and −1, no change being represented by 0 and a 50% reduction by − 0.33).

A further problem in the use of seizure frequency is the non-random nature of seizure occurrence. Many patients show clustering in the pattern of their seizures. Thus, the probability of a seizure is dependent upon when the last seizure occurred [9]. The less random the occurrence of seizures, the longer a patient should be followed before changes in seizure frequency become meaningful. Clustering of seizures presents one argument for ensuring that the periods of time over which seizure frequency is assessed in baseline and treatment phases of studies should be the same length (which is often not the case).

Flurries of seizures present problems for seizure frequency calculation. These may be seen in some patients in whom seizures may be too frequent to count over a given period of time. Patients with a history of status or flurries may be best excluded from studies in which seizure frequency is a primary outcome. Calculation of seizure frequency data for intent-to-treat analyses is also problematic. While it may be possible to extrapolate seizure frequencies once a minimum period of drug exposure has occurred, what should be done with patients exposed to the drug but withdrawn from treatment before such a time?

In spite of these problems, measures of change in seizure frequency are useful in populations of patients with chronic refractory epilepsy in whom seizures are relatively frequent and remissions exceptionally uncommon. Most studies of new AEDs would seem to indicate that an active compound may result in a 15–40% median reduction in seizure frequency compared with a 5–20% median reduction seen in placebo groups in parallel group studies.

A second approach is to reduce seizure frequency, or changes in it, to a binary or categorical outcome. Thus, in new AED studies the proportion of patients showing a 50% reduction in seizure frequency in a given unit of time is often presented, possibly with information about smaller numbers of patients who achieve 75% reduction or who become seizure-free.

The occurrence of seizures within units of time also lends itself to actuarial life table approaches. This has the virtue of allowing variable periods of follow-up and maximising the amount of data that each patient contributes to an outcome. Annegers and colleagues [10] used time to achieving remission within community-based studies, but such data also lend themselves to comparisons in longer-term clinical trials [11]. Thus in newly diagnosed patients, the proportion of patients remaining seizure-free or achieving periods of remission of 6, 12 and 24 months may also be used. These usually represent clinically important end-points as they most closely approximate to clinically acceptable control of seizures or indeed to cure of epilepsy. Life table techniques have also been used to measure shorter-term outcomes. The time to a first seizure following randomisation will usually represent a measure of efficacy that is least confounded by drop-outs due to intolerablity, while at the same time giving valuable information on the proportion of patients remaining seizure-free at any point in time following randomisation. It is, however, potentially confounded by starting dose and rate of titration. Shofer et al. [12] also examined the value of time to nth seizure in patients with more frequent seizures. The use of this outcome to define treatment failure has become popular recently and is helpful in potentially limiting the period of time that patients might be exposed to a new AED of uncertain safety within phase II studies. Thus, time to a fourth seizure following randomisation has been used in studies of patients undergoing presurgical evaluation. Pledger and colleagues (personal communication) have demonstrated that even in refractory patients entering new drugs studies, an outcome of time to a second or fourth seizure would allow the detection of statistically significant differences between placebo and active drug.

Whatever the measure of seizure frequency, the confounding by regression to the mean, or the median, should not be underestimated. Spilker and

Segreti [13] demonstrated in data from eight randomised studies that patients with higher than average seizure frequency tended to improve on placebo compared with baseline periods, while those with lower than average seizure frequencies tended to exhibit an increased seizure frequency on placebo as compared with baseline periods. Many add-on AED studies in refractory patients require seizure frequency above a predefined eligibility frequency for entry, a fact which guarantees an apparent response in untreated or placebo groups. A proportion of patients entering the study may only achieve this threshold seizure frequency during "unusual" periods of time and they will be expected on average, therefore, to improve in any subsequent period, be they treated with placebo or an active drug. The meta-analysis of Marson and colleagues [14] demonstrated that 50% responder rates in placebo-treated groups and studies of new AEDs may vary anywhere between 5% and 30%. This underlines the absolute requirement for a control group in order to draw any conclusion about treatment effects. In uncontrolled reports there can be no certainty about whether an observed change represents regression to the mean, a true placebo effect, or a treatment effect or to what extent it is contributed to by all three factors.

Seizures and Seizure Severity

For patients with chronic refractory epilepsy the expectation of complete remission or significant reduction in seizure frequency may be relatively low. A reduction in the severity of seizures may, however, be clinically important and correlate well with an improvement in quality of life [15]. As many AEDs block the propagation of seizure discharge from abnormal to normal brain, effective AEDs commonly reduce seizure severity. A practical example of this is the patient who presents in early or middle life with their first one or two tonic-clonic seizures. However, for many years they may have had more typical brief complex partial seizures during the day but never sought attention for them. AEDs commonly prevent further secondarily generalised tonic-clonic seizures. They often reduce and sometimes completely abolish complex partial seizures. Many patients do, however, continue to have the auras that they previously associated with their complex partial seizures and which continue as simple partial seizures. Thus, whilst there may be little change in seizure frequency overall, the switch from complex partial and secondarily generalised seizures to simple partial seizures may be of considerable clinical value.

In this respect, the classification of seizures along the lines of the International Classification [16] may in itself be an excellent measure of seizure severity, and is certainly valuable information in addition to total seizure counts derived from all seizure types.

In recent years more formalised methods of assessing seizure severity by patient enquiry have been developed and validated [17,18]. These use a battery of questions with Likert scale responses to assess the severity of the results of seizures, including falls, incontinence, injury and recovery time. They reliably detect differences between seizure types. The sensitivity of these measures to change within clinical trials remains much more controversial.

Health-Related Quality of Life

There is an increasing demand to show that treatment interventions not only affect clinical outcome but that this in turn feeds through to improvement in patient-perceived quality of life (QOL). Certainly, such measures would be expected to allow patients to measure an improved clinical outcome on the one hand against adverse effects of the treatment on the other. Epilepsy is a therapeutic area that is no exception and the number of papers on QOL in epilepsy and the number of tools available to assess it have increased very considerably.

The approaches used vary considerably from the development of novel tools to the application of tools validated in other areas and having generic properties. Because of the unusual impact of epilepsy on QOL, a combination of generic and disease-specific approaches seems most satisfactory. Jacoby [19] has reviewed the large number of tools currently available. The measures on one scale tend to correlate highly with those on others [20]. There does, however, seem to be very clear correlation between QOL measures and seizure-free states and chronic epilepsy [21].

At present there is uncertainty as to whether QOL measures might add sensitivity to other outcome measures in clinical trials and there is little or no evidence of their ability to measure change with sensitivity. Indeed, QOL measures might be expected to be insensitive to changes within the true frame of a conventional RCT, given that the impact of, for example, becoming seizure-free on employment, driving and self-confidence are likely to lag behind the onset of the effects of a therapeutic intervention. At best, they currently provide additional descriptive information for a secondary outcome measure.

Health Economic Outcomes

Health economic study of epilepsy is in its infancy. Most studies have been simple burden of disease studies [22,23] and there have been a few attempts to produce models to assess the cost-effectiveness of new treatments. The authors are unaware of any RCTs of AEDs which have used economic outcomes.

Tolerability

Pharmacological interventions in epilepsy are well recognised to be associated with a number of adverse effects that include dose-related, largely central nervous system effects, idiosyncratic toxicity, chronic toxicity and teratogenicity. While RCTs are rarely likely to be long enough or have sufficient power to discriminate the risks for the latter three, they can reliably detect and quantify tolerability. The tolerability of a drug usually reflects dose-related adverse effects. The recording of adverse events in drug trials generally is poor, and epilepsy is no exception to this. Many clinical trial protocols fail to describe a satisfactory methodology for reporting adverse effects. Many studies have simply used incidence reporting after passive enquiry. There is a strong case for some form of standardised interview or checklist to be used. Whilst crude incidence counts are reported, it is almost always impossible to gauge the prevalence of particular adverse events. The severity and transience of drug-related symptoms are often difficult to assess, though the important outcome of withdrawal due to side-effects is usually readily available, although potentially confounded by interaction with lack of efficacy.

The Veterans Administration (VA) multicentre studies of AEDs [24] used a toxicity score to describe the burden of side-effects. This scored symptoms, signs and laboratory test abnormalities. The validity and weighting of this summation is uncertain, and it has not been used in other RCTs.

Compound Outcomes

Effectiveness may be defined as a measure encompassing efficacy, safety and tolerability. It is most commonly measured by the time to withdrawal from a study because of inadequate efficacy, unacceptable tolerability or a combination of the two. It is clearly a clinically important end-point as it defines drug failure and particularly lends itself to use in pragmatic studies (see below). It was first used by the large VA studies in the United States [4]. Where it is used, however, it is important to understand the relative contributions of efficacy and tolerability to the overall outcome. The VA collaborative group developed a scoring system that arithmetically combined toxicity scores and a seizure occurrence score [24]. Again the validity of this scoring system is uncertain.

Types of RCT

Explanatory Clinical Trials

Explanatory clinical trials are well understood. They are essentially scientific and address a limited question concerning a mechanism of effect or proof of efficacy of an individual drug or dosage. They can be contrasted with pragmatic RCTs (see below).

The great majority of clinical trials in epilepsy are explanatory. They have been sponsored by the pharmaceutical industry to provide proof of efficacy of individual drugs and different doses of these drugs. An example of this kind of trial [25] is one in which patients were randomised to the addition of placebo or two different doses of gabapentin. The study was blinded to both patient and observer, the treatment protocols and particularly the doses were predefined and fixed, inclusion and exclusion criteria were tightly defined, there was a limited treatment period (12 weeks) and the primary outcomes were differences in change of seizure frequency and the proportion of patients in each group showing a 50% reduction in seizures. While this type of trial can provide proof of efficacy and examine the dose-response relationship for the drug and by doing so satisfy regulatory requirements, the study does little to inform clinical practice for the following reasons:

1. The comparison is against placebo. As Bradford Hill [26] pointed out "the essential medical question is how a new treatment compares with an old one, not whether the new treatment is better than nothing". This study makes no comparison of the new drugs with any other commonly used treatment in epilepsy.
2. Explanatory studies, by having tightly defined entry criteria in order to reduce heterogeneity and sample size, immediately call into question their relevance to more heterogeneous groups of patients with epilepsy. Because of the need to detect efficacy in as short a period as possible, so as to reduce risk, patients with high seizure counts need to be recruited. These are usually very atypical patients drawn from those with the most severe disease.
3. The fixed dose regimens depart very significantly from clinical practice, which conventionally involves a "start low and go slow" system of drug titration.
4. The study uses what amount to "surrogate" outcome measures (median change in seizure frequency) which have the power to provide statistical significance but are of little or no clinical relevance.

A number of different designs for RCTs have been used in explanatory RCTs in epilepsy:

Crossover Designs

Crossover designs, in which patients are randomised to a sequence of treatments in a two-way or multiple crossover, are attractive in epilepsy because each patient serves as their own control thereby reducing variance of outcome and addressing the important issues of heterogeneity in the disorder of interest. Hence, crossover trials have the advantage of requiring considerably fewer patients than parallel trials of similar power. Lamotrigine and vigabatrin used crossover designs extensively in their early development programme (see [14]). While such studies are efficient in terms of the number of patients to be recruited, they do have a number of disadvantages:

1. They require exposure to two or more treatment periods so that patients remain in a study for longer. Patients have the opportunity to compare what may be a less effective treatment with fewer side-effects (particularly in placebo-controlled studies) with more effective treatment possibly with more side-effects. It is therefore easy for patients and observers to be unblinded in such studies.
2. Patients who enter a study and receive active drug first may note a worsening of symptoms when a placebo or less active compound is substituted. They may well withdraw from a study without completing all the treatment periods giving rise to a "loss to follow-up" bias. While such patients are of obvious clinical importance, their data may be excluded from data analysis.
3. The interpretation of crossover studies may be compromised by carry-over or sequence effects. Conventionally, wash-out periods are included which take account of at least the known pharmacokinetics of compounds used. However, they may fail to take account for longer-term pharmacodynamic carry-over effects. Because crossover studies include relatively small numbers of patients they do not possess satisfactory power to exclude the presence of carry-over effects [27]. Sequence effects can be examined in studies that have more than two treatment periods, but once again the power to exclude sequence effects will be strictly limited.

Whilst it is not unreasonable to use crossover designs in explanatory clinical trials the assessments of treatment effects in epilepsy, which is a chronic condition, in studies which are by definition (because of the necessary crossover) short term, makes crossover designs of little practical clinical relevance. For this reason, there has been a steady switch to the use of parallel group studies even for regulatory purposes. Certainly, parallel group studies will always be the "gold standard" for studies seeking real clinical relevance.

Conditional Crossover Designs

Conditional crossover designs represent a hybrid between crossover and parallel group designs. Only patients judged not to respond to the randomised treatment during the first period are crossed over to the alternative treatment. This is said to represent an ethical compromise. There are, however, considerable difficulties with the statistical approach, which has not been widely tested [28], and considerable uncertainty about powering of these studies. Inevitably, those patients who do cross over are selected and not randomised. A study comparing valproate and ethosuximide in the treatment of absence seizures is an example of this design [29] and Loiseau [30] used a similar design in comparing carbamazepine and valproate in patients with newly diagnosed partial epilepsy.

Enrichment Designs

Enrichment designs are also conditional crossover studies but conversely only apparent responders are randomised [31]. This approach was used in a first study of a new AED, tiagabine [32]. All patients were exposed to open-label treatment with the drug as add-on therapy and the dose was titrated to a maximum tolerated dose. Following an observation period, patients showing a 25% or greater reduction in seizure frequency from the baseline period were then randomised to either continued treatment or withdrawal to placebo so as to test whether the apparent effect was due to a drug effect. This represents a very efficient design in ensuring that the initial patients providing information about dose tolerability of a drug can also contribute meaningful data on efficacy.

The difficulties with this type of study is that it can be very difficult to define the numbers of patients who will have to be exposed to open-label treatment to provide enough apparent responders for randomisation.

Pragmatic Clinical Trials

Pragmatic clinical trials, in contrast to explanatory studies, study treatment policies rather than limited questions of efficacy of a particular treatment. They seek to replicate everyday clinical practice and its uncertainties. Entry criteria are often based on clin-icians' varying "grey areas of uncertainty" and they therefore recruit more heterogeneous groups of patients. An example of a pragmatic clinical trial in epilepsy is the current MRC study of early epilepsy and single seizures. The aim of the study is to compare both short- and long-term outcomes of immediate versus deferred treatment in patients diagnosed with single seizures or epilepsy for the first time. This has now randomised over 1200 patients, making it the largest RCT in epilepsy. Clinicians are asked to randomise any patients whom they are uncertain whether they should treat. This includes individuals with single spontaneous seizures, with infrequent seizures, and those with seizures with minor symptomatology. Paediatricians become uncertain whether to treat after two or three seizures whereas neurologists with adult patients will usually be certain that they must treat after two or three seizures but be uncertain after a first or second seizure. At randomisation to immediate or deferred treatment the clinician is able to choose the drug that he or she regards as optimal for the individual patient and then uses the dose and the period of treatment that represent his or her usual clinical practice. The study is unblind. The MRC's study of AED withdrawal in patients with epilepsy in remission is another example of this type of trial [33].

Equivalence Trials

Whilst regulatory agencies may only feel confident to attribute efficacy to a treatment where the treatment shows a superiority (as judged by a statistically significant difference) over placebo or some active treatment, in clinical practice equivalence of outcome may be an important concept. It is certainly true that even relatively large comparative studies of AEDs find it difficult to differentiate between their efficacy [4,5]. Certainly, if a new AED were equivalent in efficacy to standard treatment but carried only half the risk of withdrawal for adverse effects then we would probably wish to use the new treatment in preference to the old. We would, however, want to be confident about equivalence of efficacy. In doing so we have to recognise that a failure to detect a difference is not the same thing as showing equivalence, the former commonly being due to inadequate powering of the study. Thus, when lamotrigine was compared with carbamazepine in newly diagnosed patients with epilepsy [34] no difference in efficacy between the doses of carbamazepine and lamotrigine used were detected. However, the hazard ratios for time to a first seizure in the study failed to exclude lamotrigine being 50% less efficacious in producing this outcome compared with carbamazepine.

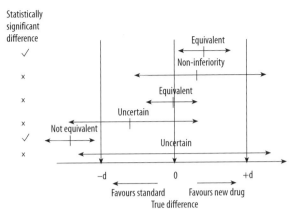

Fig. 21.1. Equivalence and definitions of minimally important differences.

Table 21.2. Example of equivalence trial power calculations

Number of patients required with an event rate of 70%			
Power (%)	Minimal important difference		
	5%	10%	20%
50%	1300	320	80
80%	2700	670	170
90%	3500	900	220
Number of Patients required with an event rate of 40%			
50%	1500	370	90
80%	3000	760	190
90%	4000	1000	250

Clinical trials can be structured and powered to establish equivalence for an outcome. The first requirement is that a clinical definition of equivalence is provided. Regulatory agencies commonly accept bio-equivalence when any difference of greater than ±20% for bio-availability can be excluded. At a clinical level we might, for instance, accept that two treatments are equivalent if we can exclude a 10% difference for a clinically important outcome such as rates at which patients become seizure-free. Clinical trials would then fulfil this requirement when the 95% confidence interval (CI) for a comparison between standard and new treatment was confined within either 0.9–1.1 (in the case of a ratio) or ±10% in the case of a difference (Fig. 21.1). More practically, it may be important to show that the new treatment is no more than 10% worse than the standard for a beneficial outcome such as efficacy non-inferiority.

Equivalence studies therefore differ from conventional difference studies in a number of important respects [35]:

* They are dependent on confidence intervals not on point estimates of difference.
* Intention-to-treat analysis is no longer conservative – protocol-correct samples should be compared.
* Poor trial design and conduct increase the likelihood of finding no difference but need to be excluded for there to be confidence about equivalence.
* They require larger numbers of patients (Table 21.2).

An example of an equivalence study is a new UK National Health Service R&D study to compare standard (carbamazepine and valproate) with new (lamotrigine, gabapentin and topiramate) AEDs. The study has been powered to detect equivalence between standard and new AEDs using a pragmatic trial design. For the seven different treatment groups in the study the requirement is for 450 patients per group.

It is likely that equivalence studies will steadily become more important in a number of fields of neurology. While the US Food and Drug Administration does not currently accept equivalence as proof of efficacy in the AED field, it does so in cancer chemotherapy and antibiotic studies where placebo controlled studies cannot ethically be undertaken.

Ethical Issues in Epilepsy RCTs

Ethical issues complicate the conduct of clinical trials in epilepsy. Basic ethical precepts do not allow people with active epilepsy to be untreated or to be exposed to only placebo preparations. This has led to considerable difficulties in proof of efficacy studies for different therapies. The AEDs Commission of the International League Against Epilepsy (ILAE) [36] has recommended that placebo-controlled add-on studies be used as initial proof of efficacy investigations. However, interpretation of such studies may be complicated by both pharmacokinetic and pharmacodynamic interactions. Further complications arise when subsequent actively controlled monotherapy studies are used to examine drug effects (see below).

Currently, most new AEDs will be licensed on the basis of placebo-controlled add-on studies in polytherapy. In the United States, the FDA historically has required evidence from two placebo-controlled trials before licensing a new compound for a particular indication. Most regulatory agencies have excluded comparative assessments against standard treatments from the regulatory process. More recently some governments have responded by requiring manufacturers to submit evidence on the comparative cost-effectiveness of their new drugs and those already used for the relevant indication.

The issue of placebo (and low-dose standard drug) controlled monotherapy studies in epilepsy is controversial, and there is increasing debate about the ethical problems of placebo controls in general [37]. The Declaration of Helsinki states unequivocally that "in any medical study, every patient – including those of a control group, if any – should be assured of the best proven diagnostic and therapeutic method". This appears to preclude placebo-controlled monotherapy trials in established epilepsy, in which the occurrence of seizures may carry risk of significant morbidity and even mortality.

It may be that placebo-controlled monotherapy studies could be undertaken ethically when genuine clinical uncertainty exists as to whether AED treatment was indicated, as might occur in the cases of patients presenting with first seizures [38] or in whom relatively few seizures occur over a prolonged time period, or in studies of patients at high risk for the development of epilepsy after head injury or neurosurgical procedures [39]. Similarly, in benign syndromes such as childhood absence epilepsy and benign Rolandic epilepsy, in which the need for active treatment in some subjects may be questioned, placebo-controlled studies might be justified. In every instance, the safety profile of a new AED should be such that it suggests a reasonable risk-benefit for the patient population.

In recent years, the FDA has accepted the use of a "low-dose standard drug" in clinical trials in which a "placebo" cannot be justified on ethical grounds. These studies randomise to what is believed to be a sub-optimal dose of an AED. It avoids the circumstances in which a patient who requires treatment is given none, but increases the chance that a difference will be detected between this arm and more optimal treatment arms. The reasoning behind this policy is that the outcome of a comparative clinical trial of a new versus a standard agent in full therapeutic doses may be difficult to interpret. Some argue that the failure to find a difference in efficacy between the two treatments does not necessarily mean that the new drug is as good as the standard drug, because the possibility that neither drug has efficacy cannot be excluded [40]. Only when a difference in favour of the test treatment is found can it be certain that the test drug has efficacy.

The most extreme examples of trials arising from this reasoning are exemplified by the presurgical paradigm. Here, patients undergoing drug withdrawal in order to record seizures for the purposes of localisation and lateralisation prior to surgery are randomised to treatment with test drug or placebo, after an adequate number of seizures have been recorded [41]. The patients are said to be protected by the use of a "time to exit" efficacy outcome. Thus patients leave the study after a number of days seizure-free, or after the occurrence of a first tonic-clonic seizure or, for example, a fourth partial seizure. Somewhat less dramatic, but as questionable, are withdrawal to monotherapy designs. In these, patients with active epilepsy who are not optimally treated with a single AED are randomised to treatment with possibly effective doses of a test drug or known suboptimal doses of a standard AED [42], or alternatively to much lower doses of the test drug. Again the primary outcome is a time to treatment "event" similar to the presurgical design.

Both these study designs are open to ethical criticism. Both fail to ensure that control patients receive optimal treatment, contrary to the Declaration of Helsinki (see above). Furthermore, the ethical requirement of equipoise [43] may be lacking, as the trials are transparently constructed with a bias to ensure that a difference is found for regulatory purposes, rather than to ask a clinically meaningful question about how an investigational drug might compare with existing optimal treatment.

One must recognise that difficulties arise in interpreting active control trials with a finding of no difference between the new drug and a recognised effective agent (active control) given at optimum doses. To be truly informative as proof of monotherapy efficacy, active control trials must have a sample size large enough to provide assurance that a clinically meaningful difference between the two treatments, if present, could have been detected (i.e. meet equivalence standard: see above) and be undertaken in a setting in which the active control has been regularly effective and for which it has been licensed by the regulatory agency to be effective and safe [44].

References

1. Coatsworth JJ. Studies on the clinical efficacy of marketed AEDs. Bethesda, MD: US Department of Health, 1971.
2. Gram L, Drachmann Bentsen K, Parnas J, Flachs H. Controlled trials in epilepsy: a review. Epilepsia 1982;23:491–519.
3. Marson AG, Chadwick DW. How easy are randomised controlled trials in epilepsy to find on medline? The sensitivity and precision of two Medline searches. Epilepsia 1996;37:377–380.
4. Mattson RH, Cramer JA, Collins JF, et al. Comparison of carbamazepine, phenobarbital, phenytoin and primidone in partial and secondary generalised seizures. N Engl J Med 1985;313:145–151.
5. Mattson RH, Cramer JA, Collins JF, et al. A comparison of valproate, with carbamazepine for the treatment of complex partial seizures and secondarily generalised tonic-clonic seizures in adults. N Engl J Med 1992;327:765–771.

6. Chiron C, Dumas C, Dulac O. Vigabatrin versus hydrocortisone as first line treatment for infantile spasms due to tuberous sclerosis. Epilepsy Res 1997;26:389–395.

7. Perucca E, Gram L, Avanzini G, Dulac O. AEDs as a cause of worsening of seizures. Epilepsia 1998;39:5–17.

8. UK Gabapentin Study Group. Gabapentin in partial epilepsy. Lancet 1990;335:1114–1117.

9. Hopkins A, Davies P, Dobson C. Mathematical models of patterns of seizures. Their use in the evaluation of drugs. Arch Neurol 1985;42:463–467.

10. Annegers JF, Hauser WA, Elveback LR. Remission of seizures and relapse in patients with epilepsy. Epilepsia 1979;20:729–737.

11. Turnbull SM, Howell D, Rawlins MD, Chadwick D. Which drug for the adult epileptic patient: phenytoin or valproate? BMJ 1985;290:815–819.

12. Shofer JB, Temkin NR. Comparisons of alternative outcome measures for AED trials. Arch Neurol 1986;43:877–881.

13. Spilker B, Segreti A. Validation of the phenomenon of regression of seizure frequency in epilepsy. Epilepsia 1984;25:443–449.

14. Marson AG, Kadir ZA, Hutton JL, Chadwick DW. The new AEDs: a systematic review of their efficacy and tolerability. Epilepsia 1997;38:859–880.

15. Smith DF, Baker GA, Dewey M, Jacoby A, Chadwick D. Seizure frequency, patient perceived seizure severity and the psychosocial consequences of intractable epilepsy. Epilepsy Res 1991;9:231–241.

16. Commission on Classification and Terminology of ILAE. Proposal for revised clinical and electroencephalographic classification of epileptic seizures. Epilepsia 1981;22:489–501.

17. Baker GA, Smith DF, Dewey M, Morrow J, Crawford P, Chadwick D. The development of a seizure severity scale as an outcome measure in epilepsy. Epilepsy Res 1991;8:245–251.

18. Duncan JS, Sander JWAS. The Chalfont seizure severity scale. J Neurol Neurosurg Psychiatry 1991;54:873–876.

19. Jacoby A. Assessing quality of life in patients with epilepsy. Pharmaco Economics 1996;9:399–416.

20. Wagner AK; Keller SD, Kosinski M, Baker GA, Jacoby A, Husu M-A, et al. Advances in methods for assessing the impact of epilepsy and antiepileptic drug therapy on patient's health-related quality of life. Quality Life Res 1995;4:115–134.

21. Jacoby A, Baker GA, Steen N, Potts P, Chadwick DW. The clinical course of epilepsy and its psychosocial correlates: findings from a UK Community Study. Epilepsia 1996;37:148–161.

22. Cockerell OC, Hart YM, Sander JWAS, et al. The cost of epilepsy in the United Kingdom: an estimation based on the results of two population-based studies. Epilepsy Res 1994;18:249–260.

23. Jacoby A, Buck D, Baker G, McNamee P, Graham-Jones S, Chadwick D. Uptake and costs of care for epilepsy: findings from a UK regional study. Epilepsia 1998;39:776–786.

24. Cramer JA, Smith DB, Mattson RH, et al. A method of quantification for the evaluation of AED therapy. Neurology 1983;33(Suppl 1):26–37.

25. US Gabapentin Study Group. Gabapentin as add-on therapy in refractory partial epilepsy: a double-blind, placebo-controlled, parallel-group study. Neurology 1993;43:228–229.

26. Hill AB. Medical ethics and controlled trials. BMJ 1963;I:1043–1049.

27. Hills M, Armitage P. The two-period crossover clinical trial. Br J Clin Pharmacol 1979;8:7–20.

28. White BG. A class of ethical designs for controlled clinical trials. Doctoral dissertation. Johns Hopkins University, Baltimore, MD, 1979.

29. Sato S, White BG, Penry JK, Dreifuss FE, Sackellares JC, Kupferberg HJ. Valproic acid versus ethosuximide in the treatment of absence seizures. Neurology 1982;32:157–163.

30. Loiseau P. Rational use of valproate: indications and drug regimen in epilepsy: Epilepsia 1984;25(Suppl 1):565–572.

31. Amery W, Dony J. A clinical trial design avoiding undue placebo treatment: J Clin Pharmacol 1975;15:674–769.

32. Richens A, Chadwick D, Duncan JS, Dam M, Gram L, Mikkelsen M, et al. Adjunctive treatment of partial seizures with Tiagabine: A placebo-controlled trial. Epilepsy Res 1995;21:37–42.

33. MRC Antiepileptic Drug Withdrawal Study Group. Randomised study of AED withdrawal in patients in remission. Lancet 1991;337:1175–1180.

34. Brodie MJ, Richens A, Yuen AWC. Double-blind comparison of lamotrigine and carbamazepine in newly diagnosed epilepsy. Lancet 1995;345:476–479.

35. Jones B, Jarvis P, Lewis JA. Trials to assess equivalence: the importance of rigorous methods. BMJ 1996;313:1169–1176.

36. Commission on Antiepileptic Drugs. Guidelines for the clinical evaluation of AEDs. Epilepsia 1989;30:400–406.

37. Rothman KJ, Michels KB. The continuing unethical use of placebo controls. N Engl J Med 1994;331:394–398.

38. First Seizure Trial Group (FIR.S.T. Group). Randomised clinical trial on the efficacy of AEDs in reducing the risk of relapse after a first unprovoked tonic-clonic seizure. Neurology 1993;43:478–483.

39. Temkin NR, Dikmen SS, Wilensky AJ, Keihm J, Chabal S, Winn HR. A randomised double-blind study of phenytoin for the prevention of post-traumatic seizures. N Engl J Med 1990;323:497–502.

40. Leber PD. Hazards of inference: the active control investigation. Epilepsia 1989;30(Suppl 1):S57–S63.

41. Bourgoise B, Leppik IE, Sackellares JC, et al. Felbamate: a double-blind controlled trial in patients undergoing presurgical evaluation of partial seizures. Neurology 1993;43:693–696.

42. Faught E, Sachdeo RC, Remler MP, et al. Felbamate monotherapy for partial onset seizures: an active control trial. Neurology 1993;43:688–692.

43. Freedman B. Equipoise and the ethics of clinical research. N Engl J Med 1987;317:141–145.

44. ILAE Commission on AEDs. Considerations on designing clinical trials to evaluate the place of new AEDs in the treatment of newly diagnosed and chronic patients with epilepsy. Epilepsia 1998;39:799–803.

22. Headache: Ethics, Outcome Variables and Clinical Studies

R. Peatfield

Introduction

There have been an enormous number of clinical trials in headache in recent years, largely as a result of the introduction of the International Headache Society diagnostic criteria for headache [1], and the development of 5-hydroxytryptamine (5HT) agonists for acute treatment, originally by one company. Interested readers are referred to an authoritative multi-author text that has recently been published [2].

This chapter will be concerned principally with functional-type headaches including migraine, cluster headache and tension-type headache. Clinical assessment and particularly recruitment for drug trials must involve the exclusion of major structural causes of headache, which include temporal arteritis, sinusitis, cervical spondylosis and post-traumatic headache; and also rarer causes (most commonly seen in emergency situations) such as subarachnoid haemorrhage and meningitis [3,4]. The treatment of these conditions is usually well established and seldom so contentious. It would be very difficult on ethical grounds, for example, to justify a trial of an alternative treatment for temporal arteritis with its risk of blindness.

Headache is a particularly subjective symptom in which the patient's description is all important, and there are no simple parameters that can be measured anatomically or radiologically. Clinicians will appreciate that the investigation of a headache patient is always intended to exclude alternative diagnoses rather than to confirm that of migraine. Clinical trials, therefore, are wholly dependent on the patient's own account of the frequency and severity of their attacks. There is a high placebo response rate in any reassuring clinical environment, which precludes meaningful open or single-blind studies except in the very earliest stages of the assessment of a new drug, and trials must have controls of some kind – it has been argued extensively that placebo-treated patients are

required at least until the earliest phase III studies [5]. Patients often seek advice for their headaches when they are at their worst, and there is a high spontaneous response rate reflecting the natural fluctuation in the frequency of attacks over months; this is particularly marked in children, in whom the improvement rate in placebo-treated patients can be so high (e.g. Forsythe et al. [6]) as to make the demonstration of statistically significant further improvement with active treatment very difficult.

Headache is among the most subjective symptoms experienced by patients; there is no simple parameter that can be measured, and assessment is totally dependent on the patient's description of their pain, which is necessarily imprecise. Absenteeism from work can be measured accurately, but loss of efficacy at work, which is much more difficult to quantify, has been shown to be about twice as significant [7].

Definition of Migraine

The definition of migraine was a particularly contentious subject until the working party of the International Headache Society published its report in 1988 [1]. Many early definitions, for example that of the Ad Hoc Committee of 1962 [8], were too vague to be useful in clinical trials at all, and there were significant difficulties with even the best definitions at the time, such as those of Vahlquist [9]. The populations studied in early trials may well be very different if a variety of diagnostic criteria were used, and in some cases these are not even made clear.

The International Headache Society criteria [1] have proved very effective in producing a defined group of patients with undoubted migraine; there is, of course, a substantial overlap with previous criteria such as those of Vahlquist [9], though the latter does tend to permit a few more patients to be diagnosed as suffering from migraine [10]. It must always be emphasised that epidemiological evidence suggests many if not most benign headache syndromes lie on a continuum with similar pathophysiology, and that the imposition of diagnostic criteria is of little relevance for routine clinical diagnosis and treatment. Migraine with aura (formerly known as classical migraine) is much less frequent than migraine without aura, though it is much easier to diagnose unequivocally [1]. It has previously been suggested that trials should be done on only one or other type of migraine, but the question of their applicability to other headache patients would then have to be raised, and it is probably better to recruit patients both with and without aura to trials, though they could be stratified. The International Headache Society has developed diagnostic criteria for cluster headache and for tension type headache [1], though it has to be admitted that all these diagnoses are still dependent on the subjective observations of the patient.

Intended Audience

When planning, performing or assessing drug trials one of the most important single considerations is the intended audience of the final report. Is the trial, for example, designed to assess efficacy and safety, specifically for regulatory authorities such as the US Food and Drug Administration or the corresponding panels in Europe, or is it intended to provide practical guidance to neurologists or general practitioners? Most trials are designed on an "intention-to-treat" basis as it is difficult to assess compliance with any reliability. Such trials, of course, give guidance to practising doctors but are perhaps less helpful in the assessment of a drug's toxicity for the regulatory authorities. There is always an uneasy balance between statistically and clinically significant results. Trials designed to satisfy regulatory authorities tend to be more concerned with whether a drug is effective in contrast to placebo, rather than with providing guidance as to whether it has advantages over existing therapies; phase III trials of *this* kind tend to be produced relatively late and are more often inconclusive because they have to be very much larger to show any significant difference between two effective therapies. Cost-effectiveness, and particularly cost advantages over existing therapies, has not been the concern of regulatory authorities, but is becoming of increasing interest to funding authorities worldwide.

Where a Trial Is Best Done

Most of the early trials in migraine were undertaken in specialist clinics. These tend to attract a hard core of intractable patients, and trial results may not have reflected the value of the drug in less highly selected patients. Although most trial protocols exclude patients who have participated in more than one previous trial it is probably better for patients to be recruited from general neurology clinics or general practice, though very large numbers of centres may need to be involved to obtain adequate numbers under these circumstances. Patients recruited from employers, general practice registers and particularly patients' self-help organisations may again be unrepresentative.

Ethical Aspects

It is not difficult to offer a placebo to migraine patients as the condition is not life-threatening. Many ethical issues can therefore be ignored, but others are thrown into sharper relief. The question, for example, of withholding successful treatment in order to start an alternative within a trial is difficult. Many patients would have to have effective treatment discontinued in order to enter a trial at all, or to start the second phase of a cross-over study.

Trials of acute treatment undertaken in hospital require patients to travel while suffering a headache; not all potential subjects may be willing to do so, particularly if they are not allowed to take any analgesia before arrival. All such trials should allow rescue medication, which may have to be given at a time when the response to placebo is still of at least potential interest.

If a trial does not include a placebo treatment group we cannot be sure either treatment is effective; whereas if it does, some patients will be left untreated.

Analgesia for Migraine

Medication for migraine is traditionally divided into treatment for acute attacks and that given to prevent attacks [5]. In recent years most of the trial work has been undertaken with analgesic agents, particularly following the very large trial programme undertaken by Glaxo before the introduction of sumatriptan [11].

Even with the use of the International Headache Society criteria for patient selection other parameters may prove contentious. Does one, for example, treat the patients in hospital or allow the patients to take treatment home, in which case they are likely to start treatment earlier in the attacks and may be treating potentially milder attacks? Is it wholly ethical to expect a patient to struggle to hospital in the middle of an attack, and then expect them to respond to treatment? The prior frequency of the attacks will need to be specified in the protocol; patients experiencing many more than 4 to 6 attacks each month may have atypical migraine; and the trial will become very prolonged if patients having attacks much less frequently than once a month are recruited, particularly as headache frequency tends to fall immediately after any patient has been assessed and reassured in an outpatient clinic. Trials should be undertaken in both sexes, covering as wide an age range as possible, conventionally 18–65 years. Separate trials may have to be undertaken later in adolescents and younger children; most pharmaceutical companies seem to feel there are too few patients over the age of 65 years in the population to justify a separate trial. Patients abusing alcohol or medications such as codeine, and those on antipsychotic and antidepressant medication, will need to be excluded, as well as pregnant women, and those with the usual range of general medical illnesses. The earlier phase II studies may need to use a very wide range of different doses to ensure that the dose range at which the clinical effect levels off can be established.

Outcome Variables

A wide variety of outcome variables were used in trials before Glaxo's sumatriptan programme. Most of these trials were very small, and the different variables make direct comparisons difficult, particularly as so many are dependent on the patients' subjective observations. Some trials, for example, state the mean percentage improvement, and others the proportion of patients who have improved more than 50%, which, it will be appreciated, is itself a vague parameter. Quantitative severity scales add further complexity and are felt to lack discriminatory power. Most trials have assessed the patients 2 h after taking treatment and some after 1 h as well – it is argued that 2 h is as long as a patient can be expected to endure a headache without the opportunity to take open escape medication. The quantitation of escape medication consumption is also used as a variable in some trials. Any trial using excessively complex quantitation is likely to have difficulty distinguishing a drug which has a mild effect on all patients from one which cures a minority, and which might, therefore, have a more significant role in routine practice.

In setting up their large assessment programme for sumatriptan, which has been a model for subsequent drug trials, Glaxo were aware of these difficulties and decided that they would only expect the patients to classify their attacks on a 4-point scale (none, mild, moderate or severe), defining those

criteria in terms of the patient's ability to function normally, or at all. The formal end-point was then the proportion of patients with a moderate or severe headache, at the time the medication was taken whose headache was mild or absent 2 h later. The trial also assessed the patients who were pain-free after 2 h, and made a similar assessment at 1 h. This design gives the advantage of producing ordinal rather than continuous data, but it makes it very difficult to assess the speed of clinical response, particularly during the first hour. The recurrence of headache after about 12 h is a substantial problem with sumatriptan, and it has been argued that counting patients who are "pain free without a later recurrence" at each end-point may be better [5,12].

Glaxo's trial design lends itself to straightforward statistical analysis (using, for example, Mantel–Haenszel chi-squared tests or linear regression) and it has become widely established for other drug companies developing alternative $5HT_{1D}$ receptor agonists, particularly as there is a need for a uniform trial design in order to produce comparative figures, which will become more necessary as these drugs are marketed. This has, of course, inhibited the development of alternative trial designs, and it is difficult to envisage substantial modifications gaining acceptance at present.

It was decided that the trials of sumatriptan would be of a parallel group rather than cross-over design because of the short-lived but definite side-effects that most patients receiving sumatriptan experienced. These include widespread paraesthesiae and ill-defined pressure sensations on the head, which are considered trivial in clinical practice but which would soon indicate to patients which drug they were receiving.

Prophylaxis of Migraine

Very few prophylactic trials have been published recently because of the great emphasis on $5HT_{1D}$ agonists. These drugs still have a major role in the management of patients with relatively frequent attacks, a common threshold being 2 per month. There is an enormous literature establishing the efficacy of such agents as methysergide, pizotifen, propranolol, amitriptyline and valproate, to take the agents in the chronological order of their development (Table 22.1) [13,14]. For example, a major recent trial of sodium valproate in patients who had had at least 2 attacks per month for the previous 3 months [15] used a 4-week single-blind run-in period, followed by a 12-week parallel group design. The mean headache frequency per month was 3.5 in those on valproate and 5.7 in those on placebo, while 48% of those on valproate and 14% of those on placebo experienced a 50% or greater reduction in headache frequency from the baseline phase.

No single trial format has been universally used in these trials, which is in complete contrast to the analgesia trials set up by Glaxo. A wide variety of different measurements have been used, and it has to be admitted that most of these are in some way imperfect [5]. Patients in the past have been recruited using a number of different definitions of migraine, though more recent trials have all used the International Headache Society criteria. The range of pre-trial headache frequency acceptable for recruitment has varied between trials; most suggest between 2 and 8 per month, and it has been recommended that these patients are stratified by baseline severity. Measurement of improvement is controversial, trials having measured attack frequency, duration and severity as well as indices and rating scales of various kinds, though a more recent authoritative discussion does not recommend these [5]. Even the assessment of frequency can prove inconsistent, particularly when some patients have relatively prolonged attacks, sometimes with recrudescences. If the absolute frequency count is recorded patients with a high attack frequency it may make a disproportionate contribution to the total reduction, whereas the reverse is true if some calculation of percentage reduction is used instead. It is possible to analyse many of the trials to determine the percentage experiencing a 50% or greater reduction in headache frequency either from the baseline phase or compared with a control group (Table 22.1).

It has been customary to offer prophylactic treatment for a minimum period of 3 months, as some drugs (particularly the calcium antagonist flunarizine, which is not available in many countries) seem to take at least as long as this to produce benefit as a result of their high lipid solubility. One has to question whether trials that record headaches over a longer period would adequately reflect normal

clinical practice. Some trials have used a placebo run-in period, usually single-blind, to try to establish a consistent headache frequency once the effect of the initial reassurance has passed, but most patients with migraine tend to improve and it can be argued that this is likely to confound interpretations of the results of longer trials.

Pharmacological Basis of Prophylaxis

Up to now there has been a tendency for each major group of drugs, almost regardless of its primary pharmacological basis, to be tried in migraine patients if only in a small trial. Several recent publications, notably that of Schmuck et al. [16], have attempted to explore the pharmacological basis of prophylaxis, demonstrating that there is a reasonable correlation between affinity of drugs at the $5HT_{2B}$ receptor and the doses conventionally required to suppress migraine. This reasoning needs to be pursued further with newer drugs developed specifically for their affinity at this receptor.

Cross-over or Parallel Group Design?

Even the most authoritative committees of the International Headache Society disagree on the relative merits of trials with cross-over or parallel group designs [5,17,18]. Cross-over studies are said to be 8 times more powerful than parallel group designs for the same number of patients, so it is difficult to envisage a parallel group trial of appropriate size being assembled from a single headache treatment centre. Although so much easier to organise and evaluate, cross-over studies have problems: the relatively prolonged study time of each individual patient will accentuate the period effect, so that the second treatment tried will often seem the more effective. Even a relatively prolonged washout period between the treatments (which would itself accentuate the drop-out rate) may not totally account for any carry-over effect from the first treatment. Evaluation of drug efficacy is, of course, more difficult, particularly in trials comparing two active treatments. Many authorities have questioned the ethics of testing a second treatment when the first proved effective, and certainly differential drop-outs may create bias. As with sumatriptan the presence of side-effects (for example bradycardia with beta blockers) may invalidate the blinding of the trial.

Compliance

The topic of compliance is seldom addressed in major trials, though it is by definition of less rele-

Table 22.1.   Migraine prophylactic medication

	Dose used in trials (mg)	Cost per month (£)	% of patients likely to make a 50% improvement compared with placebo
Propranolol	240	0.63	34
Atenolol	100	1.50	33
Pizotifen	3	15.56	28
Methysergide	6	16.08	30
Valproate	1000	9.60	34
Amitriptyline	c. 100	0.59	32

vance in pragmatic, "intention-to-treat" studies. It is difficult to monitor: one can require the patient to return unused tablets for counting (assuming they are not aware of the purpose of this), and for many agents a drug level or a physiological parameter, such as the pulse rate, can be measured. Pfaffenrath et al. [19], in a trial of amitriptyline in tension headache, added riboflavin to all the tablets as a marker substance, but they do not give the results in any detail. Steiner et al. [20] used pill boxes fitted with a device which recorded every time they were opened; in their study there were only 4 evaluable patients, who actually took the medication three times daily as instructed on only between 16% and 79% of days. This emphasises the unreliability of pill taking in most if not all of the population. Compliance is likely to be a much bigger problem in trials comparing active treatments, when it may be different in different patient groups according to the side-effects. A high drop-out rate in any trial can invalidate its conclusions, particularly if it varies between patient groups.

Cluster Headache

Although good trials have been done of inhaled oxygen [21] and subcutaneous sumatriptan [22,23] for the acute management of cluster pain, the most effective medication for this condition is prophylactic [24]. The placebo effect is believed to be small, but it is thought that placebos can be justified if only for a short period, perhaps a week or so. In cluster headache it is particularly important to control for the natural history of the attacks, and it is now recommended that patients should only be recruited if their bouts of pains can be expected to last for at least a month [25]. A good controlled trial has been published on the use of verapamil for the prevention of this condition [26]; the evidence in favour of corticosteroids, lithium, methysergide and ergotamine is rather older and less secure [24,27].

Tension-Type Headache

Tension-type headache is far more prevalent in the general population, but the sheer difficulty of designing adequate trials has meant that very few have been published [28]. Many of these patients have continuous pain and there is therefore no headache frequency to measure [29]. Trials have been undertaken of both acute and prophylactic treatment; for analgesics visual analogue scales correlate well with verbal rating scales and global ratings [30]. In one

trial, for example, Schachtel and Thoden [31] compared 400 mg ibuprofen with placebo in 70 patients with episodic tension-type headaches using a visual analogue scale. They were able to show a clear, statistically significant discrimination after 15 min, which was more marked at 30 min and later. Surprisingly little spontaneous improvement, however, was seen in the placebo-treated group, even after 2 h. Similar trials, again using rating scales, have confirmed the superiority of naproxen over paracetamol or placebo.

Prophylaxis is even more difficult to assess; simple assessment of the number of headache days can conceal too wide a spectrum of severity to be valid, particularly as many are relatively mild. Visual analogue scales may also conceal useful information. Trials of amitriptyline and other tricyclics are reviewed by Couch and Micieli [32]. More recently, in a trial in 40 patients with chronic tension-type headache, the selective serotonin reuptake inhibitor citalopram did not prove as effective as amitriptyline [33].

Further Difficulties

A major topic in clinical headache research is the proper independence of the trialists from commercial influences. The largest trials have all been sponsored by industry, and great expertise has been established within several pharmaceutical companies. This has required the pooling of data from many centres working to a common protocol, which makes it difficult for participants to have any say in the design of the study. In many studies the data are analysed centrally and their objectivity may be open to question. The World Federation Research Group on Migraine and Headache feels that independent assessment and statistical analysis are essential to ensure that trials are not unduly influenced by commercial considerations. It remains important to ensure that negative trials are also published. Trials should be published in peer-reviewed journals rather than sponsor's supplements which often preclude any independent assessment of the data. Partial publications by individual centres and the re-publication of results as more patients are accrued are also potential difficulties.

Unanswered Questions

There are a number of clinical questions which regularly tax the practising neurologist undertaking the routine care of patients complaining of headache, over and above the obvious quests for a more rapid and effective analgesic agents, and for the perfect prophylactic agent which suppresses all attacks without side-effects.

Analgesic Abuse

The anecdotal clinical evidence in favour of analgesic abuse is now overwhelming. It has been recognised for many years that taking ergotamine on a daily basis can perpetuate headache, and patients are much improved if this drug is discontinued [34]. The same seems to apply to codeine- and perhaps caffeine-containing analgesics as well, though the pharmacological basis of this is poorly understood. Analgesic abuse is probably the most common cause of secondary chronic headache in migraine patients [35,36]. The benefits of withdrawal of codeine-containing drugs has never been proven by a double-blind trial, though this could easily be undertaken with double-blind placebo substitution in a proportion of the patients. Clearly all these patients have benefited from reassurance and the offering of alternative analgesic drugs, but the effect of discontinuing codeine alone, while still taking all other medication, should be the subject of a clinical trial.

The Contraceptive Pill

Many women report that their headaches are worsened by the contraceptive pill, and it is standard practice to suggest that the pill is discontinued in patients who have sought advice about their headaches. This applies particularly if they have focal cortical symptoms, as there is believed to be an increased risk of cerebral infarctions under these circumstances [37]. No formal study of this has been undertaken, nor of alternative methods of contraception such as the progesterone-only pill which seems, anecdotally at least, to have an intermediate risk of exacerbating migrainous headaches. It would be difficult to arrange a trial in which the progesterone-only pill or a placebo was substituted for the combined pill on a double-blind basis, as one cannot imagine many patients co-operating with the necessary contraceptive precautions. The benefit of stopping the combined contraceptive pill may be delayed and the social and personal disadvantages are obvious – one may question the ethics of insisting the patient stop the pill before starting prophylactic treatment, but one may equally question whether it is appropriate to give prophylaxis to patients remaining on an agent which so often seems to be the major cause of their headaches. Should prophylactic trials be stratified into patients who are and are not taking the pill?

Conclusions

Headache is perhaps the most subjective neurological symptom and therefore the most difficult to analyse in the context of a clinical trial. There can be no doubt from the enormous number of headache trials in the published literature, however, that many treatments are effective, and yet there is ample scope to provide better treatment both analgesic and prophylactic. Although all these trials are open to criticisms of various kinds it is important to provide the best data available for the practising clinician, even if it is imperfect.

References

1. Headache Classification Committee of the International Headache Society. Classification and diagnostic criteria for headache disorders, cranial neuralgias and facial pain. Cephalalgia 1988;8(Suppl 7).
2. Olesen J, Tfelt-Hansen P (eds). Headache treatment: trial methodology and new drugs. New York: Lippincott-Raven, 1997.
3. Peatfield R. Headache. Berlin: Springer, 1986.
4. Silberstein SD, Lipton RB, Goadsby PJ. Headache in clinical practice. Oxford: ISIS Medical Media, 1998.
5. IHS Committee on Clinical Trials in Migraine. Guidelines for controlled trials of drugs in migraine. Cephalalgia 1991; 11:1–12.
6. Forsythe WI, Gillies D, Sills MA. Propranolol ("Inderal") in the treatment of childhood migraine. Dev Med Child Neurol 1984;26:737–741.
7. Lipton RB, Stewart WF, von Korff M. Burden of migraine: societal costs and therapeutic opportunities. Neurology 1997; 48(Suppl 3):4–9.
8. Ad Hoc Committee. Classification of headache. JAMA 1962;179:717–718.
9. Vahlquist B. Migraine in children. Int Arch Allergy 1955; 7:348–355.
10. Metsähonkala L, Sillanpää M. Migraine in children: an evaluation of the IHS criteria. Cephalalgia 1994;14:285–290.
11. Pilgrim AJ. Methodology of clinical trials of sumatriptan in migraine and cluster headache. Eur Neurol 1991;31:295–299.
12. Goadsby PJ. A triptan too far? J Neurol Neurosurg Psychiatry 1998;64:143–147.
13. Olesen J, Tfelt-Hansen P. Methodology of clinical trials in migraine. In: Capildeo R, Orgogozo JM, editors. Methods in clinical trials in neurology: vascular and degenerative brain disease. London: Stockton Press, 1988:85–109.
14. Tfelt-Hansen P, Olesen J. Methodological aspects of drug trials in migraine. Neuroepidemiology 1985;4:204–226.
15. Mathew NT, Saper JR, Silberstein SD, Rankin L, Markley HG, Solomon S, et al. Migraine prophylaxis with divalproex. Arch Neurol 1995;52:281–286.
16. Schmuck K, Ullmer C, Kalkman HO, Probst A, Lübbert H. Activation of meningeal 5-HT$_{2B}$ receptors: an early step in the generation of migraine headache? Eur J Neurosci 1996;8:959–967.
17. Lewis JA. Migraine trials: crossover or parallel group? Neuroepidemiology 1987;6:198–208.
18. Jones B, Lewis JA. Cross-over trials versus parallel-group trials. In: Olesen J, Tfelt-Hansen P, editors. Headache treat-

ment: trial methodology and new drugs. Philadelphia: Lippincott-Raven, 1997:35–43.

19. Pfaffenrath V, Diener H-C, Isler H, Meyer C, Scholz E, Taneri Z, et al. Efficacy and tolerability of amitriptylinoxide in the treatment of chronic tension-type headache: a multi-centre controlled study. Cephalalgia 1994;14:149–155.

20. Steiner TJ, Catarci T, Hering R, Whitmarsh T, Courturier EGM. If migraine prophylaxis does not work, think about compliance. Cephalalgia 1994;14:463–464.

21. Fogan L. Treatment of cluster headache: a double-blind comparison of oxygen vs air inhalation. Arch Neurol 1985;42: 362–363.

22. Sumatriptan Cluster Headache Study Group. Treatment of acute cluster headache with sumatriptan. N Engl J Med 1991;325:322–326.

23. Ekbom K. Treatment of cluster headache: clinical trials, design and results. Cephalalgia 1995;Suppl 15:33–36.

24. Krabbe AA. Cluster headache: a review. Acta Neurol Scand 1986;74:1–9.

25. International Headache Society Committee on Clinical Trials in Cluster Headache. Guidelines for controlled trials of drugs in cluster headache. Cephalalgia 1995;15:452–462.

26. Bussone G, Leone M, Peccarisi C, Micieli G, Granella F, Magri M, et al. Double blind comparison of lithium and verapamil in cluster headache prophylaxis. Headache 1990;30:411–417.

27. de Carolis P, de Capoa D, Agati R, Baldrati A, Sacquegna T. Episodic cluster headache: short and long term results of prophylactic treatment. Headache 1988;28:475–476.

28. International Headache Society Committee on Clinical Trials. Guidelines for trials of drug treatments in tension-type headache. Cephalalgia 1995;15:165–279.

29. Göbel H, Hamouz V, Hansen C, Heininger K, Hirsch S, Lindner V, et al. Chronic tension-type headache: amitriptyline reduces clinical headache-duration and experimental pain sensitivity but does not alter pericranial muscle activity readings. Pain 1994;59:241–249.

30. Mathew NT. Tension-type headache, cluster headache, and miscellaneous headaches: acute pharmacotherapy. In: Olesen J, Tfelt-Hansen P, Welch KMA, editors. The headaches. New York: Raven Press, 1993:531–536.

31. Schachtel BP, Thoden WR. Onset of action of ibuprofen in the treatment of muscle-contraction headache. Headache 1988;28: 471–474.

32. Couch JR, Micieli G. Prophylactic pharmacotherapy. In: Olesen J, Tfelt-Hansen P, Welch KMA, editors. The headaches. New York: Raven Press, 1993.

33. Bendtsen L, Jensen R, Olesen J. A non-selective (amitriptyline), but not a selective (citalopram), serotonin reuptake inhibitor is effective in the prophylactic treatment of chronic tension-type headache. J Neurol Neurosurg Psychiatry 1996;61:285–290.

34. Meyler WJ. Side effects of ergotamine. Cephalalgia 1996; 16:5–10.

35. Pfaffenrath V, Niederberger U. What kind of drugs are taken by patients with primary headaches? In: Diener H-C, Wilkinson M, editors. Drug-induced headache. Berlin: Springer, 1988:44–62.

36. Walker J, Parisi S, Olive D. Analgesic rebound headache: experience in a community hospital. South Med J 1993;86: 1202–1205.

37. Tzourio C, Tehindrazanarivelo A, Iglésias S, Alpérovitch A, Chedru F, d'Anglejan-Chatillon J, et al. Case-control study of migraine and risk of ischaemic stroke in young women. BMJ 1995;310:830–834.

23. Headache: Basic Trial Designs, Sample Sizes and Pitfalls

H. Angus-Leppan

Introduction

In clinical trials in headache research, the primary question – can we get rid of the headache? – seems simple but is complex. There are general issues involved in all clinical trials, and specific issues in headache research affecting trial design, sample size, analysis and interpretation of results. These confounding issues are introduced first. Specific designs, and their potential role in headache trials, are discussed and illustrated next, with reference to the guidelines of the International Headache Society (IHS) on trial design. A discussion on determination of sample size follows. Finally, pitfalls in design, analysis and interpretation are highlighted, with examples.

Confounding Issues

This section summarises specific issues to be considered in designing headache trials. These include definition and classification of headache, treatment modalities and specific ethical issues.

Defining Headache and Headache Types

Headache is a subjective experience and most headaches do not have a well-defined cause. There are no objective measures or specific investigations for migraine and tension-type headaches, the most common types. Definitions are purely descriptive. Attempts to reach consensus on headache classification date back to at least 1962 [1]. A detailed attempt to classify headache, allow structured and detailed analysis and facilitate accurate comparison within and between trials comes from the widely used IHS classification [2], due for revision in 2000. This classification has spawned dozens of papers pointing out its deficiencies and exceptions (for example [3]), as

well as potential sources of unreliability [4]. For migraine, the IHS definitions are detailed and rigid, and do not address the issue of "interval headaches" – those occurring between headaches defined as migraine [2].

Types of Headache Examined in Trials

Headaches cover the full spectrum of disease severity, prognosis, mortality and morbidity. The majority of headaches are benign but have no specific aetiology. Acute headache, associated with life-threatening conditions such as subarachnoid haemorrhage and meningitis, requires emergency treatment of the underlying cause. When correctly diagnosed, such groups are fairly homogeneous. The time scale of treatment, modalities used and outcome measures (for example mortality) are very different from those appropriate for benign chronic or intermittent headache. Other headaches are self-limiting and little studied, such as headache associated with an acute viral illness.

Difficulties arise in studies of heterogeneous headaches as a single group, when they have been linked because they share a trigger or one feature in common. For example, post-ictal headaches may be due to migraine, minor trauma, major trauma, or to the underlying cause of the seizure, such as tumour. It will be difficult to draw any conclusions from treatment studies in such a group. Similar problems arise in studies of headache following lumbar puncture [5] and headaches in patients with HIV infection [6].

Treatment Modalities and Timing

Potential treatment modalities in headache include oral and parenteral medications, "alternative medicines", physical therapies such as physiotherapy, acupuncture, aromatherapy, reflexology, behavioural therapy and biofeedback techniques (Table 23.1).

Table 23.1. Modalities of treatment in headache research

Medications
"Alternative" medicines
   Herbal medicines
   Homeopathy
Physical therapies
   Physiotherapy
   Acupuncture
   Aromatherapy
   Reflexology
Behavioural therapy/biofeedback
Psychotherapy

Table 23.2. Grading of headache severity

0 = no headache
1 = mild headache, allowing normal activity
2 = moderate headache, disturbing but not prohibiting normal activity; bed rest is not necessary
3 = severe headache, normal activity has to be discontinued; bed rest may be necessary

As recommended in IHS guidelines [2].

Most trials have studied medications, although alternative medicines are also widely used [7] and headache is a very common reason for people to use herbal remedies [8].

The timing of treatment influences the design: Is the treatment primary, rescue or prophylactic?

Outcome Measures

The principal aim of treatment is headache relief, which can only be measured by report, and must be subjective. Total headache relief is the most obvious primary outcome measure. The IHS subcommittee on clinical trials in migraine recently suggested that pain-free response at 2 h should be the primary efficacy parameter in migraine trials [9]. This committee commented also that complete response (defined as no headache at 2 h and no recurrence or drug intake within 24 h) was a parameter with low power, despite being an intuitively useful clinical measure.

Many studies use a grading system recommended by the IHS committee (Table 23.2). Success is often graded on a 4-point scale of headache pain: as none, mild, moderate or severe [10]. Some studies have used the grading scale and do not define relief or headache recurrence in absolute terms. For example, in Winner et al. [11], headache relief is defined as none or mild, and recurrence as an increase in severity of pain (from a state of relief, that is mild or no pain) at least 2 h after discharge from the clinic. This affects the power of the study, the statistical measures appropriate and the accuracy of self-reporting. In short, the non-linear grading system means that power is reduced and non-parametric statistics should be used. It is likely that self-reporting may be more variable with the grading system than it would be with a dichotomous (yes–no) system. Comparisons between trials, and in particular meta-analysis, are complicated by the differences in measures used.

If the headache grading system is coupled with a functional measure, as recommended by the IHS guidelines, the two internal measures may not always correlate. For example this grading scheme defines "mild" as "mild headache with little functional disability". There may be circumstances where the headache is mild but the clinical disability severe, and then the grading system is problematic. In many trials, the headache pain grading is used without the functional measure.

In attempts to make outcome measures more robust, secondary and surrogate outcome measures have been studied. Some of these are clinically based measures, aimed to increase validity, for example functional status [12]. These measures have not been rigorously evaluated or standardised. Some measures are physiological. The more objective these surrogate measures, the further removed they become from the starting problem and aim, and questions of validity arise. For example, the nitrous oxide model of induced headache with monitoring of cerebral blood flow [13] allows recording of an objective change (dilatation of temporal, radial and middle cerebral arteries). However, this model is not directly correlated with spontaneous headache. Peripheral vascular effects have been used to assess the effects of anti-migraine drugs, on the basis that serotonin agonists may exert part of their effect through constriction of arteriovenous anastomoses and similar vascular changes occur in the fingertips. The validity of this model is uncertain [14]. Neurophysiological techniques suffer similar drawbacks. For example, while medication modifies measures of temporal muscle activity in humans, the changes do not correlate with the degree of pain or pain relief [15].

Specific Ethical Issues Affecting Trial Design

It has been suggested that there are no specific ethical issues involved in trials for benign headache such as migraine [10]. The arguments against this are outlined below and they affect the design of trials.

Safety Issues in a Benign Condition

The level of acceptable treatment risk for a benign condition, such as migraine, is low. Neither patients, doctors nor the pharmaceutical industry would knowingly accept potential for serious adverse drug reactions (ADRs) in such a setting. In contrast, patients and doctors are likely to accept a higher level of risk for potential benefit in fatal conditions such as motor neurone disease. If ADRs are predictable and common, this is straightforward, but even large randomised trials are unlikely to detect ADRs with a frequency of less than 1 in 300 [16]. Side-effects may not become evident until many subjects have been exposed, or have had prolonged exposure, or both. For example, methysergide produced retroperitoneal fibrosis in 2 of 1000 patients treated for up to 6 years by Lance [17], while Graham [18] found reports of the problem in 100 of 500 000 treated, equivalent to a rate of 1 per 5000 and therefore well below the level usually detectable in randomised controlled trials (RCTs). A recent example of a drug causing idiosyncratic side-effects appearing at Phase IV of development is the anti-convulsant felbamate [19]. The potential in the field of headache for serious side-effects and iatrogenic harm in a benign condition must be considered and suggests that existing treatments should be rigorously tested to establish effectiveness before exposing subjects to an unknown risk.

Resource Issues

New treatments for any condition are almost always more expensive than existing treatments. Active control groups with "the best" established treatments, especially when the condition treated is benign, are desirable. If this is not done, results interpreted as showing success with a new treatment may result in the unnecessary introduction of a more expensive treatment, and diversion of funding from other areas. Poorly designed or executed trials waste resources, are unethical [20] and misleading.

Treatment of a Painful Condition

Although chronic or intermittent headaches are generally benign, they are painful, and trial design must take this into account. They must consider whether a placebo treatment group can be justified, how long it is reasonable to allow the headache to continue

without rescue medication and what form the rescue medication will take.

Basic Designs

Sackett and Wennberg [21] argue that unnecessary effort has been expended in arguing over a "gold standard" of research technique rather than "focusing on methods rather than questions". They make the important point that a trial design must be tailored to the specific questions asked. The design must ensure integrity (the data really represent what happens to the patient when they receive the drug) and validity (that studies performed have relevance to clinical practice) [22].

In the remainder of this section, a broad view of potential approaches is taken and both qualitative and quantitative research designs are examined. Most of the studies considered are drug trials, and most are phase III trials.

Qualitative Designs

Case Reports

Case reports may provide preliminary information on treatment of uncommon conditions, such as chronic paroxysmal hemicrania [23]. Despite the current emphasis on "evidence-based medicine", doctors often use empiric treatment. Patients can hardly be asked to wait until treatment has been proven in a randomised controlled trial (RCT) if they have a painful and debilitating condition. For certain headaches such as trigeminal neuralgia or sudden unilateral neuralgic pain with conjunctival injection and tearing (SUNCT), where pain is severe, the treating doctor will generally try all standard and then non-standard remedies until there is improvement. In this situation, case reports on treatment may have validity. Case reports may generate hypotheses for further testing. There is a danger, however, that they may encourage therapeutic nihilism, as for example in SUNCT where many reports are negative regarding treatment [24]. The value of case reports in common headache syndromes such as migraine will be very limited as there are better techniques available to test treatments, as discussed below.

In-depth Interviews to Saturation

Questions related to patient preference of treatments are probably best tested by in-depth interviews to the point of redundancy and saturation [21]. These studies are time-consuming, and highly dependent on the skills of the interviewer.

Quantitative Studies

Retrospective Versus Prospective Studies

Retrospective studies are hampered by selection bias, and of limited use. They give some information about adverse reactions and potential benefits. Examples include Ford and Ford [25].

Prospective Trials

Prospective trials are preferred over retrospective trials because they reduce the potential for selection bias.

Withdrawal Studies

Withdrawal studies may be used in chronic conditions, when patients are taken off treatment, and response to withdrawal is compared with those continuing on the medication. This design may be suitable for assessing efficacy of an intervention in long-standing use but never conclusively shown to be effective. This technique studies only a highly selected group, and in general only those seen to benefit, or at least who had no severe side-effects, will be on the treatment. Withdrawal studies will only be valid if randomisation, blinding, unbiased assessments and proper data analysis are performed. The applicability of this design to clinical trials in headache is very limited.

Open-Label Long-Term Studies

These phase IV studies are case reports on a large scale. For example, Zagami [26] studied 2058 patients with repeated use of zolmitriptan over 1 year, treating a total of 31 579 (but only 24 161 evaluable) headaches. Such studies represent a formalisation of post-marketing surveillance and are crucial in detecting rare idiosyncratic drug reactions or those occurring only after prolonged exposure, and unsuspected drug interactions. Such information cannot come from RCTs [16,21].

Non Randomised Concurrent Controlled Studies

Controls in this study design are subjects treated without the new intervention at approximately the same time as the intervention group. The advantages of this are patient and investigator acceptance, relative simplicity and lower cost than controlled trials. The major problem is whether the two groups are truly comparable. This problem cannot be eliminated by analysis, as there may be unknown but important differences between the two groups as well as the obvious factors. Given the high placebo rate in headache trials, this sort of unblind trial has almost no role in headache research, certainly not in trials of migraine [10] or tension-type headache [27].

Randomised Controlled Trials (RCTs)

RCTs are often considered the gold standard [28], and are generally the preferred option for answering questions such as the effectiveness of a treatment in migraine or tension-type headache. Randomisation removes potential bias in subject allocation. This bias can arise from the investigator or the subject and can influence results in unpredictable ways. The second advantage of a RCT is that it produces comparable groups – the independent covariates tend to be equally divided between the two groups. Sometimes stratification is used to guard against and adjust for unbalanced randomisations. It has been suggested that stratification on the basis of headache frequency (fewer than or more than three attacks every 4 weeks) should be used in trials of prophylactic medications used in migraine [10], because of correlation between efficacy and frequency of headache in some studies [29]. Stratification is probably not needed in acute trials. If randomisation is successful then the validity of statistical tests of significance is guaranteed.

Trials Using Placebo Control Versus Active Control

Placebo-controlled trials are suited to crossover design (see below), but active control groups have advantages, allowing comparison with long-standing treatments that are usually cheaper and have a clearly established side-effect profile. Although many of the treatments have been in clinical use since the 1930s [30], clinical trials of their efficacy began only relatively recently and some of the most commonly used medications in clinical practice are little studied and their efficacy anecdotal rather than proven.

Crossover Design

Crossover design is a form of RCT, allowing each subject to act as their own control. The design reduces variability and the sample size needed. The design requires that treatments are effective in reasonably short treatment periods, treatment is not curative and the condition remains relatively stable over the time studied. These conditions apply to migraine and tension-type headache. This design should be applied when drop-out rate does not increase over time [31], a factor very difficult to assess in headache trials. It is not a suitable technique for assessing multiple treatments.

This technique is recommended [10] for acute trials in migraine because it is assumed, although unproven, that power will be increased. For prophylactic medications, it is estimated that the crossover design is 8 times more powerful [32].

Crossover trials take longer to perform and require careful monitoring of the washout period. The underlying assumption is that the effect of the first period will not carry over into the second period, or that statistical methods can overcome problems of carry-over effect. Grizzle's method [33] attempts to check whether there is a period–treatment interaction by comparing the mean AB response with the mean BA response, but is not infallible. Sibbald and Roberts [34] point out the shortcomings of statistical methodology in dealing with carry-over effects.

An example of appropriate crossover design is the placebo-controlled study of sumatriptan for acute migraine [35]. There is no reason to suspect carry-over effect in this design. Study numbers were small, and 20 of the 61 patients did not complete the target of treatment of four migraine attacks, but efficacy was shown. The findings, however, which were analysed on a per-protocol basis, include that sumatriptan is "virtually free of substantial side-effects", but the numbers studied were inadequate for this conclusion.

Crossover design is unsuitable if spontaneous remission is likely during the study period. For example cluster headache often remits after several weeks [36] and would not be suitable for study by this technique.

Cluster Randomised Control Designs

Cluster randomised control designs are a modification of a RCT that involves allocation of a treatment to a group (cluster) of people, with either a cluster or individuals in the control group. When subjects in both the intervention and control arms are groups, it is sometimes known as group allocation or composite randomisation. It is particularly useful for diffuse interventions (such as promoting lifestyle changes or disseminating information) when there may be "leakage" of effect to those not intended to receive it [37]. It may be used where it is difficult to approach patients about randomisation, but this relates closely to the inherent ethical difficulties in the design and conduct of cluster randomised controlled trials. It is most commonly used for public health or educational interventions and there is almost no experience of this sort of trial in headache research.

Zelen Modification

Zelen modification [38] assigns subjects to groups before informing them, and only those assigned to the active intervention are asked if they wished to participate. This method does not allow blinding, depends on the rate of acceptance in the intervention group and involves ethical problems about the control group being left uninformed.

Multiple Treatments and Factorial Design

The traditional experimental design alters one factor at a time. The factorial design aims to increase efficiency and study interactions. The allied disadvantage of this design is that there is the potential for interaction between the concurrent treatments. To assess interactions, groups with multiple treatments and groups with the single components of treatment are needed.

If there are no comparative groups with treatments given singly as well as in combination the trial is not factorial. In a comparison of oral sumatriptan and ergotamine/caffeine [39] similar efficacy was found, but it remains unclear whether the effects of ergotamine and caffeine were antagonistic, additive or multiplicative. Similarly, a comparison of oral sumatriptan and aspirin plus metoclopramide [40] gives information only about the combined effects of aspirin and metoclopramide.

Multicentre Trials

Multicentre trials allow a large sample size to be attained, but increase the variability of assessment techniques. For benign headache syndromes, variability may arise in definition of headache [4], in the style and depth of follow-up, in instructions to subjects about administration and timing of medication and rescue medication, and in reporting of the degree of headache relief.

Hybrid Designs

Hybrid designs combine historical controls with randomised subjects. The aim is to reduce the number of subjects required, with resultant savings in cost and time. To do this the data from historical controls must be fairly recent, and entry criteria and subject recruitment comparable. If not, then more subjects may be needed to compensate than would otherwise have been required in a randomised trial. The second potential advantage of this design is that all subjects receive the new intervention and this increases acceptance amongst subjects and the treating physicians. Conversely if there are serious ADRs this design increases the number of subjects exposed. Historical control trials are non-randomised and non-concurrent; therefore the major problems with this design are whether the control and active groups are truly comparable with regard to collection, accuracy, validity and applicability of data from historical controls. With the passage of time, there have been changes in definitions of headache [2] and there may also be changes in the natural history and incidence of certain conditions, although there is little information about this in the field of headache research. This design has little application to trials in the common headache syndromes.

Meta-analysis

Meta-analysis and systematic reviews are often considered to be the most reliable evidence on which to base decisions about clinical treatments [28]. Meta-analyses usually exclude all but RCTs. As always for meta-analysis in subjective conditions such as pain, comparisons between trials are difficult, because global measures are inexact. For example McQuay et al. [41] used the measure of numbers needed to treat for "effectiveness" as well as side-effects. Of the studies within this meta-analysis which examined trigeminal neuralgia, a variety of measures for pain relief were made including trigeminal neuralgia symptom score [42–44], introducing considerable variability into already subjective scores.

Sample Size

The required sample size is determined by the design of the trial, the major objective, the level of significance to be achieved, the level of confidence with which negative results are to be reported and the variability of end-point measures.

Trial Design

For the common benign headaches such as migraine and tension-type headaches, RCT will be the design chosen, and relatively large numbers of subjects employed. In headache trials, investigators usually choose a standard (explanatory) trial determining whether the test treatment is better, worse or the same as the control treatment [45]. There is almost no experience with pragmatic trials [10]. The calculation of the power of the study and the number of subjects in each arm is of great importance in the standard trial. The clinician must obviously consider whether it will be possible to recruit sufficient numbers for the chosen design. For example, it is unlikely that sufficient numbers of patients could be recruited at a single centre for a RCT on cluster headache, and this would be difficult even with a multi-centre trial.

The Major Objective

In trials, the major objective will be the difference to be detected between the intervention and control group or groups. This must have both clinical and statistical validity. Previous studies in new and established medication provide the basis for estimations of a realistic major objective, and therefore are critical in determining the sample size required. They are an imperfect basis, as previously mentioned, as many of the commonly used medications have not been tested in a RCT, partly because they were introduced before the use of RCTs, and in times of less sophisticated statistical methods. Selby [30] estimates, based on controlled trials and clinical experience, that established drugs are capable of a reduction of frequency and severity of symptoms in subjects in the order of 60%. The larger the difference to be detected, the smaller the numbers needed in the trial, but the higher the chance of a type II error.

Statistical Significance

A test of significance provides a measure of the chance that treatments will appear different when in fact they are equivalent. This must be chosen arbitrarily at the 5% or 1% level at the time of design of the trial in order to calculate the sample size.

Variability of End-points

In RCTs in acute headache research the major end-point is usually a qualitative or discrete measure of pain, usually expressed as a percentage of patients with relief of headache or of graded improvement. The investigator is usually interested in determining whether the test treatment is better, worse or the same as the control treatment (that is, a standard design). In general, as measures are not linear and not of normal distribution, a larger sample size will be needed in acute headache than in quantitative studies such as cardiovascular studies of arterial hypertension. In prophylactic studies of chronic headache, quantitative measures of headache frequency may be useful. If there are a number of parameters measured this will necessitate larger numbers to enable adequate power and a Bonferroni correction if needed. Continuous response variables allow a smaller sample size to be used [46] but have not been successfully applied in answering the primary question in headache research because no valid surrogate response variable has been found. If a multi-centre trial is contemplated this will increase variance and larger numbers of subjects will be needed than in a single-centre trial.

Drop-outs and Sample Size

If drop-outs are excluded from analysis (per-protocol analysis), then the initial sample size must be increased. Attempts to assist in adjusting for drop-out rates date back at least 30 years (for example, [47]). If intention-to-treat analysis is followed, any treatment effect may be distorted by the drop-out rate and this effect will be magnified if numbers are small.

Power Calculations

The power of a study reflects the probability that a type II error will be avoided, expressed as a percentage chance. Power calculations require an estimate of confidence with which a negative result can be held. Once power is specified, sample size must be calculated to achieve the desired power. Unlike the level of significance there is little consensus on what is an appropriate level of power, with some writers suggesting a power as low as 50% to be adequate [48]. Most, however, would consider that a minimum power of 80% is required.

Of recent studies, many include power calculations in their stated methodology (for example, [11,49]), with the latter study being one of the few to specifically calculate and adjust sample size for expected drop-out rate. In Winner et al. [11] power calculations are made and the rationale explained in the methodology. The sample size is calculated based on an assumed 15% difference between dihydroergotamine and sumatriptan. One hundred and fifty patients in each group would ensure a power of 80% to detect this difference using a two-tailed test with a type I error of 0.05. Therefore a sample size of 300 was chosen. In fact 310 patients were recruited and only 295 evaluable. The end result was the same outcome at 3 h, more recurrence with sumatriptan, and more prolonged action of dihydroergotamine. The power chosen for the study is relatively low, and therefore type II error possible. The choice of detection of a relatively small difference between the two treatment groups (15%) meant that an increased power would have substantially increased the required sample size, and increased difficulties with recruitment.

In a carefully designed study comparing lysine acetylsalicylate and metoclopramide with sumatriptan for migraine [49], sample size calculations were based on expected response rates of 55–70% for oral sumatriptan, 50–55% for lysine acetylsalicylate and metoclopramide, and 20–37% for placebo. In order to detect a 15% difference between treatments (with type I risk set at 5% and type II risk at 20% with bilateral testing) the minimum size of each treatment group was estimated at 127 evaluable patients. Expecting a 10% drop-out rate a total of 420 patients were included, and the drop-out rate calculation was very accurate in this trial.

Cutler and colleagues [50] studied three dosages for sumatriptan in acute migraine but state that the

study was not powered to compare differences between sumatriptan doses. This significantly reduced the potential yield from the study. Another study, again with Dr R. Davis as one of the authors [51] used the same design and also compared three doses of sumatriptan with insufficient power of the study to compare differences of sumatriptan dosages. It is unfortunate that this work was divided and published as two studies.

Pitfalls in Clinical Trials of Headache
(Table 23.3)

Problems Related to Design

Inadequate Background Data

If clinical trials of new agents follow carefully designed animal studies, and early phase studies, designs can be optimised. If there are insufficient data on safety from animal studies, potential toxicity of new agents in humans will be difficult to predict. If phase I studies (assessing the pharmacology of compounds in volunteer subjects) and dosage studies are inadequate, phase III studies will falter. For medications in long-standing use, this

Table 23.3. Pitfalls in clinical trials in headache

Problems related to design
Inadequate background data
Choosing the question
Outcome measures
Definitions, inclusion and exclusion criteria and applicability
Power and sample size calculations
Choosing the control group (placebo or standard best treatment)
Optimising administration of treatment and control
Randomisation methods
Blinding methods
Crossover designs
Multiple concurrent treatments

Data collection problems
Methods of measurement
Details of data collection

Analysis problems
Correct statistical methods
Drop-outs and intention to treat
Placebo issues
Type I and type II errors

Application of results
Clinical utility
Selective reporting and interpretation of results
Publication bias
Vested interests and fraud

formalised backround information is lacking. On the other hand, there is the advantage of long clinical experience in thousands of patients, meaning that adverse drug reactions are usually well known, even for rare events; and optimal dosage has been established through extensive clinical experience.

Choosing the Question

Given the resources required, it is important that the design of a headache trial starts with clearly defined primary and secondary questions with importance scientifically, medically or for public health purposes that have not been previously answered. Primary and secondary end-points may be based on different response variables. For example, the primary end-point is headache relief, while the secondary end-point may be relief of other symptoms, such as nausea, vomiting or photophobia.

The second sort of question is a subgroup hypothesis. If attempts are made to correlate response to clinical factors, such as analysing response rates of migraine with and without aura, this analysis should be specified before data collection starts, based on reasonable expectations, and be limited in number to avoid type I errors.

Outcome Measures

Directly related to the end-points, the outcome measures should be clearly defined, valid and reproducible. Given the subjective nature of pain, this is difficult. It becomes more so if pain relief is defined by grade rather than in terms of absolute relief, as a "mild" headache is more difficult to define than no headache. If multi-centre trial design is employed variability is likely to increase, with a resultant need to increase sample size.

Definitions, Inclusion and Exclusion Criteria and Applicability

There have been vigorous attempts to standardise definitions and format of headache and clinical trials [10] with the aim of improving the quality of headache research. They are relatively recent and their impact remains uncertain.

Headache trials usually exclude women "at risk" of pregnancy, subjects over the age of 65 years, as well as those at high risk of developing a contraindicating condition or likely to die of another condition in the meantime. This is common to most areas of clinical research and has clear reasons, but has a particular impact in the field of headache, as young women of childbearing age are the most common group to have headaches. In general elderly people are underrepresented in clinical trials [52]. Although migraine gen-

erally affects young women, other headaches such as trigeminal neuralgia and cluster headache occur frequently in the elderly. Volunteer subjects in headache trials may not represent the average patient, therefore reducing the clinical applicability of results. They may take part in more than one trial. Results are often subsequently applied to a wider group than in the trial, and clinical validity may be reduced because of the above-mentioned factors.

Power and Sample Size Calculations

Obviously the larger the sample size the greater the power, but this relationship is not linear. Rather, sample size varies with the inverse square of the difference detected. Therefore to increase power 10-fold, sample size must be increased 100-fold [53].

The higher the incidence of an event in a group, for example number of headaches per month, the lower the number of subjects that will be required, but the more difficult it will be to recruit subjects. To overcome recruitment difficulties, a headache frequency of 1–6 monthly in studies of prophylaxis for migraine [10] has been recommended, but this means a considerable range of headache severity is included and raises the need for stratification, as discussed earlier.

A common problem with headache trials is inadequate power because of inadequate sample size. Ford and Ford [25] studied two modalities of the same compound, continuous and intermittent dihydroergotamine in treatment of intractable headache in a total of 171 subjects. End-points measured were headache freedom and time in hospital. Their conclusion that treatments are equivalent may be a type II error. Because the same drug was studied, any difference in effect is likely to be small and therefore a large sample size needed to show any real difference in treatments. The sample size is probably too small to draw conclusions of equivalence.

Methodology, including power calculations, is the same in the two publications of efficacy of naratriptan by Klassen et al. [54] and Mathew et al. [55], sponsored by the same pharmaceutical company. It is regrettable that this study was divided into two publications, and the power of each half reduced.

Choosing the Control Group (Placebo or Standard Best Treatment)

As discussed in the introduction, best use of resources and ethical considerations often support the use of active control groups. However, given the high placebo rate, placebo control groups can be justified, as long as the provision for rescue medication is adequate.

Optimising Administration of Treatment and Control

Not only must the intervention be clearly defined, the potential benefit must be maximised. This depends on careful and detailed dosage studies of new medications. This aspect is underestimated in difficulty (P. Roland, personal communication 1998), but recent guidelines devised to aid design and analysis of clinical trials [10] emphasise the importance of dosing and pilot studies. Timing is also critical. For example, subcutaneous sumatriptan shows no efficacy against subsequent headache if given during the aura phase [56], and therefore must be given once headache has developed, ideally when at least moderate, for maximum efficacy. In contrast, ergots are most effective at the onset of headache.

There is no consensus on whether migraine prophylaxis should be continued during acute headache trials, with continuation in some studies [35] and cessation 2 weeks prior in other studies [50,51].

Randomisation Methods

As pointed out by McQuay et al. [41] and many others, randomisation may be appropriate (for example the use of random number tables) or inappropriate (alternate allocation). Therefore it is not enough to describe a study as randomised: the methods of doing so must be described. Many studies do not describe the method of randomisation, one study that does used an appropriate computer-generated randomisation code [57].

Crossover Designs

Crossover designs have two major potential problems. Firstly there may be carry-over effect and it has been argued that pre-testing the data for evidence of carry-over is seriously flawed by the limited power of such tests and the potential for type II error [58].

Multiple Concurrent Treatments

Bonuccelli et al. [59] studied the effectiveness of combined treatment with amitriptyline and dexamethasone in drug-induced headache. In fact there were four treatments (the two stated as well as sumatriptan and stopping medications). There were no controls for the study, and the total number of subjects was 17, making interpretation difficult.

Data Collection Problems

Methods of Measurement

It is likely that if a subject has to grade the degree of headache relief verbally, there will be more variability than if they have to report a yes–no phenomenon (headache relief). Frequent checking by investigators may improve compliance with self-reporting, but is likely to increase the placebo response. Some authors claim increased reliability for pain visual analogue scales with access to past results [60], but these have not been validated in the field of headache research.

Details of Data Collection

The demands of accuracy and care in trials must be balanced against the tedium for the subject and the investigator of collecting vast amounts of data. Quality of data collection may deteriorate if the quantity to be collected is excessive [61].

Analysis Problems

Correct Statistical Methods

Most primary end-points of headache research will be discrete or non-uniform, and require non-parametric statistics. Mistakes are sometimes made in this area, for example using parametric statistics when analysing non-uniformly spread data points which have been inappropriately averaged.

Drop-outs and Intention-to-Treat

Intention-to-treat analysis is a safe way of avoiding bias but has two major disadvantages. If the trial is small, this form of analysis will seriously distort results. In long-term trials some patients in the active group may actually receive control medication and vice versa. In view of this Bulpitt [62] and others recommend analysis on both intention-to-treat and per-protocol bases. If the number of drop-outs is high then the assumption that the initial randomisation yielded balanced groups still holds cannot be accepted without further tests. Further, the intention-to treat-methodology [63] was designed to compare two treatments in practice but not to prove efficacy of a drug, as it is increasingly and inappropriately being used for.

Placebo Issues

The very high placebo rate in headache trials is not fully understood but affects analysis, and distorts results if blinding is incomplete. It has led to measures designed to exclude placebo rate, such as therapeutic gain [64] (see also Chapter 24). The placebo rate is also highly variable between studies, ranging from 10% [35] to 38% [50]. Blinding is a major issue in headache trials because of the high placebo rate. It must be described in the methodology and must remain throughout the trial. Measures of the efficacy of blinding are uncommon and rarely reported [53].

Type I and Type II Errors

Type I errors may be compounded by multiple analyses. Type I errors are less common [65] than type II errors. The most common reason for type II errors is recruitment of too few subjects for the trial, either because sample size was inadequate, power poorly calculated, or there was failure to adjust for drop-out rate.

Application of Results

Study findings may not be applied to clinical practice because they are not clinically useful or practical, because interpretation of results may be faulty or because the results conflict with previous studies. Conversely, results may be applied to clinical practice because of publication bias or vested interests. Fraud may influence results overtly or covertly.

Clinical Utility

The finding of statistical significance does not necessarily imply clinical significance and vice versa. Study findings may be rejected because individual clinicians are conservative, because the findings are at variance with previous publications, or because clinicians find existing treatments satisfactory and may have had decades of experience with them. Some clinicians prefer to await post-marketing surveillance studies before trying a new medication, fearing rare adverse events. New medications may be expensive and the clinician may feel the extra margin of benefit does not warrant the extra cost. Adverse reactions or difficulties may discourage clinicians. Adoption of new medications will be influenced by government restrictions, advertising, education and demand.

Selective Reporting and Interpretation of Results

It is more common for investigators to conclude too much than too little from their results. Emphasis in results and discussion may be selective. Cady et al. [66] studied subcutaneous sumatriptan and concluded that it was effective "with lasting effects for up to 24 hours". They fail to mention that 34% of patients remain headache free at 24 h, compared with 11% of placebo-treated patients. No statistical analysis of this is reported, although the original response to sumatriptan (69% versus 22% placebo response) is reported as statistically significant. In the same report, the side-effects of ergotamine are emphasised, but the basis of this is largely case reports,

dating back to the early 1970s. This mixture of statistical analysis and anecdotal evidence gives a false impression of scientific validity.

Publication Bias

The evidence that negative results tend not to be published [67] is of great concern. This problem faces all clinical treatments. Attempts to overcome type II error (false negative results) by meta-analysis compound rather than reduce this problem by magnifying this bias in the published randomised trials [53]. In an attempt to address the problem of publication bias, there has been a drive to retrospectively identify negative unpublished trails, and projects for the prospective registration of controlled trials [68]. Interestingly, Chalmers [68] argues that much of the reason for publication bias rests with the investigators who do not attempt to publish negative findings, rather than with reluctant editors. Prospective registration has found support from the IHS [20], but is not yet operational in clinical trials in headache trials [20]. The standard notation for the relative weight of different types of studies rates systematic reviews and meta-analyses as the most useful [28], but this does not take into account the problem of publication bias. This notation devalues most information not derived from RCTs.

Vested Interests and Fraud

The expense of large-scale RCTs, with the necessary careful preparation, liaison between clinicians and statisticians and use of multiple centres, means that many are funded by pharmaceutical companies with obvious commercial interests. Declaration of funding and rigorous peer review aim to protect against potential bias but this may not be enough. The problem of analyst bias and validity of mathematical models used is being increasingly considered. Unfortunately there are no regulations to ensure that statistical processing of the data from trials should be done by groups independent of the investigators and the funding agencies. There are few examples of such independent data analysis in the RCT literature.

Increasing pressure to produce results and publications creates the temptation to fabricate results [53]. There are no data on whether this is a problem in headache trials.

Conclusions

Headaches cover the clinical spectrum of severity, incidence and type. Most are benign, and the most commonly studied are migraine and tension-type headaches. There are difficulties in defining heada-che, ethical issues in exposing a usually benign con-dition to potentially dangerous treatments, and in treatment of a painful condition with placebo. Both the definition of most headaches and the primary outcome of pain relief are highly subjective.

This chapter deals with choices of designs and the advantages and disadvantages of each. For the common benign headaches, the design choice will usually be a randomised controlled double-blind study. Long-term open studies do have an important role in detecting rare adverse drug events. Some headaches are rare, and case reports and small-scale trials will be the only practical methodology. The International Headache Society has been very active in attempts to standardise definitions of headache and establish guidelines for thoughtful and careful trials in common headaches. These have already had an impact on the design of headache trials but many challenges remain. The determination of power and sample size, and the extent of the placebo effect and blinding remain problematic. Headache research shares the problem of publication bias with many other areas of clinical research. Clinicians involved in clinical trials have much to gain from the advice of statisticians, but must always maintain an indepen-dent perspective to ensure the clinical validity and relevance of the results presented. Investigators must guard against undue influence from vested interest groups. This is a particular challenge in the field of headache, a common condition with large commer-cial potential.

References

1. Ad Hoc Committee on classification of headache. Classifica-tion of headache. Arch Neurol 1962;6:173–176.
2. Headache classification committee of the international headache society. Classification and diagnostic criteria for headache disorders, cranial neuralgias and facial pain. Cepha-lalgia 1988;8(Suppl 7):1–96.
3. Pfaffenrath V, Rath M, Pollman W, Keeser W. Atypical facial pain – application of the IHS criteria in a clinical sample. Cephalalgia 1993;Suppl 12:84–88.
4. Lipton RB, Stewart WF, Merikangis KR. Reliability in headache diagnosis. Cephalalgia 1993;Suppl 12:29–33.
5. Kuntz KM, Kokmen E, Stevens JC, Miller P, Offord KP, Ho MM. Post-lumbar puncture headaches: experience in 501 consecu-tive procedures. Neurology 1992;42:1884–1887.
6. Singer J, Kim J, Fahy-Chandon B, Datt A, Tourtellotte WW. Headache in ambulatroy HIV-1 infected men enrolled in a longitudinal study. Neurology 1996;47:487–494.
7. MacLennan AH, Wilson DH, Taylor AW. Prevalence and cost of alternative medicine in Australia. Lancet 1996;347:569–573.
8. Astin JA. Why patients use alternative medicine. Results of a national study. JAMA 1998;279:1548–1553.
9. Minutes from the meeting of the International Headache Society subcommittee on clinical trials in migraine, London, 3 September 1998.
10. International Headache Society committee on clinical trials in migraine. Guidelines for controlled trials of drugs in migraine, 1st edition. Cephalalgia 1991;11:1–12.
11. Winner P, Ricalde O, Le Force B, Saper J, Margul. A double blind study of subcutaneous dihydroergotamine vs subcuta-neous sumatriptan in the treatment of acute migraine. Arch Neurol 1996;53:180–184.
12. Osterhaus JT, Townsend RJ, Gandek B, Ware JE. Measuring the functional status and well-being of patients with migraine headache. Headache 1994;34:337–343.
13. Iverson HK. Experimental headache in humans. Cephalalgia 1995;15:281–287.
14. van Es NM, Bruning TA, Cams J, Chang PC, Blauw GJ, Ferrari MD, Saxena PR. Assessment of peripheral vascular effects of antimigraine drugs in humans. Cephalalgia 1995;15:288–291.
15. Bendtsen L, Jensen R, Olesen J. Amitriptyline, a combined serotonin and noradrenaline reuptake inhibitor, reduces exte-roceptive suppression of temporal muscle activity in patients with chronic tension-type headache. Electroencephalogr Clin Neurophysiol 1996;101:418–422.
16. Bulpitt CJ. Screening for adverse drug reactions. Br J Hosp Med 1977;18:329–334.
17. Lance JW. Interval therapy in migraine. Med J Aust 1972;Suppl 2:29–32.
18. Graham JR. Cardiac and pulmonary fibrosis during methy-sergide therapy for headache. Am J Med Sci 1967;254:23–34.
19. Leppik IE. Felbamate. In: Shorvon S, Dreifuss F, Fish D, Thomas D, editors. The treatment of epilepsy. Oxford: Black-well, 1996:421–428.
20. Ethics subcommittee of the International Headache Society. Ethical issues in headache research and management. Cepha-lalgia 1998;18:505–529.
21. Sackett DL, Wennberg JE. Choosing the best research designs for each question. BMJ 1997;315:1636.
22. Vanderburg MJ. An introductory guide. Good clinical practice for investigators. Essex, UK: Medical and Clinical Bookshop, 1990:11–12.
23. Antonaci F, Sjaastad O. Chronic paroxysmal hemicrania (CPH): a review of the clinical manifestations. Headache 1989; 29:648–656.
24. Pareja JA, Sjaastad O. SUNCT syndrome. A clinical review. Headache 1997;37:195–202.
25. Ford RG, Ford KT. Continuous intravenous dihydroergota-mine in the treatment of intractable headache. Headache 1997; 37:129–136.
26. Zagami AS. 311C90: long-term efficacy and tolerability profile for the acute treatment of migraine. Neurology 1997;48(Suppl 3):S25–S28.
27. IHS committee on clinical trials. Guidelines for trials of drug treatments in tension-type headache, 1st edition. Cephalalgia 1995;15:165–179.
28. Guyatt GH, Sackett DL, Sinclair JC, Hayward R, Cook DJ, Cook RJ. Users guide to the medical literature. IX. A method for grading health care recommendations. JAMA 1995;274:1800–1804.
29. Sorensen P, Hansen K, Olesen J. A placebo-controlled, double-blind, crossover trial of flunarizine in common migraine. Cephalalgia 1986;6:7–14.
30. Selby G. Migraine and its variants. Sydney: ADIS Health Science Press, 1983.
31. Bulpitt CJ. Randomised controlled clinical trials. The Hague: Martinus Nijhoff, 1983:118–135.
32. Tfelt-Hansen P, Nielsen SL. Patient numbers needed in pro-phylactic migraine trials. Neuroepidemiology 1987;6:214–219.
33. Grizzle JE. The two period change-over design and its use in clinical trials. Biometrics 1965;21:467–480.
34. Sibbald B, Roberts C. Crossover trials. BMJ 1998;316:1719.

35. Goadsby PJ, Zagami AS, Donnan GA, Symington G, Anthony M, Bladin PF, Lance JW. Oral sumatriptan in acute migraine. Lancet 1991;338:782–783.

36. Kudrow L (1980) Cluster headache. Mechanisms and management. New York: Oxford University Press.

37. Edwards SJL, Braunholtz DA, Lilford RJ, Stevens AJ. Ethical issues in the design and conduct of cluster randomised controlled trials. BMJ 1999;388:1407–1409.

38. Zelen M. A new design for randomized clinical trials. N Engl J Med 1979;307:1242–1245.

39. The multinational oral sumatriptan and ergotamine/caffeine comparative study group. A randomised, double blind comparison of sumatriptan and ergotamine/caffeine in the acute treatment of migraine. Eur Neurol 1991;31:314–322.

40. The oral sumatriptan and aspirin plus metoclopramide comparative study group. A study to compare oral sumatriptan with oral aspirin plus metoclopramide in the acute treatment of migraine. Eur Neurol 1992;32:117–184.

41. McQuay H, Carroll D, Jadad AR, Wiffen P, Moore A. Anticonvulsant drugs for management of pain: a systematic review. BMJ 1995;311:1047–1052.

42. Lechin F, van der Dijs B, Lechin ME, Amat J, Lechin AE, Cabrera A, et al. Pimozide therapy for trigeminal neuralgia. Arch Neurol 1989;46:960–963.

43. Lindstrom P, Lindblom U. The analgesic effect of tocainamide in trigeminal neuralgia. Pain 1987;28:45–50.

44. Vilming ST, Lyberg T, Lataste X. Tizanidine in the management of trigeminal neuralgia. Cephalalgia 1986;6:181–182.

45. Schwartz D, Lellouch J. Explanatory and pragmatic attitudes in therapeutic trials. J Chron Dis 1967;20:637–648.

46. Friedman LM, Furberg CD, DeMets DL. "What is the question?" In: Fundamentals of clinical trials. St Louis: Mosby, 1985:11–22.

47. National Diet-Heart Study Report. Appendix Aa-c. Sample size estimates for medical trials. Circulation 1968;37:1279–1308.

48. Clark CJ, Downie CC. A method for the rapid determination of the number of patients to include in a controlled clinical trial. Lancet 1966;II:1357–1358.

49. Tfelt-Hansen P, Henry P, Mulder LJ, Scheldewaert RG, Schoenen J, Chazot G. The effectiveness of combined oral lysine acetylsalicylate and metoclopramide compared with oral sumatriptan for migraine. Lancet 1995;346:923–926.

50. Cutler N, Mushet GR, Davis R, Clements B, Whitcher L. Oral sumatriptan for the acute treatment of migraine: evaluation of three dosage strengths. Neurology 1995;45(Suppl 7): S5–S9.

51. Sargent J, Kirchner JR, Davis R, Kirkhart B. Oral sumatriptan is effective and well tolerated for the acute treatment of migraine. Neurology 1995;45(Suppl 7):S10–S14.

52. Avorn J. Including elderly people in clinical trials. BMJ 1997;315:1033–1034.

53. Ellis SJ, Adams RF. The cult of the double-blind placebo-controlled trial. Br J Clin Pharmacol 1997;51:36–39.

54. Klassen A, Elkind A, Asgharnejad M, Webster C, Laurenza A on behalf of the Naratriptan S2WA3001 study group. Naratriptan is effective and well tolerated in the acute treatment of migraine. Headache 1997;37:640–645.

55. Mathew NT, Asgharnejad M, Peykamian M, Laurenzia A on behalf of the naratriptan S2WA3003 study group. Naratriptan is effective and well tolerated in the acute treatment of migraine. Neurology 1997;49:1485–1490.

56. Bates D, Ashford E, Dawson R, Ensiink F-B M, Gilhus NE, et al. for the sumatriptan aura study group. Subcutaneous sumatriptan during the migraine aura. Neurology 1994;44:1587–1592.

57. The subcutaneous sumatriptan international study group. Treatment of migraine attacks with sumatriptan. N Engl J Med 1991;325:316–321.

58. Sibbald B, Roberts C. Understanding controlled trials – crossover trials. BMJ 1999;316:1719.

59. Bonuccelli U, Nuti A, Lucetti C, Pavese N, Dell'Angelo G, Muratorio A. Amitriptyline and dexamethasone combined treatment in drug induced headache. Cephalalgia 1996;16: 198–200.

60. Scott J, Huskisson EC. Accuracy of subjective measurements made with or without previous scores: an important source of error in serial measurement of subjective states. Ann Rheum Dis 1979;38:558–559.

61. Wright P, Haybittle J. Design of forms for clinical trials. BMJ 1979;II:529–530.

62. Bulpitt CJ. Randomised controlled clinical trials. The Hague: Martinus Nijhoff, 1983:179–193.

63. Peto R, Pike MC, Armitage P, Breslow NE, Cox DR, Howard SV, et al. Design and analysis of randomized clinical trials requiring prolonged observation of each patient. II. Analysis and examples. Br J Cancer 1977;35:1–39.

64. Laupacis A, Sackett DL, Roberts RS. An assessment of clinically useful measures of the consequences of treatment. N Engl J Med 1988;318:1728–1733.

65. Maxwell C. Clinical trials, reviews and the journal of negative results. Br J Clin Pharmacol 1981;1:15–18.

66. Cady RK, Wendt JW, Kirchner JR, Sargent MD, Rothrock JF, Skaggs H. Treatment of acute migraine with subcutaneous sumatriptan. JAMA 1991;265:2831–2835.

67. Easterbrooke PJ, Berlin JA, Gopalan R, Matthews DR. Publication bias in clinical research. Lancet 1991;337:867–872.

68. Chalmers I. Cranberry juice and the Cochrane library. MRC News 1998;79:17–19.

24. Headache: Experience with Large Multicenter Trials in the Treatment of Migraine Attacks

P. Tfelt-Hansen and K. Seidelin

Introduction

In this chapter we will discuss experiences with randomised controlled trials (RCTs) in the acute treatment of migraine. With the introduction of the new 5-hydroxytryptamine $(5HT)_{1B/1D}$ receptor agonist sumatriptan [1], the first drug developed specifically for migraine, and recently other triptans, the focus in RCTs in migraine has overwhelmingly been on acute migraine treatment. Only one prophylactic drug, the antiepileptic drug sodium valproate, has been introduced in recent years [2–5]. This chapter is based partly on our personal experience with multicenter RCTs in acute migraine treatment ($n = 6$) in recent years, partly on what we have perceived as problems in published multicenter RCTs. More systematic reviews on RCTs in migraine therapy are available [5–17].

Relatively large multicenter trials ($n = 400 - 1100$ [18,19]) are needed in order to define the dose-response curve and comparative efficacy of a new specific drug being developed for the treatment of migraine attacks. Previously, new drugs introduced in migraine treatment (e.g. NSAIDs) were originally used for other disorders and then used in migraine treatment. For this purpose only relatively small RCTs were needed since the profile of the drug was known [20].

Large multicenter RCTs in migraine are, in contrast to, for example, some multicenter RCTs in stroke, today totally dominated by trials sponsored by the pharmaceutical industry. It is also generally the industry which designs the RCTs; only a few trials have been conceived and designed originally by investigators (e.g. [21–23]), but they were still sponsored by the industry. The industry seems, of course, mostly interested in RCTs for registration purposes. This has resulted, so far, in relatively few comparative RCTs comparing a triptan with previously accepted standard treatments such as ergot alkaloids. Such comparative RCTs are often, however, the most interesting from a clinical point of view.

In the following, some general experience and problems with multicenter RCTs in acute migraine treatment will be dealt with. Guidelines for how to conduct migraine trials can be found in the recommendations of the International Headache Society [24] and the checklists given therein should be consulted before participating in a RCTs in migraine. These guidelines were worked out before the occurrence of large multicenter industry-sponsored RCTs and are currently being revised, taking this new situation into account. In addition, some specialized issues regarding our personal experiences with patients, probably overlooked by "central trialists", will be mentioned.

Experiences with and Problems in Multicenter RCTs in Migraine

Some of the problems in multicenter RCTs in acute migraine treatment and our personal recommendations concerning these problems are presented in Table 24.1. In the following these items will be expanded and discussed, and additional items will be presented.

General Problems

When presented with a protocol for a large multicenter RCT in acute migraine treatment one should look for the aim of the study. The aim is often stated vaguely as: we want to compare the new drug A with placebo, for efficacy and adverse events. However, the easiest way to deduce the real aim of the trial is to look at the power calculations. There, an expected difference in success rates between drug A and placebo is given; and the aim is of course to demonstrate superiority of drug A over placebo. Similarly,

Table 24.1. Some problems in multicenter randomised controlled trials in acute migraine treatment, and our recommendations for how to deal with them (for more detailed discussion, see text)

Problem	Our recommendations
General problems	
Aim of study usually vaguely stated, e.g. "to compare drug A with placebo for efficacy and adverse events"	As is evident from power calculations in the protocol, the aim is to demonstrate the superiority of drug A. This should be stated outright
Sponsors control what RCTs are performed. Too few comparative RCTs are done with current treatment options other than triptans	Health authorities should finance independent RCTs conceived by investigators
Selection of patients	
Selected patients from clinics used in most RCTs in migraine	Use population-based methods or recruit patients from general practice
Trial design	
Most RCTs are parallel group comparisons in which the benefit/risk ratio is difficult to evaluate	The crossover design should also be used. In these RCTs patients can be asked to give their preference among the treatments
Up to three attacks treated by patients with the same treatment, probably to have more exposure to the drug	Special RCTs should be performed concerning consistency of response
Tendency to start out with high doses in order to prove efficacy. Later smaller doses are often found to be optimal	Explore the whole range of the of the dose-response curve and define the minimum effective dose
Use of escape medication postponed for up to 4 h "in order to explore the full therapeutic potential of the drug"	Escape medication should be permitted after 2 h (for problems with escape medication, see text)
Evaluation of results	
Use of the Glaxo criterion for success: severe or moderate head pain reduced to none or mild. Patients do not find a decrease from moderate to mild clinically relevant	Define success as the patient being pain free after 2 h
Presentation of results, and publication policy	
Success rates vary considerably in RCTs, the higher ones commonly being used for marketing	Use "therapeutic gain" instead of success rate (see text)
It is often stated that the results can be published after the sponsor has had a certain time to review them	A publication committee should be agreed upon before the start of the trial (see text)

in comparative studies of drug A versus drug B, one can deduce from the power calculations whether the aim is to demonstrate comparability, e.g. with 95% confidence intervals (CI) of $\pm 10\%$ for the difference between A and B and a significant difference from placebo, or to demonstrate that drug A is better than drug B and placebo.

Large multicenter RCTs in migraine therapy are expensive to conduct; therefore the pharmaceutical industry sponsors them and is, in most cases, in control of what RCTs are performed. As mentioned in the Introduction, very few RCTs have been conceived by investigators. Most RCTs are concerned with finding the optimal dose, both benefit and risk being taken into account, but there is an apparent lack of interest in conducting comparative RCTs with other current and cheaper treatment options. Such RCTs are the most relevant from a clinical point of view.

Oral sumatriptan has been compared with ergotamine plus caffeine, Cafergot [25], aspirin plus metoclopramide [26], lysine acetylsalicylate plus metoclopramide [18], rapid release tolfenamic acid

[27] and diclofenac potassium [28]. Subcutaneous sumatriptan has been compared with subcutaneous dihydroergotamine (DHE) [29] (and for registration purposes with intranasal DHE [30]), whereas sumatriptan suppositories were compared with Cafergot suppositories [31]. An overview of these comparative RCTs is given in Table 24.2. *Note that the standard treatments in six of eight RCTs published so far (reference [31] was found on the Internet) were comparable to sumatriptan.* The new triptans, zolmitriptan [11,12], naratriptan [15], rizatriptan [13,14,32] and eletriptan [35], have so far, to our knowledge, been compared with non-triptan drugs other than sumatriptan in one only trial [34]. We recommend that health authorities should request more comparative RCTs in migraine and should fund RCTs conceived and designed by independent clinical investigators.

Selection of Patients

The diagnosis of migraine should be according to the operational diagnostic criteria of the

Table 24.2. Comparative RCTs comparing sumatriptan with standard treatments for migraine attacks

Reference	No. of patients	Dosage (mg)	Success rate (%)		Adverse events (%)
			At 2 h	At 4 h	
Oral sumatriptan					
[25]	220	S100	66**		45
	246	E2 + C200	48		39
[26]	133	S100	56		42**
	138	A900 + M10	45		29
[18]	119	S100	53[†]		28**
	133	LAl620 + M10	57[†]		18
	124	P	24		13
[27]	43	TA200 + TA200	77[†]		30
	42	S100	79[†]		41
	41	P	29		19
[28]	131	DIC-K 50	−17[‡]		19
	122	DIC-K 100	−19[‡]		15
	130	S100	−15[‡]		26
	131	P			20
Subcutaneous sumatriptan					
[30]	133	S6	80		43**
	133	DHE1 + DHE1[n]	50		22
[29][a]	158	S6	85**	83	?
	152	DHE1 + DHE1[s]	73	86	?
Rectal sumatriptan					
[31][b]	251	S2	63		(2[c])
	251	E2 + C100 + E2 + C100	73*		(14[c])**

S, sumatriptan; E, ergotamine; C, caffeine; A, aspirin; M, metoclopramide; LA, lysine acetylsalicylate; P, placebo; TA, rapid release tolfenamic acid; DIC-K, diclofenac potassium; DHE, dihydroergotamine.
**,* Statistically significant differences at $p < 0.01$ and $p < 0.05$, respectively. [†] Statistical significant difference from placebo at $p < 0.01$; [‡] difference from placebo in millimeters on a 100 mm visual analog scale at 2 h.
[a] headache recurred significantly less often after DHE (18%) than after sumatriptan (45%); [b] 44% preferred sumatriptan and 37% preferred Cafergot (E + C) in this crossover RCT; [c] only nausea and/or vomiting are given as adverse events; [n] Intranasal DHE; [s] subcutaneous DHE.

International Headache Society [35] and in our experience this does not cause any problems. However, migraine patients participating in RCTs are most often selected from patients in special clinics or are self-selecting by responding to advertisement. They are thus not representative of the whole migraine population. This can be illustrated by the female/male sex ratio in RCTs, which is often 8 to 2 [18,19], whereas in the general population the sex ratio is 2.5 to 1 [36]. Thus in migraine RCTs female patients tend to enter more often than male patients. In some RCTs, however, a high proportion of female patients are included because of inadequate use of contraceptives; and in one recent RCT we excluded 32 females and 10 males due to this factor.

Another possible selection bias is the choice of escape medication. If a drug A is on the market and this is recommended as escape medication, patients knowing that drug A is not effective for the treatment of their migraine attacks are less likely to participate than patients who have experienced that drug A is effective (see below for other problems with escape medication). The problems with selection bias cannot be overcome totally, but a more representative sample of patients can obtained by using population-based samples of patients [23,37] or by recruiting patients directly from general practice [21,22].

The exclusion criteria in the current RCTs often exclude normal persons by the very strict criteria used. Thus even minor nonsignificant electrocardiographic changes or abnormalities in laboratory tests can exclude patients; and it can be quite difficult to explain a patient that owing to the electrocardiography results she is not allowed to participate but should not worry because she is quite normal. It is our policy to state at the start of the screening "that it is more difficult to enter a RCT than to get a flight certificate".

Trial Design

The overwhelming majority of RCTs conducted in acute migraine treatment use a parallel group comparison [6–17]. It has been argued that this design is most suitable for the development of these drugs [38]. With this design, however, two treatments are compared for benefit (success rates) and risk (adverse events) without, in our view, the benefit/risk ratio being properly evaluated. The groups are compared for success rates (normally being defined as a decrease in head pain from severe or moderate to none or mild: for detailed discussion, see later) and the total percentage of adverse events, most often irrespective of the impact on the patients of these adverse events. Thus many migraine patients will endure minor transient adverse events if the treatment is effective. One way to evaluate this benefit/risk aspect is to ask the patients whether they would take the treatment again, and then compare these answers among treatment groups. An alternative and probably more powerful way to compare treatments is to ask for preferences, and for this the crossover design is needed. With this design it was shown that 35% preferred 100 mg sumatriptan, and 31% and 21% preferred 50 mg and 25 mg, respectively [39]. We recommend this design for evaluating patients' opinions on the benefit/risk ratio.

In some early RCTs [19,25,26] patients were asked to treat up to three attacks with the same treatment, either active drug or placebo, only the results for the first attack being used as the primary parameter and compared among treatment groups. The rationale for treating three attacks is not clear. Assessing consistency of response could be a reason for treating three attacks, and this was evaluated in one RCT [19], where it was found that only 47% of patients responded to sumatriptan in all three attacks. In one RCT [26] comparing sumatriptan and aspirin plus metoclopramide there was no significant difference between the two treatments for the first attack, the primary efficacy parameter, whereas sumatriptan was superior to the combination for the second and third attacks treated. Such results are very difficult to interpret. We recommend that only one attack of migraine should be treated, as has been the trend recently, and that consistency should be evaluated in specially designed RCTs, e.g. [40,41].

As in trials of drugs for many other disorders there seems to be a constant tendency in the development program of the triptans to start out with rather high doses in phase II in order to prove efficacy. For example, oral sumatriptan was first tested in 100 mg, 200 mg and 300 mg doses [19], whereas then current recommended dose in Europe is only 50 mg [39].

Similarly, zolmitriptan was used in phase II in a dose up to 25 mg, while the current recommended dose, with the apparent best benefit/risk ratio, is 2.5 mg [11,12]. Also rizatriptan was compared with sumatriptan in a high dose of 40 mg which caused too many adverse events [32]. The recommended dose of rizatriptan is now 5–10 mg [13,14]. In our experience several patients have had to endure sedation or drowsiness that inhibited normal activity after taking test medication, and we advise patients not to drive after taking study medication. When investigators are asked to participate in RCTs on triptans they should request that the lower part of the dose-response curve be explored and the minimum effective dose defined.

In some recent RCTs, e.g. [42,43], the use of escape medication, normally allowed 2 h after oral administration of a drug, has been postponed to 4 h, probably "in order to explore the full therapeutic potential of the drug". However, patients with migraine attacks prioritize quick onset of action [44] and, in our opinion, escape medication should be allowed after 2 h.

The use of placebo in acute migraine RCTs is necessary, even in comparative RCTs, but its use causes an as yet unrecognized problem for some patients. The use of placebo is often justified by the possibility of using escape medication after 2 h. However, usually only analgesics are allowed, and not triptans or ergotamine. This is due to the fear of an additive vasoconstrictive effect of a test drug and a triptan or ergotamine, which are thus not permitted for 24 h. For many patients sumatriptan or ergotamine are the only effective treatments for their migraine attacks. These patients who experience no effect of analgesics have in reality no effective escape medication and have to endure a migraine attack untreated for 24 h. Depending on the duration of the vasonconstrictive effect of the triptan being studied, e.g. for sumatriptan less than 4 h [45], escape medication with these specific drugs should be allowed earlier than 24 h.

Recurrence of headache after a primary successful treatment with an antimigraine drug occurs in 30–40% of attacks treated in RCTs [6–17], though less frequently with naratriptan [15] and DHE [29], both of which have a longer half-life than sumatriptan, zolmitriptan and rizatriptan [17]. Recurrence is also a major problem in clinical practice, and it cannot be prevented by giving a second dose of sumatriptan [46], but when it occurs it can be treated successfully with a second dose of sumatriptan and rizatriptan [17,47]. In our experience it is difficult for patients to understand that what we try to describe as a new effective drug for migraine can result in recurrences. Patients clearly want a drug that is quickly effective without the risk of recurrence – from a clinical point of view a very reasonable objective for future drugs in migraine treatment.

Evaluation of Results

In all recent RCTs on acute migraine treatment the "Glaxo criterion" of success has been used: a decrease from severe (3) or moderate (2) head pain to none (0) or mild (1). The clinical relevance of this definition of success has been questioned [48] and most migraine patients do not consider a decrease from 2 to 1 as a good result [49]. In addition, it has been shown that the success rates for the combination of lysine acetylsalicylate plus metoclopramide, and placebo, were significantly higher than for sumatriptan when a moderate headache was treated than when a severe headache was treated [50]. The most obvious reason for this is that it is more difficult to induce a decrease from 3 to 1 or 0 (a two-step decrease) than a decrease from 2 to 1 (a one-step decrease). In different RCTs different proportions of patients with severe or moderate headache have been included and part of the variation in reported success rates can result from this (for the use of therapeutic gain, see later). A clinically more relevant way to define success is no headache after 2 h. This is often used as a secondary parameter in current RCTs, but it should be the primary parameter. This parameter will, however, also have inherent problems (e.g. whether a decrease from 3 to 0 is comparable to a decrease from 2 to 0), and its use will increase the number of patients that need to be included in RCTs by probably 50% because of its reduced power compared with the "Glaxo criterion" [51].

Presentation of Results, and Publication Policy

Published success rates for triptans vary considerably. Thus, for subcutaneous sumatriptan the extremes are 86% [52] and 56% [21], the former being most likely to be used for marketing. However, if one looks at the placebo response in these two RCTs they were 37% in the inpatients study [52] and 8% in the study in general practice [21]. If one calculates the "therapeutic gain" (success rate for active drug minus success rate for placebo) one gets quite similar results: 49% and 48%, respectively. Thus one suitable way to correct for the variation in placebo response among different RCTs is to calculate this "therapeutic gain". This is easily done, and we recommend its use instead of success rates when results are reported [53].

Concerning publication it is often stated that the results of an RCT can be published after the sponsor

has had a certain time to review it. Currently, the authors of papers on RCTs in this field are a mixture of clinical investigators and industry employees, but there is seldom an agreed publication policy in the protocol. We recommend that before agreeing to participate in a RCT investigators should insist on a clearly stated publication policy. This should, as a minimum, define how the publication committee will be formed and its responsibilities. Furthermore, it should be stated that the RCT, whatever the results, will published in a peer-reviewed journal within a reasonable time limit.

Conclusions

In recent years the pharmaceutical industry has recruited for large multicenter randomised controlled trials (RCTs). These RCTs are really multicenter and often multinational. The number of centers can be large, both in inpatient studies, e.g. 54 [54] and 58 [55] centers, and in outpatient studies, e.g. 46 [43], 51 [19] and 68 [18] centers. With so many centers, which are in addition geographically separated, it is impossible for most investigators to have any influence on the trial design and the publication of the RCT. However, with many pharmaceutical firms in the field investigators have the opportunity to choose among RCTs presented to them. They should choose to participate in RCTs that are clinically relevant, they should ask for comparative trials, and they should insist on a clearly stated publication policy. In Table 24.3 we present our personal checklist for judging a RCT in the acute treatment of migraine.

Table 24.3. Suggested checklist for investigators before considering participating in a multicenter RCT in migraine

Aim of study clearly stated?
Simple design with relevant primary efficacy parameter?
1. Pain free after 2 h?
2. Success rate after what time?
3. Onset of action?
4. Prevention of recurrence?
Placebo included?
Appropriate doses used?
Benefit/risk ratio evaluated properly?
Power of the study?
Publication policy stated?
1. Review panel defined?
2. Will the RCT be published?
Can sufficient patients be recruited?[a]

[a] Remember the law of disappearing disease.

References

1. Humphrey PPA, Feniuk W, Marriott AS, Tanner RJN, Jackson MR, Tucker ML. Preclinical studies on the anti-migraine drug, sumatriptan. Eur Neurol 1991;31:282–290.
2. Jensen R, Brinck T, Olesen J. Sodium valproate has a prophylactic effect in migraine without aura: A triple-blind, placebo-controlled crossover study. Neurology 1994;44:647–651.
3. Mathew NT, Saper JR, Silberstein SD, Rankin L, Markley HG, Solomon S, et al. Migraine prophylaxis with divalproex. Arch Neurol 1995;52:281–286.
4. Klapper J, on behalf of the Divalproex Sodium in Migraine Prophylaxis Study Group. Divalproex sodium in migraine prophylaxis: a dose-controlled study. Cephalalgia 1997;17:103–108.
5. Steiner TJ, Tfelt-Hansen P. Antiepileptic drugs in migraine prophylaxis. In: Clesen J, Tfelt-Hansen P, Welch KMA, editors. The headaches. 2nd ed. Philadelphia: Zippincott Williams & Wilkins, 2000:483–487.
6. Tfelt-Hansen P. Sumatriptan for the treatment of migraine attacks: a review of controlled clinical trials. Cephalalgia 1993;13:238–244.
7. Plosker GL, McTavish D. Sumatriptan. A reappraisal of its pharmacology and therapeutic efficacy in the acute treatment of migraine and cluster headache. Drugs 1994;47:622–651.
8. Pilgrim AJ, Blakeborough P. The clinical efficacy of sumatriptan in the acute treatment of migraine. Rev Contemp Pharmacother 1994;5:295–309.
9. WiZkinson M, Pfaffenrath V, Schoenen J, et al. Migraine and cluster headache: their management with sumatriptan. A critical review of the current clinical experience. Cephalalgia 1995;15:337–357.
10. Perry CN, Markham A. Sumatriptan. An updated review of its use in migraine. Drugs 1998;55:889–922.
11. Palmer KJ, Spencer CM. Zolmitriptan. CNS Drugs 1997;7:468–478.
12. Rolan PE, Martin GR. Zolmitriptan: a new acute treatment for migraine. Exp Opin Invest Drugs 1998;7:633–652.
13. Dahlöf C, Lines C. Rizatriptan: a new 5-HT$_{1B/1D}$ receptor agonist for the treatment of migraine. Exp Opin Invest Drugs 1999;8:671–686.
14. Dooley M, Faulds D. Rizatriptan: a review of its efficacy in the management of migraine. Dugs 1999;58:699–723.
15. Gunasekara NS, Wiseman LR. Naratriptan. CNS Drugs 1997;8:402–408.
16. Saxena PR, Tfelt-Hansen P. Triptans, 5-HT$_{1B/1D}$ receptor agonists, in the acute treatment of migraine. In: Olesen J, Tfelt-Hansen P, Welch KMA, editors. The headaches. 2nd ed. Philadelphia: Lippincott Williams & Wilkins, 2000:411–438.
17. Tfelt Hansen P, De Vries P, Saxena PR. Triptans in migraine: a comparative review of their pharmacology, pharmacokinetics and efficacy. Drugs, in press.
18. Tfelt-Hansen P, Henry P, Mulder K, Scheldewaert RG, Schoenen J, Chazot G. The effectiveness of combined oral lysine acetylsalicylate and metoclopramide compared with oral sumatriptan for migraine. Lancet 1995;346:923–926.
19. Oral Sumatriptan Dose-defining study Group. Sumatriptan: an oral dose-defining study. Eur Neurol 1991;31:300–305.
20. Tfelt-Hansen P, McEwen J. Nonsteroidal antiinflammatory drugs in the acute treatment of migraine. In: Olesen J, Tfelt-Hansen P, Welch KMA, editors. The headaches. 2nd ed. Philadelphia: Lippincott Williams & Wilkins, 2000:391–397.
21. Russel MB, Holm-Thomsen OE, Nielsen MR, Cleal A, Pilgrim AJ, Olesen J. A randomized, double-blind, placebo-controlled crossover study of subcutaneous sumatriptan in general practice. Cephalalgia 1994;14:291–296.
22. Jensen K, Tfelt-Hansen P, Hansen EW, Krpis EH, Pedersen OS. Introduction of a novel self-injector for sumatriptan: a con-trolled clinical trial in general practice. Cephalalgia 1995;15:423–429.
23. Brennum J, Brinck T, Schriver L, Wanscher B, Soelberg Sørensen P, Tfelt-Hansen P, Olesen J. Sumatriptan has no clinically relevant effect in the treatment of episodic tension-type headache. Eur J Neurol 1996;3:23–28.
24. International Headache Society Committee on Clinical Trials in Migraine. Guidelines for controlled trials of drugs in migraine. 1st ed. Cephalalgia 1991;11:1–12.
25. Multinational Oral sumatriptan and Cafergot Comparative Study Group. A randomized, double-blind comparison of sumatriptan in the acute treatment of migraine. Eur Neurol 1991;31:314–322.
26. Oral Sumatriptan and Aspirin plus Metoclopramide Comparative Study group. A study to compare oral sumatriptan with oral aspirin plus oral metoclopramide in the treatment of migraine. Eur Neurol 1992;32:177–184.
27. Myllylä VV, Havanka H, Herrala L, Kangasneimi P, Rautakorpi I, Turkka J, Vapaatalo H, Eskerod O. Tolfenamic acid rapid release versus sumatriptan in the acute treatment of migraine: comparable effect in a double-blind, randomised, controlled, parallel-group study. Headache 1998;38:201–207.
28. The Diclofenac-K/Sumatriptan Migraine Study Group. Acute treatment of migraine attacks: efficacy and safety of a nonsteroidal anti-inflammatory drug, diclofenac-potassium, in comparison to oral sumatriptan and placebo. Cephalalgia 1999;19:232–240.
29. Winner P, Ricalde O, Le Force B, Saper J, Margul B. A double-blind study of subcutaneous dihydroergotamine vs subcutaneous sumatriptan in the treatment of acute migraine. Arch Neurol 1996;53:180–184.
30. Touchon J, Bertin L, Pilgrim AJ, Ashford E, Bes A. A comparison of subcutaneous sumatriptan and dihydroergotamine nasal spray in the treatment of acute migraine. Neurology 1996;47:361–365.
31. http://www.mpa.se/sve/mono.imig.sht (Monograph in Swedish on sumatriptan suppositories published on the Internet by the Swedish Medical Products Agency.)
32. Visser WH, Terwindt GM, Reines SA, Jiang K, Lines CR, Ferrari MD, for the Dutch/US Rizatriptan Study Group. Rizatriptan vs sumatriptan in the acute treatment of migraine. A placebo-controlled, dose-ranging study. Arch Neurol 1996;53:1132–1137.
33. Goadsby PJ, Ferrari MD, Clesen J, Stovner LJ, Senard JM, Jackson NC, Poole PH, for the Eletriptan Steering Committee. Electriptan in acute migraine: a double-blind, placebo-controlled comparison to sumatriptan. Neurology 2000;54:156–163.
34. Reches A, on behalf of the Electriptan Steering Committee. Comparison of the efficacy, safety and tolerability of oral eletriptan and Cafergot for the acute treatment of migraine. Cephalalgia 1999;19:355.
35. Headache Classification Committee of the International Headache Society. Classification and diagnostic criteria for headache disorders, cranial neuralgias and facial pain. Cephalalgia 1988;8(Suppl 7):1–96.
36. Rasmussen BK. Epidemiology of headache. Cephalalgia 1995;15:45–68.
37. Stewart WF, Lipton RB. Population-based clinical trials in headache. In: Olesen J, Tfelt-Hansen P, editors. Headache treatment: trial methodology and new drugs. New York: Lippincott-Raven, 1997:65–70.
38. Pilgrim A. Methodology of clinical trials of sumatriptan in migraine and cluster headache. Eur Neurol 1991;31:295–299.
39. Salonen R, Ashford EA, Hassani H and The S2EM11 Study Group. Patients preference for oral sumatriptan 25, 50 or 100 mg in the acute treatment of migraine: a double-blind, randomized, crossover study. Int J Clin Pract 1999; Suppl 105:16–24.

40. Rederich G, Rapoport A, Cutler N, Hazelrigg R, Jamerson B. Oral sumatriptan for the long-term treatment of migraine: clinical findings. Neurology 1995;45(Suppl 7):S15–S20.

41. Kramer M, Matzura-Wolfe D, Polis A, et al. A placebo-controlled crossover study of rizatriptan in the treatment of multiple attacks. Neurology 1998;51:773–781.

42. Mathew NT, Asgharnejad M, Peykamian M, Laurenza A, on behalf on the Naratriptan S2Wa3003 Study Group. Naratriptan is effective and well tolerated in the acute treatment of migraine: results of a double-blind, placebo-controlled crossover study. Neurology 1997;49:1485–1490.

43. Rapoport AM, Ramadan NM, Adelman JU, Mathew NT, Elkind AH, Kudrow DB, et al., on behalf of the 017 Clinical Trial Study Group. Optimizing the dose of zolmitriptan (Zomig, 311C90) for the acute treatment of migraine: a multicenter, double-blind, placebo-controlled, dose range-finding study. Neurology 1997;49:1210–1218.

44. Göbel H, Petersen-Braun M, Heinze A. Which properties do patients expect of new and improved drugs in the treatment of primary headache disorders? In: Olesen J, Tfelt-Hansen P, editors. Headache treatment: trial methodology and new drugs. New York: Lippincott-Raven, 1997:93–97.

45. Tfelt-Hansen P, Sperling B, Winter PDO'B. Transient additional effect of sumatriptan on ergotamine-induced constriction of peripheral arteries in man. Clin Pharmacol Ther 1992;51:149.

46. Rapoport AM, Visser WH, Cutler NR, Alderton CJ, Paulsgrove LA, Davis RL, Ferrari MD. Oral sumatriptan in preventing headache recurrence after treatment of migraine attacks with subcutaneous sumatriptan. Neurology 1995;45:1505–1509.

47. Ferrari MD, James MH, Bates D, Pilgrim AJ, Ashford EA, Anderson BA, Nappi G. Oral sumatriptan: effect of a second dose, and treatment of headache recurrence. Cephalalgia 1994;14:330–338.

48. Tfelt-Hansen P. How to define the best efficacy parameters for migraine. Cephalalgia 1997;17(Suppl 17):6–9.

49. Massiou H, Tzourio C, El Amrani M, Bousser MG. Verbal scales in the acute treatment of migraine: semantic categories and clinical relevance. Cephalalgia 1997;17:37–39.

50. Tfelt-Hansen P, Schoenen J, Lauret D. Success rates of combined oral lysine acetylsalicylate and metoclopramide, oral sumatriptan, and placebo depend on initial headache severity. In: Olesen J, Tfelt-Hansen P, editors. Headache treatment: trial methodology and new drugs. New York: Lippincott-Raven, 1997:103–106.

51. Tfelt-Hansen P. Complete relief (IHS criterion) or no or mild pain (Glaxo criterion)? Estimation of relative power in placebo-controlled clinical trials of sumatriptan. In: Olesen J, Tfelt-Hansen P, editors. Headache treatment: trial methodology and new drugs. New York: Lippincott-Raven, 1997: 157–160.

52. Cady RK, Dexter J, Sargent JD, Markley H, Osterhaus JT, Webster CJ. Efficacy of subcutaneous sumatriptan in repeated episodes of migraine. Neurology 1993;43:1363–1368.

53. Tfelt-Hansen P. Efficacy and adverse events of subcutaneous, oral, and intranasal sumatriptan used for migraine treatment: a systematic review based on number needed to treat. Cephalalgia 1998;18:532–538.

54. Cady RK, Wendt JK, Kirchner JR, Sargent JD, Rothrock JF, Skaggs H. Treatment of acute migraine with subcutaneous sumatriptan. JAMA 1991;265:2831–2835.

55. Subcutaneous Sumatriptan International Study Group. Treatment of migraine attacks with sumatriptan. N Engl J Med 1991;325:316–321.

25. Parkinson's Disease: Outcome Variables and Clinical Scales

E.D. Playford

Introduction

Parkinson's disease is a progressive disorder characterised by tremor, rigidity, bradykinesia and postural instability. The aetiology, pathophysiology and clinical features all have a bearing on the selection of appropriate outcome measures and will be discussed briefly.

Aetiology

Parkinson's disease manifests itself clinically when 50% of nigral neurones and 80% of striatal dopamine are lost [1]. The nature of the pathological process underlying clinical deterioration in Parkinson's disease is unknown. Neuronal loss in normal ageing is not sufficient to cause Parkinson's disease but it has been suggested that Parkinson's disease may be due to accelerated ageing [2,3], or alternatively that Parkinson's disease is a biphasic illness [4]. The first phase, an acute illness early in life, sharply depletes neuronal reserves. The second phase, normal ageing, causes further losses resulting in clinical Parkinson's disease. Another view is that the onset and progression of Parkinson's disease represents a novel ongoing degeneration [5,6]. Both these hypotheses feature a suspected preclinical period, although estimates of duration vary from 4 to 40 years.

Diagnosis

The gold standard for diagnosis of Parkinson's disease is the pathological finding of a specific degeneration of nigral and other pigmented brainstem nuclei, with a characteristic inclusion, the Lewy body, in remaining nerve cells [7]. The substantia nigra, the largest of the mesencephalic nuclei, is divided into two. The dorsal part of the nucleus, the pars compacta, contains high concentrations of dopamine and is the principal source of striatal dopamine. Current evidence suggests that the basal ganglia and their cortical connections may be viewed as forming loops [8,9]. These circuits are largely segregated from each other both structurally and functionally. There are least four of these circuits: motor, oculomotor, prefrontal and limbic. Thus, lesions within the basal ganglia, such as the decreased dopamine release in the putamen in Parkinson's disease, result in motor, cognitive and behavioural changes.

Most patients presenting with a tremulous akinetic-rigid syndrome will have the characteristic pathology at post-mortem examination. However, diagnosis is complicated by the fact that there are a number of other disorders that can present with an akinetic-rigid syndrome [10]. These disorders often have disease that is unresponsive to treatment, are particularly difficult to distinguish from Parkinson's disease at onset and may account for up to one-quarter of all patients [11,12]. Unilateral onset, classic rest tremor and a pronounced response to levodopa therapy are the best predictors of Lewy body disease [1]. The absence of rest tremor, no response to levodopa, early falls, dementia, swallowing difficulties, pronounced autonomic symptoms, a supranuclear gaze palsy, cerebellar and pyramidal signs all make an alternative diagnosis more likely. These criteria have been formally stated in the United Kingdom Parkinson's Disease Brain Bank Criteria for idiopathic Parkinson's disease [11] and criteria of this type should be employed in clinical studies in order to minimise diagnostic uncertainty. It is clear that between 16% and 24% of patients included in trials of Parkinson's disease will not have Parkinson's disease [11,12]. This will decrease the sensitivity of any study that is specific for Parkinson's disease, and the greater the diagnostic inaccuracy the more significant the problem. However, if the accuracy is higher than expected then any cost-benefit analysis may not apply to the wider community of parkinsonian patients.

Prognosis

Parkinson's disease is a relentlessly progressive disorder. Prior to the use of levodopa more than one-third of patients had advanced disease within 5 years of onset, and by 10 years the proportion was nearly two-thirds [13]. The DATATOP study which followed drug-naive patients demonstrated that motor function as measured using the UPDRS motor section deteriorated by 8–9% per year [14]. This type of progression would lead to severe disability after more than 10 years of untreated disease. However, much slower rates of decline of the order of 3% per year are found in the early stages of Parkinson's disease in patients treated with levodopa [15]. Both Hoehn and Yahr's original study [13] and two more recent studies by Bonnet et al. [16] and Goetz et al. [17] suggest that progression is more rapid in the first few years of the disease. However, the use of levodopa does influence both the natural history and mortality of the disorder resulting in a reduction of mortality ratio from about 3.0 to 1.5 [15,18]. This benefit has been noted particularly in patients in whom levodopa therapy was started early.

Clinical Features

The characteristic early signs of Parkinson's disease are tremor, rigidity and bradykinesia. The first manifestation of Parkinson's disease is often an intermittent unilateral rest tremor of the fingers, the "pill rolling" tremor. This 3–5 Hz rest tremor is characteristic of Parkinson's disease although it may be absent in both the early and advanced stages of the disease.

Rigidity describes a resistance to passive movement of equal degrees in opposing muscle groups. It is uniform throughout the entire range of movement leading to the description of "lead pipe rigidity". Movements are characteristically difficult to initiate (akinetic), slow (bradykinetic) and have a tendency to diminish with time (hypokinetic). Tremor, rigidity and bradykinesia all tend to start in one arm and later spread to involve the leg and then become bilateral. Bradykinesia is commoner than rigidity or tremor, and because all the muscles in the body can be involved, results in many of the typical features of Parkinson's disease including a blind-like face, monotonous speech, poor armswing and limited dexterity.

As the disease progresses both gait and posture become disturbed. Initially patients complain of slowness of walking; later a shuffling gait appears and this is followed by freezing, often at the sight of an obstacle such as a doorway, and festination where the gait accelerates. Posture also changes. Initially there is flexion at the elbows but later there is flexion at the neck, trunk and knees as well. As a result of these postural abnormalities and the gait disturbance patients are vulnerable to falls. Later in the disease disorders of autonomic function occur, leading to postural hypotension, constipation, bladder difficulties, and finally neuropsychiatric changes including dementia in up to 20% [19] and depression in 20–60% [20].

All these factors should be considered when designing studies of Parkinson's disease, but it is also important to remember that many features of Parkinson's disease are not only extremely variable but can also be affected by mood, diet and attention. These factors are particularly important where function is one of the outcomes.

Medical Treatment

The early stages of Parkinson's disease respond well to treatment by levodopa that is the gold standard of treatment. Unfortunately, more often than not the therapeutic efficacy is limited to 3–5 years, after which the parkinsonian symptoms re-emerge and the long-term side-effects of treatment develop. These include involuntary movements, dyskinesias, fluctuating responses including on–off phenomena, and changes in mentation and behaviour [21]. Many studies have concentrated on diminishing the severity of these side-effects by using different therapeutic approaches. The rationale behind many of these approaches is that there is a pharmacodynamic interaction between the administration of levodopa and the underlying pathophysiological substrate that leads to a loss in therapeutic effectiveness [22]. This loss in therapeutic usefulness has lead to a recent re-examination of surgical treatments, including fetal cell implants, pallidotomy and deep brain stimulation techniques.

Fetal Cell Implants: Ethical Issues

In January 1988 Madrazo and colleagues reported the first use of fetal tissue striatal implantation for the treatment of Parkinson's disease [23]. Subsequent studies have demonstrated this to be a useful treatment for individual patients with severe Parkinson's disease [24]. The principal practical difficulty is that each fetal donor provides a small number of cells so that multiple donors are required [25]. For this and other reasons (infection, chromosomal abnormality), fetal tissues from spontaneous abortions and ectopic pregnancy are limited as feasible sources for human transplantation [25]. Thus tissue from elective abortion is needed. Provided the fetus is dead the use of this tissue could be considered analogous to the use of tissues from dead people, but there are a number of other considerations, in particular the relationship between the aborted fetus and the mother.

Throughout the world societies' expectations and the laws regulating abortion differ. As a result there is no uniform code on the retrieval and use of human embryonal and fetal material for experimental or clinical research. To overcome these problems a Network of European CNS Transplantation and Restoration (NECTAR) was established to develop efficient, reliable, safe and ethically acceptable transplantation therapies for neurodegenerative conditions, based on the principles of autonomy, beneficence, non-maleficence, equality and respect for human rights [26].

These guidelines propose that tissue may be obtained from dead embryos or fetuses where the death results from either legally induced or spontaneous abortion, but that the embryo and fetus may not be kept alive artificially to develop to the most appropriate stage for implantation. Artificial rearing violates respect for the potential human being and reduces the embryo to the level of laboratory material. The guidelines also state clearly that there must be no link between the decision to terminate the pregnancy and the proposed use of the fetus, because it may influence the decision to terminate the pregnancy. In particular there should be no link between the donor and recipient. The timing and nature of the abortion procedure should not be influenced by the requirements of the transplantation when this would increase conflict with the mother's or fetus's interests. However, consent is required from the woman both for the use of the fetal material and to screen her for infectious diseases.

Another issue that has been raised is the possibility of personality transfer [27]. Although there is little doubt that certain animal experiments result in personality change, and that patients with Parkinson's disease undergo personality changes that may be changed further by certain treatments, it seems unlikely that personality can be transferred without the transplantation of large pieces of intact fetal brain which could integrate with the existing brain. Despite this NECTAR chose to adopt a cautious approach and recommended that only cell suspensions or small fragments of brain be used for transplantation. Finally all members of hospital and research staff must be kept fully informed, the procurement of fetal or embryonal tissue must not involve profit or remuneration (this may be of relevance in countries with a low abortion rate hoping to obtain fetal tissue abroad), and all projects involving the use of embryos or fetal tissue must be approved by local ethics committees.

This debate may eventually be eased by the replacement of primary fetus-derived tissue with cells grown in vitro, genetic therapy or alternative surgical procedures. It is therefore important that all such procedures are subjected to a rigorous evaluation.

Outcome Measures

The outcome of any study may be considered in terms of the pathology, impairment, disability, handicap or quality life [28]. Because different scales measure these different aspects of the same disease it is perfectly possible for a patient to improve on one scale while deteriorating on another [29]. When choosing an outcome the reason for the study is paramount. For example a physiotherapy study would be expected to concentrate on measures of mobility and disability whereas a study of a putative neuroprotective agent may wish to concentrate on direct measures of pathology or impairment. In all studies the impact of the intervention should be considered in terms of the patient's quality of life. If the intervention results in a long-term decrease in the patient's quality of life then it should be abandoned.

As has been described, Parkinson's disease has fluctuating motor, behavioural, function and cognitive features complicated by the side-effects and long-term complications of treatment. No single test can cover all these areas and thus the choice of test depends upon the reason for its use. Timing of administration of any test also needs careful consideration. The measure must also be used in such as a manner as to minimise the effects of daily fluctuations in disease activity. Ideally measurements should be made during the "best on" and "worst off" periods, but withdrawing medication for a prolonged period may be considered unethical. A pragmatic solution is to assess patients in the morning some 12 h after last dose of levodopa. In addition the duration of time spent in both states should be recorded.

A large number of scales are available that assess impairment and disability, but detailed reliability and validity studies are not always available. To be reliable these scales need clear descriptions of the meaning of individual points on the scale. There is evidence that idiosyncrasies of performance represent a major source of variability in rating scales. Henderson et al. [30] suggest that careful selection of test items, standardisation of their manner of execution, the clarification of rating criteria and the removal of contextual cues seem more likely to improve reliability than does the selection of raters on the basis of experience. Clinical rating scales in Parkinson's Disease are also discussed in Chapter 27.

In addition there has been interest in the accurate quantitation and detection of changes associated with Parkinson's disease. Electronic or mechanical devices might reasonably be expected to be more sensitive, more consistent (provided they are calibrated regularly) and, in certain circumstances, more informative than clinical measures. Such devices could be used to screen the general population and identify those with "preclinical" changes at risk of developing Parkinson's disease. They might also be used to separate Parkinson's disease from its more common differential diagnoses. In addition, these quantitative measures could assess severity, measure drug responses, ensure the compatibility of results in different centres and monitor disease progression. Examples of such tests include recordings of reaction times [31], portable devices for quantifying wrist rigidity [32], gait analysis and accelerometry [33]. A number of reviews of these objective methodologies have been published [34–36].

Pathology

Direct measurement of the extent of the pathology is often impossible, but often there are biological markers of the disease activity. In many diseases impairment is commonly used as a marker of the underlying disease process, but the validity of this approach may be confounded by treatment such as drug administration or compensatory mechanisms such as the up-regulation of D_2 receptors [37]. It is not possible to measure neuronal numbers and dopamine levels directly in the brain in vivo. Direct study of the dopaminergic system in disease has, until recently, been restricted to post-mortem examination of cerebral tissue. Positron emission tomography (PET) and single photon emission computed tomography (SPECT) are in vivo imaging techniques which enable the examination of both the pre-synaptic and post-synaptic dopminergic system in vivo, and allow repeat studies to assess disease progression [38]. The pre-synaptic metabolism of dopa in human striata was first visualised in life by Garnett et al. [39], who examined three healthy laboratory staff after intravenous injection of [^{18}F]dopa. At 3 h the tracer was seen to concentrate mainly within the caudate nuclei and putamen.

There is now considerable evidence to suggest that [^{18}F]dopa PET both correlates with disability and is an objective means of revealing the underlying rate of progression in pathology in Parkinson's disease. This evidence derives from several sources. The first is the detection of preclinical Parkinson's disease by Vingerhoets et al. [40] in subjects exposed to MPTP but who had not developed clinical parkinsonism. The second is the detection of subclinical changes in apparently healthy primates that had been treated with MPTP [41]. It has also been demonstrated that the severity of the Parkinson's disease as measured both using the Hoehn and Yahr scale and the Unified Parkinson's Disease Rating Scale (UPDRS) can be shown to correlate with the [^{18}F]dopa uptake in the putamen [42,43], and in individuals progressive disease is associated with a decrease in [^{18}F]dopa uptake [44]. In patients with striatal implants, the [^{18}F]dopa uptake increases as function improves on the treated side while being shown to decrease on the untreated side [45]. Finally there are now some studies which demonstrate that human post-mortem cell counts and dopamine levels correlate well with [^{18}F]dopa uptake and the UPDRS score [46]. [^{18}F]dopa PET is a reproducible technique and studies have demonstrated that mean variation in mean putamen measurements is 8% (this will probably decrease with modern-generation three-dimensional scanners). Recent studies demonstrate that the rate of disease progression in parkinsonian putamen is 12.5% per year [44]. Based on this work it has been possible to show that to demonstrate a neuroprotective effect by decreasing the rate of progression to 0.0004 min^{-1} per year with 80% power and 5% significance would require 65 patients in each group [47].

Impairment

Wade [48] suggests that in clinical practice the most useful tests to assess impairment in Parkinson's disease are the Hodkinson Mental Test [49] or the Short Orientation–Memory–Concentration test [50] with the McDowell Impairment Index [51]. The Hodkinson Mental Test has been validated for use with the elderly although not specifically in Parkinson's disease. It tests memory and orientation in a crude fashion and can detect only severe disorientation. It is insensitive to frontal lobe problems, and may be of limited value in younger patients with Parkinson's disease. The McDowell Impairment Index uses a 3-point scale (0 = absent, 1 = present, 2 = markedly present) for symptoms and signs which are then weighted. No explanation of the various weightings is given but it has face validity, though inter-rater reliability has been reported to vary by up to 40% [51]. It is, however, able to detect improvements produced by levodopa.

There are a number of other scales designed specifically to measure impairment in Parkinson's disease, including the Columbia Rating scale [52], Lieberman's Index [53], Hoehn and Yahr grades [13], the Webster Rating scale [54], the New York Rating scale [55] and the UPDRS [56] (see also Chapter 27, Appendices A, B, C). In some of these scales changing disease leads to a deterioration in one part of the scale (e.g. rigidity) but an improvement in another (e.g. tremor) with no overall change in score. Of these the Webster scale and the Columbia scales have been used most widely. The Webster Rating scale consists of 10 items, of which one item is a global score of disability, scored from 0 to 3 (absent, mild, moderate, severe). Each item is clearly described [54], and in 1981 the scale was recommended for use in combination with the Hoehn and Yahr, and the North Western University Disability scale by Marsden and Schachter [34]. The Columbia scale consists of 25 items divided in to four sections; tremor, rigidity, bradykinesia and functional performance. The last section comprises assessment of rapid sequential movements, facial expression, seborrhoea, sialorrhoea and speech, and thus, depite its title, focuses mainly on impairment [52]. Although intra-rater reliability is good, inter-rater reliability has been shown to be poor [57]. The New York scale has not been fully evaluated for reliability and mixes disability and impairment [55]. The Hoehn and Yahr remains a useful shorthand for describing a patient's clinical severity but is otherwise of limited use.

The need for a common and uniform method for the evaluation of Parkinson's disease prompted the formation of the Unified Parkinson's Disease Rating Scale Development Committee in 1985 [56]. The UPDRS is the scale most studied and most widely used in a study setting (see Chapter 27, Appendix B). It was developed to unify the features of the Hoehn and Yahr (see Chapter 27, Appendix A), Columbia, New York and Webster scales. It has four subsections: mentation, activities of daily living (ADL), motor, and side-effects. The motor and ADL subscales have been studied in some detail and have been shown to be valid, reliable and responsive in the hands of expert neurologists [58]. In addition the ADL section has been shown to be reliable when self-administered [59]. It is probably the preferred scale for impairment-based research but is rather long for everyday practice, taking 10–15 min to apply. The first section of the UPDRS relates to secondary features of the disease and Wade suggests that these may be better measured using short specific scales [48]. The scale mixes impairment and disability. The ADL section includes some impairments (for example

tremor) which also occur in the third section. Conversely the third section, which concentrates on motor impairments, also includes some disabilities (e.g. gait) which are covered in the second section. It does not have a behavioural subscale to cover items such as sleep patterns, depression, anxiety, psychosis and dementia.

The UPDRS has good criterion-related validity using the Hoehn and Yahr classification and timed tests, although the choice of the Hoehn and Yahr could be criticised because of its relative insensitivity [56,60]. the discriminant ability of the scale with relation to the Hospital Anxiety and Depression scale [61] and the Mini-Mental State Examination [62] is relatively low but this may in part be because the mentation subscale covers similar items [60]. The convergent validity when compared with the Intermediate Scale for the Assessment of Parkinson's Disease (ISAPD) is excellent. The internal consistency of the scale has been shown to be high (Cronbach's alpha = 0.96), but the effects of redundancy, with several items based on the same aspect of the construct, may contribute to this figure. The items related to tremor, depression and motivation appear to be poorly related [60,63]. The inter-rater reliability is also good, and there was a high correlation of the UPDRS with timed tests of finger tapping and rising from a chair. The ADL scale is really an interview and is therefore subject to interpretation, which could lead to a drop in reliability and validity.

In addition there are a number of other limitations in the scale. It does not cope well with fluctuations because it is time-consuming. It does not allow for the relative difference in contribution made to disability by impairments of the same type on either the dominant or non-dominant side.

Both simpler [64] and more complex versions of the scale exist, for example CAPIT, which was developed for surgical trials [65] (see Chapter 27, Table 27.1). However, all longitudinal studies use the UPDRS so it would be unwise to shorten the data set for such studies as later data may not be comparable with other such data sets. The total UPDRS score has been shown to correlate well with simpler scales such as the Hoehn and Yahr [13], with [^{18}F]dopa isotope uptake studies [44], neuronal cell counts and dopamine storage [46] in the basal ganglia in postmortem studies.

Disability

As described above the UPDRS covers both impairments and disability. There are also a number of other scales designed to measure disability in Parkinson's disease. These include the North Western University Disability Scale [66], the McDowell Disability Index [51] and the self-assessment

Parkinson's disease disability scale [67], which may be particularly useful in an outpatient or community setting. The North Western University Disability Scale covers five ADL items which, although not specific to Parkinson's disease, are important in this condition. The original study reported good reliability which a coefficient of concordance of 0.95 representing a mean percentage disagreement of 3.3%. It has been widely used, being recommended by Marsden and Schachter [34]. the McDowell Disability Index consists of 11 ADL items some of which are particularly relevant to the problems experienced by those with Parkinson's disease, such as getting out of bed, getting out of a chair, turning in bed and handwriting. Like the McDowell Impairment Index these items are weighted but no explanation of the various weightings is given. Once again it has face validity; inter-rater reliability has been reported to vary by up to 40% but it is, however, able to detect improvements produced by levodopa.

Wade [48] suggests that in many situations more generic measures of disability may be adequate. The Barthel Index is the most commonly used assessment of disability [68,69]. It has been well studied in a number of settings (but not specifically Parkinson's disease) and its general validity has been well established. It correlates well with clinical impression, with motor loss after stroke and with scores on other ADL scales. It is reliable, and simple to use. Its sensitivity is, however, limited by floor and ceiling effects and it is relatively unresponsive to small changes. If a scale of instrumental ADL is required the Nottingham Extended Activities of Daily Living is probably the most useful [70]. It has been shown to be reliable and valid in stroke patients, but no specific assessment has been performed for Parkinson's disease, or other progressive diseases. Nevertheless it has face validity and may be useful in this group of patients.

These scales can only be used to complement other, more directly quantifiable motor tasks such as the timed motor tasks like the stand–walk–sit test, usually over a distance of 7 or 10 m; a standardised tapping test; or a peg-board test such as the 9-hole peg test [71]. The stand–walk–sit task is a simple, reproducible measure suitable for the assessment of physiotherapy interventions aimed at improving mobility. In this test the patient rises from a chair, walks 7 m, pivots and comes back to sit down. Each element can be individually timed as demonstrated by Yekutiel et al. [72]. The total number of steps taken during this task provides a simple measure of quality which overcomes the potential problems of propulsion and festination. Other functional mobility tasks include rising from lying on a bed/plinth to standing, and rising from lying on the floor. Again each element of these tests can be timed. One criticism of these tests is that they are relatively short and do not mimic more complex everyday situations such as walking round a crowded room, in the street and through doorways. Further tests should be developed which have ecological validity, such as the obstacle course used by Nieuwboer et al. [73].

Handicap/Quality of Life

Handicap is the disadvantage for a given individual, resulting from impairment or disability that limits or prevents the fulfilment of a role that is normal for that individual [28]. Measurement can be difficult because it relates to the expectations of an individual person. The domains usually considered include orientation, physical independence, mobility, occupation of time, social integration and economic self-sufficiency. There are a number of scales which aim to examine handicap in different conditions, e.g. the Environmental Status Scale in multiple sclerosis [74], but none that has been developed for use in Parkinson's disease. In practice, the best way to record handicap is with a verbatim record of the patient's own account of their handicap.

Another way to consider handicap is as a change in a patient's quality of life. There is increasing interest in the use of measures of well-being in chronic degenerative disease. A number of instruments have been used in Parkinson's disease to measure health status and health-related quality of life, including the Nottingham Health profile [75,76] and the SF36 [77,78]. The Nottingham Health Profile has been well studied for validity and reliability and has been used in Parkinson's disease. However, it may simply be recording mood rather than a more global concept of the quality of life.

The SF36 health survey questionnaire is a short 36-item general measure of health status that can be used to assess functioning and well-being in any population group or sample. However, these scales do not address areas relevant and unique to Parkinson's disease, such as disturbance of or difficulty with concentration, and unusual bodily symptoms of discomfort, and may demonstrate ceiling effects when the disability is marked. To increase the responsiveness the content has to be modified to be of particular relevance to one patient group. In view of this the PDQ39 was developed [79,80]. In order to ensure that it had high content validity it was developed following detailed interviews with people with Parkinson's disease, and subsequently was shown to have satisfactory internal and test–retest reliability and construct validity in relation to other measures. Earlier work had shown that even in the presence of depression and cognitive impairment patients report accurately on their disability and thus this scale was developed as a self-report scale. Further work will aim to demonstrate its responsiveness to changing disease over time.

The methods and rating scales described above provide a number of different approaches to measuring pathology, impairment, disability, handicap and quality of life in Parkinson's disease. When choosing one of these measures it important to establish that the measure chosen can provide the information that is needed. Thus a measure may be valid, reliable and responsive yet inappropriate to the situation under consideration. Different types of trials demand the use of different outcome measures. The next sections will address some of the varying outcome measurement issues raised by drug, surgical and rehabilitation studies.

Drug Studies

The majority of current drug studies have one of several aims: to delay the onset of, or the severity of, motor fluctuations in patients with Parkinson's disease; to spare the use of levodopa because of the theoretical concern that free radicals generated from the the oxidative metabolism of dopamine might accelerate the degeneration of residual dopamine neurones; or to delay the underlying progression of the pathological process.

These different types of study need to be clearly differentiated. Studies which aim to improve the physical manifestations of the disease and alleviate the symptoms and signs are usually pragmatic studies [81]. In terms of the international classification of impairments, disabilities and handicaps they will use measures of impairment and disability as an outcome. Studies which aim to delay the progression of the underlying pathological process are efficacy trials [81] and in these studies a biological marker for the pathological process will be the appropriate measure.

Because of the nature of Parkinson's disease, with its tendency to progress and manifold clinical manifestations, pragmatic trials of drug therapy will usually be multicentre trials. These studies need valid, reliable, responsive and clinically useful measures of outcome. Scales which take 30 min or more to apply will be of limited use in this situation.

The size of an efficacy trial will depend far more on the accuracy of the biological markers for the underlying disease process. Where it is possible to measure this accurately studies may be small. If there is variability in the relationship between the marker and the pathology then the study will have to be large enough to take account of this. Neuroprotective agents will act by slowing the rate of loss of dopaminergic neurones. If the neuroprotection is less than 100% then there will be continued, albeit slowed deterioration of the parkinsonian symptomatology. At an advanced stage there will be no feasible treatments unless there is to be some form of neuroregeneration. Neuroprotection trials should therefore be carried out as early as possible to maximise the probability of showing protection. This means using surrogate markers of disease, but no reliable marker for the pathological process in Parkinson's disease has been found apart from the functional imaging techniques described earlier, which are both labour-intensive and expensive.

The DATATOP study was the first which aimed to examine the effects of two putative neuroprotective agents: selegiline (deprenyl) and vitamin E [14]. In this study 800 previously untreated patients were randomised to receive either selegiline, tocopherol, tocopherol and selegiline or placebo. The primary end-point was the decision to initiate levodopa treatment. Other indices of treatment effect were termed secondary response variables and included measures of motor impairment, physical disability and mental state. Analysis showed that in the selegiline-treated patients the primary end-point was delayed by about 9 months. Secondary response variables showed improvement at 1 and 3 months (wash-in effect) but only mild deterioration after stopping selegiline (wash-out). Mean rate of change of these variables was significantly lower in the treatment group.

The DATATOP study had a number of important design features. It was a multicentre study, which enabled recruitment of sufficient numbers of patients and also ensured that the results would be widely applicable. Multicentre studies can also be used to develop more complex study designs, such as the 2×2 design in which combinations of two drugs both with each other and with placebo permit a factorial analysis that enables multiple questions to be asked. Until the DATATOP study most pharmacological studies examined outcome at a fixed end-point, but the DATATOP trial changed this approach by assuming that when disease progression reaches a threshold a measurable end-point occurs. Such end-points, or outcomes, include death, the occurrence of adverse events, and the transition from one stage to another. However, in this study subsequent analysis showed that the end-point chosen could also be delayed as a result of a quantal reduction in impairment following which the rate of deterioration is unchanged [82].

The exact extent to which neuroprotection is differentiated from a symptomatic effect depends on two issues related to trial design: first whether or not disease progression was validly measured and second whether the duration of follow-up was adequate. The primary end-point, the need for levodopa treatment, was based on the subjectively perceived needs of the patient rather than objective measurements such as motor speed. The subjective impact is a notoriously poor predictor of severity. This primary end-point provided only a weak indication of the rate of progression of neuronal dysfunction. It would have been preferable to use reliable valid serial measurement of biologically based impairment.

The second issue relates to duration of follow-up. If this is too short any therapeutic efficacy will be overestimated. This occurs because only the most severely affected cases will reach the end-point and these are relatively rare. In addition, there will be a lag period between the first untreated patients passing the end-point and the treated patients beginning to do so, such that the rate of treated to untreated patients at that point in time will be distorted in favour of the treatment group. One of the problems with providing an adequate wash-out period is that if it is too long then it may be that the vulnerable cells are those that are most protected by the neuroprotective agent. When this is withdrawn one may see catch-up cell loss which may confound the results in a direct way.

It is now accepted that the DATATOP study provided clear evidence for the fact that selegiline has a symptomatic therapeutic effect in Parkinson's disease and that this alone was sufficient to explain the probability of reaching an end-point.

In contrast to studies which aim to explore the potential neuroprotective role of drugs are those which aim either to spare the use of levodopa or to control the severity of motor fluctuations in patients with Parkinson's disease, i.e. pragmatic studies. The nature of Parkinson's disease with its wide range of clinical features, variable course and day-to-day fluctuations means that studies need to be conducted on a multicentre basis to provide definitive answers. For example the information provided by studies on pergolide has been confusing. In patients with stage III and IV Hoehn and Yahr disease, several small studies suggested that pergolide leads to an improvement in parkinsonian symptoms so that the total levodopa dosage can be decreased [83,84]. However, a number of other studies failed to demonstrate any such benefit, and suggested that the side-effect profile included cardiotoxicity [85]. A multicentre study of 376 patients with stage II to IV Parkinson's disease randomised in a prospective, double-blind, placebo-controlled trial demonstrated that a mean dose of 2.94 mg of pergolide permitted a 24.7% reduction in the dose of levodopa, and that adverse reactions were mild and reversible [86].

Surgical Studies

Over the last decade there has been a re-examination of the role of surgery in the management of Parkinson's disease. This was, in part, stimulated by the first reports of successful intracerebral transplantation. The Core Assessment Program for Intracerebral Transplantation (CAPIT) was published in 1993 to standardise the diagnosis and evaluation of patients with Parkinson's disease undergoing experimental implantation [65]. The key features of this assessment included core inclusionary criteria, recommendations for a clinical assessment battery with recommendations for the timing and number of such evaluations, issues relating to fetal age, and the use of imaging including MRI and PET. The clinical assessment battery includes the UPDRS, Hoehn and Yahr staging and a dyskinesia scale score. It is also suggested that the patients should keep a self-report diary for at least a week prior to each assessment in which they should report their condition hourly using symbols to record one of five conditions: complete "on", "on" with dyskinesias, partial "on", complete "off" and sleep. There are also four timed tests to be recorded in "best on" and practically defined "off" conditions. These tests include the pronation–supination test, hand/arm movement between two points, a finger dexterity test and a stand–walk–sit test. The stand–walk–sit test is from a non-rocking or tilting seat with the seat located 45 cm from the floor. The time required to stand, walk 7 m, turn, walk back to the chair and sit is recorded.

Since the publication of CAPIT surgical treatment of Parkinson's disease has been widely re-evaluated and a number of new techniques developed, including pallidotomy, deep brain stimulation and lesions of the subthalamic nucleus [87]. CAPIT has been used in many of these studies as a "gold standard" in the evaluation of Parkinson's disease. Inevitably there have been criticisms of the program, particularly over the timed testing section where it has been suggested that the finger dexterity test be dropped and another timed method used to assess finger dexterity, such as the Purdue peg-board; the guidelines for the hand pronation–supination test be formalised and validated; and the number of steps in the stand–walk–sit test be recorded, possibly in the form of the step × seconds product [88].

Rehabilitation/Therapy Studies

It is clear that rehabilitation studies are all pragmatic studies. No-one expects that therapy will have any effect on underlying neuronal degeneration; here the aim is to see whether function can in some way be improved. Physiotherapy involves management of a movement deficit. It aims to improve mobility and function through physical re-education of the patient. Similarly, occupational therapy aims to restore daily function through activities important to the patient. These aims should influence the choice of outcome. The outcomes measures in these studies should primarily examine mobility and disability, not impairment. If for example, the aim is to improve dressing, the 9-hole peg test should not be regarded as the primary outcome.

Many general criticisms can be levelled at rehabilitation studies. There is often a poor description of the nature and purpose of the intervention. There is often no control group, and perhaps because of the intensive and expensive nature of the intervention, most studies are of small numbers with little effort to estimate the power of the study. Often the outcome appears only indirectly related to the primary intention of the intervention, e.g. quality of life gains in a study aimed primarily at improving gait. Indeed one issue seems to be that there is no consensus about the best way to measure gait in Parkinson's disease.

A study by Yekutiel and colleagues [72] describes an educational approach to physiotherapy in Parkinson's disease where patients learn to replace automatic movements with conscious movement strategies. In this study 12 patients were treated twice a week for 3 months. The evaluation was standardised, with the tests involved having clear face validity and being demonstrated to be reliable and responsive to change, particularly in the more disabled patients. The measures included timing the following movements; rising from a chair, walking to and around another chair and sitting down on the first chair; rising to standing from lying supine (divided into two components of first floor contact and remainder); and rising to standing from lying supine on the floor (divided into reaching feet-only contact with the floor and the remainder). These standardised mobility tests were performed before and after treatment and showed a statistically significant decrease of over 40% in total test time.

There are also number of studies which use an understanding of the pathophysiological basis of the disease to explore in detail the efficacy of specific interventions. These studies use measures of impairment and disability as outcome measures. For example, Morris and her colleagues [89] have conducted a series of experiments in which they examined the relationship between stride length, cadence and velocity in normal subjects and patients with Parkinson's disease. They demonstrated that although the Parkinson's disease patients retained the capacity to vary their gait velocity in a similar manner to controls, the range of response was reduced. When walking slowly, Parkinson's disease patients could vary their speed of walking by adjusting cadence and to a lesser extent stride length. However, when the speed of walking was controlled the stride length was found to be shorter and the cadence higher than in controls. Stride length could not be upgraded by internal control mechanisms in response to a fixed cadence; in contrast cadence was readily modulated by external cues and internal control mechanisms when the stride length was fixed. Thus Morris et al. concluded that regulation of stride length is the fundamental problem in gait and suggested that movement rehabilitation strategies could have the potential to assist Parkinson's disease patients to achieve a more normal step size, perhaps by using visual cueing. The rationale for these approaches lies in the understanding that predictive external sensory cues can trigger the switch from one movement component in a movement sequence to another and thus by-pass defective internal pallidocortical projections, possibly via the lateral premotor cortex which receives information in the context of externally guided movements. Thus the use of impairment-based measures such as stride length and cadence, as well as disability measures such as gait velocity, is entirely justified.

The studies mentioned above clearly demonstrate short-term gains but do not examine long-term gains such as delayed onset of falls, delay in onset of freezing, or even the role of exercise as an adjunct to delay treatment with levodopa. Such studies will need to be larger and may well need a multicentre approach. Few centres in the UK have the physiotherapy staff available to participate in such a study but one approach would be for rehabilitation studies in Parkinson's disease to be conducted within a series of structured guidelines which include diagnostic and inclusion criteria and outcome measures [90]. This would enable a series of centres to perform sequential studies in a similar manner which would then be suitable for meta-analysis.

Despite the large number of measures now available, the accurate assessment and measurement of outcome in Parkinson's disease remains a formidable problem. The careful use of accurate diagnostic criteria and the development of standardised outcome measures will allow comparisons between studies to be made. Further development of appropriate outcome measures which are used widely will permit continuing progress in this challenging field.

References

1. Marsden CD. Parkinson's disease. Lancet 1990;335:948–952.
2. Mann DMA, Yates PO. Possible role of neuromelanin in the pathogenesis of Parkinson's disease. Mechanisms Ageing Dev 1983;21:193–203.
3. Barbeau A. Aetiology of Parkinson's disease: a research strategy. Can J Neurol Sci 1984;11:24–28.
4. Koller WC, Langston JW, Hubble JP, Irwin I, Zack M, Golbe L, et al. Does a long preclinical period occur in Parkinson's disease? Neurology 1991;41(Suppl 2):8–13.
5. McGreer PL, et al. Rate of cell death in Parkinsonism indicates active neuropathological process. Ann Neurol 1988;24:574–576.
6. Fearnley JM, Less AJ. Ageing and Parkinson's disease: substantia nigra regional selectivity. Brain 1991;114:2283–2301.
7. Gibb WRG, Lees AJ. The significance of the Lewy body in the diagnosis of idiopathic Parkinson's disease. Neuropathol Appl Neurobiol 1989;15:27–44.
8. Alexander GE, DeLong MR, Strick PL. Parallel organisation of functionally segregated circuits linking basal ganglia and cortex. Annu Rev Neurosci 1986;9:357–381.
9. Alexander GE, Cruthcher MD, DeLOng MR. Basal ganglia thalamo-cortical circuits: parallel substrates for motor, oculomotor, "prefrontal" and "limbic" functions. Prog Brain Res 1990;85:119–146.
10. Duvoisin RC. The differential diagnosis of parkinsonism. In: Stern G, editor. Parkinson's disease. London: Chapman and Hall Medical, 1990:431–466.
11. Hughes AJ, Daniel SE, Kilford L, Lees AJ. Accuracy of clinical diagnosis of idiopathic Parkinson's disease: a clinico-pathological study of 100 cases. J Neurol Neurosurg Psychiatry 1992;55:181–184.
12. Ansorge O, Lees AJ, Daniel SE. Update on the accuracy of clinical diagnosis of idiopathic Parkinson's disease. Mov Disord 1997(Suppl):359.
13. Hoehn MM, Yahr MD. Parkinsonism: onset, progression and mortality. Neurology 1967;17:427–442.
14. The Parkinson Study Group. Effect of Deprenyl on the progression of disability in early Parkinson's disease. N Engl J Mcd 1989;321:1364–1371.
15. Poewe WH, Wenning GK. The natural history of Parkinson's disease. Neurology 1996;47:(Suppl 3):S146–152.
16. Bonnet AM, Loria Y, Saint-Hilatre, Lhermitte F, Agid Y. Does long term aggravation of Parkinson's disease result from non-dopaminergic lesions? Neurology 1987;37:1539–1542.
17. Goetz CG, Tanner CM, Shannon KM. Progression of Parkinson's disease without levodopa. Neurology 1987;37:695–698.
18. Ben Shlomo Y, Marmot MG. Survival and cause of death in a cohort of patients with parkinsonism: possible clues to aetiology. J Neurol Neurosurg Psychiatry 1995;58:293–299.
19. Brown RG, Marsden CD. Neuropsychology and cognitive function in Parkinson's disease: an overview. In: Marsden CD, Fahn S, editors. Movement disorders 2. London: Butterworth 1987.
20. Gotham AM, Brown RG, Marsden CD. Depression in Parkinson's disease: a quantitative and qualitative analysis. J Neurol Neurosurg Psychiatry 1986;49:381–389.
21. Marsden CD, Parkes JD. On-off effects in patients with Parkinson's disease on chronic levodopa therapy. Lancet 1976;I:292–296.
22. Juncos JL, Engber TM, Raisman R, Susel Z, Thibaut F, Ploska A, et al. Continuous and intermittent levodopa differentially affect basal ganglia function. Ann Neurol 1989;25:473–478.
23. Madrazo I, et al. Transplantation of fetal substantia nigra and adrenal medulla to the caudate nucleus in two patients with Parkinson's disease. N Engl J Med 1988;332:1118–1124.
24. Lindvall O, Widner H, Rehncrona S, et al. Transplantation of foetal dopamine neurones in Parkinson's disease: one year clinical and neurophysiological observations in two patients with putaminal implants. Ann Neurol 1992;31:155–165.
25. Harby K. Using fetus derived tissues for molecular medicine: tension between research and ethics. Mol Med Today 1996; 2:326–329.
26. Boer GJ. Ethical guidelines for the use of human embryonic or foetal tissue for experimental and clinical neurotransplantation and research. Network of European CNS Transplantation and Restoration (NECTAR). J Neurol 1994;242:1–13.
27. Northoff G. Do brain tissue transplants alter personality? Inadequacies of some standard arguments. J Med Ethics 1996; 22:174–180.
28. World Health Organization. International classification on impairments, disability and handicaps. Geneva: WHO, 1980.
29. Diamond SG, Markham CH. Evaluating the evaluations: or how to weigh the scales of parkinsonian disability. Neurology 1983;33:1098–1099.
30. Henderson L, Kennard C, Crawford TJ, et al. Scales for rating motor impairment in Parkinson's disease: studies of reliability and convergent validity. J Neurol Neurosurg Psychiatry 1991;54:18–24.
31. Ward CD, Sanes JN, Dambrosia JM, Calne DB. Methods for evaluating treatment in Parkinson's disease. In: Fahn S, Calne DB, Shoulson I, editors. Experimental therapeutics of movement disorders. Advances in neurology 37. New York: Raven Press, 1983.
32. Caligiuri MP. Portable device for quantifiying parkinsonian wrist rigidity. Mov Disorders 1994;9:57–63.
33. Jankovic J, Frost JD. Quantitative assessment of parkinsonian and essential tremor: clinical application of tri-axial accelerometry. Neurology 1980;30:393.
34. Marsden CD, Schachter M. Assessment of extrapyramidal disorders. Br J Clin Pharmacol 1981;11:129–151.
35. Jankovic J, Lang AC, Fahn S. High technology in the quantitation of movement disorders. Ninth international symposium on Parkinson's disease, 1988.
36. Lakke JPWF. Assessment and measurement. In: Stern G, editor. Parkinson's disease. London: Chapman and Hall Medical, 1990:467–491.
37. Brooks DJ, Ibanez V, Sawle GV, Playford ED, Quinn N, Bannister R, et al. Striatal D_2 receptor status in Parkinson's disease, striatonigral degeneration, and progressive supranuclear palsy, measured with ^{11}C-raclopride and PET. Ann Neurol 1992;31:184–192.
38. Playford ED, Brooks DJ. In vivo and in vitro measurements of the dopaminergic system in movement disorders. Cerebrovasc Brain Metab Rev 1992;4:144–171.
39. Garnett ES, Firnau G, Nahmias C. Dopamine visualised in the basal ganglia of living man. Nature 1983;305:137–138.
40. Vingerhoets FJG, Snow BJ, Tetrud JW, Langston JW, Schulzer M, Calne DB. Positron emission tomographic evidence for progression of human MPTP induced dopaminergic lesions. Ann Neurol 1994;36:765–770.
41. Pate BD, Kawamata T, Yamada T, McGreer EG, Hewitt KA, Snow BJ, et al. Correlation of striatal fluorodopa uptake in the MPTP monkey with dopaminergic indices. Ann Neurol 1993;34:331–338.

42. Brooks DJ, Salmon EP, Mathias CJ, Quinn N, Leenders KL, Bannister R, et al. The relationship between locomotor disability, autonomic dysfunction and the integrity of the striatal dopaminergic system in patients with multiple system atrophy, primary autonomic failure and Parkinson's disease studied with PET. Brain 1990;113:1539–1552.

43. Takikawa S, Dhawan V, Chaly T, Robeson W, Dahl R, Zanzi I, et al. Input functions for 6-(fluorine-18)fluorodopa quantitation in parkinsonism: comparative studies and clinical correlations. J Nucl Med 1994;35:955–963.

44. Morrish PK, Sawle GV, Brooks DJ. An [^{18}F]dopa-PET and clinical study of the rate of progression in Parkinson's disease Brain 1996;119:585–591.

45. Sawle GV, Bloomfield PM, Bjorklund A, et al. Transplantation of foetal dopamine neurones in Parkinson's disease: PET [^{18}F]6-L-fluorodopa studies in two patients with putaminal implants. Ann Neurol 1992;31:166–173.

46. Snow BJ, Tooyama I, Mcgreer EG, et al. Correlations in humans between postmortem PET fluorodopa uptake, postmortem dopaminergic cell counts and striatal dopaminergic levels. Ann Neurol 1993;34:324–330.

47. Altman DG. Practical statistics for medical research. London: Chapman and Hall, 1991:456.

48. Wade DT. Measurement in neurological rehabilitation. Oxford: Oxford University Press, 1992.

49. Hodkinson HM. Evaluation of a mental test score for assessment of mental impairment in the elderly. Age Ageing 1972;1:233–238.

50. Katzman R, Brown T, Fuld P, Peck A, Schecter R, Schimmel H. Validation of a short Orientation-Memory-Concentration test of cognitive impairment. Am J Psychiatry 1983;140:734–739.

51. McDowell F, Lee JE, Swift T, Sweet RD, Ogsbury JS, Kessler T. Treatment of parkinson's syndrome with L-dihydroxyphenylalanine (levodopa). Ann Intern Med 1970;72:29–35.

52. Yahr MD, Duvoisin RC, Schear MJ, et al. Treatment of Parkinsonism with levo-dopa. Arch Neurol 1969;21:343–354.

53. Lieberman AN. Parkinson's disease: a clinical review. Am J Med Sci 1974;267:66–80.

54. Webster DD. Critical analysis of the disability in Parkinson's disease. Mod Treatment 1968;5:257–282.

55. Alba A, Trainor FS, Ritter W, Dacso MM. A clinical rating scale for Parkinson patients. J Chron Dis 1968;21:507–522.

56. Fahn S, Elton RL, and members of the UPDRS Development Committee. In: Fahn S, Marsden CD, Calne DB, Goldstein M, editors. Recent developments in Parkinson's disease, vol 2. Florham Park, NJ: MachMillan Health Care Information, 1983:153–165.

57. Hely MA, Chey T, Wilson A, et al. Reliability of the Columbia scale for assessing signs in Parkinson's disease. Mov Disord 1993;8:466–472.

58. Richards M, Marder K, Cote L, Mayeux R. Interrater reliability of the Unified Parkinson's Disease Rating Scale Motor Examination. Mov Disord 1994;9:89–91.

59. Louis ED, Lynch T, Marder K, Fahn S. Reliability of patient completion of the historical section of the unified Parkinson's disease rating scale. Mov Disord 1996;11:185–192.

60. Martinez-Martin P, Gil-Nagel A, Morlan Gracia L, Balseiro Gomez J, Martinez-Sarries J, Bermejo F, and the Co-operative Multicentric Group. Unified Parkinson's disease rating scale characteristics and structure. Mov Disord 1994;9:76–83.

61. Zigmond AS, Snaith RP. The Hospital Anxiety and Depression Scale. Acta Psychiatr Scand 1983;67:361–370.

62. Folstein MF, Folstein SE, McHugh PJ. "Mini-mental state": a practical method for grading the cognitive state of patients for clinicians. J Psychiatr Res 1975;12:189–198.

63. Reynold NC, Montgomery GK. Factor analysis of Parkinson's impairment: an evaluation of the final common pathway. Arch Neurol 1987;44:1013–1016.

64. Van Hilten JJ, van der Zwan AD, Zwinderman AH, Roos RA. Rating impairment and disability in Parkinson's disease: evaluation of the Unified Parkinson's Disease Rating Scale. Mov Disord 1994;9:84–88.

65. Langston JW, Widner H, Goetz CG, et al. Core Assessment Program for Intracerebral Transplantation (CAPIT). Mov Disord 1992;7:2–13.

66. Canter GJ, De la torre R, Mier M. A method for evaluating disability in patients with Parkinson's disease. J Nerv Ment Dis 1961;133:143–147.

67. Brown RG, MacCarthy B, Jahanshahi M, Marsden CD. Accuracy of self reported disability in patients with parkinsonism. Arch Neurol 1989;46:955–959.

68. Mahoney FI, Barthel DW. Functional evaluation: the Barthel Index. Maryland State Med J 1965;14:61–65.

69. Wade DT, Collin C. The Barthel ADL index: a standard measure of physical disability? Int Disability Studies 1988;10:64–67.

70. Nouri FM, Lincoln NB. An extended activities of daily living scale for stroke patients. Clin Rehabil 1987;1:301–305.

71. Mathiowetz V, Weber K, Kashman N, Volland G. Adult norms for the nine hole peg test of finger dexterity. Occup Ther J Res 1985;5:24–37.

72. Yekutiel MP, Pinhasov A, Shahar G, Sroka H. A clinical trial of the re-education of movement in patients with Parkinson's disease. Clin Rehabil 1991;5:207–214.

73. Nieuwboer A, et al. Is using a cue the clue to the treatment of freezing in Parkinson's disease? Physiother Res Int 1997;2:125–132.

74. A symposium on the minimal record of disability. Acta Neurol Scand 1984;101(Suppl):167–207.

75. Hunt SM, McKenna SP, McEwan J, et al. A quantitative approach to perceived health status: a validation study. J Epidemiol Community Health 1980;34:281–286.

76. Schindler JS, Brown R, Welburn P, Parkes JD. Measuring the quality of life in patients with Parkinson's disease. In: Walter SR, Rosser R, editors. Quality of life: assessment and application. Lancaster: MTP Press, 1987:223–234.

77. Jenkinson C, Coulter A, Wright L. Short form 36 (SF36) health survey questionnaire: normative data for adults of working age. BMJ 1993;306:1437–1440.

78. Garratt AM, Ruta DA, Abdalla MI, Buckingham JK, Russell IT. The SF36 health survey questionnaire: an outcome measure suitable for routine use within the NHS. BMJ 1993;306:1440–1444.

79. Peto V, Fitzpatrick R, Jenkinson C. Self reported health status and access to health services in a community sample with Parkinson's disease. Disabil Rehabil 1997;19:97–103.

80. Jenkinson C, Peto V, Fitzpatrick R, Greenhall R, Hyman N. Self reported functioning and well-being in patients with Parkinson's disease: comparison of the short-form health survey (SF36) with the Parkinson's disease questionnaire (PDQ 39). Age Ageing 1995;24:505–509.

81. Schwartz D, Flanmant R, Llelouch J. Clinical trials. New York: Academic Press, 1991.

82. Ward CD. Does selegiline delay progression of Parkinson's disease? A critical re-evaluation of the DATATOP study. J Neurol Neurosurg Psychiatry 1994;57:217–220.

83. Lang AE, Quinn N, Brincat S, Marsden CD, Parkes JD. Pergolide in late stage Parkinson's disease. Ann Neurol 1982;12:243–247.

84. Tanner GM, Goetz CG, Glantz RH, Glatt SL, Klawans HL. Pergolide mesylate and idiopathic Parkinson disease. Neurology 1982;32:1175–1179.

85. Lieberman A, Goldstein M, Leibowitz M. The effect of pergolide on the cardiovascular system of forty patients with Parkinson's disease. Adv Neurol 1984;37:121–130.

86. Olanow CW, Fahn S, Muenter M, et al. A multicenter double blind placebo-controlled trial of Pergolide as an adjunct to Sinemet in Parkinson's disease. Mov Disord 1994;9: 40–47.

87. Obeso JA, Guridi J, DeLong M. Surgery for Parkinson's disease. J Neurol Neurosurg Psychiatry 1997;62:2–8.

88. Lang AE, Benabid A-L, Koller WC, Lozano AM, Obeso JA, Olanow CW, Pollak P. The Core Assessment Program for Intracerebral Transplantation [letter]. Mov Disord 1995;10: 527–528.

89. Morris ME, lansek R, Matyas TA, Summers JJ. The pathogenesis of gait hypokinesia in Parkinson's disease. Brain 1994;117:1169–1181.

90. Margitic SE, Morgan TM, Sager MA, Furberg CD. Lessons learned from a prospective metanalyis. J Am Geriatr Soc 1995;43:435–439.

26. Parkinson's Disease: A Review of Drug Trials

S.B. Blunt

Introduction

There has been a huge amount of research into neurodegenerative diseases in the past 30 years. In Parkinson's disease, the research has been fruitful, demonstrating amongst many other findings that the main biochemical abnormality in the brain is a loss of striatal dopamine which results from a progressive degeneration of the nigrostriatal pathway. This neuronal loss is associated with an abundance of activated microglia within the substantia nigra; elevated levels of iron in the nigra; biochemical changes to suggest oxidative stress; and evidence of mitochondrial dysfunction. Whilst the primary cause of these changes is unknown, a great amount can be done to alleviate the symptoms by replacing the loss of dopamine or stimulating its receptors within the brain. The manner in which dopamine is replaced can have considerable impact on the natural history of the patient's illness. Because of the limitations of dopaminergic treatment other approaches with both drug treatment and surgical methods have been studied.

As in all areas of medicine, treatments in Parkinson's disease have emerged by all manner of routes. Some treatments have been introduced as a result of fortuitous or incidental observation, some by logical empirical and anecdotal trial in single or small numbers of patients, and others by a spectrum of clinical trials in larger groups. Judging the efficacy of a particular treatment, or comparing its profile with that of another, can be difficult, especially in Parkinson's disease where the initial diagnosis is sometimes uncertain, and where clinical features, even for a "typical case", are so varied and variable even within a single patient on stable drug treatment. Judgements of the efficacy of a treatment are made even more difficult where the effect of a treatment is likely to be subtle (such as in slowing progression of disease), and a chance of obtaining a clear answer can only be hoped for if carefully controlled trials of large numbers of appropriately characterised patients are undertaken.

With the ever-increasing choice of treatments in the current medical armamentarium, proper investigation is required to see whether they are of genuine benefit to patients. The randomised controlled clinical trial has become widely regarded as the main method of obtaining reliable assessment of effect of a particular treatment, be it drug, surgical or behavioural. There is an enormous amount of trial data available to the practitioner, from which he or she must decide whether to alter their practice accordingly. In an ideal world, the correct practice of medicine must derive from the information available, but only that which has been properly demonstrated to be effective (evidence-based medicine), and the findings then incorporated as appropriate into medical practice. An appreciation of how clinical trials are and should be conducted is therefore of obvious benefit, as is the ability to "keep up" with the plethora of published medical research. The proper use of statistical methods in both planning and interpretation of results is also crucial in understanding the usefulness of any clinical trial. The value of systematic reviews such as those undertaken by the Cochrane Collaboration (see Chaper 4) for these purposes cannot be overemphasised.

Ways in Which Treatments Can Be Evaluated

It is important to remember that whilst the clinical trial is now accepted as the optimal way of assessing a new treatment, not all treatments (in Parkinson's disease) that are now widely used established their place in medical practice in this way; indeed, the success of many antiparkinsonian medications became incorporated into clinical practice before results from clinical trials became available, and often before the mechanism of action was understood. Ideally, though, with any new treatment, particularly with the use of drugs that are "me too" types, their individual value must be rigorously assessed.

Case studies describe the effects of a treatment on the course of one patient's disease, but such results cannot be extrapolated to the general population. Clinical trials inevitably require groups of patients – generally, the larger the better.

The efficacy of some treatments has been deduced in some cases by retrospective studies. In these, the outcome of particular treatments on past patients is examined. These unplanned, observational, surveys of treatments have serious potential biases (for example treatments that are in fact less effective being given to patients with milder disease, and thus appearing wrongly to have a better outcome). These studies should be referred to with extreme caution and rarely make a reliable contribution to the evaluation of treatments. These types of surveys do not constitute clinical trials.

In this chapter the results from studies of novel surgical treatments such as pallidotomy, thalamotomy, subthalmic lesioning, or grafting of tissue will not be discussed. I will summarise the types of clinical trials that have been used in the assessment of medical treatment for Parkinson's disease and discuss their appropriateness in design and interpretation.

Rationale for Use of Particular Treatments in Parkinson's Disease

Treatment for Parkinson's disease has come a long way since the historic book written by James Parkinson in which he (admittedly not very enthusiastically) recommended trials of bleeding "from the upper part of the back of the neck", vesicatories and purging from the bowels. Parkinson also felt that internal treatments would be "scarcely warrantable" and a "highly nutritious diet" not helpful. Since then, trials of treatments have progressed from, at one extreme, anecdotal experiments through the gamut of methods mentioned above to the opposite extreme of multicentre full-scale clinical trials.

Anticholinergic Drugs

The first specific drugs to be used in the treatment of Parkinson's disease with any beneficial effect were the natural anticholinergic agents. In his 1867 doctoral thesis Charcot's student Ordenstein reported

that, amongst other experimental trials in patients, hyoscine temporarily reduced the tremor. Later trials towards the end of the nineteenth century experimented with almost all known medicinal preparations of plant origin, including belladonna alkaloids, veratrum, ergot, strychnine, opium, coniine, curare, gelsemium and many others. It was only the belladonna alkaloids which received widespread recognition of their modest palliative effects, well before their anticholinergic properties were known.

A further flurry of activity in experimental anecdotal treatment emerged during the period of the post-encephalitic parkinsonian epidemic of encephalitis lethargica between 1916 and 1927. Whilst drugs such as nicotine, curare and bullbocapnine were tried, the most effective again appeared to be extracts of the *Atropa belladonna* root [1]. Indeed, very high doses of atropine were subsequently found to be effective in reducing not only the extrapyramidal motor syndrome but also the tics, behavioural abnormalities and oculogyric crises. Indeed a variety of proprietary preparations of belladonna root were produced, including delightful concoctions such as a wine made from the Bulgarian plant (which was believed to be particularly efficacious) and which was marketed in Europe as Bulgakur. Tablets of the belladonna root were also used, and suggested dosage regimens of such natural alkaloids were mentioned even as late as 1955, in the neurological text by Merritt [2].

The natural products were superseded in the 1950s by a range of synthetic anticholinergic drugs. Early investigations of clinical efficacy of various anticholinergic agents (paticularly the piperidine derivatives such as benzhexol), reported a significant benefit in most patients. These studies were poorly controlled by modern standards. In an open trial of trihexyphenidyl in 69 patients with Parkinson's disease, a dramatic improvement in 77% of patients was noted, but this was based on descriptive letters from the patient, their relatives or the family doctor! Later open trials relied mainly on physical examination and functional capacity over long periods and convincingly demonstrated an improvement following treatment with anticholinergic drugs, especially in rigidity and tremor [3–7].

Results of double-blind, placebo-controlled studies were not as consistent, some reporting no improvement while others noted small but significant benefit. However, the differences could be explained by the fact that different drugs, doses, patient selection or methods of assessment were used [8–14].

Finer analysis of the effects of anticholinergic agents on specific parkinsonian features again led to inconsistency. It was suggested that they were most effective in the treatment of tremor and rigidity, with little effect on akinesia [15–17]; however, this selective action is not accepted by everyone [18,19]. One of the difficulties in this type of evaluation is that different signs in Parkinson's disease are not equally amenable to objective assessment. Tremor is the most amenable to mechanical quantification and, using accelerometers or modified electromyographic equipment, most investigators found that it was this feature that seemed to be improved most by anticholinergic treatment [14,20–23], but these findings may simply be because tremor was easier to quantify in those early days than akinesia and rigidity! In 1956, measurements of rigidity improved with the introduction of a strain gauge assembly, but using this technique one group found an improvement of 55% after treatment [20] while another found no change [10].

After the clinical efficacy of levodopa was recognised in the late 1960s, anticholinergics were no longer actively studied as sole treatment, but were seen more as adjunctive to first line treatment. Most investigators in controlled trials found that anticholinergics enhanced the efficacy of levodopa [14,24–26]. These were double-blind crossover trials with placebo control assessed with qualitative and quantitative measures of outcome.

Based on a combination of empirical, experimental and clinical trial data, the general recommendation is that anticholinergic drugs are useful as sole therapy in patients with mild Parkinson's disease. Tremor and rigidity may respond best. Patients with more severe axial problems and akinesia are likely to require dopaminergic treatment, but adjunctive treatment with anticholinergic drugs may reduce the total dopaminergic dose required, and may also be beneficial for dystonia. Occasionally, where one anticholinergic drug fails to produce benefit, changing to another can help [27,28]. Others noted that combinations of anticholinegic drugs could be beneficial, although these suggestions have not been based on clinical trials [3–9].

Anticholinergic drugs remained the mainstay of the medical treatment of parkinsonism for over 100 years – between the first observation of the palliative effect of hyoscine in 1867, to the introduction of levodopa in the late 1960s.

Amantadine

A chance observation by Schwab et al. [29] in 1969 that amantadine resulted in symptomatic improvement in a parkinsonian patient given the drug as prophylaxis against the 'flu, led to clinical trials that confirmed the initial observations [30–32]. Schwab et al. [29] treated 163 Parkinson's disease patients

with amantadine in an uncontrolled study; 66% of patients treated with a maximum daily dose of 200 mg showed improvement consisting of a reduction in akinesia and rigidity and lessening of tremor. Longer-term outcome studies suggested that the effect declined after 4–8 weeks in a third of patients. Side-effects were noted in 22% of patients. Subsequent trials are difficult to derive conclusions from because open trials tended to give more favourable results; furthermore, in most of the trials, as was the case in Schwab et al.'s original paper, patients took standard antiparkinsonian drugs as well (e.g. anticholinergics and antihistamines), making it impossible to assess the effect of amantadine as monotherapy.

Trials of Amantadine Versus Placebo as Monotherapy

Mann et al. [33] conducted a double-blind study assessing the effect of amantadine after discontinuation of all previous antiparkinsonian drugs. Amantadine was found to be superior to placebo in reducing functional disability, but the trial was only 4 days long. Bauer and McHenry [34], in the second phase of a double-blind study, discontinued use of conventional drugs and assessed the effect of amantadine during a 3 week period. Amantadine produced a 21% improvement in motor scores over baseline but this part of the study was not blinded. Perhaps the best-conducted trial was by Butzer et al. [35], who undertook a double-blind, placebo-controlled crossover study in 26 patients with only 3 continuing on other antiparkinsonian medication; amantadine provided a statistically significant (12%) overall improvement over placebo and a 13% improvement over baseline disability scores. The majority of the patients selected amantadine for long-term usage before codes were broken. Another double-blind, crossover study, by Gilligan et al. [36], compared placebo and amantadine in 33 patients, each of whom was given the drug for 3 weeks. Improvements for most patients were subjective although significant objective improvement was noted in tremor.

Trials of Amantadine Versus Placebo in Patients Already Taking Anticholinergics

Parkes et al. [37] performed a double-blind crossover trial of amantadine and placebo each given for 2 weeks to patients on anticholinergics. They found a significant improvement in scores in patients receiving amantadine, but there was no interaction with anticholinergics. Hunter et al. [38] in a double-blind placebo-controlled study of amantadine versus placebo showed a small sustained beneficial effect on physical signs but none on disability. Dallos et al. [39] undertook a double-blind trial over 4 weeks and observed a modest but significant effect in the amantadine-treated patients with a favourable drug effect profile in most patients. Appleton et al. [40] undertook a patient and observer scored study comparing amantadine with placebo and again indicated on both assessments a beneficial effect of the drug.

Jorgenssen et al. [41] conducted a multicentre double-blind trial assessing the effects of amantadine in patients on anticholinergics. Improvement was seen in 56% of patients, with more severely affected patients benefiting most.

Amantadine Compared with Anticholinergics or Levodopa

Walker et al. [42] compared baseline Parkinson's disease scores in patients on anticholinergics compared with amantadine and single therapy in a double-blind manner. Although few of the differences were statistically significant, it was their impression that patients on amantadine did as well or better than those on anticholinergics on almost every qualitative or quantitative measure performed. Parkes et al. [43] compared benzhexol alone, amantadine alone, or both together in 40 drug-naive patients who were mildly disabled; in this randomly assigned double-blind crossover trial they found that each drug alone produced a 15% reduction in functional disability but that the combination produced a 40% reduction.

Koller [44] compared amantadine with an anticholinergic or levodopa in patients with unilateral tremor. Each drug was administered for 2 weeks in a double-blind manner. The conclusion was that amantadine reduced tremor but to a lesser degree than the anticholinergic; interestingly patients preferred the anticholinergic.

An interesting study by Fieschi et al. [45] compared amantadine with levodopa in a double-blind crossover study (2 weeks drug, 1 week placebo, 2 weeks drug). Improvement in motor scores was much less with amantadine than with levodopa, but there was a strong correlation between patient responsiveness to the two drugs. Following in this vein, Parkes et al. [46] suggested that levodopa and amantadine had a similar spectrum of activity but that use of 200 mg amantadine was a less effective dose than the optimal dosage of levodopa. In a subsequent non-blind long-term trial by the same group it was noted that the response to levodopa could be predicted by the response to amantadine; both drugs improved all the symptoms of Parkinson's disease but the effects of amantadine were

mild on akinesia and rigidity, better on tremor and posture.

In a double-blind placebo-controlled study Barbeau et al. [47] compared amantadine with levodopa in an open study in which all patients were assessed by the same observers and using the same battery of tests. The conclusion was that levodopa was far superior to amantadine, and in contrast to the studies mentioned earlier, there was no correlation between levodopa and amantadine responsivity.

What can be concluded from these short-term clinical trials? Amantadine has a useful if modest antiparkinsonian effect which is clearly less than that of levodopa but possibly similar to that of the anticholinergics. Concurrent use of anticholinerics does not seem to interfere with the benefit gained from amantadine, apart from one study which demonstrated a synergistic effect between the two drugs. In the studies which provided this information, it seems that the drug is well tolerated by patients; improvement in functional disability was greater than objective signs. Amantadine seems to improve all aspects of the parkinsonian picture, although the extent to which this occurs showed disparate results [29,35,36,40,43,46]. No conclusion can be drawn as to which type of patient responds best. Several studies have reported the decline in efficacy of the drug over time.

Amantadine Combined with Levodopa

The clinical efficacy of amantadine and levodopa has not been rigorously tested in clinical trials, but long experience with both drugs has shown them to have a useful role in Parkinson's disease. Several investigators have sought to assess whether the amantadine response is a predictor of levodopa responsiveness: Is there any interaction or potentiation between the two drugs on parkinsonian features; Can amantadine improve levodopa-related fluctuations?

Most of the studies addressing these questions have been short-term (2 months), non-controlled and non-blind; most patients were also already receiving conventional antiparkinsonian medications. Whilst results from the different studies have varied, some showed that addition of levodopa to amantadine showed a clear improvement [34,47,48], whilst others showed no added benefit of using amantadine as well as levodopa [46].

Fahn et al. [49] looked at the effect of amantadine in patients with Parkinson's disease before and after 5 and 11 months of continuous levodopa treatment. They found that the response to amantadine was not consistent during this period. Whilst 50% of patients benefited from amantadine after 1 year, many of those who showed a beneficial effect at earlier time points failed to do so in the longer term.

Studies looking at the addition of amantadine to levodopa have been conflicting or yielded insufficient data. Thus, Fieschi et al. [45] found amantadine helpful in more than 50% of patients on levodopa, but this study was very short (2 weeks), consisted of 20 patients and was non-blind. Walker et al. [42] undertook a double-blind crossover trial over 3 weeks in 28 patients in which addition of amantadine to patients on stable levodopa doses was compared with placebo; whilst all objective parkinsonian scores improved in patients on combined treatment, the functional disability scores were not improved. Fehling [50] found similar results in a double-blind crossover placebo-controlled trial in 21 patients of 1 month's duration. The failings of these studies are that they were all short and in small numbers of patients.

Some studies have attempted to address whether addition of amantadine to levodopa can improve motor fluctuations. De Deviitis et al. [51] studied the effect of amantadine given to 19 patients with predictable levodopa-related afternoon motor fluctuations. On the whole this study demonstrated a reduction or abolition of motor fluctuations, and an improvement in parkinsonian features.

In conclusion, the studies looking at combined amantadine and levodopa treatment do not allow clear recommendations to be made. The conclusions that can be drawn are that amantadine has an antiparkinsonian effect with a profile similar to levodopa; the drug is well tolerated; its effect, especially in early Parkinson's disease, is at least equal to that of anticholinergics; and it may allow for a delay in introduction of levodopa. However, the beneficial effects tend to lessen with time and the addition of amantadine to levodopa has questionable value, but it adds few side-effects.

More recently an impression has been emerging, based not on any form of clinical trial but on anecdotal experience, that amantadine may be of benefit in patients with atypical parkinsonism.

Levodopa

Levodopa is found in a large variety of natural compounds including various bean plants such as the broad or fava bean. The role of dopamine in the human brain and its relevance to parkinsonism did not begin to emerge until 1957 [52–54]. Bertler and Rosengren [55] first attributed the striatal dopamine to control of motor function and the relevance of dopamine to Parkinson's disease emerged in 1960 with the work of Ehringer and Hornykiewicz [56].

These findings led to the suggestions that levodopa might be useful in the treatment of parkinsonian patients [52,57]. Initial use of the drug was undertaken by intravenous injection [57,58] resulting in a striking "abolition or substantial relief of akinesia". Further empirical trials occurred with DL-dopa [59] together with pyridoxine with little obvious effects; this may have been because pyridoxine (unbeknown to these workers at the time) blocks the effects of L-dopa. Barbeau et al. [60] undertook short-term open trials with oral D- and L-dopa in a small group of Parkinson's disease patients; they studied the time course and extent of effect and subsequently undertook long-term studies. Several more studies took place between 1963 and 1966 to evaluate the effects of dopa on Parkinson's disease [61–65]. With few exceptions, e.g. [65,66], these trials were not blinded or placebo controlled.

In 1966, Fehling conducted a full double-blind trial of L-dopa [65]. She found no difference in response at all between L-dopa and placebo except that several patients developed nausea on L-dopa. Another double-blind trial in 1968 [66] had similar disappointing results. Surprising as it may seem now, conclusions about the effects of L-dopa were therefore mixed, with many neurologists failing to be convinced of its benefits. However, these views were based on studies which were by today's standards poorly designed, dosage of drug was inadequate, and the optimal form of the drug was not yet realised. Furthermore, the confounding effects of additional drugs (including pyridoxine) were not appreciated.

Trials Consolidating Oral L-DOPA Use in Parkinson's Disease

In 1967, Cotzias et al. [67] gave a racemic mixture of DL-dopa orally to 16 Parkinson's disease patients only; unlike in previous studies, the doses used were high, at between 3 and 16 g daily. Dramatic beneficial effects were observed on the parkinsonian features, and the previously recognised side-effects of nausea, faintness and vomiting could be avoided or reduced with slow increments in dose. Dyskinetic movements were noticed for the first time, at high doses. These anecdotal reports showed conclusively that dopa had pronounced central effects at high dosage [67].

Between 1967 and 1970, several further reports confirmed these findings [68–75]. Regardless of whether the trials were open, single- or double-blind, the outcome was universal: high-dose oral levodopa treatment produced a dramatic symptomatic improvement in approximately 80% of patients, and the dopa effect far exceeded that seen with anticholinergics. However, even in those early days, associated effects of levodopa including motor fluctuations, on–off effects and dyskinesias were beginning to be noted by several neurologists.

Introduction of Dopa Decarboxylase Inhibitors

In 1969, Birkmayer [76] discussed the use of a dopa decarboxylase inhibitor in Parkinson's disease, aimed at reducing the total dose of levodopa needed and also at reducing the peripheral side-effects of the drug. In 1971, Yahr, in an open study, and Calne et al. in a double-blind trial [77,78], found that use of a peripheral dopa decarboxylase inhibitor reduced the required levodopa dose by 75%. Many later open [79–81] and double-blind trials [82] of benserazide, and open [83] and double-blind studies of carbidopa [84–86] supported these initial results. One study directly compared these two decarboxylase inhibitors and found little difference between benserazide and carbidopa when combined with levodopa [87].

As a result of empirical studies followed by varyingly rigorous trials, combined oral levodopa and peripheral decarboxylase treatment was established as the mainstay of treatment of Parkinson's disease worldwide and its place still remains to be usurped!

Studies Triggered by Recognition of Motor Fluctuations and Acknowledgement of Long-Term Levodopa Side-effects and Limitations

Within a very short time of use of levodopa, side-effects were already being observed: the development of motor fluctuations, wearing off and dyskinesias were already being mentioned at a symposium in 1969 [88]. However, the relationship of such fluctuations and excessive movements to the use of lev odopa has been controversial [89–93]. Because of the short half-life of levodopa and the variability in its absorption from the gut, plasma levels (and presumably brain levels) can fluctuate wildly. One hypothesis is that it is these fluctuations in plasma levels that result in the development of motor fluctuations.

A number of rational approaches have been tried in attempts to "smooth out" the plasma levodopa level profile, and thus, it is hoped, reduce motor fluctuations. These include use of intravenous infusion (used mainly to investigate the pathophysiology and exact role of plasma levels of levodopa on motor fluctuations rather than as a proposed treatment); slow-release preparations; and inhibition of dopa or dopamine-metabolising enzymes. Other approaches have been aimed at by-passing the standard usage of levodopa as a precursor for dopamine, and have con-

centrated on direct stimulation of the post-synaptic receptors with dopamine agonists.

Studies of Levodopa Infusion

In 1974, it was shown that variation in plasma levodopa levels during oral treatment correlated to some extent with patients' motor symptoms [94]. Levodopa infusions reduced the fluctuations in blood levels at the same time as improving motor activity; it was thus suggested that many of the motor abnormalities in Parkinson's disease could be due to fluctuations in levodopa levels.

Apart from the investigational studies in single patients mentioned above, therapeutic studies have included a double-blind crossover trial [95] demonstrating that the infusions were well tolerated; compared with oral therapy there was a 36% improvement in antiparkinsonian response and a 42% reduction in response variability; there was no consistent effect on dyskinesias; patients with wearing off phenomena were too few to draw conclusions from.

Long-Acting Levodopa Preparations

The combination of levodopa and a peripheral decarboxylase inhibitor remains the mainstay of treatment for Parkinson's disease. However, long-term observations of patients, with retrospective analyses, showed that the panacea of beneficial effects resulting from this treatment are not maintained. Thus, the response declines with time, motor performance begins to fluctuate and side-effects, particularly dyskinesias, develop [89,90]. The proportion of patients developing such effects is around 50%. Factors influencing gastric emptying, absorption and diet all tended to aggravate the unpredictability of plasma levels resulting from oral levodopa [96,97]. Whilst intravenous levodopa studies demonstrated that many of the motor fluctuations could be reduced by maintaining a stable plasma level, this approach was clearly not practicable for most patients.

Initially one approach was to increase the frequency of levodopa oral doses but reduce the size of each dose. An alternative and more acceptable approach was to produce a preparation which resulted in a slower or controlled release (CR) of levodopa/carbidopa, whereby tablets could be of higher dose and spaced out over the day. In relation to the use of slow-release preparations, clinical studies and experience have shown that there are a number of potential uses for these preparations. The first aim was to establish that they are effective in the treatment of parkinsonian features; the second was to assess whether they improve the profile of the motor response, which is the main rationale for studying them; the third is to establish how best to use them in the context of other available drugs. All these points have been addressed to some extent in clinical trials, but some aspects of the role of these drugs have emerged with experience rather than formal trial.

Most trials looking at the effects and role of CR preparations have been with small samples, and comparisons between trials have been difficult to make because of the variation in patient groups. For example, patients included in some studies have had mild disease whilst in others they have had severe motor fluctuations.

There have been a number of clinical trials assessing the efficacy of CR preparations, comparing different dose combinations and comparing these drugs with standard levodopa/carbidopa preparations. The formulation of the early CR preparations varied and these early studies laid the ground for the further study of the formulation that is currently marketed as Sinemet CR (Du Pont). Hutton et al. [98] conducted a double-blind crossover study of a CR Sinemet (100/25) in 20 parkinsonian patients and compared the efficacy with standard Sinemet 125. Efficacy measures consisted of standardised clinical scales and a physiological measure of tremor severity. All measures showed the CR preparation to be less efficacious than the standard preparation; there was also no difference in adverse reactions.

Two later studies compared different doses, proportions of the drug components and release matrix of the two CR preparations (Sinemet CR-2 and CR-3) in a two-way double-blind crossover study and compared with the standard preparations [99]. Twenty patients were studied and efficacy was assessed by standard scales and physiological measures of tremor bradykinesia and hand movements. There were no significant differences between the different treatments as far as efficacy measures showed, but both CR formulations resulted in a gentler rise to peak plasma level and a more uniform pharmacokinetic curve than with the standard preparation. Whilst these better plasma profiles were not associated with improved efficacy measures, this may be simply because this was not the best patient group to study: ideally patients with pronounced motor fluctuations should have been used.

Subsequent trials focused on patients with motor fluctuations. Using Sinemet CR-3 (200/50), Nutt et al. [100] found that CR preparations resulted in higher plasma levodopa concentrations but variations in level and motor fluctuations were no better than with the standard preparation; they also found that the optimal CR dose was 3 times that of the standard preparation. In two open-label studies [101,102],

Sinemet CR-3 was shown to produce high plasma levels with mild improvements in response fluctuations, but due to the poor bioavailability of the formulation and its unpredictable plasma level it was not chosen for further study. In contrast, Sinemet CR-2 (a different release matrix from CR-3), which resulted in less effective clinical improvement, had resulted in predictable plasma levodopa levels, so the CR-2 formulation was chosen to study a drug with a higher dose: Sinemet CR-4, the current Sinemet CR.

Studies with Sinement CR

In pharmacokinetic studies, Sinemet CR has been shown to produce consistent rises in plasma levodopa levels which are maintained for 3–4 h longer than those of standard Sinemet preparations [103], and which are more stable [104,105]. Open-label studies showed that Sinemet CR allows a significant reduction in number of daily doses, reduction in time "off" and improvement in disability scores [103–105].

In a double-blind study of 20 patients, Goetz et al. [105] compared Sinement CR (given twice daily) with standard Sinemet (given four times a day) in patients with mild, non-fluctuating Parkinson's disease. Patients on Sinement CR showed more stable and smoother plasma levodopa curves, and a reduced total daily dose requirement for similar efficacy compared with standard Sinemet. Whilst no differences in clinical disability were found, the majority of the patients preferred to stay on the CR preparation.

Hutton et al. [106] conducted a double-blind crossover comparison of Sinemet CR and standard Sinemet in 21 patients with motor fluctuations. There was an initial open-label dose finding period. Subsequently, using this "best dose" regimen, patients received either Sinemet CR or standard Sinemet for 8 weeks in random order. During each 8 week period patients took two types of tablets – one identical in appearance to Sinemet CR the other to standard Sinemet – but only one tablet type was active. Efficacy measures included the UPDRS, physician and patient evaluations, and daily diaries kept by the patients of their motor fluctuations. During the last 2 weeks of the double-blind periods, patients on Sinemet CR required just over 50% of the number of daily doses of standard Sinemet, although the mean amount of Sinemet CR required was greater. Efficacy measures were generally better with Sinemet CR during the open-label phase of the study, although no significant differences emerged during the blinded period. This negative finding might be attributable to the relatively small sample size and the variation in

Table 26.1. Results of a multicentre study comparing Sinemet CR with standard Sinemet[107]

	Sinemet CR as compared with standard Sinemet
Dose frequency	33%
Total daily dose	25%
Global ratings	
Patient	Mean scores better in "on" and "off"
Physician	Mean scores better in "on" and "off"
Motor fluctuations	Better
Helpfulness of medication	Better
Adverse effects	No difference
Tablet preference	90%

scores within groups. This single study was part of a multicentre trial summarised next.

Multicentre CR Study

Eight centres in the United States participated in a multicentre CR study and 220 patients were enrolled [107]. Patients were divided between Hoehn and Yahr stages II and IV. Average duration of disease was 10 years, and all patients showed motor fluctuations. The results of the study are summarised in Table 26.1.

Long-Term Follow-up of Patients on Sinemet CR

Several retrospective studies have shown that Sinemet CR is well tolerated in the long term and that it remains efficacious [108–111]. One 2 year study demonstrated that patients on Sinemet CR had more time "on" and fewer side-effects compared with those on standard Sinemet [111].

Studies with CR Levodopa/Benserazide

The combination of CR levodopa and benserazide is marketed outside the USA as Madopar HBS (Roche). There have been few studies looking at the effects of this formulation on efficacy and on motor fluctuations, and it is difficult to draw conclusions regarding the role of this preparation in Parkinson's disease [112–114].

Conclusions

These various studies demonstrate that CR Sinemet can result in a reduction in total daily dose frequency, but with an increase in total daily levodopa dose without a reduction in efficacy. There is considerable evidence to support the suggestion that CR preparations produce a smoother motor response profile. However, one drawback of this drug commonly reported by patients, and not formally studied in trials, is the lack of initial "kick-start" with these preparations.

Clinical Trials Using Dopamine Agonists

Dopamine agonists were first introduced with the aim of using them in patients with advanced disease. The exact role of these drugs in the treatment of Parkinson's disease has been difficult to establish, and is still unclear, due to the variety of published reports on their effects. Many of the early reports were not based on double-blind prospective controlled trials. Here I will summarise the main trials looking at the role of the three commonly used dopamine agonists: bromocriptine, pergolide and lisuride. Further dopamine agonists have entered clinical use recently (nopininole, pramipexole and cabergoline).

Establishing the Efficacy of Dopamine Agonists

Bromocriptine was first used in patients with advanced Parkinson's disease who were no longer responding well to levodopa. There have been many studies which sought to assess the role of bromocriptine in the treatment of Parkinson's disease. These studies have differed in many ways. Patients were first selected for agonist treatment for many reasons including declining response to levodopa, motor fluctuations or intolerance. In some bromocriptine was chosen as first drug. The studies have varied in how efficacy was evaluated, the dose of drugs used (e.g. low- or high-dose bromocriptine), evaluation of motor oscillations and adverse reactions records.

In four double-blind studies totalling 79 patients with mild to moderate disease, assessing the role of bromocriptine monotherapy [115–118], low-dose bromocriptine resulted in improvement in 58% of patients; 9% experienced side-effects leading to drug withdrawal. Other studies assessing higher starting doses of bromocriptine led to the notion that whilst this had greater antiparkinsonian effect than lower starting doses, many patients could not perservere with the drug because of the side-effects. In an attempt to establish the minimum dose of bromocriptine required and the speed of increase in dosing, 134 drug-naive patients were recruited to a multicentre double-blind study comparing two dose regimes: a low-slow technique, increasing to a maximum of 25 mg/day; and a high-fast regime increasing to a maximum of 100 mg/day over 26 weeks [119]. The conclusions, which still hold today, were that bromocriptine is an effective first line treatment but that the high-fast treatment regime is less well tolerated while the low-slow regime is limited by the long delay before patients reach an effective dose.

The efficacy of other dopamine agonists has also been studied in various ways. Short-term trials testing the efficacy of pergolide as an adjunctive therapy to levodopa have included five open-label trials [120–124] and four double-blind placebo-controlled studies [125–128]. In the open-label trials, reliable data are available on 113 patients, of whom 80% showed symptomatic improvement with the addition of pergolide. A total of 100 patients were studied in the double-blind protocols. Three studies showed improvement with addition of pergolide, but the fourth (20 patients) showed improvement which was no better than the placebo control.

Lisuride as monotherapy was first studied in an open non-randomised study in previously untreated patients [129]; it was reported that efficacy of lisuride was equal to that of bromocriptine and there were fewer dyskinesias than with bromocriptine and fewer cardiovascular side-effects than with pergolide. This study had many drawbacks, not the least being the small number of patients studied in each group, so the findings could be relied on only as preliminary tendencies. Later studies [130,131] in small numbers of patients suggest that lisuride is effective in the short term but that later addition of levodopa is usually required.

There are very few studies comparing the efficacy of these dopamine agonists. In a prospective, double-blind randomised crossover trial of lisuride versus bromocriptine, Le Witt et al. [132] concluded that the response profile was similar for the two drugs. In an open study [130,133] Lieberman compared lisuride with bromocriptine and pergolide and confirmed that with lisuride the improvement in parkinsonian features was similar or superior to that with bromocriptine, whilst pergolide had similar effects, possibly with more "on" time than lisuride. One open, controlled and prospective study assessed the value of adding lisuride or pergolide to levodopa treatment in 49 patients [134]. The conclusion was that lisuride and bromocriptine could allow a reduction in levodopa dose without loss of functional benefit; lisuride was more effective than bromocriptine but also caused more side-effects.

Dopamine Agonists and Motor Fluctuations

Early studies using bromocriptine suggested that dopamine agonists used alone do not result in response fluctuations or dyskinesias [135–138]. Studies also conclude that agonists used alone result in less benefit than levodopa, and most patients require the addition or substitution of levodopa

within a year or so [139]. Other studies have suggested that in patients with levodopa-associated fluctuations and dyskinesias, these can be reduced by the total or partial replacement of dopa with an agonist [140]. As a result of such studies, it has been suggested that dopamine agonists should be used earlier in the disease [140–143].

Rinne reported several open-label trials of bromocriptine [143], lisuride [129] and pergolide [144] compared with historical controls of levodopa alone. He reported that a dopamine agonist alone or used with levodopa early in the disease resulted in less motor fluctuation than in those treated with levodopa alone, but whilst obtaining the same degree of benefit. The clear drawbacks of these studies centre on the use of historical controls rather than randomised assignments of treatments, and on the lack of double-blind protocols. Montastruc et al. [145] undertook a randomised study of bromocriptine alone versus levodopa in 28 de novo patients. A dose-finding initial period was employed. This study suggested that efficacy was similar; dyskinesias occurred in 3 patients on levodopa and none on bromocriptine, pyschosis in one patient on bromocriptine, and lack of efficacy in 3 patients on bromocriptine and none on levodopa.

A multicentre, double-blind randomised trial of 4 years' duration compared bromocriptine alone, bromocriptine with levodopa and levodopa alone. One of the centres has separately reported its findings: Weiner et al. [146] treated 22 patients with early Parkinson's disease and showed no advantage of one treatment over another. In fact the combination of drugs resulted in a higher percentage of patients developing motor fluctuations than levodopa alone. This study is clearly too small to draw firm conclusions, but it does raise doubt over whether early combination should be advocated.

The question of whether dopamine agonists have a role in modifying motor fluctuations associated with use of levodopa has been studied better in the last 15 years with pergolide, providing useful conclusive results. In five open studies and four double-blind studies [120–128], pergolide reduced motor fluctuation by decreasing "off" time and/or increasing "on" time. With one exception [126] numbers of hours "off" or "on" were significantly improved by 50% or more when patients were on pergolide. The response to pergolide of the other individual parkinsonian features such as bradykinesia, gait, tremor and rigidity varied, and there is no uniform conclusion between the studies.

A very well designed study assessed the role of lisuride in patients who had developed wearing off or motor fluctuations on long-term levodopa [147]. This was a controlled randomised prospective study in which patients were treated at random with either the addition of lisuride or an increase in levodopa dose. After 6 months it was shown that not only was the addition of lisuride more effective in improving parkinsonian features, but motor fluctuations improved. This study was extended to 4 years [148], and whilst smaller numbers of patients remained, the effects of lisuride with levodopa was still superior to that of levodopa alone. These beneficial effects of lisuride on motor fluctuations associated with levodopa were confirmed by Lees and Stern [149] who treated 12 patients with end-of-dose deterioration in a single-blind placebo-controlled trial.

More recently there has been evidence that dopamine agonists may be neuroprotective. Experimental studies in rat models of Parkinson's disease showed that pergolide, bromocriptine, apomorphine and pramipexole can reduce the production of free radicals in vitro and in vivo [150–153]. Convincing clinical studies are now needed to establish whether dopamine agonists have a similar neuroprotective role in Parkinson's disease.

In conclusion, a very mixed bag of studies have tended to suggest that dopamine agonists have a role to play in Parkinson's disease. In the first instance, provided adverse effects can be avoided by using low-slow dose regimes, these drugs can have useful DOPA-sparing effects in early disease. More recent trials have raised the possibility that these drugs may be useful in preventing the development of motor fluctuations if used earlier, and they may also have a role once such effects have developed.

Selegeline (Deprenyl)

The first clinical trials of deprenyl in Parkinson's disease were by Birkmayer et al. [154,155]. In an open study of 223 patients they showed that deprenyl combined with levodopa improved disability scores and they raised the question of deprenyl having a protective effect on remaining dopamine neurones [155].

Later, Lees et al. [156] showed in a double-blind crossover study of 41 patients receiving maximum doses of levodopa with or without carbidopa, that addition of deprenyl reduced end-of-dose akinesia and wearing-off effects. A reduction of the dopa dose was also possible. This study also showed an increase in drug-induced dyskinesias. A further short-term controlled study [157] demonstrated the efficacy and safety of deprenyl. Open long-term studies in 381 patients [158] and 79 patients [159] confirmed improvement in motor fluctuations and wearing-off phenomena in patients receiving levodopa and carbidopa.

Whilst it is accepted that deprenyl has a role in patients with end-of-dose deterioration and wearing-off phenomena, there has been considerable debate about whether this drug has a role in slowing the progression of the disease. This topic has attracted such interest that it is not possible to summarise fully the literature on the subject. This idea emerged following the first studies of Birkmayer mentioned above, and later was reinforced by experimental studies which suggested selegeline could protect against certain neurotoxins. In 1985, Birkmayer et al. [160] reported that treatment with selegeline in addition to levodopa-benserazide increased life expectancy in 564 patients. But this study was open, uncontrolled and retrospective.

Against this background, Tetrud and Langston [161] started a double-blind placebo-controlled study with the aim of establishing whether selegeline could delay the need for levodopa by slowing disease progression. Fifty-four patients were randomly assigned and the outcome was that the need for levodopa was delayed in patients on selegeline. In 1987, the DATATOP study [162] began, in which 38 physicians in the United States and Canada participated. This was a double-blind, multicentre placebo-controlled trial and included over 800 patients. The study was terminated prematurely because of the interim findings that selegeline significantly increased the time before levodopa needed to be added.

Whilst there is little disagreement regarding the evidence that selegeline monotherapy can delay the need for levodopa in early untreated patients, the reason for this, i.e. whether this is a simple symptomatic effect or whether it truly slows the disease progression, is very controversial [163–166]. The final report of the DATATOP study was published in 1993. At this point the conclusion was that the observed benefit of selegeline was related simply to a symptomatic amelioration of symptoms. This study demonstrates the pitfalls of designing a trial where assumptions of drug effects are based on earlier studies, which suggested that selegeline monotherapy results in no symptomatic improvement in patients with early Parkinson's disease. In summary, whilst there is evidence for a role of deprenyl in wearing-off phenomena, there is no convincing evidence at present that it has any effect on the course of the disease.

Newer Drugs Currently Under Investigation in Parkinson's Disease

A number of newer agents are currently in the early stages of study in Parkinson's disease. These include the selective dopamine agonists, such as ropinirole, cabergoline and pramipexole, and the catechol-O-methyl transferase inhibitors such as (drug withdrawn recently) entacapone. The reported literature and experience with these drugs are still in their infancy and beyond the scope of this chapter.

In conclusion, the medical treatment of Parkinson's disease is as much a science based on clinical trial data (of varying quality) in patient groups, anecdotal report or long-term experience as it is an art based on judging the response of individual patients. A firm place for anticholinergics, amantadine, levodopa, selegeline and dopamine agonists exists, but no hard and fast recommendations can be made on their exact roles and places in relation to each other in the treatment of patients with Parkinson's disease.

References

1. Von Witzleben HD. Methods of treatment in postencephalitic parkinsonism. New York: Columbia University Press, 1939: 48–82.
2. Merritt HH. Textbook of neurology. Philadelphia: Lea & Febiger, 1955:332–334.
3. Doshay LJ. Five-year study of benztropine (Cogentin) methanesulfonate. JAMA 1956;162:1031–1034.
4. Strang RR. Experiences with Cogentin in the treatment of parkinsonism. Acta Neurol Scand 1965;145:413–418.
5. Doshay LJ, Constable K, Fromr S. Preliminary study of a new antiparkinsonian agent. Neurology 1952;2:233–243.
6. Doshay LJ, Constable K. Treatment of paralysis agitans with orphenadrine (Disipal) hydrochloride. JAMA 1957;163: 1352–1357.
7. Burns D, DeJong D, Solis-Quiroga OH. Effects of trihexyphenidyl hydrochloride (Artane) on Parkinson's disease. Neurology 1964;14:13–23.
8. Strang RR. Double-blind clinical evaluation of UCB 1549 in treatment of Parkinson's disease. BMJ 1966;II:112–113.
9. Livanainen M. KR 339 in the treatment of parkinsonian tremor. Acta Neurol Scand 1974;50:469–477.
10. Brumlik J, Canter G, La Torre R, Mier M, Petrovick M, Boshes B. A critical analysis of the effects of trihexyphenidyl (Artane) on the components of the parkinsonian syndrome. J Nerv Ment Dis 1964;138:424–431.
11. Norris JW, Vas CJ. Methixene hydrochloride and parkinsonian tremor. Acta Neurol Scand 1967;43:535–538.
12. Timberlake WH. Double-blind comparison of levodopa and procyclidine in parkinsonism, with illustrations of levodopa-induced movement disorders. Neurology 1970;20:31–35.
13. Gillespy RO, Ratcliffe AH. Treatment of parkinsonism with a new compound (BS 5930). BMJ 1995;II:352–355.
14. Koller W. Pharmacologic treatment of parkinsonian tremor. Arch Neurol 1986;43:126–127.
15. Ebling P. The medical management of Parkinson's disease before the introduction of L-dopa. Aust NZ J Med 1971;Suppl 1:35–38.
16. Williams A, Calne DB. Treatment of parkinsonism. In: Barbeau A, editor. Disorders of movement. Lancaster: MTP Press, 1981:171–189.
17. Obeso JA, Martinez-Lage JM. Anticholinergic and amantadine. In: Koller W, editor. Handbook of Parkinson's disease. New York: Marcel Dekker, 1987:309–316.
18. Duvoisin RC. A review of drug therapy in parkinsonism. Bull NY Acad Med 1965;41:898–910.
19. Yahr M, Duvoisin RC. Medical therapy of parkinsonism. In: Vinken PJ, Bruyn GW, editors. Disease of the basal ganglia.
20. Agate FJ, Doshay LJ, Curtis FK. Quantitative measurement of therapy in paralysis agitans. JAMA 1956;160:353–354.
21. Clarke S, Hay GA, Vas CJ. Therapeutic action of methixene hydrochloride on parkinsonian tremor and a description of a new tremor-recording transducer. Br J Pharmacol 1966;26: 345–350.
22. Shahani B, Young RR. Physiologic and pharmacological aids in the differential diagnosis of tremor. J Neurol Neurosurg Psychiatry 1976;39:772–783.
23. Martin WE, Loewenson RB, Resch JA, Baker AB. A controlled study comparing trihexyphenidyl hydrochloride plus levodopa with placebo plus levodopa in patients with Parkinson's disease. Neurology 1974;24:912–919.
24. Parkes JD, Baxter RC, Marsden CD, Rees JE. Comparative trial of benzhexol, amantadine, and levodopa in the treatment of Parkinson's disease. J Neurol Neurosurg Psychiatry 1974;37:422–426.
25. Tourtellotte WW, Potvin AR, Syndulko K, Hirsch SB, Gilden ER, Potvin JH, et al. Parkinson's disease: Cogentin with Sinemet, a better response. Prog Neuropsychopharmacol Biol Psychiatry 1982;6:51–55.
26. Bassi S, Albizzati MG, Calloni E, Sbacchi M. Treatment of Parkinson's disease with orphenadrine alone and in combination with L-dopa. Br J Clin Pract 1986;40:273–275.
27. Hurtig HI. Anticholinergics for Parkinson's disease. Ann Neurol 1980;5:495.
28. Calne DB. The role of various forms of treatment in the management of Parkinson's disease. Clin Neuropharmacol 1982;5(Suppl 1):538–543.
29. Schwab RS, England AC Jr, Pokanzer DC, Young RR. Amantadine in the treatment of Parkinson's disease. JAMA 1969;208:1168–1170.
30. Dallos V, Heathfield K, Stone P, Allen FAD. Use of amantadine in Parkinson's disease: results of a double blind trial. BMJ 1970;IV:24–26.
31. Parkes JD, Zilkha DK, Calver DM, et al. Controlled trial of amantadine hydrochloride in Parkinson's disease. Lancet 1970;I:259–262.
32. Fahn S, Isgreen WP. Long term evaluation of amantadine and levodopa combination in parkinsonism by double-blind crossover analysis. Neurology 1975;25:695–700.
33. Mann DC, Pearce LA, Waterbury LD. Amantadine for Parkinson's disease. Neurology 1971;21:958–962.
34. Bauer RB, McHenry JT. Comparison of amantadine, placebo, and levodopa in Parkinson's disease. Neurology 1974;24:715–720.
35. Butzer JF, Silver DE, Sahs AL. Amantadine in Parkinson's disease: a double blind, placebo-controlled cross-over study with long term follow-up. Neurology 1975;25:603–606.
36. Gilligan BS, Veale J, Wodak J. Amantadine hydrochloride in the treatment of Parkinson's disease. Med J Aust 1970;2: 634–637.
37. Parkes JD, Zilkha KJ, Calver DM, Knill-Jones RP. Controlled trial of amantadine hydrochloride in Parkinson's disease. Lancet 1970;I:1130–1133.
38. Hunter KR, Stern GM, Laurence DR, Armitage P. Amantadine in parkinsonism. Lancet 1970;I:1127–1129.
39. Dallos V, Heatherfield K, Stone P, Allen FAD. Use of amantadine in Parkinson's disease: results of a double blind trial. BMJ 1970;IV:24–36.
40. Appleton DB, Eadie MJ, Sutherland JM. Amantadine hydrochloride in the treatment of parkinsonism: a controlled trial. Med J Aust 1970;2:626–629.

41. Jorgenssen PB, Bergin JD, Haas L, et al. Controlled trial of amantadine hydrochloride in Parkinson's disease. NZ Med J 1971;73:263–269.

42. Walker JE, Albers JW, Tourtellotte WW, et al. A qualitative and quantitative evaluation of amantadine in the treatment of Parkinson's disease. J Chron Dis 1972;25:149–182.

43. Parkes JD, Baxter RC, Marsden CD, Rees JE. Comparative trial of benzhexol, amantadine and levodopa in the treatment of Parkinson's disease. J Neurol Neurosurg Psychiatry 1974;37: 422–426.

44. Koller WC. Pharmacologic treatment of parkinsonian tremor. Arch Neurol 1986;43:126–127.

45. Fieschi L, Nardini M, Casacchia M, Tedone ME. Amantadine for Parkinson's disease. Lancet 1970;I:945–946.

46. Parkes JD, Baxter RCH, Curzon G, et al. Treatment of Parkinson's disease with amantadine and levodopa. Lancet 1970;I:1083–1087.

47. Barbeau A, Mars H, Botez MI, et al. Amantadine-HCl (Symmetrel) in the management of Parkinson's disease: a double-blind cross-over study. Can Med Assoc J 1971;105:42–46.

48. Godwin-Austen RB, Frears CC, Bergmann S, Parkes JD, Knill-Jones RP. Combined treatment of parkinsonism with L-dopa and amantadine. Lancet 1970;II:383–385.

49. Fahn S, Isgreen WP. Long term evaluation of amantadine and levodopa combination in parkinsonsim by double-blind cross-over analyses. Neurology 1975;25:695–700.

50. Fehling C. The effect of adding amantadine to optimum L-dopa dosage in Parkinson's syndrome. Acta Neurol Scand 1973;49:245–251.

51. De Deviitis E, D'Andrea F, Signorelli CD, Cerillo A. L'amantadine nel trattamento dell'ipokinesia transitoria di pazienti parkinsoniani in corso di terapia con L-dopa. Minerva Med 1972;409:4007–4008.

52. Hornykiewicz O. From dopamine to Parkinson's disease: a personal research record. In: Samson F, Adelman G, editors. The neurosciences: paths to recovery, II. 1991:125–146.

53. Montagu KA. Catechol compounds in rat tissues and in brains of different animals. Nature 1957;180:244–245.

54. Weil-Malherbe H, Bone AD. Intracellular distribution of catecholamines in the brain. Nature 1957;180:1050–1051.

55. Bertler A, Rosengen E. Occurrence and distribution of dopamine in brain and other tissues. Experientia 1959;15: 10–11.

56. Ehringer H, Hornykiewicz O. Verteilung von Noradrenalin und Dopamin (3-Hydroxytyramin) im Gehirn des Menschen und ihr Verhalten bei Erkrankungen des extrapyramidalen Systems. Klin Wochenschr 1960;38:586–587.

57. Carlsson A. The occurrence, distribution, and physiological role of catecholamines in the nervous system. Pharmacol Rev 1959;11:490–493.

58. Birkmayer W, Hornykiewicz O. Der L3,4-dioscyphenylalanin (=DOPA)-Effekt bei der Parkinson-Akinese. Wien Klin Wochenschr 1961;73:787–788.

59. McGeer PL, Boulding JE, Gibson WC, Foulkes RG. Drug induced extrapyramidal reactions: treatment with diphenhydramine hydrochloride and dihydroxyphenylalanine. JAMA 1961;177:665–670.

60. Barbeau A, Sourkes TL, Murphy GF. Les catecholamines dans la maladie de Parkinson. In: De Ajuriaguerra J, editor. Monoamines et système nerveux central. Paris: Masson, 1962:925–927.

61. Friedhoff AJ, Hekimian L, Alper M. Dihydroxyphenylalanine in extrapyramidal disease. JAMA 1963;184:285–286.

62. Greer M, Williams CM. Dopamine metabolism in Parkinson's disease. Neurology 1963;13:73–76.

63. McGeer PL, Zeldowicz LR. Administration of dihydroxyphenylalanine to parkinsonian patients. Can Med Assoc J 1964;90:463–466.

64. Birkmayer W, Hornykiewicz O. Weitere experimentelle Untersuchugen über beim Parkinson-syndrom und Reserpin-parkinsonismus. Arch Psychiatr Zeitschr Neurol 1964;206:367–381.

65. Fehling C. Treatment of Parkinson's syndrome with L-dopa: a double blind study. Acta Neurol Scand 1966;43:367–372.

66. Rinne UK, Sonninen V. A double-blind study of L-dopa treatment in Parkinson's disease. Eur Neurol 1968;1:180–191.

67. Cotzias GC, Van Woert MH, Schiffer LM. Aromatic amino acids and modification of parkinsonism. N Engl J Med 1967;276:374–379.

68. Cotzias GC, Papavasiliou PS, Gellene R. Modification of Parkinson's disease: chronic treatment with L-dopa. N Engl J Med 1969;280:337–345.

69. Cotzias GC, Papavailiou PS, Gellene R. L-Dopa in Parkinson's disease [letter]. N Engl J Med 1969;281:272.

70. Yahr MD, Duvosin RC, Schear MJ, Barrett RE, Hoehn MM. Treatment of parkinsonism with levodopa. Arch Neurol 1969;21:343–354.

71. Godwin-Austen RB, Tomlinson EB, Frears CC, Kok HWL. Effects of L-dopa in Parkinson's disease. Lancet 1969;II: 165–168.

72. Calne DB, Spiers ASD, Stern GM, Laurence DR, Armitage P. L-Dopa in idiopathic parkinsonism. Lancet 1969;II:973–976.

73. ••.

74. Paulson GW, Wiederholt WC, Allen JN, Shuttleworth EC, Friedman HM. The use of L-dopa in parkinsonism. Ohio State Med J 1969;65:995–999.

75. Barbeau A. L-Dopa therapy in Parkinson's disease: a critical review of nine years' experience. Can Med Assoc J 1969;101:59–68.

76. Birkmayer W. Clinical effects of L-dopa plus Ro 4-4602. In: Barbeau A, McDowell FH, editors. L-Dopa and parkinsonism. Philadelphia: FA Davis, 1970:53–54.

77. Yahr MD, Duvoisin RC, Mendoza MR, Schear MJ, Barrett RE. Modification of L-dopa therapy of parkinsonism by alpha-methyldopa hydrazine (MK-486). Trans Am Neurol Assoc 1971;96:55–58.

78. Calne DB, Reid JL, Vakil SD, et al. Idiopathic parkinsonism treated with an extracerebral decarboxylase inhibitor in combination with levodopa. BMJ 1971;III:729–732.

79. Dupont E, Hansen E, Melsen S, Pakkenberg H, Holm P. Treatment of parkinsonism with a combination of levodopa and the decarboxylase inhibitor Ro-4-4602 (a comparison with levodopa treatment alone). Acta Neurol Scand Suppl 1972;51:115–117.

80. Holmsen R, Kvan L, Presthus J, Thoresen GB. Treatment of parkinsonism with a compound of L-dopa (Laradopa) and a decarboxylase inhibitor (Ro 4-4602). Acta Neurol Scand Suppl 1972;51:121–122.

81. Miller EM, Wiener L. Ro 4-4602 and levodopa in the treatment of parkinsonism. Neurology 1974;24:482–486.

82. Rinne UK, Birket-Smith E, Dupont E, et al. Levodopa alone and in combination with a peripheral decarboxylase inhibitor benserazide (Madopar) in the treatment of Parkinson's disease. J Neurol 1975;211:1–9.

83. Marsden CD, Barry PE, Parkes JD, Zilkha KJ. Treatment of Parkinson's disease with levodopa combined with L-alpha-methyldopahydrazine, an inhibitor of extracerebral DOPA decarboxylase. J Neurol Neurosurg Psychiatry 1973;36:10–14.

84. Schwartz AM, Olanow CW, Spencer A. A double-blind controlled study of MK-486 in Parkinson's disease. Trans Am Neurol Assoc 1973;98:301–303.

85. Markham CH, Diamond SG, Treciokas LJ. Carbidopa in Parkinson's disease and in nausea and vomiting of levodopa. Arch Neurol 1974;31:128–133.

86. Lieberman A, Goodgold A, Jonas S, Leibowitz M. Comparison of dopa decarboxylase inhibitor (carbidopa) combined

with levodopa and levodopa alone in Parkinson's disease. Neurology 1975;25:911–916.

87. Korten JJ, Keyser A, Joosten EMG, Gabreels FJM. Madopar versus Sinemet: a clinical study on their effectiveness. Eur Neurol 1975;13:65–71.

88. Barbeau A, McDowell FH, editors, L-Dopa and parkinsonism. Philadelphia: FA Davis, 1970.

89. Rinne UK, Sonninen V, Siirtola T. Plasma concentration of levodopa in patients with Parkinson's disease: response to administration of levodopa alone or combined with a decarboxylase inhibitor and clinical correlations. Eur Neurol 1973;10:301–310.

90. Yahr MD. Variations in the "on-off" effect. Adv Neurol 1974;5:397–399.

91. Rossor MN, Watkins J, Brown MJ. Plasma levodopa, dopamine and therapeutic response following levodopa therapy of parkinsonian patients. J Neurol Sci 1980;46: 385–392.

92. Tolosa ES, Martin WE, Cohen HP, Jacobson RL. Patterns of clinical response and plasma levels in Parkinson's disease. Neurology 1975;25:177–183.

93. Muenter MD, Tyce GM. L-Dopa therapy of Parkinson's disease: plasma L-dopa concentration, therapeutic response, and side effects. Mayo Clin Proc 1971;46:231–239.

94. Shoulson I, Glaubiger GA, Chase TN. On-off response: clinical and biochemical correlations during oral and intravenous levodopa administration in parkinsonian patients. Neurology 1975;25:1144–1148.

95. Juncos JL, Mouradian MM, Fabbrini G, et al. Levodopa methyl ester treatment of Parkinson's disease. Neurology 1987;37:1242–1245.

96. Fahn S. Fluctuations of disability in Parkinson's disease: pathophysiology. In: Marsden CD, Fahn S, editors. Movement disorders. Boston: Butterworth Scientific, 1982:123–145.

97. Fabrini G, Juncos JL, Mouradian MM, et al. Levodopa pharmacokinetic mechanisms and motor fluctuations in Parkinson's disease. Ann Neurol 1987;21:370–376.

98. Hutton JT, Dippel RL, Bianchine JR, Strahlendorf HK, Meyer PG. Controlled-release carbidopa/levodopa in the treatment of parkinsonism. Clin Neuropharmacol 1984;7: 135–139.

99. Hutton JT, Albrecht JW, Roman GC, Kopetzky MT. Prolonged serum levodopa levels with controlled-release carbidopa-levodopa in the treatment of Parkinson's disease. Arch Neurol 1988;45:55–57.

100. Nutt JG, Woodward WR, Carter JH. Clinical and biomedical studies with controlled-release levodopa/carbidopa. Neurology 1986;36:1206–1211.

101. Cedarbaum JM, Breck L, Kutt H, McDowell FH. Controlled-release levodopa/carbidopa. I. Sinemet CR-3 treatment of response fluctuations in Parkinson's disease. Neurology 1987;37:233–241.

102. Juncos JL, Fabrini G, Mouradian MM, Serrati C, Kask AM, Chase TN. Controlled release levodopa treatment of motor fluctuations in Parkinson's disease. J Neurol Neurosurg Psychiatry 1987;50:194–198.

103. Goetz CG, Tanner CM, Klawans HL, Shannon KM, Carroll VS. Parkinson's disease and motor fluctuations: long-acting carbidopa/levodopa (CR-4-Sinemet). Neurology 1987;37: 875–878.

104. Cedarbaum JM, Breck L, Kutt H, McDowell FH. Controlled-release levodopa/carbidopa. II. Sinemet CR-4 treatment of response fluctuations in Parkinson's disease. Neurology 1987;37:1607–1612.

105. Goetz CG, Tanner CM, Shannon KM, et al. Controlled-release carbidopa/levodopa (CR4-Sinemet) in Parkinson's disease patients with and without motor fluctuations. Neurology 1988;38:1143–1146.

106. Hutton JT, Morris JL, Roman GC, Imke SC, Elias JW. Treatment of chronic Parkinson's disease with controlled-release carbidopa/levodopa. Arch Neurol 1988;45:861–864.

107. Hutton JT, Morris JL, Bush DF, Smith ME, Liss CL, Reine S. Multicentre controlled study of Sinemet CR vs Sinemet (25/100) in advanced Parkinson's disease. Neurology 1989; 39(Suppl 2):67–72.

108. Aarli JA, Gilhus NE. Sinemet Cr in the treatment of patients with Parkinson's disease already on long-term treatment with levodopa. Neurology 1989;39(Suppl 2):82–85.

109. Bush DF, Liss CL, Morton A, et al. An open multicentre long-term treatment evaluation of Sinemet CR. Neurology 1989;39(Suppl 2):101–104.

110. Rondot P, Ziegler M, Aymard N, Teinturier A. Effect of controlled-release carbidopa/levodopa on motor performance in advanced Parkinson's disease. Neurology 1989;39(Suppl 2):74–77.

111. Goetz CG, Tanner CM, Gilley DW, Klawans HL. Development of progression of motor fluctuations and side effects in Parkinson's disease: comparison of Sinemet CR versus carbidopa/levodopa. Neurology 1989;39(Suppl 2):62–63.

112. Rinne UK. Madopar HBS in the long-term treatment of parkinsonian patients with fluctuations in disability. Eur Neurol 1987;27(Supple 1):120–125.

113. Jensen NO, Dupont E, Hansen E, Middelsen B, Mikkelson BO. A controlled release form of Madopar in Parkinsonian patients with advanced disease and marked fluctuations in motor performance. Acta Neurol Scand 1988;77:422–425.

114. Pacchetti C, Martignoni E, Sibilla L, Bruggi P, Turla M, Nappi G. Effectiveness of Madopar HBS plus Madopar standard in patients with fluctuating Parkinson's disease: two years of follow-up. Eur Neurol 1990;30:319–323.

115. Goodwin-Austen RB, Smith NJ. Comparison of the effects of bromocriptine and levodopa in Parkinson's disease. J Neurol Neurosurg Psychiatry 1997;44:4479–4482.

116. Grimes JD, Hassan MN. Bromocriptine in the long-term management of advanced Parkinson's disease. Can J Neurol Sci 1983;10:86–90.

117. Rinne UK, Martilla R. Brain dopamine receptor stimulation and the relief of parkinsonism: relationship between bromocriptine and levodopa. Ann Neurol 1978;4:263–267.

118. Teychenne PF, Bergsrud D, Racy A. Bromocriptine: low dose therapy in parkinsonism. Neurology 1982;32:577–583.

119. UK Bromocriptine Research Group. Bromocriptine in Parkinson's disease: a double blind study comparing "low-slow" and "high-fast" introductory dosage regimens in de novo patients. J Neurol Neurosurg Psychiatry 1989;52:77–82.

120. Lees AJ, Stern GM. Pergolide and Lisuride for levodopa-induced oscillations. Lancet 1981;I:577.

121. Lieberman A, Goldstein M, Leibowitz M, Neophytides A, Kupersmith M, Pact V, et al. Treatment of advanced Parkinson's disease with pergolide. Neurology 1981;31:675–682.

122. Lang AE, Quinn N, Brincat S, Marsden CD, Parkes JD. Pergolide in late-stage Parkinson disease. Ann Neurol 1982;12:243–247.

123. Lieberman A, Goldstein M, Gopinathan G, Leibowitz M, Neophytides A, Walker R, et al. Further studies with pergolide in Parkinson disease. Neurology 1982;32:1181–1184.

124. Tanner CM, Goetz CG, Glantz RH, Glatt SL, Klawans HL. Pergolide mesylate and idiopathic Parkinson disease. Neurology 1982;32:1175–1179.

125. Saje JI, Duvoisin RC. Pergolide therapy in Parkinson's disease: a double-blind, placebo-controlled study. Clin Neuropharmacol 1985;8:260–265.

126. Diamond SG, Markham CH, Treciokas LJ. Double-blind trial of pergolide of Parkinson's disease. Neurology 1985;35:291–295.

127. Jankovic J, Orman J. Parallel double-blind study of pergolide in Parkinson's disease. In: Yahr MD, Bergmann KJ, editors. Advances in neurology. New York: Raven Press, 1986:551–554.

128. Olanow CW, Alberts MJ. Double-blind controlled study of pergolide mesylate as an adjunct to Sinemet in the treatment of Parkinson's disease. In: Yahr MD, Bergmann KJ, editors. Advances in neurology. New York, Raven Press, 1986:555–560.

129. Rinne UK. Lisuride, a dopamine agonist in the treatment of early Parkinson's disease. Neurology 1989;39:336–339.

130. Lieberman AN, Goldstein M, Gopinathan G, Neophytides A, Leibowitz M, Walker R, et al. Lisuride in Parkinson's disease and related disorders. In: Calne DB, Horowski R, McDonald RJ, Wuttke W, editors. Lisuride and other dopamine agonists. New York: Raven Press, 1983:419–429.

131. Giovannini P, Scigliano G, Piccolo I, Soliveri P, Suchy I, Caraceni T. Lisuride in Parkinson's disease: 4 year follow-up. Clin Neuropharmacol 1988;11:201–211.

132. LeWitt PA, Gopinathan G, Ward CD, Sanes JN, Dambrosia JM, Durso R, et al. Lisuride versus bromocriptine treatment in Parkinson's disease: a double-blind study. Neurology 1982; 32:69–72.

133. Lieberman AN, Leibowitz M, Gopinathan G, Walker R, Hiesiger E, Nelson J, et al. Review: the use of pergolide and lisuride, two experimental dopamine agonists, in patients with advanced Parkinson's disease. Am J Med Sci 1985; 290:102–106.

134. Caraceni T, Giovannini P, Parati E, Scigliano G, Grassi MP, Carella F. Bromocriptine and lisuride in Parkinson's disease. Adv Neurol 1984;40:531–535.

135. Lieberman AN, Goldstein M. Bromocriptine in Parkinson disease. Pharmacol Rev 1985;37:217–227.

136. Lieberman AN, Goldstein M, Leibowitz M. Treatment of advanced Parkinson disease with pergolide. Neurology 1981;31:675–682.

137. Lieberman AN, Goldstein M, Gopinathan G. Further studies with lisuride in Parkinson's disease. Eur Neurol 1983; 22:119–123.

138. Calne DB, Williams AC, Neophytides A. Long term treatment of parkinsonism with bromocriptine. Lancet 1978;I:735–738.

139. Lesser RP, Fahn S, Spider SR, Cote LJ, Isgreen WP, Barrett RE. Analysis of the clinical problems in parkinsonism and the complications of long-term L-DOPA therapy. Neurology 1979;29:1253–1260.

140. Rinne UK. Early contribution of bromocriptine and levodopa in the treatment of Parkinson's disease: a 5-year follow-up. Neurology 1987;37:826–828.

141. Olanow CW. A rationale for dopamine agonists as primary therapy for Parkinson's disease. Can J Neurol Sci 1992;19: 108–112.

142. Lieberman A. Dopamine agonists used as monotherapy in de novo PD patients: comparisons with selegiline. Neurology 1992;42(Suppl 4):37–40.

143. Rinne UK. Early combination of bromocriptine and levodopa in the treatment of Parkinson's disease: a 5 year follow-up. Neurology 1987;37:826–828.

144. Rinne UK. Early dopamine agonist therapy in Parkinson's disease. Mov Disord 1989;4(Suppl 1):S86–S94.

145. Montastruc JL, Rascol O, Rascol A. A randomised controlled study of bromocriptine versus levodopa in previously untreated parkinsonian patients: a 3 year follow up. J Neurol Neurosurg Psychiatry 1989;52:773–775.

146. Weiner WJ, Factor SA, Sanchez-Ramos JR, Singer C, Sheldon C, Cornelius L, et al. Early combination therapy (bromocriptine and levodopa) does not prevent motor fluctuations in Parkinson's disease. Neurology 1993;43:21–27.

147. Rabey JM, Treves T, Streifler M, Korzyn AD. Comparison of efficacy of lisuride hydrogen maleate with increased doses of levodopa in parkinsonian patients. Adv Neurol 1986; 45:569–572.

148. Rabey JM, Streifler M, Treves T, Korczyn AD. Long-term lisuride in Parkinson's disease. Ital Neurol Sci 1987;5(Suppl):55.

149. Lees AJ, Stern GM. Pergolide and lisuride for levodopa-induced oscillations. Lancet 1981;II:577.

150. Opacka-Juffry J, Wilson AW, Blunt SB. Effects of pergolide treatment on in vivo hydroxyl free radical formation during infusion of 6-OHDA in rat striatum. Brain Res 1998; 810:27–33.

151. Hall ED, Andrus PK, Oostveen JA, Althaus JS, Von Voigtlander FF. Neuroprotective effects of the dopamine D2–D3 agonist pramipexoie against postischemic of methamphetamine induced degeneration of nigrostriatal neurons. Brain Res 1996;742:80–88.

152. Liu XH, Kato H, Chen T, Kato K, Itoyama Y. Bromocriptine protects against delayed neuronal death of hippocampai neurons following cerebral ischemia in the gerbil. J Neurol Sci 1995;129:9–14.

153. Gassen M, Glinka Y, Pinchasi B, Youdim MB. Apomorphine is a highly potent free radical scavenger in rat brain mitochondrial fraction. Em J Pharmacol 1996;308:219–225.

154. Birkmayer W, Riederer P, Youdim MBH, Linaur W. Potentiation of anti-akinetic effect after L-dopa treatment by an inhibitor of MAOB, I-deprenyl. J Neural Transm 1975; 36:303–323.

155. Birkmayer W, Riederer P, Ambrozi L, Youdim MBH. Implications of combined treatment with "Madopar" and deprenyl in Parkinson's disease: a long term study. Lancet 1977; I:434–443.

156. Lees AJ, Shoaw KM, Kohout LJ, et al. Deprenyl in Parkinson's disease. Lancet 1977;I:791–795.

157. Presthus J, Hajba A. Deprenyl (selegeline) combined with levodopa and decarboxylase inhibitor in the treatment of Parkinson's disease. Acta Neurol (Scand) 1983;Suppl 95:127–133.

158. Birkmayer W, Knoll J, Riederer P, Youdim MBH. Deprenyl leads to prolongation of L-dopa efficacy in Parkinson's disease. Mod Prob Pharmacopsychiatry 1983;19:170.

159. Yahr MD, Mendoza MM, Moros P, Bergmann KJ. Treatment of Parkinson's disease in early and late phases: use of pharmacological agents with special reference to deprenyl (selegeline). Acta Neurol Scand 1983;Suppl 95:95–102.

160. Birkmayer W, Knoll J, Riederer P, Youdin MBH, Hars V, Marton J. Increase life expectancy resulting from addition of L-deprenyl to Madopar treatment in Parkinson's disease: A long term study. J Neurol Transm 1985;64:113–127.

161. Tetrud JW, Langston JW. The effect of deprenyl (selegiline) on the natural history of Parkinson's disease. Science 1989;245:519–522.

162. The Parkinson Study Group. DATATOP: a multicenter controlled clinical trial in early Parkinson's disease. Arch Neurol 1989;46:1052–1060.

163. Zweig RM, Carmichael JM, Morrill GB. Deprenyl for the treatment of early Parkinson's disease. N Engl J Med 1989;322:1526.

164. Landau WM. Clinical neuromythology. IX. Pyramid sale in the bucket shop: DATATOP bottoms out. Neurology 1990;40:1337–1339.

165. Kofman OS. Deprenyl: protective vs symptomatic effect. Can J Neurol Sci 1991;18:83–85.

166. Lieberman A, Fahn S, Olanow CW, et al. Does selegiline provide a symptomatic or a neuroprotective effect? Neurology 1992;42(Suppl 4):41–48.

27. Parkinson's Disease: Experience with Large Multicentre Trials

C.E. Clarke

Parkinson's Disease and Current Treatments

Although potentially treatable causes of parkinsonism can be identified relatively easily in the clinic (e.g. neuroleptic therapy, multiple cerebral infarct state), differentiating idiopathic Parkinson's disease (IPD) from other neurodegenerative conditions such as multiple system atrophy (MSA) and progressive supranuclear palsy (PSP) can be difficult. In addition to parkinsonism in MSA, autonomic and/or cerebellar features occur, whereas in PSP early impairment of balance and a supranuclear eye movement disorder are found. Recent neuropathological studies have shown that the clinical diagnosis of IPD may be wrong in 24% of cases [1,2]. This has a considerable impact on clinical trials in Parkinson's disease, particularly long-term studies where a significant drop-out rate must be expected due to diagnostic error.

Early treatments such as anticholinergic agents and amantadine have a relatively low efficacy and high side-effect profile. The monoamine oxidase B inhibitor selegiline (US: deprenyl) has poor symptomatic effects. Initial claims that it was neuroprotective [3–5] have now been questioned [6].

The gold standard therapy for Parkinson's disease remains levodopa, which is converted in the striatum to the deficient neuromodulator dopamine. The beneficial effects of levodopa are marred by long-term side-effects which develop in around 50% of patients after 6 years of treatment [7] and 100% of younger patients after a similar period [8]. More recent strategies have been to use dopamine agonists, not as an adjunctive therapy late in the disease as in the past, but at the outset to delay the introduction of levodopa and thus its side-effects. Such agonists act directly on dopamine receptors in the striatum. Although there appears little to choose between them in later disease, few are licensed for early treatment.

Undoubtedly, new approaches to the prevention and management of the long-term complications of levodopa therapy are required. This has spurred the development of other dopamine agonists and catechol-O-methyltransferase inhibitors. Glutamate antagonists such as remacemide are commencing trials and may be able to prevent or treat levodopa complications. Surgical procedures are enjoying a revival now the neural mechanism of Parkinson's disease is understood in greater detail. Pallidotomy may reduce dyskinetic movements and subthalamic stimulation may also relieve parkinsonian symptoms, but the cost of the procedure and the associated hardware may be prohibitive. Fetal midbrain transplants into the striatum continue to be developed. Transplantable genetically engineered cell lines which manufacture tyrosine hydroxylase will be the next great step in this field.

Potential Problems with Trials in Parkinson's Disease

General

The strength of the *placebo effect* in Parkinson's disease trials is considerable. This is largely due to the psychological effects of participation in the study. It may be attributable to the positive attitude that many have to participation in a trial with a novel drug, small patient support groups forming within the trial or a supportive research nurse. *Bias* can be introduced at any stage of a trial. In Parkinson's disease studies care must be taken to ensure patients are properly randomised to avoid bias in the initial allocation of study medication. For example, if the age ranges in the study arms are considerably disparate, this may influence the outcome of the study. Similarly, minor antiparkinsonian agents such as the anticholinergics, amantadine and selegiline may influence the way subsequent preparations act; therefore these must be balanced between the study arms. Some bias is almost inevitable in the selection of patients for a study. Most investigators in the field have a particular interest in Parkinson's disease and their clinics are consequently highly specialised with a bias towards younger and perhaps more difficult cases. Study populations recruited in this manner will not necessarily be representative of Parkinson's disease in the community.

Specific to Parkinson's Disease

The *lack of definitive diagnostic criteria* for IPD can lead to difficulties in long-term studies; potentially up to 24% of patients may drop out of the trial due to a change in diagnosis [1,2]. IPD is a *progressive condition*, a fact which must also be taken into consideration in long-term work. Later in the condition, patients naturally undergo *fluctuations in the response to medication*, particularly levodopa preparations. For this reason, most studies choose to examine efficacy in either an "off" period, when the patient has been without medication overnight, or a set period after medication ingestion, when they are likely to be in their best "on" phase. These are the most reproducible times for assessments to be performed.

Another difficult problem with trials in Parkinson's disease is *measuring the severity of the condition*. Numerous timed tests and automated analysers have been invented over the years, but trialists continue to return to clinical rating scales as a reliable, reproducible and inexpensive way of measuring the response to medication. The details of many of these rating scales are examined below, but they lead to further problems in that investigators used different scales for many years. To avoid this difficulty, the Unified Parkinson's Disease Rating Scale (UPDRS) has now been developed which forms the core of most modern trials [9]. Similar considerations apply to the *measurement of dyskinesia*, with several rating scales being available. *Measurement of the duration of the total daily "on" period* depends on patient diaries. Fortunately, these have been standard for many years, but they rely on patients being well tutored in their use and on an unhealthy degree of attention to the phase of their condition.

Basic Design of Trials in Parkinson's Disease

Trial designs aim to minimise the problems outlined above. By far the most popular design is the *parallel group randomised controlled trial* (RCT) in which the study population is randomly allocated to different interventions. These may be two or more active agents or one active agent versus placebo. This is superior to the *crossover design*, in which patients act as their own controls, since the progression of Parkinson's disease will act as a time-dependent confounding variable with this design in anything but very short studies. One crucial aspect of RCTs is the precise *method of randomisation*. Each patient must have the same chance of receiving each of the interventions which is independent of any other individual's chance of receiving the intervention. This may be achieved by a centralised randomisation scheme, a randomisation scheme controlled by pharmacy, numbered or coded containers in which capsules from identical-looking numbered bottles are administered sequentially, an on-site computer system where allocations are in a locked unreadable file or sequentially numbered sealed envelopes [10]. Quasi-random allocation uses methods which are not strictly random such as date of birth, day of the week, medical record number, month of the year and order of entry (e.g. alternation). The method used to randomise patients in a study must be described in the trial report in detail.

Although randomisation reduces the potential for confounding variables at the beginning of a study, *blinding* should be employed to prevent unwanted influences during the work. Many large multicentre studies in Parkinson's disease, particularly those involving pharmaceutical manufacturers, use the gold standard *triple blinding* method. In this, the patient, the investigator and the person(s) analysing the results are blinded to the intervention in the individual case. When this is not possible, a *double-blind* technique is employed in which the patient and the investigator are blinded. This requires matching interventions, so that no difference can be detected between the intervention in question and the older agent or placebo. Designing identical tablets or capsules for each arm of a trial is not sufficient in this regard. All interventions must taste alike as patients often chew their medication. Any adverse response to taking the interventions must also be considered. If the active agent changes the colour of the patient's urine, this may potentially unblind at least the investigator. Nausea, vomiting, hypotension and increased dyskinesia are common side-effects of antiparkinsonian medication and may make it clear to an investigator that the patient is not receiving an inactive placebo. Where such effects are suspected, the investigators and patients should be asked at the end of the study to guess what medication they were receiving. If the guess rate is significantly higher than that expected by chance, the study cannot be said to have been performed in a truly blinded fashion. Where difficult titration of study medication is required, a *blinded rater* technique can be used. Here the patient and the chief investigator are not blinded but the person assessing the outcome measures of the study is blinded to the medication the patient is receiving. For example, this can be achieved by a research nurse performing rating scales and adverse event recording, while dosing is controlled by the investigator. The potential for patients unblinding the "blinded rater" in this situation is high and an end-of-study question regarding blinding should be included in the case record form. *Open designs*, in which both the patient and the investigator are unblinded, are often employed in post-marketing phase IV studies. They are less expensive than blinded trials and therefore lend themselves to large multicentre studies where finance is limited [6]. They can be of great value but are open to criticism regarding various forms of bias. If such a method is employed, it is imperative that the randomisation technique is rigorous as this will protect against many confounding variables at the outset.

Measurement Methods

The variability in the severity of Parkinson's disease and the complications of its treatment mean that any assessment must be carried out under conditions which have been standardised as far as possible. This usually entails measurement in the "off" phase, after withdrawal of medication overnight, and in the "on" phase, after a set period following dosing.

Quantitative Methods

Quantitative measurement methods have the advantages of giving the investigator a precise numerical result using a continuous variable which allows the use of parametric statistical methods when analysing the results. They are subject to little inter- and intra-investigator variability and they are also more sensitive than clinical rating scales. However, the more sophisticated quantitative techniques require detailed electrophysiological measures and thus equipment which may not be suitable or affordable for larger multicentre studies.

Simple Timed Motor Tasks

A number of simple timed motor tasks have been used over many years to quantify the motor deficits in Parkinson's disease and to follow them in response to medication. In the standardised "off" or "on"

period, the patient is asked to perform the task a set number of times which is timed with a stop watch [11]. In the *pronation–supination test*, the patient alternately taps the palm and dorsum of the hand on the knee whilst sitting for 20 cycles, one cycle consisting of a palm and dorsum tap. This is performed twice for each hand and the better of the measurements recorded for each hand. In the *hand movement between two points test*, the patient taps the index finger between two points set 30 cm (12 inches) apart for 20 taps. Again, this should be performed twice for each hand and the better measurement recorded for each hand. In the *finger dexterity task*, the patient is required to tap the thumb against the index finger and then each of the other fingers in turn for a total of 10 cycles. The better result of two trials for each hand should be noted. In the commonly used *stand–walk–sit test*, the patient is timed whilst they rise from a chair, walk 7 m (23 feet), turn, walk back to the chair and sit down. The chair should be firm and armless with four legs and a seat which is 45 cm in height (18 inches). The better of two trials should be recorded, along with the number of freezing episodes.

Electrophysiological Measures

Electrophysiological measures of disability in Parkinson's disease are rarely used in clinical trials since the equipment required is not easily available or is difficult to access in the clinic. However, they have proved invaluable in investigating the neural mechanism of the condition.

The slowness of movement in Parkinson's disease, or *bradykinesia*, can be assessed by measuring reaction and movement times [12]. These techniques require a queuing device, such as a computer, which presents a visual or audible queue to the patient. They are then required to perform a motor task, such as moving a handle and pointing device a set distance with the forearm fixed so that movement can only occur at the wrist. Surface electromyography (EMG) is used to detect the first sign of movement. The time between the start queue and the first EMG activity is the reaction time, whereas the time from the start of movement to its completion is the movement time. Movement time measures bradykinesia and is more frequently abnormal in Parkinson's disease. Reaction time reflects central processing and the generation of a motor programme and is abnormal in late Parkinson's disease.

Rigidity can be measured by passively moving a joint such as the elbow using a torque motor [12]. A plot of the angular position of the joint versus the torque developing in the arm, measured by strain gauges, allows the compliance of the limb to be measured. Tremor can be measured using accelerometers attached to any limb or surface EMG electrodes attached to the flexors and extensors of a joint [12]. These will demonstrate the 4–5 Hz rest tremor and 5–6 Hz postural tremor seen in Parkinson's disease. To date, measures of rigidity and tremor have rarely been used in clinical practice.

Clinical Rating Scales

A confusing number of clinical rating scales have been used to assess the severity of Parkinson's disease and its complications over the last 40 years. It is important to understand that these measure different aspects of the condition. Some reflect the overall stage of the disease the patient has reached, others measure motor impairments, whilst yet others measure the degree to which the patient is handicapped in their activities of daily living. Older studies often used different scales, so that comparison of their results or meta-analysis is virtually impossible. In future studies, a standard battery of scales should be used based on the instruments described below.

Stage of the Disease

Since its introduction in 1967, the Hoehn and Yahr scale has become the cardinal method for quantifying the stage which a patient with Parkinson's disease has reached [13]. This is a useful way of ensuring before a trial that the patients entered are all in a mild early stage of the disease or later in the course of the illness. It is also useful at the end of a study to ensure that the overall severity of the disease in the different arms of a trial was similar. It can also provide a way of dividing up patients according to the stage of the disease to compare the effects of different treatments at different stages.

The details of the scale are given in Appendix A. The clinical features used in the scale, such as unilateral versus bilateral disease and the presence or absence of balance disturbance, can be quickly assessed by even relatively inexperienced observers and the patient staged accordingly.

Disability Measures

It is important to differentiate measures of disabilities caused by Parkinson's disease from measurements of the handicaps it produces [14]. A disability may be defined as the failure to perform a specific task to a "normal" level. Various disabilities act together to produce handicap or disadvantage because the patient has problems with everyday life.

Clinical rating scales measuring disabilities in Parkinson's disease will be dealt with in the present section, whereas those dealing with handicaps or difficulties with activities of daily living will be covered in the next section.

The first disability scale was introduced in 1961. The *Northwestern University Disability Scale* (NUDS) used precise definitions of each score to measure dressing, hygienic care and speech (10 points each) along with eating and feeding (5 points each) [15]. In 1968, *Webster* published a more extensive 10-item scale with definitions of the 4 points (0 to 3) to be used for each item [16]. The scale measured bradykinesia, rigidity, posture, arm swing, gait, tremor, facies, seborrhoea, speech and self-care. The *Columbia* scale was introduced in 1971 and was comprised of the same items as the Webster scale but included salivation, rising from a chair, postural instability and rapid movement of the fingers, hands and feet and utilised a 5-point scale [17]. Various adaptations of these scales have appeared, usually named after the institution in which the investigators worked – hence, the *Kings College Hospital* and *NYU* scales [18,19]. A further development was the weighting of certain items in this type of scale; motor functions scores were considered more important and thus were given more weight [20]. The justification for such weighting seems tenuous.

Although such scales proved invaluable in the clinic, investigators often used different scales, which made comparisons of the results and meta-analysis impossible. Also the reliability, validity and responsiveness of the scales was rarely established [21]. As a result, the *Unified Parkinson's Disease Rating Scale* (UPDRS) was conceived at a workshop in Bermuda in October 1984 and version 3.0 finalised in February 1987 [9]. The UPDRS has become the standard disability measure in Parkinson's disease research. It has been found to be a highly reliable and valid measure of the condition [9,22], although some work suggests that it could be simplified [23].

The UPDRS scores each item on a 5-point scale (0 to 4). It is divided into four sections (Appendix B): In Section I, four items cover mental aspects of the condition. In Section II, the patient rates 13 of their disabilities themselves, whereas in Section III the examiner rates 14 different motor disabilities. For Sections II and III, scores in the "off" and "on" phases should be recorded and the mean calculated prior to addition to the other scores if necessary. In Section IV, 11 complications of therapy are scored by the examiner after discussion with the patient. Traditionally, the Hoehn and Yahr score and the Schwab and England Activities of Daily Living score (see below) should also be recorded, along with the patient's weight, sitting and standing blood pressure, and pulse [9].

In spite of the widespread acceptance of the UPDRS, most investigators choose to use the items within it separately rather than produce a total score. For example, it is common practice to use the mean change in the motor score (Section III), or a 20–30% improvement in this, as the primary efficacy measure in a trial.

Handicap Measures

England and Schwab [24] first introduced a measure of activities of daily living in 1956 to quantify the effects of thalamotomy. Originally, there were no definitions for each point on the scale. This was resolved in the *Schwab and England scale* which was published in 1969 [25]. This assesses the patient's activities of daily living on a scale from 100% (normal) to 0 (complete dependence), with 10% increments which have clear definitions. This is usually now used in the modified form which was introduced with the UPDRS (Appendix C) [9]. Interpolation in 5% points between the 10% points of the scale is allowed, thereby doubling the sensitivity. Its was also suggested in these modifications that the patient, the patient's family and the examiner score the patient's handicap using the scale and that this should be performed in both the "on" and "off" states. No method of averaging these scores has been provided but, in practice, most patients, their relatives and the examiner agree on ratings in each phase, so there seems little to be gained by recording more than the examiner's conclusions in the "on" and "off" state. Interestingly, the Schwab and England scale had the highest concordance rate for inter-rater reliability when the components of the UPDRS were assessed, closely followed by the motor examination (Section III) [9].

The so-called activities of daily living part of the UPDRS (Section II) should not be mistaken for a measure of handicap. This requires the patient to score various of their disabilities.

Dyskinesia and Motor Fluctuations Rating Scales

Unfortunately, there is little agreement on the way that dyskinesia and motor fluctuations should be measured. Whilst the complications of therapy form part of the UPDRS (Section IV) and the latter does provide one means of crudely assessing these problems, it is common in clinical trials in later Parkinson's disease to include an additional scale to monitor dyskinesia. These continue to vary, so it is suggested that the scale adopted as part of the Core Assessment Program for Intracerebral Transplanta-

tions (CAPIT) is used [11]. This was adapted from the work of Obeso and scores the intensity of dyskinesia (0 = absent, 1 = minimal, 2 = patient conscious of dyskinesia but no interference with voluntary movement, 3 = dyskinesia impairs voluntary movements but patient can undertake most motor tasks, 4 = intense interference with movement control and activities of daily life greatly limited, 5 = violent dyskinesias, incompatible with any motor task) and its duration (0 = none, 1 = only present when carrying out motor tasks, 2 = present 25–50% of waking hours, 3 = present 51–75% of waking hours, 4 = present 76–99% of waking hours, 5 = continuous throughout the day). More recently, this scale has been simplified to use only 5 points to measure severity when assessing four standard activities: walking, drinking from a cup, putting on a coat and buttoning clothing [26]. This proved to have a high inter- and intra-rater reliability, but further modifications were suggested to standardise the phrasing of the categories (Modified Dyskinesia Scale version 2) [26].

The best method of measuring the disabling "off" periods patients suffer is the *patient diary*. The patient or carer is required to record whether the patient is "on", "off" or asleep at 30 or 60 min intervals throughout 2 or 3 days prior to a visit to the investigator. This should be performed during baseline assessments and repeated after active intervention. The improvement in the mean daily "off" time can then be compared between the interventions. This requires a considerable amount of training of the patient or carer before the study and a large commitment on the patient's behalf to ensure the data are accurate. Compliance with these diaries can be a significant problem, so sufficient attention must be given to this area of any trial.

Quality of Life Scales

Parkinson's disease can lead to a significant reduction in the patients quality of life. In a postal questionnaire in 1982 of patients and carers who had been in contact with the UK Parkinson's Disease Society, Oxtoby [27] found that patients had numerous problems with functional, emotional and social well-being. Few changes had occurred by 1994 when a similar questionnaire was administered to 72 parkinsonian patients [28]. It is therefore appropriate to measure quality of life in clinical trials and this is rapidly becoming standard practice.

For the purposes of a trial, quality of life should be measured using a standardised instrument which has undergone rigorous reliability testing and validation. These may be generic scales such as the *Sickness Impact Profile* (SIP) [29] and *Short Form 36*

(SF36) [30,31]. More recently, a disease-specific scale has been developed, the *Parkinson's Disease Questionnaire-39* (PDQ-39) [32]. These are self-administered and take a short time to complete, so they can be fitted into a study visit. The PDQ-39 includes questions about the patient's disabilities, so there is overlap with Section II of the UPDRS.

Depression Scales

Depression occurs in 40–50% of patients with Parkinson's disease at some point during their illness [33]. The brief measures of mood included in the UPDRS Section I are often supplemented with a generic depression rating scale such as the *Hamilton Depression Scale* [34]. However, in the author's experience it is unusual for there to be any significant change in depression scores in short-term trials with anti-parkinsonian agents up to 6 months. This is more likely in long-term trials, in which the possibility of depression being a confounding factor must be considered.

Economic Evaluations

The financial pressures on health care systems in recent years has given rise to considerable interest in the cost-effectiveness of all interventions. The health care economics of Parkinson's disease and its treatment has received little attention thus far. In one such study it was shown that the long-term complications of levodopa therapy increase the cost of treatment, so approaches to minimise these may reduce the overall costs of Parkinson's disease to the community [35].

Mortality Studies

From recent reviews of cohort and case–control studies, it has been concluded that patients with Parkinson's disease continue to die at twice the rate of their peers [36,37]. It is imperative that new treatments are examined for their potential neuroprotective role and, it is hoped, some effect on mortality. This requires long-term studies of over 5 years or more and large numbers of patients in view of the small differences in mortality which must be detected. Few pharmaceutical manufacturers are willing to invest the large sums of money required for such work, so consequently this often falls to large groups of investigators, such as the Parkinson's Disease Research Groups of the United Kingdom (UKPDRG) and the United States. Examples of such work include the DATATOP study, which ultimately failed to prove that selegiline and vitamin E had any neuroprotective properties [3,4], and the UKPDRG Study 1, which found an excess of deaths in patients

Table 27.1. The Core Assessment Program for Intracerebral Transplantations (CAPIT)

Unified Parkinson's Disease Rating Scale
Hoehn and Yahr Stage
Dyskinesia Rating Scale (see text)
"On"/"off" diary
Timed tests
Pronation–supination test
Hand/arm movement between two points
Finger dexterity
Stand–walk–sit test
Levodopa challenge
Above tests at 20 min intervals after patient's usual levodopa dose

From [11].

taking selegiline and Madopar compared with those taking Madopar alone [6].

Test Batteries

In spite of the launch of the UPDRS in 1987, the wave of transplantation studies in the early 1990s used varying rating scales and other assessment methods. It was therefore decided by a large number of the workers in the movement disorders field to draw up a core of assessments which should be used in all transplant studies, to which other tests may be added at the investigator's discretion [11]. The Core Assessment Program for Intracerebral Transplantations (CAPIT) includes many of the methods described above (Table 27.1). It was suggested that these assessments be performed at 3 monthly intervals after transplantation, with two assessments at 3 and 6 months pre-operatively. For the 3 months prior to the procedure, the patient's medication should remain unchanged. Pre- and post-operative magnetic resonance imaging and positron emission tomography (fluorodopa uptake) was also recommended.

Whilst the CAPIT recommendations are a useful starting point for anyone designing a trial in parkinsonian patients, it is suggested that the other assessment methods outlined above should be considered. Not all the CAPIT measures may be necessary. For example, many trialists omit timed tests from their assessment battery. The scales used must depend on a critical appreciation of the condition, the likely effects of the intervention(s) to be used and their complications.

Statistical Considerations

The statistical principles governing clinical trials have been considered elsewhere. This section will therefore deal with particular pitfalls in Parkinson's disease trials. It must be stressed at the outset that a statistician should be consulted at the planning stage of any trial to decide on the most appropriate statistical techniques.

The statistics employed in a trial will depend on the types of outcome variables chosen. In the author's experience this is a common mistake in many studies in this field. The majority of pharmacological studies in Parkinson's disease are parallel group, double-blind randomised controlled trials. The commonly used outcome variables are derived from clinical rating scales, such as mean change in UPDRS motor score. These are *ordinal variables* which are descriptive and ordered. This ranking does not produce a continuum: the difference of one point between Stage 1 and 2 on the Hoehn and Yahr scale is not the same as the difference between Stage 4 and 5 disease. Thus, the use of means and standard deviations is not appropriate and *non-parametric techniques* should be used for analysis of differences between medians, such as the Mann–Whitney U (Wilcoxon rank-sum) test. Outcome variables derived from actual measurements such as timed tests (e.g. stand–walk–sit test, "on" time from daily diaries) are *continuous variables* which in most cases are normally distributed. The mean and standard deviation are appropriate in this case and *parametric statistics* should be used. Thus, in a trial with two arms, a Student's t-test is appropriate, whereas if there are three or more arms, ANOVA should be employed. With a dichotomous outcome variable, such as the presence or absence of dyskinesia by the end of the study, in a trial with two arms then a chi-squared test should be used.

Another mistake is to omit a *sample size estimate* from the initial planning of a trial. Usually, previous work has examined similar agents using the same outcome variables, so some assumptions about the effect size and variability in outcome can be made. Decisions regarding the size of type 1 error (false positive) and type 2 error (false negative) that will be acceptable should then be made. This information can then be used to calculate the sample size required. Additional patients will be required over and above this calculation to account for drop-outs and non-compliance.

An *intention-to-treat analysis* should be the preferred approach to the analysis of the results of the study. This maintains the benefit of randomisation so that non-compliant patients are not allowed to bias the results. However, particularly in long-term studies, a high drop-out rate may mean a *per-protocol analysis* is also appropriate.

It is not uncommon for the report of a trial to include multiple *subgroup analyses* which were not planned in advance. This must be avoided as chance associations will be found in 1 in 20 analyses using $p < 0.05$.

In long-term trials, *early stopping rules* are often employed. These are usually administered by a panel independent of the original investigators who remain unaware of the precise results of any interim analysis, unless it is terminated, so as to avoid the introduction of bias. If the study terminates early, such rules may reduce the cost of the work but, more importantly, may lead to the earlier introduction of the intervention into clinical practice. However, performing multiple analyses of the data throughout a trial can lead to false positive results. It has been shown in simulation studies that, with three interim analyses and one terminal analysis at the $p < 0.05$ level of significance, 17% of studies will produce a false positive conclusion compared with the 5% expected [38]. This can be avoided by using smaller significance levels in earlier interim analyses. One technique would use p values of less than 0.001, 0.004, 0.018 and 0.042 in four interim analyses to maintain the overall significance level at $p < 0.05$ with a low risk of inappropriate early termination of the study [38].

Conduct of the Trial

Studies funded by the pharmaceutical industry are usually designed in-house with advice from one or more external experts in the field. The draft protocol is then discussed with the investigators recruited for the work. This *consultation process* is often late in the design process and, if some investigators have already submitted the protocol to their ethics committee, belated amendments must also be submitted which may delay the start of the study. A suggested plan for the study *protocol* is shown in Table 27.2. The details required in *ethics committee submissions* vary considerably in the UK and there is currently a debate over their remit. In general, well-designed pharmaceutical trials with multi-investigator input and a potential benefit to patients are likely to be approved quickly.

The majority of investigators taking part in Parkinson's disease studies run specialised *Movement Disorders clinics*. It can be argued that these are tertiary referral centres and that the patients do not represent the burden of the disease in the community. However, this is the best way of running the service for these patients and it can provide a large number of patients for clinical trials in a short space of time. Many investigators perform trials with the assistance of *research nurses*. The latter rapidly become expert in performing such studies and can

Table 27.2. Protocol design

Summary
Flow chart
Introduction
Objectives
Study design
Patient population (including inclusion and exclusion criteria)
Trial medication
Observations and methods (including efficacy and safety measures)
Conduct of the trial
Statistics
Documentation (including case record forms)
Quality assurance
Publication strategy
Ethical considerations
References
Appendixes (including rating scales, dosing regimes and Declaration of Helsinki)

be relied upon to perform rating scales, other efficacy measures, phlebotomy and electrocardiography. Trial protocols should be written so that these roles can be fulfilled by the nurse rather than the investigator.

The first line of *quality control* in large pharmaceutical trials is the study monitor, who visits individual sites periodically to check the case record forms (CRF). The majority of the problems identified at these visits are minor and can be rectified in discussion with the research nurse or the investigator. More formal auditing of individual centres may be internal, conducted by the sponsor's quality assurance unit, or external, conducted by a Drug Regulatory Agency (e.g. the US Food and Drug Administration). Although further queries may be found, these are usually minor in centres with long experience of conducting such work.

It is usual in trials sponsored by the pharmaceutical industry for there to be regular *meetings* during the study. After the first to ratify the protocol, one or more may be held during the study to update investigators on drop-outs and pre-planned interim analyses. These are often at major neurosciences meetings. A further meeting should be held to discuss the results of the work and to nominate a publication committee.

It should be considered unethical not to *publish* the results of any well-designed study, positive or negative, for fear of others replicating the work unnecessarily. Usually this will be performed by a panel of investigators with experience in the field along with any pharmaceutical manufacturer involved. Clear guidelines now exist for the reporting of randomised controlled trials [39,40]. The *CONSORT Statement* emerged from a series of meetings of the Standards of Reporting Trials group from 1993 onward. This provides a checklist of items which should be included in the report. The major changes from present practice include better reporting of the methods of randomisation and blinding, inclusion of a trial profile detailing the numbers of patients present throughout the trial and the use of summary statistics in sufficient detail to allow alternative assessments such as meta-analysis [39]. The last point is now of considerable importance as the *Cochrane Movement Disorders Group* will be performing systematic reviews of all interventions in Parkinson's disease. Initially this will be retrospective but, in the future, the results of RCTs will be added to the existing Movement Disorders module on the Cochrane Database of Systematic Reviews as soon as possible after publication.

Future Developments

The standard of pharmaceutical trials in Parkinson's disease increased considerably in the 1990s with the general acceptance of the randomised controlled trial, the adoption of a small number of clinical rating scales and the availability of a small number of investigators dedicated to research in movement disorders. It is hoped that further improvements will emerge from acceptance of the CONSORT guidelines.

Numerous techniques continue to enter everyday practice without rigorous evaluation. Although there is considerable evidence that pallidotomy may be an effective treatment for Parkinson's disease from work in experimental models of parkinsonism, trials in the human condition have been small open-label studies with no control group. The ultimate abandoning of adrenal medulla transplants in Parkinson's disease occurred only after rigorous examination of the technique in multiple centres. This should be a lesson to us all. Large multicentre randomised controlled trials are the way forward in movement disorders research.

Appendixes

Appendix A. Modified Hoehn and Yahr Staging [13]

Stage 0   No signs of disease
Stage 1   Unilateral disease
Stage 1.5 Unilateral plus axial involvement
Stage 2   Bilateral disease, without impairment of balance

Stage 2.5 Mild bilateral disease, with recovery on pull test

Stage 3 Mild to moderate bilateral disease; some postural instability; physically independent

Stage 4 Severe disability; still able to walk or stand unassisted

Stage 5 Wheelchair-bound or bed-ridden unless aided

Appendix B. Unified Parkinson's Disease Rating Scale [9]

Section I. Mentation, Behaviour and Mood

1 Intellectual impairment
0 = None
1 = Mild. Consistent forgetfulness with particular recollection of events and no other difficulties
2 = Moderate memory loss, with disorientation and moderate difficulty handling complex problems. Mild but definite impairment of function at home with need of occasional prompting
3 = Severe memory loss with disorientation for time and often to place. Severe impairment in handling problems
4 = Severe memory loss with orientation preserved to person only. Unable to make judgements or solve problems. Requires much help with personal care. Cannot be left alone at all

2 Thought disorder (due to dementia or drug intoxication)
0 = None
1 = Vivid dreaming
2 = "Benign" hallucinations with insight retained
3 = Occasional to frequent hallucinations or delusions; without insight; could interfere with daily activities
4 = Persistent hallucinations, delusions, or florid psychosis. Not able to care for self

3 Depression
0 = Not present
1 = Periods of sadness or guilt greater than normal, never sustained for days or weeks
2 = Sustained depression (1 week or more)
3 = Sustained depression with vegetative symptoms (insomnia, anorexia, weight loss, loss interest)
4 = Sustained depression with vegetative symptoms and suicidal thoughts or intent

4 Motivation/initiative
0 = Normal
1 = Less assertive than usual; more passive
2 = Loss of initiative or disinterest in elective (non-routine) activities
3 = Loss of initiative or disinterest in day-to-day (routine) activities
4 = Withdrawn, complete loss of motivation

Section II. Activities of Daily Living (for both "on" and "off")

5 Speech
0 = Normal
1 = Mildly affected. No difficulty being understood
2 = Moderately affected. Sometimes asked to repeat statements
3 = Severely affected. Frequently asked to repeat statements
4 = Unintelligible most of the time

6 Salivation
0 = Normal
1 = Slight but definite excess of saliva in mouth; may have night-time drooling
2 = Moderately excessive saliva; may have minimal drooling
3 = Marked excess of saliva with some drooling
4 = Marked drooling, requires constant tissue or handkerchief

7 Swallowing
0 = Normal
1 = Rare choking
2 = Occasional choking
3 = Requires soft food
4 = Requires nasogastric tube or gastrostomy feeding

8 Handwriting
0 = Normal
1 = Slightly slow or small
2 = Moderately slow or small; all words are legible
3 = Severely affected; not all words are legible
4 = The majority of words are not legible

9 Cutting food and handling utensils
0 = Normal
1 = Somewhat slow and clumsy, but no help needed
2 = Can cut most foods, although clumsy and slow; some help needed
3 = Food must be cut by someone, but can still feed slowly
4 = Needs to be fed

10 Dressing
0 = Normal
1 = Somewhat slow but no help needed

2 = Occasional assistance with buttoning, getting arms in sleeves

3 = Considerable help required, but can do some things alone

4 = Helpless

11 Hygiene
0 = Normal

1 = Somewhat slow, but no help needed

2 = Needs help to shower or bathe, or very slow in hygienic care

3 = Requires assistance for washing, brushing teeth, coming hair, going to bathroom

4 = Foley catheter or other mechanical aids

12 Turning in bed and adjusting bed clothes
0 = Normal

1 = Somewhat slow and clumsy, but no help needed

2 = Can turn alone or adjust sheets, but with great difficulty

3 = Can initiate, but not turn or adjust sheets alone

4 = Helpless

13 Falling (unrelated to freezing)
0 = Normal

1 = Rare falling

2 = Occasional falls, less than once per day

3 = Falls on average once daily

4 = Falls more than once daily

14 Freezing when walking
0 = Normal

1 = Rare freezing when walking; may have start-hesitation

2 = Occasional freezing when walking

3 = Frequent freezing. Occasional falls from freezing

4 = Frequent falls from freezing

15 Walking
0 = Normal

1 = Mild difficulty. May not swing arms or may tend to drag leg

2 = Moderate difficulty, but requires little or no assistance

3 = Severe disturbance of walking, requiring assistance

4 = Cannot walk at all, even with assistance

16 Tremor (symptomatic complaint of tremor in any part of body)
0 = Absent

1 = Slight and infrequently present

2 = Moderate; bothersome to patient

3 = Severe; interferes with many activities

4 = Marked; interferes with most activities

17 Sensory complaints related to parkinsonism
0 = None

1 = Slight and infrequently present

2 = Frequently has numbness, tingling or aching; not distressing

3 = Frequent painful sensations

4 = Excruciating pain

Section III. Motor Examination

18 Speech
0 = Normal

1 = Slight loss of expression, diction and/or volume

2 = Monotone, slurred but understandable; moderately impaired

3 = Marked impairment, difficult to understand

4 = Unintelligible

19 Facial expressions
0 = Normal

1 = Minimal hypomimia, could be normal "poker face"

2 = Slight but definitely abnormal diminution of facial expression

3 = Moderate hypomimia; lips parted some of the time

4 = Marked or fixed facies with severe or complete loss of facial expression; lips parted $\frac{1}{4}$ inch ($\frac{1}{2}$ cm) or more

20 Tremor at rest
0 = Absent

1 = Slight and infrequently present

2 = Mild in amplitude and persistent; or moderate in amplitude but only intermittently present

3 = Moderate in amplitude and present most of the time

4 = Marked in amplitude and present most of the time

21 Action or postural tremor of hands
0 = Absent

1 = Slight; present with action

2 = Moderate in amplitude; present with action

3 = Moderate in amplitude with posture holding as well as action

4 = Marked in amplitude; interferes with feeding

22 Rigidity
(Judged on passive movement of major joints with patient relaxed in sitting position; ignore cog-wheeling)

0 = Absent

1 = Slight or detectable only when activated by mirror or other movements

2 = Mild to moderate

3 = Marked, but full range of motion easily achieved

4 = Severe, range of motion achieved with difficulty

23 Finger taps
(Patient taps thumb with index finger in rapid succession with widest amplitude possible, each hand separately)

0 = Normal

1 = Mild slowing and/or reduction in amplitude

2 = Moderately impaired. Definite and early fatiguing. May have occasional arrests in movement

3 = Severely impaired. Frequent hesitation in initiating movements or arrests in ongoing movements

4 = Can barely perform the task

24 Hand movements
(Patient opens and closes hands in rapid succession with widest amplitude possible, each hand separately)

0 = Normal

1 = Mild slowing and/or reduction in amplitude

2 = Moderately impaired. Definite and early fatiguing. May have occasional arrests in movement

3 = Severely impaired. Frequent hesitation in initiating movements or arrests in ongoing movement

4 = Can barely perform the task

25 Rapid alternating movements of hands
(Pronation–supination movements of hands, vertically or horizontally, with as large an amplitude as possible, each hand separately)

0 = Normal

1 = Mild slowing and/or reduction in amplitude

2 = Moderately impaired. Definite and early fatiguing. May have occasional arrests in movement

3 = Severely impaired. Frequent hesitation in initiating movements or arrests in ongoing movement

4 = Can barely perform the task

26 Leg agility
(Patient taps heel on ground in rapid succession, picking up entire leg; amplitude should be about 3 inches (1.2 cm))

0 = Normal

1 = Mild slowing and/or reduction in amplitude

2 = Moderately impaired. Definite and early fatiguing. May have occasional arrests in movement

3 = Severely impaired. Frequent hesitation initiating movements or arrests in ongoing movement

4 = Can barely perform the task

27 Arising from chair
(Patient attempts to arise from a straight-back wood or metal chair with arms folded across chest)

0 = Normal

1 = Slow; or may need more than one attempt

2 = Pushes self up from arms of seat

3 = Tends to fall back and may have to try more than one time, but can get up without help

4 = Unable to arise without help

28 Posture

0 = Normal erect

1 = Not quite erect, slightly stooped posture; could be normal for older person

2 = Moderately stooped posture, definitely abnormal; can be slightly leaning to one side

3 = Severely stooped posture with kyphosis; can be moderately leaning to one side

4 = Marked flexion with extreme abnormality of posture

29 Gait

0 = Normal

1 = Walks slowly, may shuffle with short steps, but no festination (hastening steps) or propulsion

2 = Walks with difficulty, but requires little or no assistance; may have some festination, short steps or propulsion

3 = Severe disturbance of gait, requiring assistance

4 = Cannot walk at all, even with assistance

30 Postural stability
(Response to sudden strong posterior displacement produced by pull on shoulders while patient erect with eyes open and feet slightly apart. Patient is prepared, and can have had some practice runs)

0 = Normal

1 = Retropulsion, but recovers unaided

2 = Absence of postural response; would fall if not caught by examiner

3 = Very unstable, tends to lose balance spontaneously

4 = Unable to stand without assistance

31 Body bradykinesia and hypokinesia
(Combining slowness, hesitancy, decreased arm swing, small amplitude, and poverty of movements in general)

0 = None

1 = Minimal slowness, giving movements a deliberate character; could be normal for some persons. Possibly reduced amplitude

2 = Mild degree of slowness and poverty of movement which is definitely abnormal. Alternatively, some reduced amplitude

3 = Moderate slowness, poverty or small amplitude of movement

4 = Marked slowness, poverty or small amplitude of movement

Section IV. Complications of Therapy (in the past week)

A Dyskinesias

32 Duration: What proportion of the waking day are dyskinesias present?
(Historical information)
0 = None
1 = 1–25% of day
2 = 26–50% of day
3 = 51–75% of day
4 = 76–100% of day

33 Disability: How disabling are the dyskinesias?
(Historical information; may be modified by office examination)
0 = Not disabling
1 = Mildly disabling
2 = Moderately disabling
3 = Severely disabling
4 = Completely disabling

34 Painful dyskinesias: How painful are the dyskinesias?
0 = No painful dyskinesias
1 = Slight
2 = Moderate
3 = Severe
4 = Marked

35 Presence of early morning dystonia
(Historical information)
0 = No
1 = Yes

B Clinical fluctuations

36 Are any "off" periods predictable as to timing after a dose of medication?
0 = No
1 = Yes

37 Are any "off" periods unpredictable as to timing after a dose of medication?
0 = No
1 = Yes

38 Do any of the "off" periods come on suddenly, e.g. over a few seconds?
0 = No
1 = Yes

39 What proportion of the waking day is the patient "off" on average?
0 = None
1 = 1–25% of day
2 = 26–50% of day
3 = 51–75% of day
4 = 76–100% of day

C Other complications

40 Does the patient had anorexia, nausea or vomiting?
0 = No
1 = Yes

41 Does the patient have any sleep disturbances, e.g. insomnia or hypersomnolence?
0 = No
1 = Yes

42 Does the patient have symptomatic orthostasis?
(Record the patient's blood pressure, height and weight on the scoring form)
0 = No
1 = Yes

Appendix C. Schwab and England Activities of Daily Living Scale [9]

(Interpolation in 5% levels between these definitions is allowed)

100%   Completely independent. Able to do all chores without slowness, difficulty or impairment. Essentially normal. Unaware of any difficulty

90%   Completely independent. Able to do all chores with some degree of slowness, difficulty and impairment. Might take twice as long. Beginning to be aware of difficulty

80%   Completely independent in most chores. Takes twice as long. Conscious of difficulty and slowness

70%   Not completely independent. More difficulty with some chores, three to four times as long in some. Must spend a large part of the day with chores

60%   Some dependency. Can do most chores, but exceedingly slowly and with much effort. Errors; some impossible

50%   More dependent. Help with half of chores, slower, etc. Difficulty with everything

40%   Very dependent. Can assist with all chores but few alone

30%   With effort, now and then does a few chores alone or begins alone. Much help needed

20%   Nothing alone. Can be a slight help with some chores. Severe invalid

10%   Total dependent, helpless. Complete invalid

0%   Vegetative functions such as swallowing, bladder and bowel functions are not functioning. Bed-ridden

References

1. Hughes AJ, Daniel SE, Kilford L, Lees AJ. Accuracy of clinical diagnosis of idiopathic Parkinson's disease: a clinicopathological study of 100 cases. J Neurol Neurosurg Psychiatry 1992;55:181–184.
2. Hughes AJ, Daniel SE, Blankson S, Lees AJ. A clinicopathologic study of 100 cases of Parkinson's disease. Arch Neurol 1993; 50:140–148.
3. The Parkinson Study Group. Effect of deprenyl on the progression of disability in early Parkinson's disease. N Engl J Med 1989;321:1364–1371.
4. The Parkinson Study Group. Effects of tocohperol and deprenyl on the progression of disability in early Parkinson's disease. N Engl J Med 1993;328:176–183.
5. Birkmayer W, Knoll J, Riederer P, Youdim MBH, Hars V, Marton J. Increased life expectancy resulting from addition of L-deprenyl to Madopar treatment in Parkinson's disease: a long-term study. J Neural Transm 1985;64:113–127.
6. Lees AJ and Parkinson's Disease Research Group. Comparison of therapeutic effects and mortality data of levodopa and levodopa combined with selegiline in patients with early, mild Parkinson's disease. BMJ 1995;311:1602–1607.
7. Rajput AH, Stern W, Laverty WH. Chronic low-dose levodopa therapy in Parkinson's disease: an argument for delaying levodopa therapy. Neurology 1984;34:991–996.
8. Quinn N, Critchley P, Parkes D, Marsden CD. When should levodopa be started? Lancet 1986;II:985–986.
9. Fahn S, Elton RL, and Members of the UPDRS Development Committee. Unified Parkinson's disease rating scale. In: Fahn S, Marsden CD, Goldstein M, Calne DB, editors. Recent developments in Parkinson's disease, vol 2. New Jersey: Macmillan Healthcare Information, 1987:153–163.
10. The Cochrane Collaboration. The Cochrane database of systematic reviews. London: British Medical Association Publications, 1996; issue 2.
11. CAPIT committee, Langston JW, Widner H, et al. Core assessment program for intracerebral transplantation (CAPIT). Mov Disord 1992;7:2–13.
12. Watts RL, Mandir AS. Quantitative methods of evaluating Parkinson's disease. In: Olanow CW, Lieberman AN, editors. The scientific basis for the treatment of Parkinson's disease. New Jersey: Parthenon, 1992:13–32.
13. Hoehn MM, Yahr MD. Parkinsonism: onset, progression, and mortality. Neurology 1967;17:427–442.
14. Ward CD. Rehabilitation in Parkinson's disease. Rev Clin Gerontol 1992;2:254–268.
15. Canter CJ, de la Torre R, Mier M. A method of evaluating disability in patients with Parkinson's disease. J Nerv Ment Dis 1961;133:143–147.
16. Webster DD. Clinical analysis of the disability in Parkinson's disease. Mod Treatment 1968;5:257–282.
17. Duvoisin RC. The evaluation of extrapyramidal disease. In: de Ajuriaguerra J, Gauthier G, editors. Monoamines noyaux gris centraux et syndrome de Parkinson. Geneva: Georg & Cie, 1971:313–325.
18. Parkes JD, Zikha KJ, Calver DM, Knill-Jones RP. Controlled trial of amantadine hydrochloride in Parkinson's disease. Lancet 1970;I:259–262.
19. Lieberman A. Parkinson's disease: a clinical review. Am J Med Sci 1974;267:66–80.
20. McDowell F, Lee JE, Swift T, Sweet RD, Ogsbury JS, Tessler JT. Treatment of Parkinson's syndrome with dihydroxyphenylalanine (levodopa). Ann Intern Med 1970;72:29–35.
21. Hobart JC, Lamping DL, Thompson AJ. Evaluating neurological outcome measures: the bare essentials. J Neurol Neurosurg Psychiatry 1996;60:127–130.
22. Richards M, Marder K, Cote L, Mayeux R. Interrater reliability of the unified Parkinson's disease rating motor examination. Mov Disord 1994;9:89–91.
23. Van Hilten JJ, van der Zwan AD, Zwinderman AH, Roos RAC. Rating impairment and disability in Parkinson's disease: evaluation of the Unified Parkinson's Disease Rating Scale. Mov Disord 1994;9:84–88.
24. England AC, Schwab RS. Post-operative evaluation of 26 selected patients with Parkinson's disease. J Am Geriatr Soc 1956;4:1219–1232.
25. Schwab RS, England AC. Projection technique for evaluating surgery in Parkinson's disease. In: Gillingham FJ, Donaldson IML, editors. Third symposium on Parkinson's disease. Edinburgh: E & S Livingstone, 1969:152–157.
26. Goetz CG, Stebbins GT, Shale HM, et al. Utility of an objective dyskinesia rating scale for Parkinson's disease; inter- and intrarater reliability assessment. Mov Disord 1994;9:390–394.
27. Oxtoby M. Parkinson's disease patients and their social needs. Parkinson's Disease Society, 1982.
28. Clarke CE, Zobkiw RM, Gullaksen E. Quality of life and care in Parkinson's disease. Br J Clin Pract 1995;49:288–293.
29. Bergner M, Bobbitt RA, Carter WB, Gilson BS. The Sickness Impact Profile: development and final revision of a health status measure. Med Care 1981;19:787–805.
30. Garratt AM, Ruta DA, Abdalla MI, Buckingham JK, Russell IT. The SF 36 health survey questionnaire: an outcome measure suitable for routine use within the NHS. BMJ 1993;306:1440–1444.
31. Jenkinson C, Coulter A, Wright L. Short form 36 (SF36) health survey questionnaire: normative data for adults of working age. BMJ 1993;306:1437–1440.
32. Peto V, Jenkinson C, Fitzpatrick R, Greenhall R. The development and validation of a short measure of functioning and well being for individuals with Parkinson's disease. Qual Life Res 1995;4:241–248.
33. Mayeux R. Depression and dementia in Parkinson's disease. In: Marsden CD, Fahn S, editors. Movement disorders. London: Butterworth, 1982:75–95.
34. Hamilton M. A rating scale for depression. J Neurol Neurosurg Psychiatry 1960;23:56–61.
35. Dodel RC, Singer M, Nuijten M, Rathay B, Scholz E, Selzer R. Parkinson's disease: an economic evaluation. Mov Disord 1996;11(Suppl 1):176.
36. Clarke CE. Does levodopa therapy delay death in Parkinson's disease? A review of the evidence. Mov Disord 1995;10:250–256.
37. Clarke CE, Pavelin AP, Carter PM, Daniel SE. Survival in 286 cases of pathologically confirmed idiopathic Parkinson's disease. Mov Disord 1997;12(Suppl 1):22.
38. Hauser RA, Olanow CW. Designing clinical trials in Parkinson's disease. In: Olanow CW, Lieberman AN, editors. The scientific basis for the treatment of Parkinson's disease. New Jersey: Parthenon, 1992:275–293.
39. Begg C, Cho M, Eastwood S, et al. Improving the quality of reporting of randomised controlled trials. JAMA 1996;276:637–639.
40. Schulz KF. Randomised trials, human nature, and reporting guidelines. Lancet 1996;348:596–598.

28. Tremor: Clinical Measurement of Impairment, Disability and Handicap

S.H. Alusi and P.G. Bain

Clinical Measurement of Tremor

Clinical methods for quantifying tremor severity are cheap, quick and easy to perform, which allows them to be more widely deployed than the physiological techniques described in the following chapter. Furthermore, these simple methods provide readily comprehensible indices of tremor severity, which is perhaps their most significant advantage over physiological techniques. Clinical instruments presently exist for documenting tremor impairment as well as its impact on the patient in terms of disability, handicap, quality of life and suffering (Table 28.1).

Subjective Clinical Measures

Tremor Rating Scales

A variety of tremor rating scale designs have been used in clinical trials for documenting changes in tremor magnitude. However, there has been little discussion about the relative merits of each design and the composition of these scales has differed considerably from trial to trial. Nevertheless certain principles should influence tremor rating scale design:

1. The severity of tremor should be related to the parts of the body that are affected.
2. The scores for each anatomical site should be kept separate and not amalgamated or averaged, because tremors affecting different body parts may respond differently to treatment.
3. The scale should score tremor magnitude separately for different tremor components (rest, postural, kinetic tremor, etc.), as these components will have different influences on the resultant disability and handicap.

4. An analogue scale has mathematical/statistical advantages over one that is based on discrete steps.
5. The number of steps within a discrete-step scale should be optimised, because the number of gradations on the scale influences reliability. Scales with few gradations (for example a 0–3 scale) are more easily scored than those with a greater number of increments (for example a 0–10 scale). However, increasing the number of steps also decreases the significance of a "unit" error, so that true score variance is altered advantageously for reliability [1–3].

Presently there is only one tremor-specific rating scale that incorporates these design features (Appendix A) [3]. This scale was designed by Bain and colleagues and was chosen after experimenting with various alternative designs because raters found it easy to use. It is an analogue (0–10) tremor impairment scale in which the magnitudes of the various tremor components are scored separately for each limb and, if appropriate, other body parts. The scale includes a supplementary mild–moderate–severe framework to facilitate scoring. It has been tested for validity and inter- and intra-rater reliability, using Cohen's kappa coefficients [3–5]. The results of these evaluations showed that the tremor scores ascribed by raters employing this scale correlated well with patient self-assessments of their own tremor-related disability and that the reliability of the scoring was good [3]. The degree of agreement between raters' scores was found to be in the moderate to almost perfect range for postural tremor of the upper limbs and head tremor [3].

One other tremor-specific rating scale, produced by Fahn, Tolosa and Marin, has been evaluated for reliability [6]. It is a complex multimodal scale that includes ratings of tremor impairment (on a discrete 5-point scale) as well as tremor-induced disability and handicap [6]. It is divided into three subsections that reflect (a) tremor impairment (intrinsically

Table 28.1. Clinical methods for assessing tremor severity

Objective functional performance tests
Water spilt from a cup
Nine-hole pegboard test
Gibson maze

Subjective clinical measures
Clinical rating scales of tremor
Rating tremor in spirals or handwriting

Impact of tremor on patients' lives
Disability scales
Handicap questionnaire
Quality of life
Overall burden of illness (suffering)

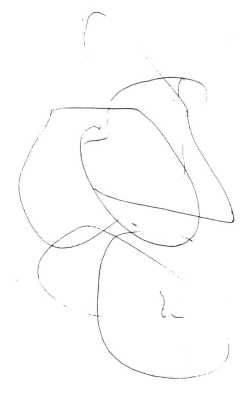

Fig. 28.1. An attempt by a patient with multiple sclerosis at drawing a spiral, illustrating the marked upper limb movement disruption that can occur in this condition. It is difficult to know from the spiral whether the patient had severe tremor, other ataxic features or a combination of the two; this makes the spiral hard to score on a 0–10 tremor scale.

weighted for upper limb tremor), (b) functional tasks (writing, drawing and pouring water) and (c) disability and handicap (Appendix B). However, this scale saturates at tremor amplitudes of greater than 2 cm and thus is unsuitable for studies involving patients with severe tremor, for example the hyperkinetic type of tremor evident in multiple sclerosis or Holmes's (rubral) tremor. This ceiling effect is much less of a problem in the scale designed by Bain and colleagues [3].

Spirography and Handwriting Analysis

It is a simple matter in routine clinical practice to obtain specimens of handwriting and spirals from tremulous patients. Therefore it would be convenient if the tremor apparent in a spiral or piece of handwriting could be scored reliably, particularly if the score correlated with tremor-invoked disability. Fortunately, this is the case for tremor caused by essential tremor or that associated with dystonia [3,5]. Typically, tremulous patients are instructed to draw a spiral (from inside to out) with each hand in turn with the pen held in a normal way, rather than at the top, this being an important technical point because spirography is rather over-sensitive to fine tremors even when the pen is held normally [4,5].

The tremor visible in a spiral can then be scored independently by blinded raters using a 0–10 subjective scoring system [3–5]. The inter- and intra-rater reliability of this method of scoring essential and dystonic tremor in spirals has been shown to be good [3]. Furthermore, the spiral scores correlated with those obtained with a tremor rating scale, patient self-assessments of tremor-induced disability and the magnitude of upper limb tremor measured by uni-axial accelerometers [3]. The system for scoring spirals can be refined by refering to a published col-

lection of previously graded tremulous spirals whilst scoring each spiral [4].

There is no advantage in rating tremor in writing rather than spirals, which raters find easier to score [3,4]. However, handwriting specimens can often be obtained retrospectively (e.g. old letters or school work), which may be particularly useful in confirming the patient's age at tremor onset, for example when looking for objective evidence of anticipation in a genetic study.

The main disadvantages with spirography are firstly that some patients with severe action tremor may be unable to put pen to paper, making it impossible to score spirals or handwriting, and secondly that it can be difficult for the rater to distinguish the effects of tremor from other ataxic movements in a spiral, which makes scoring problematic. This problem is exemplified in the spirals drawn by some patients with multiple sclerosis (Fig. 28.1). It should also be noted that passive transmission of tremor from other parts of the body (for example head or trunk) may disrupt handwriting or spiral specimens.

Objective Functional Performance Tests

The most commonly deployed objective functional performance tests used for assessing tremor are the volumetric method, maze test and the nine-hole pegboard test. All these methods provide objective measures of impaired upper limb function (focal disability).

Volumetric Method

There are two variants of the volumetric method: (a) pouring water from one cup to another (a bimanual kinetic tremor test) [6] or (b) simply holding a full cup of water for 1 min (which tests for unilateral postural tremor) [4,5,7] . In the latter version of this test the patients are asked to hold a 100 ml plastic beaker full of water between the thumb and fingers with the elbow supported and flexed by about 20°, with the forearm in a semi-prone position and slightly elevated, as though about to raise the cup to drink. The volume of water remaining in the beaker after 1 min is measured. The assessment is usually carried out three times for each hand and the means for each hand recorded [4]. The volumetric method allows start-up time (the time from the start of the test to first spilling water) to be measured, which provides insight into the patient's ability to suppress their tremor in the temporal domain (a characteristic of parkinsonian tremor) [5]. Furthermore, the method has been validated for patients with essential tremor as the data obtained by this method correlated with those obtained by rating spirals and accelerometry [5]. However, the volumetric method is insensitive to fine tremors and there is a ceiling effect that appears when all the water is spilt [4,5,7]. Other practical disadvantages are that it can be quite messy when applied to patients with severe tremor and it is sensitive to other impairments, for example myoclonic jerks.

The Nine-Hole Pegboard Test

The nine-hole pegboard test is a reliable test of upper limb function (focal disability). The results can be recorded as the time taken to insert all the pegs or the time taken to place each peg into a hole, the latter being preferable. Normal controls average about 2 seconds to place each peg [8]. It is particularly useful for documenting the impact on arm function of mild to moderate action tremors. However, the results are influenced by factors other than tremor and patients with severe action tremor may be unable to pick up or place a single peg.

The Gibson Maze Test

The Gibson maze test, which is a form of quantifiable spiral, has been used widely in clinical trials to quantify tremor [9,10]. The patient is instructed to draw a line through a printed spiral maze, starting at the arrow in the centre and aiming to get out via the maze's pathway without touching the spiral's printed boundaries or circular obstacles. The number of times a patient's drawn line touches these obstructions is counted, which gives the test its objectivity. However, like the peg-board test and volumetric method it is useless for patients with severe action tremors or marked hand weakness and like the other measures of focal disability is sensitive to other movement disorders as well as tremor.

Assessing the Impact of Tremor on Patients' Lives

The impact of tremor on patients' lives can be assessed in a variety of ways, including measures of disability, handicap, quality of life or burden of illness (Table 28.1). Although these entities do not measure tremor magnitude directly, from a clinical perspective the effect of tremor on patients' lives is ultimately more important. Furthermore, the patients' views on changes in their own state of health are likely to be highly influential on whether or not they comply with therapy. Nevertheless a generic problem with this type of assessment is that all the tests are affected by concurrent symptoms or illness. In addition the distinction between measures of disability, handicap and quality of life are not clear-cut. Conventionally, disability is the difficulty that a patient encounters in performing their daily living activities (the loss of function caused by an impairment) and can be quantified using either generic or disease-specific disability questionnaires, the latter tending to be more sensitive to their target condition.

Disability Questionnaires

Finding practical ways of assessing tremor severity which relate to disability is a major problem in trial design, because otherwise the measure becomes an abstraction and of no practical importance to patients. The most direct method of ascertaining whether or not a specific treatment has helped a patient is the use of a disability questionnaire. However, the reliability of this type of questionnaire depends on patients being able to give an accurate account of their own physical disability; this is usually the case provided no concurrent mental illness is present [11].

Comparison of activity of daily living questionnaires designed specifically for tremulous patients reveals that the main conundrum inherent in this method of assessment is what items should be incorporated within the questionnaire [3,4,6]. In particular, is any specific item a good indicator of tremulous patients' overall disability or are several items required to assess this? Is utilisation of all the item (elemental) scores and their addition to give a "total" score appropriate? Does the utilisation of a scale having several interrelated items increase the reliability of the overall score? What proportions of the questionnaire should reflect dominant hand function, bimanual function, toiletting, mobility or other disabilities and how should these be relatively weighted? Thus the main practical problem for the tremor expert is to provide patients with a questionnaire that is readily understood, and which can be transcribed into numerical values for statistical analysis. There have been two attempts to achieve this aim: one of these is a tremor-specific disability self-questionnaire shown in Appendix C and the other comprises section C of the Fahn, Tolosa and Marin scale (see Appendix B) [6].

Handicap

Handicap, which is the social and societal consequences of having a specific set of disabilities, can also be quantified and, as far as the patient is concerned, determines the real severity of a tremor, as patients can have significant handicap in spite of relatively minor disability – a not infrequent occurrence in clinical practice. Only one handicap instrument has been specifically developed for the study of tremulous patients. It is largely qualitative and was used in a study of hereditary essential tremor to explore whether or not patients thought that they were handicapped by the physical disability or embarrassment caused by their tremor (see Appendix D) [3,4,12].

Quality of Life Measures

Whether or not quality of life is a different entity to disability or handicap is a matter of debate. There does not appear to be a unifying concept underlying the most commonly deployed quality of life instruments, which include categorically different components [13]. However, it would be reasonable to propose that the term quality of life is used to represent the patients' subjective impressions of their own state of affairs whilst handicap could be considered as the objective or externally assessed social consequences of an illness. Thus quality of life would differ meaningfully from handicap because of the influence of the patients' internal personality domains. If this definition were to be generally accepted it would exclude most of the presently available quality of life instruments, which firstly impose the designer's sense of values onto patients (i.e. measure handicap) and secondly include items that address disability. However, there is one instrument (SEIQoL-DW) which allows patients to choose their own assessment domains and apportion weight to them according to their own sense of perspective [14].

Burden of Suffering

There is one interesting instrument (the pictorial representation of illness and self-measure: PRISM which has recently been developed for quantifying the total burden of suffering caused by an illness, although it has not yet been used to evaluate tremulous patients in the setting of a formal clinical trial [15]. In the PRISM task the patient is asked to imagine that a small board represents his or her life and a fixed disc on an A4-sized board represents his or her self. The task consists of placing another disc (representing the illness) on the board to reflect the current importance of the illness in the patient's life. The main outcome measure is simply the distance between the self and illness discs, which tends to be shorter when the burden of suffering is greater.

The Detractor Effect

A comprehensive review of the published data on controlled therapeutic trials involving patients with essential tremor showed that the effect of medication (including primidone and propranolol) on tremor may have been overestimated, as a 50% reduction in acceleration did not appear to translate into a similar alleviation of disability or handicap [16]. Furthermore, there was a progressive decline in the apparent benefit produced by anti-essential tremor medications when the benefit was measured in terms of handicap, disability or functional performance tests compared with electrophysiological parameters or clinical ratings of impairment [16]. This fall off in efficacy as the measurement instrument becomes more realistic was termed a "detractor" effect, a term that describes the relationships between an impairment (tremor) and the objective disability or handicap that it produces [16]. A detractor may have complex shape depending on the precise behavioural characteristics of the specific tremor involved. In order to understand the impact of tremor upon patients more fully the shapes of the detractors pertaining to each type of tremor require further study. In the meantime clinical trials that use multi-dimensional evaluations are to be strongly commended.

Conclusion

Tremors are highly complex phenomena that vary continuously with the state of activity of the patients. The parameters of tremor alter from beat to beat and from minute to minute, making assessment of severity extremely difficult. However, some method of quantifying tremor severity is necessary if the natural histories of tremors are to be understood and the influence of drugs comprehended. There are advantages and disadvantages to each of the techniques commonly employed and there is no single ubiquitous solution. It is now possible to measure tremor and its impact on the patient in a multi-dimensional way that includes electrophysiological techniques, clinical rating scales, simple objective tests of limb function, and measures of disability, handicap, quality of life and total burden of illness.

Patient disability self-questionnaires provide the most meaningful results in terms of deciding whether or not a particular treatment has actually helped tremulous patients with their activities of daily living, although handicap is perhaps the most important measure from the patient's perspective. In spite of the importance of these measures a great deal of further research is required to produce optimal disability and handicap questionnaires for tremulous patients. Similarly the design of tremor rating scales needs further scrutiny and the scales carefully evaluated for intra- and inter-rater reliability prior to their use in clinical trials. The advantage of these simple measures over physiological techniques is that statistically significant changes are likely to be meaningful and real.

Selection of an optimal physiological technique to accompany the simple clinical methods of measuring tremor magnitude depends critically on the type of tremor being assessed: Accelerometry is a reasonable way of quantifying essential tremor or similar-magnitude postural tremors but would be inappropriate for the intention or hyperkinetic tremors associated with multiple sclerosis, which [providing that displacement is less than 30 cm] would be better captured with a motion analysis system, such as the Polhemus device [17]. Long-term electromyography (EMG) techniques may be a useful way of quantifying tremor in parkinsonian patients [18–20], whilst primary orthostatic tremor and primary writing tremor are probably best quantified

by systems based on EMG and digitising tablets respectively [21–23].

The presence of the detractor effect in therapeutic trials means that simple clinical assessment methods (including estimates of tremor severity, functional performance tests and tremor-dependent disability) should always support electrophysiologically derived data because the latter may lead to an overestimate of the actual benefit of treatment for patients, providing a distorted impression of the effect of an intervention.

Appendices

Appendix A. The Tremor-Specific Rating Scale Designed by Bain and Colleagues [3]

The scale has been assessed for reliability and validity.

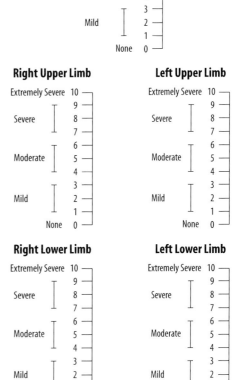

Appendix B. The Tremor Severity Scale Designed by Fahn, Tolosa and Marin [6]

The scale has been assessed for reliability and validity.

Items 1–21 are all scored on a 0–4 scale [6]. The maximum possible score is 144.

Part A. Tremor Impairment

Tremor of	Rest	Posture	Act/Int	Total
1 Face				
2 Tongue				
3 Voice				
4 Head				
5 R arm				
6 L arm				
7 Trunk				
8 R leg				
9 L leg				
Subtotal A				

Part B. Handwriting, Drawing and Pouring

Handwriting:
10 A dated sample of the patient's best handwriting.
Drawings:
11–12 Draw a spiral on the paper provided, without crossing the lines, with the right and then left hand.
13 Draw 3 straight lines on the paper provided, without crossing the lines, with the right and then left hand.
Pouring:
14 Pour water from one cup to another.

	Right	Left	Total
10 Handwriting		dominant only	
11 Drawing A			
12 Drawing B			
13 Drawing C			
14 Pouring			
Subtotal B			

Part C. Functional Disabilities due to Tremor

15 Speaking	
16 Eating	
17 Drinking	
18 Hygiene	
19 Dressing	
20 Writing	
21 Working	
Subtotal C	

Global Assessment by Examiner

0: no functional disability
1: mild disability (1–24% impaired)
2: moderate disability (25–49% impaired)
3: marked disability (50–74% impaired)
4: severe disability (75–100% impaired)

Global Assessment by Patient

0: no functional disability
1: mild disability (1–24% impaired)
2: moderate disability (25–49% impaired)
3: marked disability (50–74% impaired)
4: severe disability (75–100% impaired)

Subjective Assessment by Patient Compared with Last Visit

+3: marked improvement (50–100% improved)
+2: moderate improvement (25–49% improved)
+1: mild improvement (10–24% improved)
0: unchanged
−1: mild worsening (10–24% worse)
−2: moderate to marked worsening (25–49% worse)
−3: marked worsening (50–100% worse)

Appendix C. Activities of Daily Living Questionnaire

The patient is asked to put a circle around the number (from 0 to 3) that most appropriately reflects the degree of difficulty encountered with each task:

Key: 0 Able to do the activity without difficulty
      1 Able to do the activity with a little effort
      2 Able to do the activity with a lot of effort
      3 Cannot do the activity by yourself

Disability Questionnaire

1 Cut food with a knife and fork	0	1	2	3
2 Use a spoon to drink soup	0	1	2	3
3 Hold a cup of tea	0	1	2	3
4 Pour milk from a bottle or carton	0	1	2	3
5 Wash and dry dishes	0	1	2	3
6 Brush your teeth	0	1	2	3
7 Use a handkerchief to blow your nose	0	1	2	3
8 Take a bath	0	1	2	3
9 Use the lavatory	0	1	2	3
10 Wash your face and hands	0	1	2	3
11 Tie your shoelaces	0	1	2	3
12 Do up buttons	0	1	2	3
13 Do up a zip	0	1	2	3
14 Write a letter	0	1	2	3

15	Put a letter in an envelope	0	1 2 3
16	Hold and read a newspaper	0	1 2 3
17	Dial a telephone	0	1 2 3
18	Make yourself understood on the telephone	0	1 2 3
19	Watch a television	0	1 2 3
20	Pick up your change in a shop	0	1 2 3
21	Insert an electric plug into a socket	0	1 2 3
22	Unlock your front door with the key	0	1 2 3
23	Walk up and down stairs	0	1 2 3
24	Get up out of an armchair	0	1 2 3
25	Carry a full shopping bag	0	1 2 3

Appendix D. Assessment of Tremor-related Handicap

The patient is asked to answer the following questions by putting a circle around the appropriate letter: A, B, C or D

Has your tremor stopped you:

1	Working?	A B C D
2	Applying for a job or promotion?	A B C D
3	Shopping by yourself?	A B C D
4	Doing your favourite hobby or sport?	A B C D
5	Travelling by public transport?	A B C D
6	Driving a car?	A B C D
7	Eating out?	A B C D
8	Going on holiday?	A B C D
9	Accepting a party invitation?	A B C D

Key:
A *No*
B *Yes*, because you are *embarrassed* by the tremor
C *Yes*, because of the *physical difficulties* produced by the tremor
D *Yes*, because of BOTH the *physical difficulties* and the *embarrassment* produced by tremor

References

1. Landy FJ, Farr JL. Performance rating. Psychol Bull 1980; 87:72–107.
2. Nunnally JC. Psychometric theory. New York: McGraw-Hill, 1978: chap 15.
3. Bain PG, Findley LJ, Atchison P, Behari M, Vidailhet M, Gresty MA, et al. Assessing tremor severity. J Neurol Neurosurg Psychiatry 1993;56:868–873.
4. Bain PG, Findley LJ. Assessing tremor severity. London: Smith-Gordon, 1993.
5. Bain PG, Mally J, Gresty MA, Findley LJ. Assessing the impact of essential tremor on upper limb function. J Neurol 1993;241: 54–61.
6. Fahn S, Tolosa E, Marin C. Clinical rating scale for tremor. In: Jankovic J, Tolosa E, editors. Parkinson's disease and movement disorders. Baltimore: Urban & Schwarzenberg, 1988: 225–234.
7. Mally J. Aminophylline and essential tremor. Lancet 1989;II: 279–279.
8. Wade DT. Measurement in neurological rehabilitation. Oxford: Oxford University Press, 1992:171.
9. Gibson HB. The spiral maze: a psychomotor test with implications for the study of delinquency. Br J Psychol 1964;55: 219–225.
10. Morgan MH, Langton-Hewer R, Cooper R. Effect of beta adrenergic blocking agent propranolol on essential tremor. J Neurol Neurosurg Psychiatry 1973;36:618–624.
11. Brown RG, MacCarthy B, Jahanshahi M, Marsden CD. Accuracy of self-reported disability in patients with parkinsonism. Arch Neurol 1989;46:955–959.
12. Bain PG, Findley LJ, Thompson PD, Gresty MA, Rothwell JC, Harding AE, et al. A study of hereditary essential tremor. Brain 1994;117:805–824.
13. Wade DT. Measurement in neurological rehabilitation. Oxford: Oxford University Press, 1992:89–96.
14. O'Boyle CA, Browne JP, McGee HM, Hickey A, Joyce CRB. Manual for the SEIQoL-DW. Dublin: Department of Psychology, Royal College of Surgeons of Ireland, 1996.
15. Buchi S, Sensky T, Sharpe L, Timberlake N. Graphic representation of illness: a novel method of measuring patients' perceptions of the impact of illness. Psychother Psychometrics 1998, in press.
16. Bain PG. The effectiveness of treatments for essential tremor. Neurologist 1997;3:305–321.
17. Spyers-Ashby JM, Stokes MJ, Bain PG, Roberts SJ. Classification of normal and pathological tremors wing a multidimensional electromagnetic system. Medical Engineering and Physics 1999;21:713–723.
18. Spieker S, Loschmann P, Jentgens C, Boose A, Klockgether T, Dichgans J. Tremorlytic activity of budipine: a quantitative study with long-term tremor recordings. Clin Neuropharmacol 1995;18:266–272.
19. Spieker S, Jentgens C, Boose A, Dichgans J. Reliability, specificity, and sensitivity of long-term tremor recordings. Electroencephalogr Clin Neurophysiol 1995;97:326–331.
20. Spieker S, Strole V, Sailer A, Boose A, Dichgans J. Validity of long term tremor electromyography in the quantification of tremor. Mov Disord 1997;12:985–991.
21. Bain PG. A combined clinical and neurophysiological approach to the study of patients with tremor. J Neurol Neurosurg Psychiatry 1993;56:839–844.
22. Elble RJ, Sinha R, Higgins C. Quantification of tremor with a digitizing tablet. J Neurosci Methods 1990;32:193–198.
23. Elble RJ, Brilliant M, Leffler K, Higgins C. Quantification of essential tremor in writing and drawing. Mov Disord 1996; 11:70–78.

29. Tremor: Natural Behaviour, Trial Design and Physiological Outcome Measures

S.H. Alusi and P.G. Bain

Tremor

General Considerations

For the purposes of neurological practice tremor is defined as an involuntary rhythmical, oscillatory movement of a body part [1]. Pathological tremors are involuntary with the possible exception of "psychogenic" tremor, in which the pathophysiological mechanisms are poorly understood [1,2]. Healthy people also have an involuntary low-amplitude physiological tremor and can voluntarily mimic large-magnitude tremors [1,3].

Tremors have been classified on an aetiological basis, by the state of activity of the tremulous body part and by the anatomical site of the causative lesion [1,4]. In the light of our present knowledge these different classification systems are in many ways both useful and complementary but have also led to confusion, and should be regarded as metaphors. Nevertheless it is necessary to adopt a common language, albeit an imperfect one, before the complexities of measuring tremors can be discussed. Consequently, we have used the terminology agreed upon in a consensus statement on tremor issued by the Movement Disorder Society (Table 29.1) [1].

Natural Tremor Fluctuation

Before discussing the intricacies of clinical trial design and the methodologies involved in assessing tremor it is useful to reflect upon the natural behaviour of unmodified pathological tremors. How do pathological tremors behave?

Firstly all pathological tremors have characteristic triggers which switch them on or off. Neurologists will be familiar with the way in which parkinsonian rest tremor comes and goes during the physical examination. Thus it is routine practice to utilise various manoeuvres to bring out rest tremor, for example by asking the patient to count down. Furthermore, tremor typically comes and goes during on/off fluctuations in the latter stages of Parkinson's disease, making quantitative studies of tremor magnitude difficult and critically dependent on the timing of medication. Certain types of tremor have very specific triggering factors, for example type A primary writing tremor is induced by the act of writing and drawing, although an attenuated tremor may be present during other fine manual tasks. Similarly, position-specific tremors may occur only when the affected limb adopts critical positions [5].

Secondly, all pathological tremors have natural amplitude and, to a lesser degree, frequency fluctuations. Beat-to-beat amplitude fluctuations are apparent in drawings of Archimedes spirals (Fig. 29.1) as well as in electromyogram (EMG) burst parameters (Fig. 29.2) [6]. In formal accelerometric test–retest studies of untreated essential tremor the amplitude varied by up to 50%, in spite of careful standardisation of the recording conditions [7]. Similarly the amplitude of other forms of tremor can vary rapidly depending on the precise circumstances. For example, in some patients with advanced multiple sclerosis the severe upper limb action tremor can be greatly influenced by certain factors, such as the precise position of the patient's shoulder (S.H. Alusi and J. Worthington, unpublished observation) and visual cues [8]. In essential tremor the frequency and amplitude characteristics have been demonstrated to change with different tasks [9,10]. Thirdly, the characteristics of tremors are influenced by a variety of complex factors including the experimental environment, the patient's physical, emotional and mental state as well as its natural perturbations. [2,11,12].

Sampling Tremor

The variability of tremor behaviour causes a problem for those wishing to measure tremor. This difficulty becomes acute when it is necessary to know whether

Table 29.1. Phenomenological classification of tremor

Tremor envelope: the profile of the visible tremor amplitude during movement, for example the finger–nose–finger test

Rest tremor: tremor which occurs in a body part that is not voluntarily activated and that is completely supported against gravity

Action tremor: any tremor that is produced by voluntary contraction of muscle. This includes postural, kinetic, intention, isometric and task-specific tremor

Postural tremor: tremor apparent whilst voluntarily maintaining a position against gravity

Kinetic tremor: tremor occurring during any type of movement

Simple kinetic tremor: tremor occurring during voluntary movements that are not target-directed

Intention tremor (tremor during target-directed movement): is present when:
(i) tremor amplitude increases during visually guided movements towards a target at the termination of a movement
(ii) the possibility of a position-specific tremor or postural tremor arising at the beginning and end of movement has been excluded

Task-specific kinetic tremor: kinetic tremor that appears or is exacerbated during specific activities

Isometric tremor: tremor occurring as the result of muscle contraction against a rigid stationary object

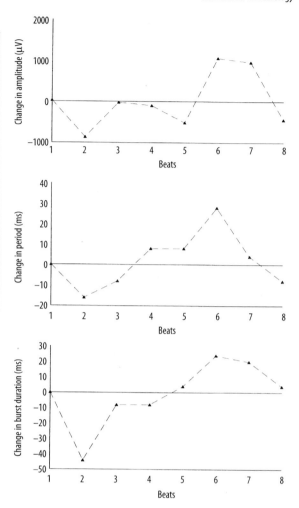

Fig. 29.2. Changes in tremor amplitude, period and burst duration in eight consecutive tremor bursts measured from the forearm flexor EMG records of a patient with a 4 Hz parkinsonian tremor.

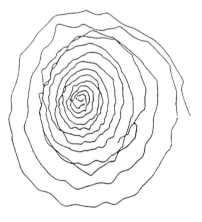

Fig. 29.1. An Archimedes spiral drawn by a patient with essential tremor showing natural fluctuations in tremor magnitude.

or not a change in tremor magnitude is the result merely of a natural fluctuation or of an intervention.

At this point it is worth considering an analogy with meteorology: How can a meteorologist determine whether a change in the weather represents normal variation or climatic change? Could measur-

ing the temperature or another variable at a specific location on two different days *prove* that the climate had changed? The answer is probably not; although an extreme change would provide good circumstantial evidence, if it was out of kilter with previous records of diurnal and seasonal variation. Even then the result may have been caused by a freak of nature. The problem for tremor experts, unlike meteorologists, is that the patterns of the natural magnitude fluctuations of tremors have not received detailed study or documentation. We do not know what governs the long-term behaviour of tremors, which raises the practical issue of how to obtain a representative tremor sample.

There is no rigorous solution to this sampling problem when dealing with tremulous individuals. In practice clinicians compare an observed change in a patient's tremor with their own experience of magnitude fluctuations in similar patients. Unfortunately, this tactic may not be possible for rare or unique tremor types. In these circumstances the patient and their entourage can be a useful resource and may be able to provide evidence from changes in their everyday activities that their tremor has altered significantly, but this information can be obscured by poor-quality observations, simultaneous changes in the non-tremulous aspects of multi-symptomatic diseases such as multiple sclerosis or Parkinson's disease, or coincidental illness.

Clinical Trial Design

The objectives of treatment are to reduce tremor magnitude, improve or restore ability and reduce social handicap whilst minimising unwanted side-effects because, presently, the treatment of tremor is entirely symptomatic. In this regard it is worthwhile reflecting on the shape of the relationships between tremor amplitude and the resultant disability and handicap. Thus the main design requirement for the majority of therapeutic trials involving tremulous patients is to obtain data that allow neurologists to put an evidence-based treatment strategy into practice.

The problems caused by spontaneous temporal fluctuations in tremor magnitude make random allocation of patients within trials a virtual necessity, if bias is to be avoided. A crossover design is advantageous because it increases statistical power, provided the pharmacokinetics of the drugs involved are established and an adequate washout period can be incorporated into the trial. There is also a strong case for including a placebo phase, even when effective treatments presently exist, as it has been demonstrated that the magnitude of untreated (essential) tremor decreases with serial assessments, perhaps because patients become more familiar and thus more relaxed in the test situation [7]. This would inevitably lead to an overestimate of the beneficial effects of trial medications unless the size of this false positive effect can be determined from the placebo phase and then subtracted from the effect of each active treatment [13]. However, a crossover design is inappropriate for treatments aimed at influencing the natural progression of a particular tremor, when randomisation into parrallel treatment/placebo limbs is necessary. Whereas for irreversible surgical interventions, for example thalamotomy or pallidotomy, randomisation of patients to groups with different waiting times allows the short-term impact of the procedures to be assessed, this does introduce another ethical issue for consideration, namely delaying treatment. For surgical treatments with the potential to progressively ameliorate

tremor, for example fetal nigral cell transplantation into the putamen of patients with Parkinson's disease, there are two options: firstly, to randomise patients to either have surgery or not; or secondly, assess the effect of an unilateral procedure by comparing the effect on the contralateral limbs with the ipsilateral limbs over time. However, this paradigm is less rigorous as surgery may cause confounding ipsilateral effects.

Ethics Involved in Trial Design

It is now widely accepted that in order to reduce the chances of producing misleading results, randomised double-blind controlled studies are necessary. New and many old putative symptomatic treatments for tremor should be carefully assessed in formal trials to: (i) protect patients from being prescribed ineffective drugs; (ii) provide reasonable estimates of what proportion of patients respond to a specific drug; (iii) determine to what extent symptomatic relief is obtained; and (iv) provide an estimate of the incidence and severity of common drug-related side-effects, although rare complications are unlikely to be identified.

Furthermore, socio-economic pressures reasonably demand that resources are not wasted on ineffective treatments or inappropriate trials. Thus the organisers of a tremor study ought to have: (i) carefully considered the present data on the relevant treatment and tremor; (ii) decided on the optimum study design/paradigm; (iii) consulted a statistician and if possible derived a power estimation before deciding the number of patients required for the study; (iv) measured the relevant tremor in an optimal way; and (v) obtained approval from the appropriate ethics committee.

Statistical Analysis

There is undoubtedly a conflict between a desire for statistical purity and a wish for obtaining as much useful clinical information as possible from a study. Statisticians prefer one outcome variable and are sceptical of data that include multidimensional evaluations that produce a series of interrelated variables with often complex and poorly understood relationships. Conversely, neurologists want to obtain as much clinical information as possible from a trial and want the "whole" picture, finding reassurance when the trend in several outcome variables is in a similar direction. There is thus a genuine culture difference between the statistician and clinician. Nevertheless statistical analysis of the data from a double-blind randomised crossover trial comparing one medical intervention with either another treatment or placebo is appropriately conducted using, for example, the Wilcoxon signed rank sum test for paired samples of data. An alternative would be the sign test, which is particularly useful if it is only known whether the patients improved, worsened or remained the same after an intervention and no quantitative data are available. The Wilcoxon signed rank sum test is a more powerful statistic than the sign test, as the former uses the magnitudes as well as the signs of the differences, and thus is the preferred method when tremor magnitudes have been measured. Both these statistical methods are distribution-free (non-parametric) tests, which make them less efficient than the corresponding standard (parametric) tests and means that for any given level of significance (e.g. $p = 0.05$) there is a greater chance of producing a type II error, namely being misled into thinking that there is no difference between two anti-tremor treatments (as beta would be greater for a non-parametric compared with a parametric test).

In studies involving surgical procedures, in which patients have been randomised to receive surgery at different post-randomisation times, it is more appropriate to use the rank sum test. The same applies to treatments that are not only symptomatic but may also influence the natural progression of tremor (for example neuroprotective drugs or cell transplantation). Again the use of a distribution-free statistic has the advantage of being more likely than an equivalent standard test to give a conservative significance level, but this has the disadvantage of also increasing the chance of making a type II error. When sequential measurements are made it is usual to present the data as an area under the curve (variable versus time) so as to avoid making multiple statistical comparisons.

Interpretation of Trial Results

Firstly, when looking at clinical-trial evidence it is useful to consider whether bias was excluded by an adequate trial design and whether the results were significant from both a statistical and a clinical perspective. Clearly statistical significance does not necessarily correlate with clinical benefit, which ultimately means improvement in patients' functional abilities and reduced social handicap. Thus, it is useful to conceptually divide the data presented in therapeutic tremor trials into six categories: (i) statistical significance; (ii) electro-physiological indices of tremor magnitude (for example accelerometeric or EMG data); (iii) impairment (i.e. tremor severity as measured by clinical rating scales, rating spiral drawings or handwriting), (iv) objective functional performance-test measurements (e.g. 9-hole pegboard test, or the amount of water spilt from a cup);

(v) disability; and (vi) social handicap. It is also necessary to be aware of other methodological issues such as the precise dosage and method of drug administration and the timing of the measurements, which all influence the results and need careful scrutiny.

One important point about the presentation of "percentage improvements" is worth careful consideration, namely that the same percentage improvements may mean quite different absolute improvements. For example, two patients (A and B) with Parkinson's disease may score 12 and then 6 (A) and 36 and then 18 (B) before and after pallidotomy in the motor examination subsection of the Unified Parkinson's Disease Rating Scale (UPDRS) (possible subscale score range: 0–56 with higher scores indicating a worse state) [14]. Each patient has improved by 50% relative to self but the absolute change is 3 times greater for patient B compared with patient A. This problem can be overcome by dividing the absolute change for each patient by the total scale range (in this case 56) before summing the results. Unfortunately, this is not customarily done and usually the individual percentage changes are summed to give an average.

Evaluation of Outcome Measures

Ideally the outcome measures deployed in a study should have been previously assessed for reliability, validity and responsiveness [15]. Reliability estimates the capacity of an instrument to measure tremor in an accurate, reproducible and consistent way. Validity, in this context, considers whether an instrument actually reflects tremor; whilst responsiveness determines whether the instrument is sensitive to clinically important changes in tremor severity.

Reliability

It is useful to know the reliability of the measurement techniques involved in a study prior to the start because this information will influence the number of patients required to show a specific size of therapeutic effect. It might also suggest to the trial organisers that specific raters are replaced or rating systems changed to more reliable ones. Reliability is not a single entity and can be usefully subcategorised into the following:

1. *Internal consistency*, which is the extent to which the items in a scale measure the same concept (a measure of the scale's homogeneity). This can be assessed by either Cronbach's alpha or Kuder-Richardson 20 statistic depending on whether the measurement scale is respectively continuous or dichotomous [16,17].

Table 29.2. Conventional interpretation of kappa scores

Kappa coefficent	Strength of agreement
<0	Poor
0–0.20	Slight
0.21–0.40	Fair
0.41–0.60	Moderate
0.61–0.80	Substantial
0.81–1.00	Almost perfect

Table 29.3. Physiological techniques for measuring tremor

Accelerometry
Displacement transducers
Electromyography (short or long term)
Mechanically coupled systems
Kinematic measurement systems
Gyroscopic techniques
Computer tracking tasks
Graphic digitising tablets

2. *Test–retest reliability*, which reflects the temporal stability of the measuring instrument and is documented by giving the measure to the same group of tremulous patients at two different times.

3. *Rater reliability*, which is divisible into intra-rater reliability (error between two separate measurements of the same tremor by a single observer) and inter-rater reliability (strength of agreement between two different observers' ratings). Both forms of rater reliability can be quantified by examining either the correlation between ratings or, respectively for continuous and dichomotous scales, the intra-class correlation coefficient or Cohen's kappa statistic [17–21]. The latter is widely acknowledged as being suitable for assessing reliability because it is distribution-free, allows credit for partial agreement between raters and corrects for agreement due to chance. It also makes use of individual items in the rating scale and corrects for differences in the raters' mean scores (Table 29.2) [20].

By allowing only one observer to make measurements in a trial the errors caused by inter-rater variation can be eliminated, which is advantageous but difficult to achieve in multi-centre studies.

Validity

Validity concerns the relationship between the concept measured (tremor) and the instrument used to assess it [22–25]. Validity (see also Chapter 2) is divisible into:

1. *Content validity*, which is the extent to which a measure is representative of the conceptual domain that it is intended to cover. This is established by putting the measure into the context of present knowledge and is not measured statistically.

2. *Criterion related validity*, namely the degree to which a measure of tremor correlates with the gold standard. However, as will become evident, there is no gold standard for measuring tremor.

3. *Construct validity*, which is the process used to establish the validity of a measurement instrument

by testing it against other measures of tremor. It examines whether an instrument (a) measures tremor, (b) does not measure something else, for example dysmetria or myoclonic jerks, (c) is able to distinguish between different tremors, and (d) produces results in line with present knowledge.

Responsiveness

In order to obtain meaningful results the instruments involved in a study must be responsive to changes in tremor severity. The responsiveness of the instruments can be determined by serial assessments of tremor over an epoch in which tremor severity is known to change. However, the responsiveness required varies considerably depending on the type of tremor and the nature of the intervention. Thus a study of diurnal changes in physiological tremor would need highly responsive electrophysiological instrumentation, whilst assessment of the effect of thalamotomy on essential tremor does not.

Measuring Tremor Severity

Tremors can be measured objectively by physiological techniques or by simple tests of the tremor's impact on function, or subjectively using clinical rating scales. Table 29.3 shows the main physiological techniques for assessing tremor severity. In addition the impact of tremor on patients in terms of disability or handicap or the effects on patients' quality of life can be quantified. In practice most tremor studies have relied heavily on accelerometry as the objective method of measurement [13,26]. This emphasis on accelerometry is reflected in Table 29.4, which shows the breakdown by measurement technique of the results of randomised controlled trials involving primidone administration to patients with essential tremor [27–33]. However, as the purpose of a clinical trial is to determine whether or not a particular anti-tremor therapy helps patients, it is vital that the outcome measures relate to

Table 29.4. Essential tremor: randomised controlled studies of primidone

Studies of primidone	No. of patients	Dosage (mg/day)	Statistical significance	Accelerometry	Impairment clinical scales	Performance tests	Disability
Findley et al. [27]	22	750	$p < 0.01$	56%	28%	24%	NA
Gorman et al. [28]	14	750	$p < 0.02$	76%	NA	NA	NA
Koller et al. [29]	12	250	$p < 0.01$	55%	NQ	0%	0%
Findley [30]	18	750	$p < 0.01$	56%	NA	NA	NA
Dietrichson and Espen [31]	13	750	$p < 0.001$	NP	NA	NA	NA
Sasso et al. [32]	13	750	$p < 0.05$	NA	16%	9%	NA
Sasso et al. [33]	15	750	$p < 0.01$	34%	NA	NA	NA

NA, not assessed; NP, not published.

disability. Otherwise, the measurements become abstractions and of no practical importance. Consequently, the validity of the results of a *therapeutic* trial depends upon the outcome measure relating, in a meaningful way, to changes in the patients' daily lives.

Physiological Outcome Measures

Accelerometry

Tremors can be quantified in terms of the frequency and magnitude of the oscillatory cycles. These parameters are usually measured using linear accelerometers, which are small piezo-resistive electronic devices that can be attached to the body. It requires at least six one-dimensional transducers to measure all the translational and rotational movement components of a limb [34,35]. Nevertheless because human tremors have higher frequency and lower amplitude characteristics than voluntary limb movements, linear accelerometers are the most widely deployed transducers for measuring tremor. Accelerometers are preferable to displacement and velocity transducers because they are more sensitive to higher-frequency vibrations and introduce less noise (which is amplified by differentiation of velocity or displacement signals) [36]. The accelerometers used in clinical practice are either uni-axial or tri-axial, the latter being preferable [37,38]. Typically their sensitivity is of the order of 0.5–5 mV/ms² with flat frequency responses from DC to >100 Hz [4,5,9,26]. Although an instantaneous output can be displayed it is customary to process the signal to produce an average of several (about 5–10) overlapping spectra derived from overlapping samples of tremor within a 1 min period which display the root mean square (rms) magnitude of frequency components as a function of frequency (Fig. 29.3) [5,8,9]. Typically the spectra

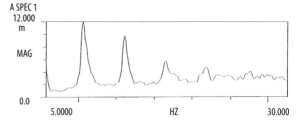

Fig. 29.3. Autospectra obtained by accelerometry from a patient with primary writing tremor, showing frequency (Hz) plotted against rms acceleration ($g \times 10^{-3}$). The accelerometer was attached to the dorsum of the patient's right hand and the record obtained during tremulous writing. The trace shows a dominant peak at a frequency of 5.6 Hz, accompanied by harmonics at higher frequencies which are multiples of the dominant peak.

range from DC to 50 Hz with 500 lines of spectral resolution and about 100 dB dynamic range. For moderate to severe tremor the averaged spectrum has a single dominant peak and the dominant frequency of the tremor is taken as the frequency of the largest peak. Similarly the magnitude of rms acceleration at the main peak is taken and can be coverted into displacement arithmetically, using the formula:

$$\text{Displacement} = \text{acceleration}/4\pi^2 f^2$$

where f is the frequency of the tremor.

However, some judgement may be necessary in identifying the principal peak, as in some cases there can be several harmonics of comparable size. For mild essential tremor the averaged spectrum typically has significant components at a broad spread of frequencies reflecting its multiple component origins, as is the case for normal physiological tremor [9,39]. In this situation it is preferable to have an estimate of all the frequency components. The total power content of the spectrum should be measured by calculating the sum of the squares of all the frequency components [40]. The spectrum can also be transformed to a velocity spectrum which has a total power content proportional to the kinetic energy dissipated by the tremor ($1/2 \times$ (mass of limb) $\times$ (velocity)^2.

Electromyographic Recordings

Short-Term Recordings

The EMG activity accompanying pathological tremor may be recorded by pairs of silver/silver chloride electrodes arranged over the surface of tremorogenic muscles. Bursts of EMG activity separated by relative quiescence occurs in all types of pathological and enhanced physiological tremor but not in normal low-magnitude physiological tremor [4,39,41,42]. Typically tremor is recorded for about 1 min and the EMG signal is amplified, filtered and, if desired, rectified before the bursts are measured from records stored on paper or computer. The amplitude of the EMG is inversely proportional to the distance between the motor unit and the electrode [43]. The resultant rectified-filtered EMG is proportional to muscle force during static and dynamic muscular contractions and is proportional to the force fluctuations caused by tremor [44–47]. However, the relationships between rectified-filtered EMG, muscle force and movement are significantly non-linear [43,48]. The extent of non-linearity is a function of the muscle type and of the measurement technique [43,48]. Thus the amplitude of the rectified-filtered (demodulated) EMG bursts is only a surrogate measure of tremor amplitude and is a reflection of the number of motor units producing tremor [49]. The signal can also be processed in a similar way to that obtained by accelerometry to produce a spectrum of the magnitude of the frequency components of the EMG against frequency [41].

Long-Term Recordings

A system using a portable cassette recorder coupled to surface EMG electrodes has been developed for obtaining 24 h EMG samples of tremor in patients with essential tremor and Parkinson's disease [49–51]. This technique attempts to overcome the problem of obtaining representative tremor samples. It can be used to measure tremor occurrence rate, which is the proportion of time that rhythmic EMG activity occurs during a specified period, as well as the average EMG magnitude and tremor frequency over a give epoch. Tremor occurrence rate has been shown to correlate with clinical ratings of essential and parkinsonian tremor severity [50–52]. The technique has the considerable merit of assessing patients during their normal activities rather than in an artificial laboratory environment, where patients may (at least initially) be unduly tense and anxious. It also allows diurnal variations of tremor magnitude to be measured.

Mechanical and Optically Based Systems

The earliest systems used for recording human tremor were mechanical and measured displacement with a tambour applied to the tremulous limb. Displacement of the tambour was transmitted through mechanical levers to produce a permanent record of the tremor on a rotating smoked drum [53]. This type of mechanical coupling system was subsequently replaced by optical techniques, which magnified the displacement of light produced by the tremulous finger or hand and recorded it on photographic paper or photosensor [54,55].

The limitations of these techniques to the measurement of rest or postural tremors led to the development of systems for studying kinetic tremor, for example that seen during the finger–nose–finger test. Holmes [56] studied the effect of cerebellar lesions on upper limb movement using a chronophotographic motion analysis system. However, Holmes could only study gross tremor as the resolution of his pioneering system was poor. Subsequent developments have led to systems (e.g. MacReflex) that deploy a minimum of two computer-controlled cameras which can produce real-time digital coordinates of the movement of several infrared or light-emitting diodes on the patient [57]. The best systems are portable and have sampling rates of 50 or 100 Hz, which is well above the required Nyquist folding frequencies for pathological human tremor and is thus sufficient to capture these tremors without aliasing. However, data analysis is time-consuming and presently there is scant experience of these systems in the field of therapeutic tremor studies.

Gyroscopic Techniques

Miniature solid state "gyroscopes" that sense rate of limb and trunk rotation have been adapted for measuring tremor [58]. One device (Systron model QRS-11) weighs 26 g and measures 40 mm in diameter and 13 mm in height. It utilises a vibrating quartz tuning fork that generates a torque when rotated around a predetermined axis (axis of symmetry). A second quartz fork is rigidly attached to the first and acts as a piezoelectric transducer that senses the torque, converting it into a voltage proportional to the rate of angular rotation and thereby acting as a gyroscope. The advantage of this method over standard accelerometry is that the latter is affected by gravity (9.81 m/s^2), because as the axes of a linear accelerometer oscillate around the gravitational vector a component of gravity is recorded at tremor frequency. This causes a measurement error, which varies according to the angle between the gravitational vector and the accelerometer's axis. However, the bulk of the Systron device makes it unsuitable for recording digital tremor. It is also quite delicate and expensive.

Computerised Tracking Tasks

Computerised tracking tasks have been used to quantify the severity of essential tremor and the action tremor of multiple sclerosis [8,9]. The tracking task was designed to provide a two-dimensional eye–hand coordination test, which involves patients tracking a target across an oscilloscope screen using a joystick control. The objective is to maintain superimposition of the tracking projectile on the target for the 1 min duration of the sweep. The joystick is mounted on the arm of a chair and is held between the thumb and fingers of the hand with the forearm supported. It is thus predominantly sensitive to a visually dependent feedback form of kinetic tremor (as there is some hand movement) which causes vertical disparity between the target and tracking projectile, the tracking error being characterised by the integral of the modulus of the distance of the tracking projectile trace from a 1 mm deep neutral zone about the target trace [9]. The technique is elegant because it measures the error produced by a tremor during a useful manual task and can be adapted to distinguish between tremor and other causes of impaired movement velocity control [8].

Digitising Tablets

The use of commercially available digitising tablets for the measurement of the frequency and severity of tremor present during writing and drawing is receiving increasing attention [59,60]. Digitising tablets are much less expensive than EMG- or accelerometry-based techniques (less than 10% of the cost) and the signal does not require amplification. It can be used to measure tremor during writing and drawing. Furthermore, the results of inter-trial variability studies performed on 87 patients with essential tremor showed that the results obtained with a digitising tablet were comparable to those produced by tri-axial accelerometry [59]. The study also confirmed the observation by Bain and colleagues [9,59] that

the frequency and amplitude of essential tremor change significantly with different tasks, with a tendency for tremor frequencies to constrict during kinetic tasks compared with a maintained posture. This fact nicely illustrates the dynamic variability of tremor.

Conclusion

There is presently no universally applicable physiological technique for measuring human tremor, as the system requirements vary according to the type of tremor under study and the experimental situation. The physiological techniques listed in Table 29.3 can all produce objective measures of tremor frequency and magnitude but all of them have specific limitations. First and foremost these systems are not widely available and are both expensive and time-consuming to operate in comparison with simple clinical methods, which immediately limits their deployment to highly specialised departments. Secondly, as discussed above, the main difficulty in measuring tremor is obtaining an appropriate sample of it. Thus there is little point, from the perspective of a therapeutic trial, in obtaining an accurate measurement of tremor magnitude over a short epoch if seconds or minutes later a measurement would be entirely different. Additionally patients with severe self-injurious action tremor are usually unwilling to allow their arms to thrash about unabated for even a few seconds, whilst it is recorded. It is this type of problem that introduces a significant subjective bias to these objective electrophysiologically based measurement techniques, and the observer is faced with one crucial problem: When should the recording device be turned on and off?

As accelerometry has several advantages over other transducer-based techniques, most published therapeutic tremor studies have used uni-axial accelerometers that record tremor in one dimension from their site of attachment [13]. However, there are several problems associated with accelerometric based measurements. Firstly, the low-frequency high-displacement components of a tremor are the events most likely to disrupt a piece of work but produce little effect on the dominant peak of averaged autospectra. Secondly, postural tremor magnitude measured by uni-axial accelerometry did not correlate with patients' self-reported disability – an observation that must put the validity of standard accelerometric techniques into question [26]. Thirdly, it is useless attempting to perform a fast Fourier transform (FFT) on a signal obtained from a patient with intention tremor; as the finger–nose–finger-test takes about 2 s to perform (providing fewer than 10 tremor cycles), during which tremor amplitude escalates. This causes a non-stationary signal and results in an inaccurate FFT – a problem compounded by the fact that intention tremors usually have low frequencies (around 3–4 Hz).

EMG-dependent methods record a surrogate marker of movement which has a complex and variable relationship with a limb's action. The resultant effect of the EMG bursts in an agonist muscle is dependent on the aggregated timing and size of the bursts in the antagonist as well as several other muscle groups. Additional complication is introduced by cross-talk from neighbouring muscles and migration of the surface electrodes off the underlying target muscle during rotational tremors. The same difficulties apply to long-term ambulatory EMG recordings. This technique, however, allows tremor to be recorded in the patient's normal environment and reduces the sampling dilemma involved in short-duration studies. The main outcome measure of this approach is tremor occurrence rate. Since tremors occur during certain states of muscle activity, tremor occurrence rate ultimately measures what proportion of time a muscle is being used or rested. Secondly, the size of an EMG burst in a particular muscle has a variable effect on disability, which depends on the state of activity of that limb. For example a parkinsonian patient may have a rest and an action tremor of similar magnitudes. The former may be present for a greater proportion of time (i.e. have a greater occurrence rate) but the latter is more likely to be incapacitating. Thirdly, the disabilities caused by different types of tremor (e.g. parkinsonian tremor, essential tremor and dystonic tremor) may depend as much on the relative extents to which they can be suppressed during functional activities as on their absolute magnitudes during posture or rest. Suppressability is the extent to which tremor amplitude can be voluntarily damped by the patient whilst performing specific tasks and the period of time that this damping can be maintained (reflected in the coefficients of amplitude and temporal suppression respectively) [9,61]. This point was nicely illustrated by Jager and King [62] who described a man with marked hereditary essential tremor who could nonetheless shoot deer with a rifle at a hundred metres. Consequently, any method that solely examines tremor occurrence rate does not account for variations in tremor magnitude when it most matters.

Gyroscopes bypass the difficulty caused by gravitational effects on accelerometers but are expensive, cumbersome and frail. The currently available devices are unsuitable for measuring finger tremor because of their bulk, which adds considerably to the overall inertia and can also interfere with fine manual activities. The sensitivities of the commercially available digitising tablets are inadequate for measurements of physiological tremor, whilst severe action tremors cause the pen to come off the tablet making analysis impossible [59]. Digitising tablets can only be used to record tremor in writing and drawing, which is inappropriate for other forms of task-specific tremor (e.g. in musicians) or tremor that affects other parts of the body (e.g. primary orthostatic tremor).

The continuing refinement of motion analysis systems (e.g. MacReflex) may lead to nicer ways of quantifying kinetic tremors, which cannot be captured accurately with accelerometers. However, at present data analysis is time-consuming and there is insufficient evidence from clinical studies to know whether these systems provide reliable, valid or responsive measures of tremor.

Conclusion

The complex movements produced by human tremors are difficult to capture with physiological techniques. The precise problems encountered vary according to the measurement technique involved and the tremor type. There is presently no universally accepted electro-physiological method for measuring tremor and thus it is unwise to base the outcome of a therapeutic trial solely on data obtained by deploying one.

References

1. Deuschl G, Bain PG, Brin M and an Ad Hoc scientific committee. Consensus-statement of the Movement Disorder Society on tremor. Mov Disord 1998;13(Suppl 3):2–23.
2. Deuschl G, Koster B, Scheidt C. Diagnostic criteria and clinical course of psychogenic tremors. Mov Disord 1998;13:294–302.
3. Britton TC, Thompson PD, Day BL, Rothwell JC, Findley LJ, Marsden CD. Resetting of postural tremors at the wrist with mechanical stretches in Parkinson's disease, essential tremor, and normal subjects mimicking tremor. Ann Neurol 1992;31:507–514.
4. Bain PG. A combined clinical and neurophysiological approach to the study of patients with tremor. J Neurol Neurosurg Psychiatry 1993;56:839–844.
5. Bain PG, Findley LJ, Britton TC, Rothwell JC, Gresty MA, Thompson PD, Marsden CD. Primary writing tremor. Brain 1995;118:1461–1472.
6. Bain PG, Findley LJ. Clinical aspects of parkinsonian tremor. In: Quinn NP, Stern G, editors. The Parkinson Papers. London: Franklin Scientific Projects, 1992.
7. Cleeves L, Findley LJ. Variability in amplitude of untreated essential tremor. J Neurol Neurosurg Psychiatry 1987;50:704–708.
8. Liu X, Miall C, Aziz TZ, Palace J, Haggard P, Stein JF. Analyis of action tremor and impaired control of movement velocity

in multiple sclerosis during visually guided wrist-tracking tasks. Mov Disord 1997;992–999.

9. Bain PG, Mally J, Gresty MA, Findley LJ. Assessing the impact of essential tremor on upper limb function. J Neurol 1993; 241:54–61.

10. Elble RJ, Sinha R, Higgins C. Quantification of tremor with a digitizing tablet. J Neurosci Methods 1990;32:193–198.

11. Bain PG, Findley LJ, Thompson PD, Gresty MA, Rothwell JC, Harding AE, et al. A study of hereditary essential tremor. Brain 1994;117:805–824.

12. Critchley M. Observations on essential (heredofamilial) tremor. Brain 1949;72:113–139.

13. Bain PG. The effectiveness of treatments for essential tremor. The Neurologist 1997;3:305–321.

14. Lang AET, Fahn S. Assessment of Parkinson's disease. In: Munsat TL, editor. Quantification of neurological deficit. London: Butterworth, 1989:49–67.

15. Hobart JC, Lamping DL, Thompson AJ. Evaluating neurological outcome measures: the bare essentials. J Neurol Neurosurg Psychiatry 1996;60:127–130.

16. Cronbach LJ. Coefficient alpha and the internal structure of tests. Psychometrika 1951;16:297–334.

17. Kuder GF, Richardson MW. The theory of estimation of test reliability. Psychometrika 1937;2:151–160.

18. Shrout PE, Fleiss JL. Intraclass correlations: uses in assessing rater reliability. Psychol Bull 1979;86:420–428.

19. Francis DA, Bain PG, Swan AV, Hughes RAC. An assessment of disability rating scales used in multiple sclerosis. Arch Neurol 1991;48:299–301.

20. Cohen J. Weighted Kappa: nominal scale agreement with provision for scaled disagreement or partial credit. Psychol Bull 1968;70:213–220.

21. Fleiss JL. Measuring nominal scale agreement among many raters. Psychol Bull 1971;76:378–382.

22. Cronbach LJ, Meehl PE. Construct validity in psychological tests. Psychol Bull 1955;52:281–302.

23. Cambell DT, Fiske DW. Convergent and discriminant validation by the multitrait–multimethod matrix. Psychol Bull 1959;56:81–105.

24. Cambell DT. Recommendations for APA test standards regarding construct, trait, or discriminant validity. Am Psychol 1960;15:546–553.

25. Messick S. Test validity and the ethics of assessments. Am Psychol 1980;35:1012–1027.

26. Bain PG, Findley LJ, Atchison P, Behari M, Vidailhet M, Gresty MA, et al. Assessing tremor severity. J Neurol Neurosurg Psychiatry 1993;56:868–873.

27. Findley LJ, Cleeves L, Calzetti S. Primidone in essential tremor of the hands and head: a double-blind controlled clinical study. J Neurol Neurosurg Psychiatry 1985;48:911–915.

28. Gorman WP, Cooper R, Pocock P, Cambell MY. A comparison of primidone, propranolol, and placebo in essential tremor, using quantitative analysis. J Neurol Neurosurg Psychiatry 1986;49:64–68.

29. Koller WC, Biary N, Cone S. Disability in essential tremor: effect of treatment. Neurology 1986;36:1001–1004.

30. Findley LJ. The pharmacology of essential tremor. In: Marsden CD, Fahn S, editors. Movement disorders 2. London: Butterworth, 1987:438–458.

31. Dietrichson P, Espen E. Primidone and propranalol in essential tremor: a study based upon quantitative tremor recording and plasma anticonvulsant levels. Acta Neurol Scand 1987;75:332–340.

32. Sasso E, Perucca E, Calzetti S. Double blind comparison of primidone and phenobarbital in essential tremor. Neurology 1988;38:808–810.

33. Sasso E, Perucca E, Fava R, Calzetti S. Quantitative comparison of barbiturates in essential hand and head tremor. Mov Disord 1991;6:65–68.

34. Padgaonker AJ, Krieger KW, King AI. Measurement of angular acceleration of a rigid body using linear accelerometers. J Appl Mech (Trans ASME) 1975;42:552–556.

35. Gilbert JA, Maxwell GM, McElhaney JH, Clippinger FW. A system to measure the forces and movements at the knee and hip during level walking. J Orthop Res 1984;2:281–288.

36. Ladin Z, Flowers WC, Messner W. A quantitative comparison of a position measurement system and accelerometry. J Biomech 1989;22:295–308.

37. Frost JD. Triaxial vector accelerometry: a method for quantitating tremor and ataxia. IEEE Trans Biomed Eng 1978;25:17–27.

38. Jankovic J, Frost JD. Quantitative assessment of parkinsonian and essential tremor: clinical application of triaxial accelerometry. Neurology 1981;31:1235–1240.

39. Marsden CD. Origins of normal and pathological tremor. In: Findley LJ, Capildeo R, editors. Movement disorders: tremor. London: Macmillan Press, 1987:37–55.

40. Gresty MA, Findley LJ. Definition, analysis and genesis of tremor. In: Findley LJ, Capildeo R, editors. Movement disorders: tremor. London: Macmillan Press, 1984:15–26.

41. Elble RJ, Koller WC, editors. Tremor. Baltimore: Johns Hopkins University Press, 1990:28–32.

42. Rothwell JC, Kachi T, Thompson PD, Day BL, Marsden CD. Physiological investigations of Parkinsonian rest tremor and benign essential tremor. In: Beneke R, Conrad B, Marsden CD, editors. Motor disturbances 1. London: Academic Press, 1987:1–17.

43. Basmajian JV, De Luca CJ. Muscles alive: their functions revealed by electromyography. Baltimore: Williams and Wilkins, 1985.

44. Lippold OCJ. The relation between integrated action potentials in a human muscle and its isometric tension. J Physiol (Lond) 1952;117:492–499.

45. Bouisset S, Maton B. Quantitative relationship between surface EMG and intramuscular electromyographic activity in voluntary movement. Am J Phys Med 1972;51:285–295.

46. Bigland B, Lippold OCJ. Motor unit activity in voluntary contraction of human muscle. J Physiol (Lond) 1954;125:322–335.

47. Elble RJ, Randall JE. Motor unit activity responsible for 8- to 12-Hz component of human physiological finger tremor. J Neurophysiol 1976;39:370–383.

48. Solomonow M, Baratta R, Zhou BH, et al. The EMG force model of electrically stimulated muscles: dependence on control strategy and predominant fiber composition. IEEE Trans Biomed Eng 1987;34:692–703.

49. Bacher M, Scholz E, Diener HC. 24 hour continuous EMG tremor quantification based on EMG recording. Electroencephalogr Clin Neurophysiol 1989;72:176–183.

50. Spieker S, Loschmann P, Jentgens C, Boose A, Klockgether T, Dichgans J. Tremorlytic activity of budipine: a quantitative study with long-term tremor recordings. Clin Neuropharmacol 1995;18:266–272.

51. Spieker S, Jentgens C, Boose A, Dichgans J. Reliability, specificity, and sensitivity of long-term tremor recordings. Electroencephalogr Clin Neurophysiol 1995;97:326–331.

52. Spieker S, Strole V, Sailer A, Boose A, Dichgans J. Validity of long term tremor electromyography in the quantification of tremor. Mov Disord 1997;12:985–991.

53. Horsley V, Schafer EA. Experiments on the character of the muscular contractions which are evoked by excitation of the various parts of the motor tract. J Physiol (Lond) 1886;7:96–110.

54. Graham JDP. Static tremor in anxiety states. J Neurol Neurosurg Psychiatry 1945;8:57–60.

55. Cooper JD, Halliday AM, Redfearn JWT. Apparatus for the study of human tremor and stretch reflexes. Electroencephalogr Clin Neurophysiol 1957;9:546–550.

56. Holmes G. The cerebellum in man. Brain 1939;63:1–30.
57. Steg G, Ingvarsson PE, Johnels B, Valls M, Thorselius M. Objective measurement of motor disability in Parkinson's disease. Acta Neurol Scand 1989;126:67–75.
58. Tetrud J, Felsing G, Sunnarborg D, Delimeier W. Assessment of tremor using a solid-state angular rate sensor. Presented at the 45th American Academy of Neurology, New York, 1993.
59. Elble RJ, Brilliant M, Leffler K, Higgins C. Quantification of essential tremor in writing and drawing. Mov Disord 1996;11: 70–78.
60. Elble RJ, Sinha R, Higgins C. Quantification of tremor with a digitizing tablet. J Neurosci Methods 1990;32:193–198.
61. Bain PG, Findley LJ, editors. Assessing tremor severity. London: Smith-Gordon, 1993.
62. Jager BV, King T. Hereditary tremor. Arch Intern Med 1955;95:788–793.

30. Multiple Sclerosis: Ethics, Outcome Variables and Clinical Scales

A.J. Coles and D.A.S. Compston

Introduction

The first randomised controlled trial in clinical medicine, of streptomycin in tuberculosis, was published in 1948 [1] and this was followed 9 years later by the first randomised placebo-controlled double-blind study in multiple sclerosis [2]. Despite this early start, clinical trials in multiple sclerosis have been beset by the difficulty of measuring treatment efficacy in a disease which has notoriously protean clinical manifestations. The advent of magnetic resonance imaging in the late 1980s seemed to offer a sensitive surrogate to clinical outcome in the assessment of putative new treatments. However, as the controversy over recent trials of interferon beta (IFNβ) clearly shows, the interpretation of changes in magnetic resonance imaging markers is not straightforward. As understanding of the immunological basis of multiple sclerosis has grown, so biological assays have increasingly been used in treatment trials. In this chapter, we review these three classes of outcome variables: clinical, radiological and immunological.

Multiple sclerosis is a common and potentially disabling disease, accounting for considerable physical, emotional and economic distress. No drug has been identified which represents a predictable, safe and widely available treatment. Every therapeutic endeavour introduces a substantial placebo effect and outcome measures are either susceptible to observer bias or of disputed relevance. All of these points have implications for the ethical justification of trials in multiple sclerosis.

There are two distinct therapeutic goals in multiple sclerosis: first, modifying the disease process (which includes abrogating the relapse, dealing with persistent symptoms and influencing the clinical course) and secondly, repair of the accumulated damage.

The Ethics of Clinical Trials in Multiple Sclerosis

The Ethical Balance and Trial Design

The ethical position of any clinical trial hinges on the balance between management of the individual participant and the potential gains to the wider community. For those trial patients taking an active agent, the possible good of a successful treatment should outweigh the potential harmful effects of the drug or disease progression. By definition, these risks are unknown before a trial so a patient's attitude to uncertainty or risk-taking and their perception of the disease process will influence their decision about participation. To the wider community of disease sufferers, there is the potential good that an effective treatment will be discovered. In addition, a well-conducted trial, irrespective of its result, should always advance understanding of the disease and so benefit a wide population. For instance, the negative result of the IFNγ trial [3] may be considered entirely ethical although the drug appeared to provoke neurological relapses in some individuals. The trial design allowed for early recognition of this adverse effect, the study was stopped and harm to the participants was minimised. The suggestion that IFNγ may promote relapses was new and led to a greater understanding of the pathogenesis of multiple sclerosis, so maximising the collective ethic.

A corollary is that a poorly designed trial that leads to an unclear conclusion loses the collective benefit and so risks being regarded as unethical. Consider the early evaluation of isoniazid as a treatment for multiple sclerosis. In 1953, an uncontrolled preliminary report suggested that isoniazid was beneficial [4], but no treatment effect was observed when a further trial adopted a blind and placebo-controlled design [2]. Despite this early demonstration of the need for randomised blinded design, many trials have since been published which fall short of this ideal, and so compromise the collective ethic. Particular pitfalls are the use of multiple treatment arms without a control group [5–7] and variation in patient selection and drug dosage within the same arm [8]. The relative weight of collective and individual ethics depends on the aims of the trial. In phase I and II trials individual ethics should predominate, as the information derived from such a trial will not be applied directly to the wider community but will lead at most to a phase III study.

A dogmatic utilitarian analysis may lead to unacceptable conclusions. For instance, because multiple sclerosis is common, it might in theory be considered permissible deliberately to disadvantage a small group of trial patients (for example withholding an efficacious treatment from the control group) because the benefit to the collective is perceived to be so great. To protect against such behaviour, utilitarian ethics should be complemented by a deontological (or rules-based) approach. Here primacy is given not to outcome or utility but to motive and ethical principles, such as those advocated by Beauchamp & Childress [9]. One such principle is that of *non-maleficence* – "first do no harm". Superficially, a strict application of this rule would disallow all clinical trials. But an appeal to the principle of *autonomy* allows that: "human dignity can be severely undermined by serious illness as well as by the human experimentation designed to eliminate such illness. There is an ethical cost attached to not doing such research as well as to proceeding with it" [10]. This is manifestly true of multiple sclerosis.

One important consequence of the principle of non-maleficence is the requirement for "treatment indifference" in clinical trials. The treating physicians, acting in the best interests of the patient, should have no preference for the agent (or placebo) that each patient will receive. Here is the protection for the individual against rank utilitarianism. However, inherent in design of the double-blind trial, there is a subtle subjugation of the individual ethic by the collective. As a single-blind trial progresses, its results gradually filter back to the observing physicians who may then develop a treatment preference on the basis of clinical judgement, a property of the individual doctor–patient relationship. So the principle of non-maleficence is breached and action should be taken. When the trial is double-blind, the treating physicians do not accumulate such experience; the unblind review committee has continuous access to the trial data, but is unlikely to act without statistical significance, which is a feature

of the collective. There is no easy resolution of these ethical tensions.

The Ethics of Outcome Measures and Patient Selection

Under the utilitarian approach a trial is most ethical when its design minimises the potential harm to the individual and maximises the good to the collective. Hence outcome measures and statistics should be devised to minimise the number of patients required to enter a trial. Thus, a sensitive outcome measure is more ethical than an insensitive one, all else being equal. Two important tests of an outcome measure are *rigour* and *relevance*. By rigour, we mean a global index of sensitivity, reproducibility and objectivity. The relevance of an outcome variable is a measure of its correlation with the underlying disease process. These tests have ethical implications. For example, measuring magnetic resonance abnormalities is more rigorous than merely using clinical scales in trials of drugs in multiple sclerosis. The increased sensitivity of magnetic resonance imaging greatly reduces the number of patients required to assess the efficacy of a drug at a given power. So the individual ethic is maximised. But the relevance of magnetic resonance imaging changes to the underlying disease is disputed and the collective ethic is therefore compromised (see below for a more detailed discussion).

For the individual, acceptable risks of an experimental drug are considered against the potential threat of the disease. Thus in early trials of a drug whose side-effect profile is little known, it may seem ethically preferable to select only very disabled patients. However, this may compromise the collective ethic in two ways. First, it may be hard sensitively to measure outcome in this group and so reach any clear conclusions. Secondly, the results of such trials can only be applied to a highly selected patient group, thus reducing the collective benefit. A more sophisticated approach is to select patients who have the highest chance of treatment failure as this reduces the sample size required to detect a given treatment effect. If treatment failure is defined in terms of the Kurtzke score, then features predictive of failure at onset are not only the patient's baseline score but also measures of specific systems in which disease activity maximises disability, for example pyramidal and brainstem function [11].

Placebo, Blinding and Consent

The usual response of the placebo group in multiple sclerosis trials is to show a partial treatment effect. In three recent multiple sclerosis trials, the annualised relapse rate was reduced by 29% (IFNβ-1b) [12], 25% (IFNβ-1a) [13] and 42% (Copolymer-1) [14]. In part, this reduction in relapse rate may reflect regression to a mean level of disease activity in a group of patients selected on the basis of a recent high relapse rate. However, comparison with historical controls (see Weinshenker [15,16]) shows a clear placebo effect in multiple sclerosis trials. Therefore a trial without a placebo control [17,18] is vulnerable to misinterpretation of the placebo effect as a true treatment effect. In trials involving patients with progressive multiple sclerosis, some investigators dispense with the control group [5]. The implicit assumption is that patients will continue to deteriorate at a steady rate, so that cessation of progression or any improvement in disability is necessarily a treatment effect. However, this assumption is not correct; Weinshenker et al. [11] have shown that 11% of progressive patients may spontaneously improve by greater than one EDSS point in the usual time period of a trial. Clearly control groups are essential. Patients and investigators should be blinded from randomisation. The standard clinical scales used in trials are very susceptible to biased interpretation. For instance, in the Canadian cyclophosphamide trial, an unblind assessor reported a positive treatment effect whereas the blind assessor did not [19].

The optimum trial design in multiple sclerosis is double-blind and randomised, but an inevitable consequence of these requirements is that recruitment of patients is jeopardised. The ethical principle of autonomy, as well as the requirements of drug regulation agencies, dictate that patients give fully informed consent to enter a randomised trial. Patients must understand that they may receive a placebo. This usually has the effect of limiting volunteers to a trial, especially when standard and experimental therapies are being compared. Several methods have been employed to circumvent this problem without compromising the principle of autonomy. Mauch et al. [20] compared the effect of low-dose cyclophosphamide in multiple sclerosis patients who asked for an experimental treatment compared with "controls" choosing steroid treatment because they felt this had been previously efficacious. Zelen [21] has proposed another technique. Patients are randomised before their first consultation. Only those so randomised are offered the experimental treatment; those who decline are treated with standard therapy. Provided the number who choose the standard therapy is low, the treatment group will not be excessively contaminated [22,23]. Both of these approaches compromise ideal trial design and so reduce the collective ethic to boost recruitment. In as common a disease as multiple sclerosis, this is hard to justify.

The Partially Effective Treatment

The introduction of IFNβ as the first drug licensed as a disease-modifying agent in patients with relapsing-remitting multiple sclerosis, and subsequently secondary progressive, has raised two important questions. First, is it now ethically acceptable to experiment with other drugs when an effective treatment is available? At first glance the principle of treatment indifference is breached. It might be argued that a reasonable physician, acting out of concern for the individual patient, should never choose to give an experimental drug of unknown qualities and withhold IFNβ. However, IFNβ is only a partially effective treatment in multiple sclerosis. Even for its licensed use, the reduction of relapse rate in relapsing-remitting patients of moderate disability (UK guidelines), it is not completely effective. A physician might reasonably regard the potential benefit of an experimental drug to be equivalent to the established modest benefit of IFNβ. Another rational view might be that halting the progression of disability in multiple sclerosis is a more important goal and here IFNβ has less to offer. So at the level of the individual ethic, the principle of treatment indifference may be maintained. For the multiple sclerosis community as a whole, there can be no doubt that more efficacious treatments are desirable and should be actively searched for.

Secondly, should all experimental drugs be compared with IFNβ rather than placebo in clinical trials? Introducing such a comparison would immediately compromise the individual ethic as sample sizes would have to increase to demonstrate an additional treatment effect. However to deliberately deny a group of patients a licensed and partially efficacious treatment is maleficent. In our opinion, there is little place for placebo groups in phase III studies of relapsing-remitting multiple sclerosis.

As well as these theoretical considerations, there are two pragmatic solutions to these questions. First, the United States' experience has been that appreciable numbers of patients treated with IFNβ outside a trial choose to discontinue it, because of adverse effects or perceived lack of benefit. These may not be a truly representative sample of patients, but this cohort would probably serve as candidates for a trial with a placebo group. Secondly, in countries such as the United Kingdom, political and economic restraints limit the access to IFNβ. This means that strict entry criteria to funded prescriptions for IFNβ treatment still leaves a substantial pool of untreated patients available for trials. Even patients eligible for IFNβ may be denied treatment because of health service rationing. There are historical precedents for exploiting this lack of availability: Sir Austin Bradford Hill pointed out that it was ethical to use streptomycin in a controlled trial because of its lack of availability even though the drug was widely believed to be efficacious; "whenever a newly introduced drug . . . is scarce in its early days, then there presents an opportunity of which immediate advantage should, if possible, be taken. With a serious disease in which the old offers very little hope of benefit, the new cannot be withheld. The chance of adequately and quickly assessing the value of the latter, if any, may never again occur" [24]. Finally it should be remembered that IFNβ has little to offer to the largest groups of patients with multiple sclerosis – those with benign or progressive disease.

Transplantation Research

When an agent is found that halts the inflammatory activity of multiple sclerosis, it will become feasible to consider techniques for restoring structure and function in the damaged brain. One approach may be to implant tissue into the central nervous system cells which have the ability to migrate, proliferate, differentiate and remyelinate [25]. This has parallels with work in Parkinson's disease and Huntington's chorea. Several potential sources of the necessary tissue are ethically contentious [26]. This is particularly true for the use of human fetuses acquired from the medical termination of pregnancy. Foremost amongst the ethical issues raised is the extent to which use of such material influences the individual's decision in favour of termination. A UK governmental report concluded that the use of fetal tissue for transplantation is acceptable provided that the contact between researchers and pregnant women considering a termination is mediated through a neutral third party [27]. In this way, direct coercion of women by investigators is rightly minimised. But such measures do not prevent the global perception of terminations being changed by the medical use of fetal material. In an emotionally fraught situation, the solace of "some good" arising from terminations might well influence a woman's decision to proceed. If that is so, then proponents of the medical use of fetal tissue cannot disengage altogether from the ethical issues surrounding abortion.

The Pharmaceutical Industry

The requirements of most trials for large numbers of patients, sophisticated laboratory monitoring and extensive data collection for regulators are beyond the financial means of most academic departments and increasingly of government research budgets. Therefore sponsorship by pharmaceutical companies is necessary; indeed an estimated 60% of medical research in the UK is directly financed by the pharmaceutical industry [28]. Whilst this involvement is actively encouraged in the UK by medical charities and governmental funding bodies, the consequent conflicts of interest should be recognised. This is most obvious when investigators stand to gain personally from a positive trial, a notorious example being the trial of tissue plasminogen activator (tPA), a thrombolytic agent, in myocardial infarction, in which the investigators held shares in Genentech, the manufacturer of tPA [29]. Concern over the potential temptation for fraud has led to the "disclosure policy" of the *New England Journal of Medicine*, now followed by many other journals, whereby all commercial associations of the authors are disclosed to the editor who may then disseminate this information [30]; or the "elimination approach" which suggests that investigators should not be allowed to deal in shares of any companies with an interest in the trial outcome [31]. A more subtle pressure on investigators is the capitation fee, which may be up to $5000, that pharmaceutical companies offer institutions for each patient recruited to a trial. Although nominally intended to cover the expenses of trial participation, an academic department may make a profit of up to $200 000 on a trial of 50 patients [32]. As soon as researchers and institutions become dependent on such inducements, their objectivity may be corroded. Colleges, medical associations and journals have all proposed ways to clarify the roles of physicians and industry in the conduct of trials [33].

The involvement of industry in clinical trials thrusts investigators into the arena of financial speculation and unscrupulous competition. For instance, a small company, Autoimmune Inc., conducted a clinical trial of bovine oral myelin, Myloral, in 500 patients with multiple sclerosis in collaboration with scientists who had been involved in oral myelin treatment of experimental allergic encephalomyelitis. The trial started in 1994 and a rise in the company's share price by $10 followed. In February 1996 a competitor, Myelin Distributors of New York, started advertising its version of oral myelin basic protein to multiple sclerosis societies in Canada, with a misleading endorsement by the National Multiple Sclerosis Society (USA). In April 1996, the Myloral trial was discussed on NBC Nightly News and The Today Show in the United States in cautiously optimistic tones and, in February 1997, senior executives of Autoimmune Inc. wrote to shareholders: "we look forward to Phase III substantiation of its [Myloral's] efficacy in reducing attack rate and slowing the progression of disability". Statements such as these encouraged speculative interest and Autoimmune's share price rose $10 again between October 1996 and May 1997 as the trial results were anticipated. On 21 April 1997 the company released preliminary results from the trial to comply with Federal Securities and Exchange Commission regulations concerning information for investors in publicly held companies: Myloral had no significant effect on the frequency of relapses or progression of disability compared with controls. Other trial data, including magnetic resonance imaging scans, had not been analysed, but Autoimmune's share price dropped $12 overnight as thousands of shares were sold. The Internet carried news of the trial within days, and the financial press reported its results that week; a peer-reviewed paper in a medical journal has yet to appear. It is hard to imagine that this turbulent and speculative environment is ideal for the disinterested assessment of a new drug.

Pharmaceutical companies have an accepted place in the continuing education of doctors, particularly by their representatives "detailing" physicians about new products. Doctors fondly imagine that they are influenced only by academic drug literature; in fact their practice suggests commercial sources of information are of at least equal influence [34]. Pharmaceutically sponsored educational courses tend to be biased in their presentation [35]. It is virtually impossible for someone active in clinical research to avoid potential conflicts of interest. We have both accepted individual and corporate hospitality from pharmaceutical companies, and not always only when actually speaking at symposia actively sponsored by those companies. To a greater or lesser extent, conflict of interest is now endemic.

Outcome Variables in Clinical Trials of Multiple Sclerosis

In the choice of outcome variable for multiple sclerosis trials, there is often a conflict between rigour and relevance. Ultimately a drug will be judged useful only if it has an impact on significant clinical events which influence the natural history of multiple sclerosis. Clinical scales are therefore rightly considered the most relevant outcome measures. But, being subjective, unreliable and insensitive, they lack rigour. In the early phase of drug development, trials may be designed to prove a therapeutic concept, to explore a dosing schedule or to demonstrate that the agent has a pharmacological effect. Here rigorous criteria are used that allow the trial to be conducted quickly on as few patients as possible, whilst accepting that their relevance to the underlying disease process may be disputed. Secondary considerations in the choice of an outcome variable are its ease of

measurement and universal acceptance; the use of novel outcome scales [6,20] compromises acceptance of trial results.

Clinical Scales

The clinical hallmarks of multiple sclerosis are that it affects disparate sites throughout the central nervous system at varying times; and the ensuing impairments may resolve (partially or completely) or may progress. Such impairments sum to cause loss of particular functions, or disabilities, that affect the patient's life as distinct handicaps. As an example of the complexity of these relationships, consider a slight impairment of manual discriminative sensation in two patients with multiple sclerosis. In one, otherwise well and employed as a teacher, this represents a trivial handicap; in the other, whose vision is already compromised and who works at a computer keyboard, the handicap may be devastating.

There are three distinct challenges for a clinical scale. First, an ideal clinical scale must reliably identify and define the status of all the protean manifestations of multiple sclerosis, including impairments in power, coordination, sensation, sphincter function, eye movements, visual acuity and cognitive function. Secondly, the ensuing disabilities and handicaps must be measured. Thirdly, the ideal scale should account for the history of the impairment. Sustained disability is of much more consequence to the patient than a transient impairment occurring in the context of a recent relapse but with the expectation of subsequent recovery. In the Copolymer-1 trial there is a significant treatment effect if one simply compares mean disability at the beginning and end of the trial. But if account is taken of relapse status and the probability of remaining free from sustained progression compared, this treatment effect disappears [14,36].

Relapse Rate or Progression of Disability?

Superficially, a relapse of multiple sclerosis is easy to define [37]. In practice, however, it is not always easy to distinguish the symptoms and signs due to new multiple sclerosis lesions from those resulting from reactivation or exacerbation of previously demyelinated lesions by temperature [38], intercurrent illness or soluble inflammatory mediators [39]. However, relapse rate is easily quantified and so it is a popular outcome variable in multiple sclerosis trials, for instance those of IFNβ-1b [12] and IFNβ-1a [13]. More credence is given to events confirmed by assessing physicians since patients may not be able to make the distinction between symptoms due to new multiple sclerosis activity and Uthoff phenomena. Pre-treatment relapse rates should not be calculated from patients' histories but from an observed run-in period in order to avoid a false positive treatment effect arising from the physician's stricter criteria for a relapse.

The most important criticism of relapse rate as an outcome measure in multiple sclerosis trials is on the grounds of relevance for the long-term course of the disease. It is clear that relapse frequency is not a reliable indicator of disability. Neurological impairment is more predictably acquired through the non-relapsing progressive phase of multiple sclerosis. Indeed, relapse frequency tends to fall during the natural history of multiple sclerosis, whereas disability accumulates. Drugs which suppress relapse frequency do not necessarily reduce the progression of disability, as the IFNβ trials have shown. It follows that relapse rate and progression of disability should be regarded as independent clinical measures. If so, which is the more important for patients? Handicap is dominated by the degree of sustained neurological impairment. Relapse rate is the more relevant outcome measure only for those patients in whom relapses are sufficient to constitute a source of handicap independent of disability, but this is a very small proportion of the multiple sclerosis population. For these reasons, there is now a consensus that the most important clinical measure in multiple sclerosis trials is progression of impairment or disability [40].

Impairment, Disability and Handicap

Combined Scales and Statistical Analysis. It is impossible to contain within a single score a quantifiable description of all the variable clinical manifestations of multiple sclerosis. There are two approaches to the problem. Distinct impairments in the same patient may be amalgamated qualitatively to give a *composite* score as in the lower grades (0–3.5) of Kurtzke's Expanded Disability Severity Score (EDSS). Alternatively, each separate impairment score may be segregated within a *multivariate* analysis: an example was used by Vandenbark et al. [41] in their trial of T-cell receptor peptide vaccination. They defined the patients' clinical outcome as "improved," "stable" or "worsened" on the basis of changes in EDSS and three separate quantitative tasks of mobility and coordination. Specific information on each impairment is lost by this approach, but each patient's global disability may be compared, albeit arbitrarily. As a composite score is necessarily ordinal, the statistical analysis must be non-parametric. The utility of any composite score depends ultimately upon the assumptions contained within the choice of unit impairments and the ways in which they are combined.

In a multivariate approach, each impairment score remains distinct. An extravagant example is given by a trial of total lymphoid irradiation, in which each patient was scored separately on the functional components and overall EDSS, an additional "functional score", a timed walk, visual analogue scores for limb and bladder function, an incapacity scale, a modified version of the environmental status scale and a battery of psychometric tests [42]. One theoretical advantage of this approach is that a treatment effect confined to isolated impairments may be elicited. For instance in a study of azathioprine combined with plasma exchange [43] patients were scored clinically by two techniques and then had tests of visual evoked potentials, somatosensory potentials and central motor conduction time. The conclusion was that the treatment increased central motor conduction. From a similarly wide battery of tests in a trial of low-dose methotrexate [44], upper limb dysfunction emerged as responsive to treatment. In fact, all these studies illustrate a common error. They fail to account for the increased likelihood of false positive results generated by the increased number of tests done in a multivariate score. This may be compensated for by applying the Bonferroni correction, which is often omitted by trialists (presumably because it reduces the power of the study accordingly). An alternative approach to either a composite or a multivariate analysis with Bonferroni correction is the *sum of the squares of the Z score*. This has higher power than a multivariate analysis but introduces the risk, as do composite scores, of including invariant dimensions which therefore dilute any real treatment effect [40].

It should be remembered that statistical and clinical significance are not equivalent. Consider the claim that "Copolymer-1 had a significant effect on neurologic disability" [14]. The mean change in EDSS scores is −0.05 in the treated group by 2 years compared with +0.21 in the placebo group. Although *p* is 0.023, this difference in disability is well below the threshold of clinical detection.

The most recently advocated composite outcome measure for clinical trials in MS is that of the National Multiple Sclerosis Society (US) Task Force [45].

Impairment. Each impairment in multiple sclerosis can be assessed by a unique clinical scale. Ideally these should be quantitative, giving increased objectivity and allowing parametric statistics. Examples of such quantitative scales are those of Tourtellotte et al. [46], and timed distance walking or tests of coordination such as the 9-hole peg board and the box-and-block tests. Some impairments may also be measured electrophysiologically; visual evoked potentials are the main outcome measure in a current trial of the remyelinating capacity of intravenous immunoglobulin organised at the Mayo Clinic. Difficult impairments to quantify are fatigue, pain and dysaesthesiae. Different impairments may give the same disability. For instance, a cerebellar lesion and a spinal cord lesion cause different impairment to limb function, but both may effectively reduce the ability of a patient to walk 100 metres.

Disability. In the 1950s and 1960s John Kurtzke analysed the systematised records of 250 World War II veterans who had been hospitalised for multiple sclerosis at the Veterans Administration Hospital in the Bronx, New York. He compiled a list of eight independent fields of impairment (roughly correlating with neurological sites) which came to be called functional systems [47,48]. The impairment in each functional system was graded independently. In some systems, such as visual function, the grades were based on objective measures. But in others, such as the pyramidal function, the grading remained qualitative and imprecise (requiring a distinction between "moderate" and "blind" paraparesis for instance). These scores are now often used to derive the final EDSS score of disability, they may be used separately, but have been used independently in some trials [49].

It is important to recognise that the EDSS is not a pure scale of disability. In the early grades (0–3.5) it is a composite impairment scale, dominated by the functional systems scores. From grade 4.0 onwards, disability and handicap are pre-eminent. For instance, the ability to "be up and about for most of the day" and "work a full day in a position of average physical difficulty", which marks grades up to 4.5, are measures of both disability and handicap. The six grades from 5.0 to 7.5 are dominated by walking distance. Here "direct observation may be required" (a pure measure of disability) but "patient's statements about walking are ordinarily acceptable" (allowing contamination by motivational factors). Beyond grade 7.5, handicap dominates, with distinctions between points resting on self-care functions. Trained paraclinical staff can reliably use the EDSS for scores over 4.0, where there is not an absolute dependence on neurological examination.

The Kurtzke scale has important flaws as an outcome measure. It is not particularly rigorous and it its relatively insensitive. In patients judged by the EDSS to be clinically stable over time, 14% were felt to have had active disease by clinical impression [50]. The subjectivity in some parts of the grading reduces its reliability, which is about 50–65% between observers and 75% by the same observer over time. Unintentional examiner bias is therefore a very real

possibility, as seen in the Canadian cyclophosphamide trial [19]. Many, including Kurtzke himself initially, have failed to realise that the EDSS is an ordinal scale and requires non-parametric statistics. The distance between steps is arbitrary and not necessarily equivalent. Indeed there are strong arguments for allowing changes by 0.5 point below scores of 6.0 to be regarded as equivalent statistically and functionally to changes by 1.0 point above this grade [11]. Despite these comments, the Kurtzke scale is of enduring value. This achievement rests largely on its simplicity, ease of use and widespread acceptance.

Handicap. Very few disease-modifying agents are tested against scales of handicap, as this outcome is felt to be distant from biological events and too easily distorted by extraneous factors such as motivation and education. The CAMBS scale does incorporate a simple visual analogue scale of handicap, as well as a summary of disability and time course [51]. Although not adopted in any trials, this scale is unique in building a statement of clinical context for current disability, impairment and handicap status but, as currently configured, it lacks sensitivity. In addition to its designers, CAMBS has some admirers (Charles Poser and John Noseworthy, personal Communication)!

Radiological Markers

The technique of magnetic resonance imaging has introduced a rigorous, objective and highly sensitive outcome measure for clinical trials in multiple sclerosis. But enthusiasm for its use has been tempered by unresolved ambiguities about the relevance of magnetic resonance imaging changes to patients' long-term experience of their disease. As Bryan Matthews warned in the early days of magnetic resonance imaging in clinical trials: "It must be hoped that in the process of counting shadows we do not neglect to ask the patients how they feel" [52]. There are many detailed accounts of the role of magnetic resonance imaging in outcome assessment in clinical trials [53–57]. We will confine ourselves here to a few general comments.

Multiple Sclerosis Activity

Gadolinium enhancement is believed to follow breakdown of the blood–brain barrier, which represents an early event in the development of the multiple sclerosis plaque. This and enlargement of T2-weighted white matter lesions are regarded as markers of recent inflammatory activity. As inflammation quietens, so these markers disappear. Demyelination develops; during or after this phase of active inflammation it may remyelinate or persist, being followed by gliosis and axon degeneration resulting in fixed and progressive disabilities, respectively. In relapsing-remitting or secondary progressive multiple sclerosis, gadolinium-enhancing and enlarging T2 lesions occur 10–20 times more frequently than clinically detectable changes. So, for a given number of patients, their use as an outcome measure markedly increases the power of a trial [53]. Furthermore magnetic resonance imaging markers are sensitive, may be fully blinded and provide a permanent record. All these attributes attest to the high degree of rigour of magnetic resonance imaging as a marker for disease activity. Despite its objectivity, controls are still required since magnetic resonance imaging markers of multiple sclerosis activity show a sinusoidal variation over time [58], reflecting the fluctuant clinical expression of the disease. If patients are selected on the basis of high activity, the expected regression to the mean may be misinterpreted as a treatment effect. An unfortunate consequence of using magnetic resonance imaging in treatment trials has been the exclusion of patients with primary progressive forms of the disease, in whom there is a low frequency of magnetic resonance imaging lesions in both the cerebrum and spinal cord.

The main objection to using magnetic resonance imaging markers of multiple sclerosis activity as an outcome measure is on the grounds of relevance. It has yet to be demonstrated that a reduction in these surrogate markers of multiple sclerosis activity has any implications for the subsequent development of disability, however appealing this notion may be intuitively. In pilot studies of new agents, where the individual ethic is dominant, the rigour of magnetic resonance imaging markers of multiple sclerosis activity commends them as outcome measures, not least because they reduce the numbers of patients exposed to a potentially harmful agent. However, in larger studies, which inform changes in clinical practice, they cannot be recommended as primary outcome measures because of disputed relevance.

Radiological Markers of Clinical Disability

The undoubted sensitivity of magnetic resonance imaging led to the hope that changes in magnetic resonance imaging markers would correlate with clinical disability. If this was to be established, then magnetic resonance imaging could become a true *surrogate marker* for disability, and the power of studies would then increase with a fall in the labour of investigating new drugs. Consequently, there has been much interest in examining the relationship between magnetic resonance imaging markers and

disability. The argument can quickly become circular, as the proposed justification for a surrogate marker of disability is the poor quality of clinical scales of disability. A poor correlation between a radiological and clinical marker of disability may therefore simply reflect deficiencies in the clinical scale.

Disability is caused in part by the accumulation of demyelination, which is usually found at sites of gliotic scarring, where axons may also be degenerating. There is no reason to expect the extent of this accumulation to be represented by evidence for inflammatory activity of multiple sclerosis and this illogicality is borne out by the poor correlation of magnetic resonance imaging markers of activity with disability; one study found a significant correlation coefficient of only 0.113 [59]. The total lesion load on T2-weighted scans is taken as an indicator of the extent of gliotic scarring and therefore theoretically is more likely to reflect disability, but in fact there is only a weak correlation – although in the IFNβ-1b trial there was a highly statistically significant correlation coefficient of $r = 0.229$ [12]. Paradoxically, the 1.6 mU dose of IFNβ had a moderate effect on the accumulation of magnetic resonance imaging lesion load and produced a dramatic reduction in new magnetic resonance imaging lesion formation, but this group reached treatment failure earlier than the control group. In the lymphoblastoid interferon trial there was "essentially no agreement between the clinically derived EDSS scores and the magnetic resonance imaging-determined lesion areas" [60].

There are many reasons for the poor correlation between T2 lesion load and clinical disability. There is a surprising fluctuation of T2 lesion load over time in relapsing-remitting patients [61]. Most importantly, radiological lesions are not weighted for the clinical eloquence of their anatomical site; for instance spinal cord lesions account for a disproportionate amount of disability, yet are ignored by most techniques used in treatment trials. Simply measuring spinal cord area, where shrinkage is taken to reflect axonal degeneration, gives a high correlation with clinical disability of $r = -0.7$ [62]. This raises a second reason for the discrepancy between lesion load and disability, namely that irreversible disability may depend much more on axonal degeneration than on demyelination or gliotic scarring measured by T2 lesions. Several novel magnetic resonance imaging techniques have been devised to detect such axon degeneration (reviewed by Miller [55,56]).

Immunological Outcome Variables

The immune system plays a critical role in the pathogenesis of multiple sclerosis. Accordingly many drugs that are tested in clinical trials act immunologically. Two types of immunological outcome variable are regularly encountered and are illustrated by a recent trial of IFNα-2a in multiple sclerosis [63]. IFNα-2a induces MHC class I antibodies and so the serum level of β2-microglobulin, a protein associated with class I, was measured as an in vivo test of the drug's *pharmacological activity* whereas the spontaneous release of IFNγ and tumour necrosis factor alpha (TNFα) from patients' lymphocytes in vitro was taken as a marker of *multiple sclerosis activity*.

Immune Markers of Multiple Sclerosis Activity and Disability

There is no established immune marker of multiple sclerosis activity, which reflects the current knowledge of the immunological mechanisms underlying the disease. Necessarily the *relevance* of all postulated markers is found wanting. Sharief et al. [64,65] have shown that TNFα is raised in serum and cerebrospinal fluid during periods of clinical activity, but this observation has not been confirmed [66]. A consistent finding in multiple sclerosis is the presence of oligoclonal immunoglobulin bands in the cerebrospinal fluid. These have been used as immunological markers in several trials; cyclosporine reduces the rate of intrathecal IgG synthesis [8], whereas this is increased by lymphoblastoid interferon [67]. Unfortunately it is impossible to interpret such results when the pathogenic role of oligoclonal immunoglobulin bands is not fully understood. The biological half-life of inflammatory mediators is usually measured in hours or days at most. Therefore, by analogy with magnetic resonance imaging markers of inflammatory activity, it is unlikely that immune markers would reflect the level of accumulated disability. It is surprising, then, to find a reasonable correlation of serum interleukin-2 levels with disability claimed in one study ($r = -0.5$ and $p = 0.009$) [68].

One futuristic role of immunological markers of multiple sclerosis activity is the prediction of relapses. Several markers are said to rise days or weeks before a clinical attack [69–71] and may conceivably prompt the administration of an agent to abort incipient disease activity. Such ideas should be tested in current therapeutic and natural history studies of multiple sclerosis.

Markers of the Aberrant Immune Profile in Multiple Sclerosis

It is clear that the clinical, radiological and immunological manifestations of multiple sclerosis fluctuate over time, in common with many other autoimmune diseases. The mechanism for this fluctuation is not clear. Perhaps each cycle of immunological activity represents loss of self-tolerance of a self-antigen and then its restoration. Different autoantigens may be involves on each occasion. Whatever the explanation, at some early stage in the pathogenesis of multiple sclerosis there must be a stable fault, a deviant *immune set*, that promotes the subsequent expression of the disease.

By way of example, patients who are allergic to bee or wasp sting. Their deviant immune set is a dramatic over-response to a specific allergen. When these patients; immune cells encounter the responsible allergen in vitro, whatever the clinical state of the patient, a deviant response is seen (in this case over-expression of interleukins IL-4 and IL-10) [72]. This immunological test may then be used to monitor the eficacy of therapy, as it predicts exactly the extent of reaction a patient would have to a sting [73]; if the causative antigen in multiple sclerosis were known, similar experiments could be done. Unfortunately this is not the situation, nor indeed is it clear that there is only one antigen. Early attempts to define the immune set of patients with multiple sclerosis circumvented this problem by measuring the proliferative response of their peripheral blood monuclear cells (PBMCs) to mitogens such as phytohaemagglutinin or pokeweed [74,75]. A more recent sophistication is to analyse the cytokines induced in such systems [76,77]. Brod et al. [78] analysed the response of PBMCs taken from patients treated with IFNβ-1b to the non-specific stimulants, OKT3 and concanavalin A. Their results were conflicting and defy easy interpretation. The relevance of such measurements to inflammatory events in white matter of the central nervous system has to be questioned. Alternatively, investigators may measure antigen-specific responses in multiple sclerosis, having first made an assumption about the identity of the causative autoantigen. For example, in a trial of T cell receptor peptide vaccination, the frequency of PBMCs responsive to myelin basic protein, and the cytokines induced by this protein, were each measured. A shift in lymphocyte phenotype was found from Th1 (pro-inflammatory) to Th2 (anti-inflammatory). The relevance of any observation on myelin basic protein-reactive lymphocytes in multiple sclerosis is undermined by the fact that normal individuals have T cells with similar reactivities [79].

Conclusions

Multiple sclerosis is a common and serious disease. Therefore the collective ethic has relative dominance in trial design, with the individual ethic protected by the principles of non-maleficence and treatment indifference. The licensing of treatments for multiple sclerosis raises questions of the ethics of placebo controls in clinical trials of relpasing-remitting multiple sclerosis. It is clear that, so far, each licensed product is at best partially effective and therefore a physician may reasonably consider the potential benefit of an experimental treatment to be greater. Furthermore, trials can be performed in patients who, though eligible for these treatments, do not receive them, for reasons of treatment drop-out or inadequate drug supply. It should be remembered that the number of patients for whom there are any useful treatments is relatively small. The choice of outcome measure in clinical trials in multiple sclerosis is a conflict between rigour and relevance. In phase III studies, clinical measures must be the primary outcome variable as these are most relevant to the patients' experience of the disease. Unfortunately the varied clinical manifestations of multiple sclerosis can only be expressed in composite or multivariate scales. These lack rigour and so are not suitable for small pilot studies where the individual ethic predominates and the risk to the study population must be minimised. Here magnetic resonance imaging markers are useful, having greater sensitivity and objectivity than clinical measures. The correlation of magnetic resonance imaging markers with clinical scales of disability is poor at present, although this may improve with new radiological techniques. Until our knowledge of the basic immunological mechanisms underlying multiple sclerosis increases, immune markers do not have a role as primary outcome measures in clinical trials in multiple sclerosis.

References

1. Medical Research Council. Streptomycin treatment of tuberculosis. BMJ 1948;769–782.
2. Veterans Administration Study Group. Isoniazid in treatment of multiple sclerosis: report on Veterans Administration Cooperative study. JAMA 1957;163:168–172.
3. Panitch HS, Hirsch RL, Haley AS, Johnson KP. Exacerbations of multiple sclerosis in patients treated with gamma interferon. Lancet 1987;I:893–894.
4. Kurtzke JF, Berlin L. The effects of isoniazid on patients with multiple sclerosis: a preliminary report. Am Rev Tuberc 1954;70:577–592.
5. Khatri BO, McQuillen MP, Hoffmann RG, Harrington GJ, Schmoll D. Plasma exchange in chronic progressive multiple sclerosis: a long-term study. Neurology 1991;41:409–414.
6. Kappos L, Patzold U, Dommasch D, et al. Cyclosporine versus azathioprine in the long-term treatment of multiple sclerosis: results of the German Multicenter Study. Ann Neurol 1988;23:56–63.
7. Weiner HL, Mackin GA, Orav EJ, et al. Intermittent cyclophosphamide pulse therapy in progressive multiple sclerosis: final report of the Northeast Cooperative Multiple Sclerosis Treatment Group. Neurology 1993;43:910–918.
8. Rudge P, Koetsier JC, Mertin J, et al. Randomised double blind controlled trial of cyclosporin in multiple sclerosis. J Neurol Neurosurg Psychiatry 1989;52:559–565.
9. Beauchamp TJ, Childress JF. Principles of Biomedical Ethics. Oxford: Oxford University Press, 1994.
10. Schafer A. The ethics of the randomized clinical trial. N Engl J Med 1982;307:719–724.
11. Weinshenker BG, Issa M, Baskerville J. Meta-analysis of the placebo-treated groups in clinical trials of progressive MS. Neurology 1996;46:1613–1619.
12. Duquette P, Despault L, Knobler RL, et al. Interferon beta-1b in the treatment of multiple sclerosis: final outcome of the randomized controlled trial. Neurology 1995;45:1277–1285.
13. Jacobs LD, Cookfair DL, Rudick RA, et al. Intramuscular interferon beta-1a for disease progression in relapsing multiple sclerosis. Ann Neuro 1996;39:285–294.
14. Johnson KP, Brooks BR, Cohen JA, et al. Copolymer 1 reduces relapse rate and improves disability in relapsing-remitting multiple sclerosis: results of a phase III multicenter, double-blind, placebo-controlled trial. Neurology 1995;45:1268–1276.
15. Weinshenker BG, Rice GP, Noseworthy JH, Carriere W, Baskerville J, Ebers GC. The natural history of multiple sclerosis: a geographically based study. 4. Applications to planning and interpretation of clinical therapeutic trials. Brain 1991;114:1057–1067.
16. Weinshenker BG. The natural history of multiple sclerosis. Neurol Clin 1995;13:119–146.
17. Carter JL, Hafler DA, Dawson DM, Orav J, Weiner HL. Immunosuppression with high-dose IV cyclophosphamide and ACTH in progressive multiple sclerosis: cumulative 6-year experience in 164 patients. Neurology 1988;38:9–14.
18. Kappos L, Heun R, Mertens HG. A 10-year matched-pairs study comparing azathioprine and no immunosuppression in multiple sclerosis. Eur Arch Psychiatry Neurol Sci 1990;240:34–38.
19. Noseworthy JH, Ebers GC, Vandervoort MK, Farquhar RE, Yetisir E, Roberts R. The impact of blinding on the results of a randomized, placebo-controlled multiple sclerosis clinical trial. Neurology 1994;44:16–20.
20. Mauch E, Kornhuber HH, Pfrommer U, Hahnel A, Laufen H, Krapf H. Effective treatment of chronically progressive multiple sclerosis with low-dose cyclophosphamide with minor side-effects. Eur Arch Psychiatry Neurol Sci 1989;238:115–117.
21. Zelen M. A new design for randomized clinical trials. N Engl J Med 1979;300:1242–1245.
22. Curran WJ. Sounding Board. Reasonableness and randomization in clinical trial: fundamental law and government regulation. N Engl J Med 1979;300:1273–1275.
23. Fost N. Sounding Board. Consent as a barrier to research. N Engl J Med 1979;300:1272–1273.
24. Hill AB. Medical ethics and controlled trials. BMJ 1963;I:1043–1049.
25. Compston A. Future prospects for the management of multiple sclerosis. Am Neurol 1994;36(Suppl):S146–50.
26. Nuffield Council on Bioethics. Animal-to-human transplants: the ethics of xenotransplantation. 1996.
27. Review of the guidance on the research use of fetuses and fetal material. Presented to Parliament, July, 1989. CM 762.
28. Collier J. Conflicts between pharmaceutical company largesse and patients' rights. Med Leg J 1992;60:243–250.
29. Anonymous. Doctors as stockholders [abstract]. Newsday 1987;1.
30. Anonymous. Information for authors. N Engl J Med 1989;320:952.
31. Healy B, Campeau L, Gray R, et al. Conflict-of-interest guidelines for a multicenter clinical trial of treatment after

coronary-artery bypass-graft surgery [see comments]. N Engl J Med 1989;320:949–951.

32. Shimm DS, Spece RG, Jr. Industry reimbursement for entering patents into clinical trials: legal and ethical issues. Ann Intern Med 1991;115:148–151.

33. Huth EJ. Conflicts of interest in industry funded research. In: Spece RG, Shimm DS, Buchanan AE, editors. Conflicts of interest in clinical practice and research. New York: Oxford University Press, 1996:389–406.

34. Avorn J, Chen M, Hartley R. Scientific versus commercial sources of influence on the prescribing behavior of physicians. Am J Med 1982;73:4–8.

35. Shimm DS, Spece RG, DiGregorio MD. Conflicts of interest in relationships between. Physicians and the pharmaceutical industry. In: Spece RG, Shimm DS, Buchanan AE, editors. Conflicts of interest in clinical practice and research. New York: Oxford University Press, 1996:321–360.

36. Wolinsky JS. Copolymer 1: a most reasonable alternative therapy for early relapsing-remitting multiple sclerosis with mild disability [editorial; comment]. Neurology 1995;45:1245–1247.

37. Poser CM, Paty DW, Scheinberg L, et al. New diagnostic criteria for multiple sclerosis: guidelines for research protocols. Ann Neurol 1983;13:227–231.

38. McDonald WI. The pathophysiology of multiple sclerosis. In: McDonald WI, Silberberg DH, editors. Multiple sclerosis. London: Butterworth, 1986:112–133.

39. Redford EJ, Kapoor R, Smith KJ. Nitric oxide donors reversibly block axonal conduction: demyelinated axons are especially susceptible. Brain 1997;120:••–••.

40. Rudick R, Antel J, Confavreux C, et al. Clinical outcomes assessment in multiple sclerosis. Ann Neurol 1996;40:469–479.

41. Vandenbark AA, Chou YK, Whitham R, et al. Treatment of multiple sclerosis with T-cell receptor peptides: results of a double-blind pilot trial. Nature Med 1996;2:1109–1115.

42. Wiles CM, Omar L, Swan AV, et al. Total lymphoid irradiation in multiple sclerosis. J Neurol Neurosurg Psychiatry 1994; 57:154–163.

43. Sorensen PS, Wanscher B, Szpirt W, et al. Plasma exchange combined with azathioprine in multiple sclerosis using serial gadolinium-enhanced MRI to monitor disease activity: a randomized single-blind cross-over pilot study. Neurology 1996;46:1620–1625.

44. Goodkin DE, Rudick RA, VanderBrug Medendorp S, et al. Low-dose (7.5 mg) oral methotrexate reduces the rate of progression in chronic progressive multiple sclerosis [see comments]. Ann Neurol 1995;37:30–40.

45. Cutter GR, Baier ML, Rudick RA, Cookfair DL, Fischer JS, Petkau J, et al. Development of a multiple sclerosis functional composite as a clinical trial outcome measure. Brain 1999 May;122 (Pt 5):871–882.

46. Tourtellotte WW, Haerer AF, Simpson JF, Kuzma JW, Sikovski J. Quantitative neurological testing. I. A battery of tests designed to evaluate in part the neurological function of patients with multiple sclerosis and its use in a therapeutic trial. Ann N Y Acad Sci 1965;122:480–505.

47. Kurtzke JF. On the evaluation of disability in multiple sclerosis. Neurology 1961;11:686–694.

48. Kurtzke JF. Further notes on disability evaluation in multiple sclerosis, with scale modifications. Neurology 1965;15:654–661.

49. Steck AJ, Regli F, Ochsner F, Gauthier G. Cyclosporine versus azathioprine in the treatment of multiple sclerosis: 12-month clinical and immunological evaluation. Eur Neurol 1990;30:224–228.

50. Noseworthy JH. Clinical scoring methods for multiple sclerosis. Ann Neurol 1994;36(Suppl):S80–5.

51. Mumford CJ, Compston A. Problems with rating scales for multiple sclerosis: a novel approach – the CAMBS score. J Neurol 1993;240:209–215.

52. Matthews WB. Treatment of multiple sclerosis. In: Matthews WB, editor. McAlpine's multiple sclerosis. Edinburgh. Churchill Livingstone, 1991:257.

53. Miller DH, Barkhof F, Berry I, Kappos L, Scotti G, Thompson AJ. Magnetic resonance imaging in monitoring the treatment of multiple sclerosis: concerted action guidelines [see comments]. J Neurol Neurosurg Psychiatry 1991;54:683–688.

54. Miller DH, Albert PS, Barkhof F, et al. Guidelines for the use of magnetic resonance techniques in monitoring the treatment of multiple sclerosis. US National MS Society Task Force. Ann Neurol 1996;39:6–16.

55. Barkhof F, Filippi M, Miller DH, Tofts P, Kappos L, Thompson AJ. Strategies for optimizing MRI techniques aimed at monitoring disease activity in multiple sclerosis treatment trials. J Neurol 1997;244:76–84.

56. Evans AC, Frank JA, Antel J, Miller DH. The role of MRI in clinical trials of multiple sclerosis comparison of image processing techniques Ann Neurol 1997;41:125–132.

57. Filippi M, Horsfield MA, Tofts PS, Barkhof F, Miller DH. Quantitative assessment of MRI lesion load in monitoring the evolution of multiple sclerosis. Brain 1995;118:1601–1612.

58. Frank JA, Stone LA, Smith ME, Albert PS, Maloni H, McFarland HF. Serial contrast-enhanced magnetic resonance imaging in patients with early relapsing-remitting multiple sclerosis: implications for treatment trials. Ann Neurol 1994;36(Suppl):S86–90.

59. Filippi M, Paty DW, Kappos L, et al. Correlations between changes in disability and T2-weighted brain MRI activity in multiple sclerosis: a follow-up study. Neurology 1995;45:255–260.

60. Kastrukoff LF, Oger JJ, Hashimoto SA, et al. Systemic lymphoblastoid interferon therapy in chronic progressive multiple sclerosis. I. Clinical and MRI evaluation. Neurology 1990;40:479–486.

61. Stone LA, Albert PS, Smith ME, et al. Changes in the amount of diseased white matter over time in patients with relapsing-remitting multiple sclerosis. Neurology 1995;45:1808–1814.

62. Losseff NA, Webb SL, O'Riordan JI, et al. Spinal cord atrophy and disability in multiple sclerosis: a new reproducible and sensitive MRI method with potential to monitor disease progression. Brain 1996;119:701–708.

63. Durelli L, Bongioanni MR, Ferrero B, et al. Interferon alpha-2a treatment of relapsing-remitting multiple sclerosis: disease activity resumes after stopping treatment. Neurology 1996;47:123–129.

64. Sharief MK, Thompson EJ. In vivo relationship of tumor necrosis factor-alpha to blood–brain barrier damage in patients with active multiple sclerosis. J Neuroimmunol 1992;38:27–33.

65. Sharief MK, Hentges R. Association between tumor necrosis factor-alpha and disease progression in patients with multiple sclerosis [see comments]. N Engl J Med 1991;325:467–472.

66. Peter JB, Boctor FN, Tourtellotte WW. Serum and CSF levels of IL-2, sIL-2R, TNF-alpha, and IL-1beta in chronic progressive multiple sclerosis: expected lack of clinical utility Neurology 1991;41:121–123.

67. Kastrukoff LF, Oger JJ, Tourtellotte WW, Sacks SL, Berkowitz J, Paty DW. Systemic lymphoblastoid interferon therapy in chronic progressive multiple sclerosis. II. Immunologic evaluation. Neurology 1991;41:1936–1941.

68. Trotter JL, Clifford DB, McInnis JE, et al. Correlation of immunological studies and disease progression in chronic progressive multiple sclerosis. Ann Neurol 1989;25:172–178.

69. Beck J, Rondot P, Catinot L, Falcoff E, Kirchner H, Wietzerbin J. Increased production of interferon gamma and tumor necrosis factor precedes clinical manifestation in multiple sclerosis: Do cytokines trigger off exacerbations? Acta Neurol Scand 1988;78:318–323.

70. Link J, Soderstrom M, Ljungdahl A, et al. Organ-specific autoantigens induce interferon-gamma and interleukin-4 mRNA expression in mononuclear cells in multiple sclerosis and myasthenia gravis. Neurology 1994;44:728-734.

71. Link J, Fredrikson S, Soderstrom M, et al. Organ-specific autoantigens induce transforming growth factor-beta mRNA expression in mononuclear cells in multiple sclerosis and myasthenia gravis. Ann Neurol 1994;35:197–203.

72. Daser A, Meissner N, Herz U, Renz H. Role and modulation of T-cell cytokines in allergy. Curr Opin Immunol 1995;7:762–770.

73. McHugh SM, Deighton J, Stewart AG, Lachmann PJ, Ewan PW. Bee venom immunotherapy induces a shift in cytokine responses from a TH-2 to a TH-1 dominant pattern: comparison of rush and conventional immunotherapy. Clin Exp Allergy 1995;25:828–838.

74. Hafler DA, Weiner HL. Immunosuppression with monoclonal antibodies in multiple sclerosis. Neurology 1988;38:42–47.

75. Hafler DA, Fallis RJ, Dawson DM, Schlossman SF, Reinherz EL, Weiner HL. Immunologic responses of progressive multiple sclerosis patients treated with an anti-T-cell monoclonal antibody, anti-T12. Neurology 1986;36:777–784.

76. Glabinski A, Mirecka M, Pokoca L. Tumor necrosis factor alpha but not lymphotoxin is overproduced by blood mononuclear cells in multiple sclerosis. Acta Neurol Scand 1995;91:276–279.

77. Navikas V, He B, Link J, et al. Augmented expression of tumour necrosis factor-alpha and lymphotoxin in mononuclear cells in multiple sclerosis and optic neuritis. Brain 1996;119:213–223.

78. Brod SA, Marshall GD Jr, Henninger EM, Sriram S, Khan M, Wolinsky JS. Interferon-beta(1b) treatment decreases tumor necrosis factor-alpha and increases interleukin-6 production in multiple sclerosis. Neurology 1996;46:1633–1638.

79. Pette M, Fujita K, Kitze B, et al. Myelin basic protein-specific T lymphocyte lines from MS patients and healthy individuals. Neurology 1990;40:1770–1776.

31. Multiple Sclerosis: Study Design, Sample Sizes and Pitfalls

B.G. Weinshenker and J.H. Noseworthy

Introduction

Rapid growth in the number, scale and quality of clinical trials in multiple sclerosis (MS) has occurred over the last decade. The recent surge of interest has resulted from a number of developments. Firstly, basic scientific inquiry in such areas as cytokine research, T cell receptor gene recombination and adhesion molecule interactions has suggested novel methods of treatment, including the use of immunoregulatory cytokines (e.g. interferon beta, transforming growth factor beta), T cell or T cell receptor peptide vaccination, and monoclonal antibodies to adhesion cell antigens expressed on the surface of lymphocytes and endothelial cells so as to block their interaction [1]. Secondly, a certain degree of optimism has developed following the report of positive results in three phase III trials of therapeutic agents [2–4], which have now been demonstrated to reduce attacks. One agent, interferon beta-la (Avonex), reduced short-term progression of neurological impairment as determined by change in terms of the Expanded Disability Status Scale (EDSS). Finally, rapid advances in magnetic resonance (MR) technology have provided a sensitive, objective, quantitative, and easily blind method for detecting treatment effects in phase I and II trials in a fraction of the time necessary for a definitive phase III clinical trial. MR technology has been proposed and widely accepted to be the primary outcome of choice for screening potential therapeutic agents for efficacy in phase I and II clinical trials [5].

However, many limitations exist in the application of these advances to clinical trials in MS. The etiology of MS is unknown, and the relevance of many observations made in experimental models, such as experimental allergic encephalomyelitis (EAE), remains uncertain. Numerous examples exist of agents, effective in EAE and other animal models, that have not been shown to be effective in MS. MS is an unpredictable disease, that evolves over decades. The relevance of treatment effects over the short term is unknown insofar as it might predict a long-term clinical benefit ("predictive validity"). Finally, the primary clinical outcome measure for long-term phase III clinical trials, the EDSS, is discontinuous, nonquantitative and somewhat insensitive. Furthermore, strategies to evaluate agents which might be effective for other therapeutic settings, such as treatment of acute attacks and reversal of fixed neurological deficits, are in early developmental stages. Designs for clinical trials for symptomatic treatments are somewhat better defined and are generally similar to strategies for symptomatic treatment in other diseases.

In this chapter, we will first classify clinical trial strategies in use for MS and briefly review important elements of study design. We will then critically discuss the pitfalls inherent in basic elements of clinical trial design in MS, including patient selection, choice of primary outcome, choice of a control group and specification of trial duration. Most of the discussion will be dedicated to clinical trials of agents designed to prevent relapses of MS and/or progression of impairment, as this strategy has attracted the most attention to date.

Classification

MS clinical trials are best classified according to the therapeutic goal or hypothesis that is being addressed. These therapeutic goals emerge from our understanding of the natural history and pathogenesis of the disease. First, we will summarize knowledge of the natural history of MS [6].

The temporal course of MS has been the major method of its classification. A recent, widely accepted classification scheme has been proposed by Lublin et al. [7]. The majority of patients with MS initially suffer from acute relapses of neurological disability

371

which can affect one or a number of neurological functional systems, such as vision, strength, coordination and bladder/bowel function. Approximately 55% of MS attacks result in mild neurological dysfunction and 45% in moderate to severe dysfunction [2]. Most attacks resolve to a large degree, many virtually completely, with or without treatment. However, an important minority of attacks leave major disability in their wake. The relapse frequency is highly variable but tends to decline over time. The majority of MS patients eventually develop progressive neurological disability without remission (secondary progressive), an average of 10 years after the first acute attack of MS. The reason the temporal profile of MS converts from relapsing-remitting to a progressive course remains poorly defined, although the best evidence from MR studies is that the number of inflammatory events detected by gadolinium-enhancing MR lesions is actually greater in patients with secondary progressive MS. Progressive axonal loss occurs both in lesional and nonlesional tissue as detected by declining MR spectroscopy-determined axonal markers such as *N*-acetylaspartate [8].

Approximately 15% of MS patients do not experience attacks but present with an insidiously developing neurological condition (primary progressive), most commonly manifest as a chronic progressive myelopathy but occasionally as a progressive cerebellar syndrome or a progressive cognitive decline. The patients who present with a chronic progressive myelopathy, while frequently manifesting MR evidence of inflammatory demyelination, generally have fewer MR lesions than patients with relapsing-remitting or secondary progressive MS and have less histological evidence of inflammation at autopsy [6]. These recent findings have led investigators to segregate this subgroup of MS patients from clinical trials for which patients with secondary progressive MS are eligible, because the pathophysiology may differ in patients with primary progressive MS sufficiently to result in a different treatment response to anti-inflammatory medications. This has not been formally addressed, but one uncontrolled study suggests differential responsiveness to global immunosuppression in patients with primary progressive MS [9].

Finally, MS patients are subject to a number of disease-related complications including fatigue and spasticity which require symptomatic treatment. Symptomatic treatments have also been the targets of clinical trials in MS.

The following is a classification of clinical trials in MS by therapeutic goal:

1. Treatment of attacks.
2. Treatment of established and fixed neurological deficits.
3. "Prevention" of MS following a monosymptomatic presentation.
4. Prevention of attacks in established clinically definite MS.
5. Prevention or slowing of progression of neurological disability.
6. Symptomatic treatments.

Each of these strategies will be discussed. The attention paid to each of these strategies by clinical investigators of MS has varied considerably, for several reasons:

1. Adequate treatment is available for some of the clinical situations but not others; spontaneous remission limits the need for additional treatments for some clinical situations, and results in insufficient power when a new treatment must outperform an established treatment that is effective.
2. The availability of promising treatments is limited for some of the therapeutic goals, in large part because the mechanisms to restore normal tissue architecture are unknown, or limited by other tissue pathology, such as gliosis.
3. Pathophysiological studies which support a role of autoimmunity have been the major focus of attention of research on the etiology and pathogenesis of MS over the last 20–30 years; this approach has led to a major interest in long-term anti-inflammatory and immunosuppressive treatments that are most applicable to prevention of attacks and preventing or slowing progression of disability.
4. Some goals have proved easier to attain than others and have more frequently produced a positive result; for example, it has generally proved easier to reduce attack frequency than to limit progression of disability.

Trials to decrease attack frequency and limit progression of disability have dominated MS clinical trials and will be discussed in greater detail in the next section. In this section, we will deal with the other types of clinical trials.

Treatment of Attacks

Attacks of MS are generally believed to result from ingress of lymphocytes and macrophages across a disrupted blood–brain barrier. These events are inflammatory and are mediated by combinations of cellular and humoral components, including cytokines, antibodies and complement. The therapeutic agents studied have generally had anti-inflammatory properties (e.g., corticosteroids) or are believed to deplete circulating humoral components which lead to increased blood–brain barrier permeability or cellular cytotoxicity and maintenance of the inflammatory response (e.g., plasma exchange). A number of new therapeutic strategies are currently under study, including agents which inhibit inflammatory cell traffic across the blood–brain barrier by interfering with endothelial–lymphocyte receptor interactions, and metalloproteinase inhibitors, which inhibit enzymes secreted by inflammatory cells to enhance their ability to penetrate the endothelial basement membrane.

Most relapses of MS remit spontaneously. Furthermore, steroids and ACTH are accepted treatments for acute attacks of MS. Accordingly, it is difficult to show a benefit of a new treatment given the generally favorable outcome of the natural history of acute attacks and results of current treatment. However, patients who suffer attacks in the setting of progressive MS, for which the results of treatment are less favorable, and patients who suffer steroid-refractory attacks, might be targeted in clinical trials. Recently completed and continuing clinical trials aimed at treatment of attacks have been designed to address the following specific hypotheses:

1. High-dose intravenous methylprednisolone results in superior (faster, more consistent) recovery than standard ACTH treatment [10,11].
2. Plasma exchange salvages patients with severe attacks who have failed treatment with a standard course of steroid therapy; another study examined plasma exchange as adjunctive treatment for acute attacks of MS [12].

Eligibility criteria are determined by the therapeutic goal. A randomized parallel group design is standard. A current study at the Mayo Clinic in patients with severe steroid-refractory attacks uses a crossover design to make the active treatment available to all patients, considering the rather desperate clinical situation of many of the participants; this design requires that the primary endpoint be evaluable by the end of the 2 week period prior to crossover. A potential difficulty with the crossover design in this setting is carryover effect into the second treatment period.

The optimum outcome measure for this type of trial is not well defined in the literature. The EDSS is the most commonly used endpoint. While the EDSS reflects the usual sequence of disabilities that develop in the context of progressive MS, it is insensitive to many manifestations of acute attacks of MS. The neurological involvement in the context of acute attacks is less predictable than it is for progressive MS, and is more in keeping with a random distribution of lesions throughout the neuraxis. For example, an attack with severe upper extremity involvement

may not be well reflected by change in the patient's EDSS, especially when the patient's ambulation is not also compromised by the relapse. At the Mayo Clinic we have used the targeted neurological deficit (TND) as the primary outcome in the study of plasma exchange in steroid-refractory severe attacks of demyelinating disease, reasoning that the most sensitive outcome is likely to be one that addresses the dominant neurological deficits(s). Usually, one deficit is dominant, but up to two may be specified in this trial. The degree of improvement may be measured semiquantitatively on the individual outcome scale appropriate to the TND, or may be categorized into mild, moderate or marked. For some expensive or toxic treatments, less than moderate improvement is deemed to be of little clinical interest.

Many trials have insufficient statistical power to demonstrate a treatment effect. There is a dearth of data about the natural history of recovery from attacks of MS. This complicates attempts to accurately estimate sample size for clinical trials. The natural history data of Kurtzke from World War II US veterans [13] are valuable, but applicable only to attacks in the early course of disease. Furthermore, in this study, recovery was expressed only in terms of the EDSS, with its inherent limitations as an outcome measure for attacks of MS, as discussed above. Other studies have suggested that recovery is less satisfactory in individuals with progressive MS who generally have MS of longer duration. Other probable determinants of the likelihood of recovery from attacks include the duration over which the attack evolves and the functional systems involved. In general, however, data which can be used for stratification or for analysis of covariation in the final analysis of the outcome are available in the literature.

The availability of adequate therapy precludes a placebo-controlled design, unless patients have failed standard therapy. A recent study in progress includes a placebo control design but allows for rescue treatment in the event patients fail. The decision to rescue is hard to standardize and control, particularly in a multicenter trial, however, and represents a difficulty of design.

Treatment of Fixed Neurological Deficit

The process of recovery from an attack of MS is rapid in the first few days and months. Steroids "seal" the blood-brain barrier as evidenced by a rapid reduction or elimination of gadolinium enhancement. Removal of inflammatory cells is probably a relatively early event. Subsequent repair likely involves physiological processes such as synthesis and spreading of depolarizing sodium channels beyond their normal location at the nodes of Ranvier, and reparative processes, especially remyelination. There is substantial pathological evidence that remyelination occurs in experimental models of immunologically mediated demyelination as well as in MS.

Trials directed at improvement of fixed neurological deficits suffer from a lack of data on which neurological outcome measures might be expected to improve in humans. Even in rodents, where remyelination can be shown histologically, success is not always evident in improvement of neurological dysfunction, but may be manifest only as slowing of the progression of neurological deficit (M. Rodriguez, Mayo Clinic, personal communication). Strategies to promote remyelination include growth factors, oligodenroglial transplants and antibody-induced remyelination [14,15].

Very few clinical trials have addressed recovery of fixed neurological deficits. Among the deficits that neurologists are best able to quantitate is visual function. In an uncontrolled trial, patients with fixed visual deficits were reported to experience significant and persistent improvement in visual acuity after treatment with intravenous immunoglobulin [16]. Investigators at the Mayo Clinic have embarked on a parallel group design, randomized, controlled clinical trial of intravenous immunoglobulin. Patients with a fixed visual deficit with a visual acuity of 20/40 or worse are eligible. The primary outcome measure is improvement in visual acuity (logMar) at 6 months [14,15].

A similar trial of intravenous immunoglobulin in patients with recently acquired (within 18 months) fixed motor deficit of at least 3 months' duration in MS patients deemed to have nonprogressive deficits and demonstrated to have a measurably stable deficit is being conducted at the Mayo Clinic. The primary outcome is the sensitive reproducible measure of quantitative strength in targeted neurological muscles as measured in a biomechanics laboratory. The data can be normalized to percent of normal strength. Other outcome measures include blinded assessment of videotaped limb-coordination tests as well as more standard clinical rating scales and functional measures such as the 9-hole peg test and box-and-blocks test [15].

"Prevention" of MS after Monosymptomatic MS-like Events

It is now well recognized that many, if not most, individuals with an isolated demyelinating event will subsequently develop further events which will lead to a clinically definite diagnosis of MS, albeit at a very variable interval from the index attack. Magnetic resonance imaging (MRI) studies clearly show that the risk of "conversion" to clinically definite MS is predictable based on whether there are lesions on the MRI scan of the head and on the number of T2-weighted lesions [5].

A follow-up of patients in the Optic Neuritis Treatment Trial [17] suggested that conversion to clinically definite MS was less frequent in those who received intravenous methylprednisolone than in patients receiving placebo. This observation suggested that conversion to MS might be "preventable" (see more detailed discussion under the subheading "Control Group"). One should point out that the evidence for dissemination by MRI was present in the majority of individuals, and it can reasonably be argued that the delay observed was only in the arbitrary requirement of observing two clinical attacks prior to confirming a diagnosis of MS. Unfortunately, this observation about the possible effectiveness of intravenous methylprednisolone has not been and is not likely to be the subject of a confirmatory clinical trial. However, this strategy has been adopted in the CHAMPS (Controlled Trial of High-Risk Subjects in a Multiple Sclerosis Prevention Study) [18]. Patients experiencing a first episode of demyelinating disease that is isolated to either one optic nerve, the brainstem or the spinal cord, who have an MRI scan revealing lesions consistent with inflammatory demyelination and who have been treated with intravenous methylprednisolone within 14 days, were randomized to treatment with interferon beta-1a (Avonex) or placebo for 3 years. This followed on the positive study which revealed that interferon beta-1a reduced the attack frequency in patients with relapsing-remitting MS.

Symptomatic Therapies

The symptoms of MS which have been studied in controlled clinical trials include fatigue, spasticity and cerebellar tremor. In these trials, the measures are specifically targeted to these neurological problems. A common approach to enhance power and reduce the impact of interindividual differences in symptom rating is to use a crossover design with an intervening washout period. A somewhat different strategy has been used to evaluate short-acting agents which act on depolarizing sodium channels, such as 3,4-diaminopyridine and 4-aminopyridine, that might reasonably be expected to have a short-term benefit on multiple diverse MS-related neurological deficits. Studies of aminopyridine have used a number of subjective and objective rating scales including blind assessments of maximum voluntary isometric contraction, grip strength (hand-held dynamometer) and blind assessments of videotaped examination.

Fatigue studies naturally involve subjective outcome measures. Global rating scales and visual analogue scales are commonly used. Several fatigue scales have been developed [19,20] which have been designed for serial follow-up of MS-related fatigue. Crossover studies between active drug and placebo, or two different active drugs with an intervening washout, allow patients to serve as their own control and represent the standard for this type of clinical trial.

Spasticity trials most often use the Ashworth Scale [21] as primary outcome, but disability scales (such as the Functional Independence Measures of FIM) [22] are important secondary measures. Physiological measurement including H-reflex [23] and pendulum biomechanics measures have been employed in some studies [24].

Studies evaluating tremor have employed ordinal ataxia scales as well as sensitive measures of tremor which are applied in motion analysis laboratories. Many agents appear to have demonstrable efficacy in reducing tremor without significant functional improvement; hence, disability and quality-of-life scales [25] are critical secondary outcomes in such trials.

Although neurogenic bladder and bowel difficulties are common in MS, no randomized clinical trials have been conducted in this area, to our knowledge. Amitriptyline has been shown to be effective for pseudobulbar hyperemotionality in MS in a crossover trial [26].

Prevention of Attacks and/or Slowing of Progression

The two therapeutic goals of prevention of attacks and/or slowing of progression are grouped together for the purpose of discussion, as most agents which are considered for one of these goals have been or might be reasonably considered for the other as well. These goals have been the target of most phase III randomized clinical trials.

The therapeutic strategies that have been or are currently being considered are diverse and have been summarized by Sriram [1]. A detailed discussion is beyond the scope of this chapter. The strategies can basically be grouped as follows:

1. Prevention of sensitization of T cells, or desensitization of T cells – e.g. selective inactivation of T cell receptors of encephalitogenic T cell clones by vaccination, modulation of T cell response with altered peptide ligands; monoclonal antibodies to co-stimulatory peptides on the surface of antigen presenting cells and lymphocytes.

2. Elimination of T cells, especially helper T cells – e.g. anti-CD4 monoclonal antibodies.
3. Reduction of lymphocyte traffic across the blood–brain barrier – e.g. corticosteroids; matrix metalloproteinase inhibitors; anti-adhesion molecule monoclonal antibodies.
4. Suppression of T cell function – e.g. global immunosuppressants; cyclosporin.
5. Alteration of cytokine milieu or profile – e.g. monoclonal antibodies to proinflammatory cytokines; immunoregulatory or immunosuppressives cytokines; inhibitors of cytokine production; therapeutic agents capable of switching from Th1 to Th2 cytokine profile.

Two different approaches have been developed to establish efficacy, which will be separately discussed. The first, which is primarily applicable to preliminary or pilot phase I and II randomized clinical trials, involves a MR-based primary outcome; the duration of such a trial is generally 6–12 months. The second approach, which applies to phase III "pivotal" clinical trials, involves a clinical primary outcome; the duration of such a trial is generally 2 or 3 years.

Phase I and II Clinical Trials

In phase I and II randomized clinical trials, the goal is to screen agents for efficacy. Given their greater sensitivity to subclinical disease activity [27,28] and the presence of significant, though imperfect, correlation with clinical deficits in MS [29,30], MR measurements have been proposed as the primary outcome measure. MR measurements, in addition to sensitivity, have the advantage of greater potential for successful blinding and probably less susceptibility to placebo effect.

The trial designs that have been considered are of two general types: crossover and parallel group design. As most MS therapies have significant potential for carryover activity, a crossover between treatment and control treatment is generally not valid; therefore, there is generally a 6 month "run-in" (no treatment) period and a 6 month treatment period. The primary outcome measure is gadolinium-enhancing lesions and/or new or active T2-weighted lesions. Most lesions which develop over prospective follow-up appear to show gadolinium enhancement if follow-up occurs with sufficient frequency (approximately once per month [28]); however, a significant minority of lesions show no enhancement with frequent serial MRI scans at approximately 1 month intervals [31]. T2-weighted image "burden of disease" or lesion volume is relegated to an optional secondary outcome measure. Given the lack of a control group, the National MS Society Task Force on

MRI Outcome Measures [5] has advised that a phase III study be considered based on the results of a crossover study only if there has been an 80% decrease in the number of lesions on treatment compared with baseline run-in. A decrease of 50–80% in the number of enhancing or new lesions should be further evaluated in a parallel group MRI-based phase I or II study. The sample size for this type of study has been estimated based on "bootstrapping techniques" that involve simulation of data in untreated cohorts based on natural history MRI data in patients who would have been eligible for these studies. Miller et al. [5] cautioned that the natural history data for MRI studies are limited and should be regarded as approximate guidelines. For a crossover design with a 6 month baseline run-in and a 6 month treatment period, 10–15 patients are sufficient to detect a 50% reduction in numbers of new or enhancing lesions.

In a parallel group design, patients are randomly assigned to treatment or placebo after a run-in period of 1–6 months. A longer run-in period or a second-tier selection criterion based on activity observed during the run-in period can enhance the power of the study. Forty patients (2 groups of 20 patients) or 80 patients (2 groups of 40 patients) are required if the run-in period is 6 months or 1 month, respectively.

Phase III Clinical Trials

Phase III clinical trials in either relapsing-remitting or secondary progressive MS are mammoth undertakings. They are generally multicenter trials. When powered to detect a clinical effect on relapse rate, sample sizes in the 200–400 range followed over 2–3 years are necessary. When powered to detect an effect on disability, the target sample size is closer to 700–1000 patients followed over 3 years. The budget of such trials to detect an effect of disability in North America is currently in the $10 million range or greater.

The general approach that has been followed is usually a parallel design clinical trial. Most randomized clinical trials have been placebo controlled in the "modern era", but the appropriateness of a placebo group is controversial, especially for relapsing-remitting MS. The is discussed in detail in the section "Control Group" below (see also Chapter 30). For agents being evaluated for efficacy in secondary progressive and primary progressive MS, placebo control groups are appropriate.

Patients are usually targeted for enrollment because of active MS. Typical entry criteria are two or more attacks in the previous 2 years for trials that target attack rate, and deterioration by 1 or more points on the EDSS in the previous 2 years in trials aimed at slowing progression of disability. More restrictive entry criteria have not enhanced the power of a clinical trial by selecting patients more likely to deteriorate. More restrictive criteria also make accrual more difficult, limit generalizability of the trial and increase the phenomenon of "regression to the mean". Regression to the mean refers to an apparent decrease in disease activity resulting simply from the fact that patients selected for an unusual degree of disease activity are more likely to return to the mean than to continue their unusually high degree of disease activity.

Patients with primary progressive MS have recently been excluded from trials targeting patients with progressive MS. Patients with primary progressive MS have relatively few lesions on MRI scans of the head and very few enhancing lesions [32]. There is less evidence of inflammation at autopsy. These characteristics have led many investigator to speculate that such patients may be less likely to respond to anti-inflammatory or immunosuppressive treatments [6].

There are advantages and disadvantages of multi-limb trials evaluating different doses. Multi-limb trials increase the required sample size and, consequently, the cost of a trial. However, if the drug is not well tolerated at one dose and this leads to excessive drop-outs in the high-dose limb, efficacy at lower doses may still be discerned. Furthermore, demonstrating dose responsiveness may further point to efficacy. For example, in the interferon beta-1b (Betaseron) study, an MRI benefit was seen at both active doses, though a significant clinical benefit was seen only at the higher dose [29].

The optimal duration of a study is 2 years for a trial evaluating relapse frequency as the primary outcome and 3 years for trials evaluating progression rate. The limitations inherent in a shorter duration of follow-up will be discussed in further detail in the section on "Pitfalls".

The primary outcome in studies targeting attack frequency is the annualized relapse rate, which should be based on the total experience of patients in the study. The primary outcome in studies targeting disability is generally the proportion of treatment failures or time-to-treatment failure by survival analysis. Mean change in EDSS is less than optimal because of the ordinal characteristics of the EDSS and because inconsequential variation in scores from visit to visit within the range of inter-rater variability may obscure a real treatment difference because they are averaged into the mean change in EDSS. The degree of deterioration considered clinically significant should be defined a priori for each baseline EDSS level. Difficulties inherent in staying times at different levels of the EDSS will be discussed later. In recent clinical trials, deterioration by 0.5 EDSS points is accepted as meeting the criterion of treatment failure when the baseline EDSS score is 6.0 or greater.

MRI is generally relegated to a secondary-outcome measure [5]. The optimal MRI measures remain controversial, but, generally, lesion burden on T2-weighted images is standard. Other parameters considered include lesion area of dark white matter on T1-weighted images ("black holes"), because these lesions may correlate better with disability than T2-weighted lesions [33]. Often a subset of patients in a phase III randomized clinical trial is assigned to have frequent (every 3 months) MRI scans to determine the effect of the therapeutic agent on the dynamic disease activity. MR spectroscopy and magnetic transfer imaging remain research-level methods, not yet regularly applied in MS clinical trials, though they each have characteristics which may make them superior in defining clinically relevant change.

Two neurologists generally evaluate patients to enhance blinding; this measure is discussed later. The usual frequency of evaluation is every 3 months for clinical assessments and once a year for MRI assessments. Neuropsychological test batteries sensitive to MS-associated cognitive dysfunction and quality-of-life assessment have become standard in phase III randomized clinical trials.

Interim analyses are generally conducted once during the course of a 3 year trial, though they do compromise the power of the study when conducted for efficacy. Several stopping rules for efficacy have been proposed [34] but, given the unpredictable course of MS, we believe that the most conservative approach for stopping a trial for efficacy is best. This is particularly true considering that the predictive validity of the primary-outcome measures remain uncertain.

Patient retention is often problematic in MS clinical trials. As patients often perceive worsening before the physician can document failure, every effort must be made to encourage participation until patients satisfy the treatment failure definition on two successive visits ("sustained change"). Accordingly, the treatment failure definition must be convincing, but not so extreme that patients are unreasonably expected to adhere to the protocol when it is clear to both them and the physician that they are failures.

The primary analysis generally evaluates the annualized attack rate or time-to-treatment failure. An intent-to-treat analysis is required. The complex relationships between relapse rate and EDSS worsening and the importance of performing an intent-to-treat analysis are considered in detail in the section on "Pitfalls".

The importance of secondary outcome measures in supporting the results of the primary outcome measure is also discussed later. MRI measurements, being perhaps the least susceptible to unblinding and the most objective and sensitive measures, provide strong support for a clinical endpoint, when the results of these studies are also positive. However, while MS disease activity is generally believed to be associated with MRI changes, it is important to recall that some agents may exert important clinical effects though they do not influence breaches of the blood–brain barrier, and their benefit may not be reflected in MR activity. A relation between disability and MR lesion volume likely exists [29,30] but it is undoubtedly weak and imperfect.

Pitfalls

Many of the problems inherent in clinical design and conduct are common to the investigation of other chronic illnesses. Others are particularly troublesome in this extraordinarily unpredictable disease.

Patient Selection

With the start of any clinical trial, investigators feel pressured to enroll patients in timely fashion. Whenever possible, it is best to rely on one's personal records to avoid the inherent problems when patients present for the first time hoping to fulfill enrollment criteria. Enrollment criteria are generally based on baseline disability and evidence of recent disease activity (e.g., two or more attacks in the previous 2 years and/or a change in the EDSS of at least 1 point over the preceding 2 years). Eligibility criteria are generally restrictive to focus the treatment to a particular subset of patients. With increasing patient awareness of enrollment criteria, some patients may embellish aspects of their history that emphasize their eligibility, including clinical features that may have escaped the attention of physicians who have documented their course previously. Enrolling physicians may be prone to the same tendency to embellish criteria for eligibility in prospective candidates, pressured by the need to identify patients for study. Clinical trials which target patients with recent disease activity (e.g., frequent relapses, abundant MRI activity) are at particular risk for these patients to "regress to the mean" after enrollment, which is problematic when the power of the study is predicated on pre-enrollment disease activity. This tendency is now broadly recognized by MS clinical trialists and is one of the major reasons why a control group is essential. The widespread use of the Internet has facilitated communication about clinical trial research opportunities but has also enhanced discussion between patients about such diverse topics as eligibility criteria, adverse effects from study drugs, personality traits of individual investigators, opinions about various treatment centers, and variability in treatment opportunities available nationwide.

Clinical trialists must be aware of the importance of disease duration and course. Typically, relapse rates fall with disease duration. This is particularly well documented to occur in the first years after diagnosis [35]. Therefore, treatment and control groups should be well matched for disease duration. Natural history studies have demonstrated that patients are not evenly distributed across all ranges of the EDSS [36]. At any one time, a relatively small percentage of patients meet the criterion of an EDSS score of between 4 and 5.5, a common target for clinical trials of MS. Treatment groups must be matched for EDSS scores at enrollment, as the probability of further progression is determined in large part by the current EDSS score. In a large natural history study, Weinshenker et al. [37] demonstrated that the length of time spent at various levels of the EDSS by patients who were observed to progress varied by as much as three-fold (e.g., [E]DSS 1.0: 4.09 years ± 0.19 SEM; [E]DSS 3.0: 1.95 ± 0.11 SEM; [E]DSS 4.0 and 5.0: 1.2 ± 0.06 SEM; [E]DSS 6.0: 3.06 ± 0.17 SEM). While differences in staying times at different levels of the EDSS may be an artifact of the way MS impairment is quantitated by the scale, the EDSS is the "gold standard" in MS clinical trials for the present. Studies targeting patients with entry EDSS scores of 3–5.5 will be more difficult to enroll than those which include patients with EDSS scores of 1–6. Conversely, sample size estimates will need to be adjusted (increased) for trials with considerable numbers of patients with these more stable baseline EDSS scores. Petkau et al. [34] have stressed the importance of comparing post-randomization behavior stratified on the EDSS at enrollment to help address this problem of a discontinuous, unevenly distributed outcome measure. The ordinal nature of the EDSS prevents the use of standard analyses of covariance to control for the effect of baseline EDSS on outcome measures.

Primary Outcome

Perhaps the most important element in the design of any clinical trial is the choice of the primary outcome measure. Clearly, this variable must reflect the underlying hypothesis of the treatment trial. As others have emphasized, the primary measure should be valid (e.g., measure what it is supposed to measure); reliable (i.e., reproducible on repeated measures); indicative of an important "distant"

change in disease course (i.e., "predictive validity"); applicable across a wide range of disabilities and avoid "ceiling and basement" effects (i.e., sensitive to improvement or worsening); noninvasive; easy to perform; and, if possible, relatively inexpensive [38]. The characteristics of the primary outcome measure determine the sample size required to show the necessary treatment effect. The sample size is influenced by the predicted behavior of the primary outcome measure (i.e., "anticipated failure" rate); the anticipated "drop-out rate"; the size of the treatment effect (e.g., 30% slowing of progression); the decision as to whether the study is asking a one-sided question (e.g., "Is treatment more efficacious than the control treatment?") versus a two-sided question (e.g., "Will treated patients do better, the same or worse than the control group?"); the statistical power to identify a treatment effect (usually set at 0.8 or 0.9). Studies designed with sufficient power to identify an effect of treatment on a common occurrence (e.g., relapse rate) may be insufficiently powered to identify an event which occurs less frequently (e.g., EDSS progression); for example, in the interferon beta-1b trial, a statistically significant decrease in attack frequency was detected but only a trend to reduced frequency of EDSS progression was observed.

The majority of recently performed MS clinical trials have selected either relapse rate or EDSS change for the primary analysis. Neurologic worsening from MS is recognized clinically as either relapse-related or relapse-independent; the latter refers to progressive neurological decline either in patients with primary progressive MS or in those who have developed secondary progressive MS after an initial relapsing-remitting course. Relapse-related worsening is often accompanied by MRI evidence of apparent disease activity (e.g., new, larger or reappearing T2 lesions: gadolinium-enhancing lesions [27,28]). Relapse-independent progressive neurological worsening may not be accompanied by changes in MRI behavior, even in patients studied carefully with serial T2, T1 and postgadolinium-T1 scanning of the entire neuraxis [39]. For patients with relapse-related worsening, relapse rate is a more responsive (sensitive) outcome measure than EDSS worsening. Unfortunately, relapse rate is incompletely correlated with what is most important to patients, namely long-term impairment progression, measured by EDSS change [29].

It may be difficult for the clinician and patient to distinguish a "relapse" from transient worsening of pre-existing symptoms and signs from an intercurrent illness ("pseudoexacerbations"). To optimize the reliability of this outcome measure, recent pivotal trials have formulated formal operational definitions for relapses, often requiring objective worsening of the neurological examination. Prior to initiating a study it is essential to reach consensus on the definition of the primary outcome, including how to deal with relapses occurring in the setting of fever or infection-related worsening, during steroid withdrawal, and the occurrence of a second apparent relapse within 4 weeks of the first event. It may be especially challenging to determine the occurrence of a relapse with certainty in the evaluation of experimental therapies which may symptomatically worsen pre-existing MS symptoms in the absence of new inflammatory activity because of fever and systemic 'flu-like symptoms (e.g., monoclonal antibodies which deplete T cells such as OKT3, interferon beta-1b, interferon beta-1a).

As mentioned above, there is considerable inter- and intra-rater variability in the use of the EDSS [40-42]. Consequently, changes of at least 1.0 point (e.g., a 2 step worsening) are generally required by trialists to conclude that a clinically significant change has occurred for patients with a baseline EDSS of <5.0. Some groups have advised that single-step changes (e.g., ≤0.5 EDSS point) are sufficient to conclude improvement or worsening for patients with EDSS scores of ≥5.5 [43]. Although the EDSS is familiar to most MS clinical trialists and has been extensively used for years, considerable care is needed at the start of a new trial to be certain that investigators use the scale identically across centers. Most "modern" trials have conducted evaluator training sessions and have written detailed instructions to enhance the reliability of the scale. Each modified version of the rating scales has addressed the troublesome differentiation between "mild," "moderate" and "severe" weakness, measurement of ataxia in the presence of major weakness, and quantitation of bladder and bowel dysfunction, for example. Trialists stress the need for an observed gait analysis in deciding the appropriate EDSS score. Patients who use an ankle-foot orthosis alone are generally not considered as needing "unilateral assistance," and those who choose to use a cane for convenience but are able to walk at least 100 meters without this device are not scored as having an EDSS of 6.0 but the EDSS dictated by the observed distance they can walk without assistance. Specific definitions of the requirements for each step have varied modestly across several large trials (e.g., need to walk a full 100 meters versus almost 100 meters to achieve a score of <6.5). Most investigators have experienced the frustration of observing a patient's gait deteriorate in terms of speed, stride length and steadiness and not see this reflected in the EDSS because the patient is still able to walk 100 meters. The chances of failure because of ambulation likely vary according to the major deficit – hemiplegia versus paraplegia versus ataxia.

There has not been an adequate study addressing the influence of trial duration on assignment of the EDSS by evaluating neurologists. Initially, the evaluator might tend to minimize the severity of clinical signs early in the course of a trial (e.g., limb ataxia rated as "mild" rather than "moderate"), and with the passage of time and repeated measures this assessment may change (worsen) without a real functional change. Presumably, this bias will be evenly distributed across treatment and control groups, however. Nonetheless, if this effect does occur, perhaps due to evaluator fatigue or pessimism, impairment scores will gradually worsen, perhaps minimizing a clinical benefit of treatment.

The EDSS is an ordinal scale and, therefore, changes in EDSS scoring should not be analyzed statistically using parametric methods (e.g., change in mean EDSS score) [44]. Most trialists, however, still report "mean change in EDSS" as a secondary analysis because this parameter is widely familiar to MS investigators. For reasons reviewed later in this chapter, most current trials use survival statistics (e.g., time to failure, Kaplan–Meier), treatment failure definitions, and changes in the primary outcome at various time intervals after enrollment (e.g., proportion of patients better, worse or unchanged at 1, 2 and 3 years) [34].

There is a need for a valid, sensitive surrogate measure of disease activity which would more quickly predict long-term clinical outcome. Such a measure would significantly shorten the time necessary for drug development and reduce the numbers of patients and duration of follow-up necessary to conduct pivotal trials. Some trials have focused on the Neurologic Rating Scale (Scripps) [45] or upper-limb function tests (e.g., 9-hole peg test, box-and-blocks test [46]) and the Ambulation Index [47] in a composite index (with or without MRI scan data). In a recent phase II, placebo-controlled, double-blind trial of oral methotrexate in chronic progressive MS, Goodkin et al. [46] used a composite index as the primary outcome in which failure of any component would be considered evidence that the patient had reached treatment endpoint (e.g., treatment failure). The composite index was comprised of tests of upper-limb function (9-hole peg test and box-and-blocks test), changes in EDSS and Ambulation Index performance, with or without evidence of MRI worsening. The authors concluded that methotrexate provided meaningful benefit to patients with chronic progressive MS, based on a statistically significant difference using this composite measure. No difference between treatment groups was seen, however, using the EDSS or Ambulation Index alone. Apparent treatment-related slowing of progression of upper-limb disability (as measured by the 9-hole peg test and box-and-block tests) accounted for the success of the composite outcome measure in detecting an apparent treatment effect. This composite outcome measure has been criticized because it is not clear that the components are mutually independent; indeed, the opposite appears likely. Other measures such as the need for steroid cointervention, hospitalization for the treatment of relapse, quantitative measures of muscle strength, quality of life measures, disability, and handicap scales (e.g., Functional Impairment Measure, Incapacity Status Scale, Environment Status Scale) are usually considered secondary outcome measures (e.g., supporting or refuting the findings of the primary analysis).

Serial MRI studies have been shown to be sensitive, objective, reliable and biologically plausible but have not yet been shown to be sufficiently predictive of impairment evaluations at 3 and 5 years to permit MS clinical trialists to conclude that short-term changes in MRI behavior will predict long-term clinical course.

Examples from recent studies will illustrate some of the difficulties with the choice of the primary outcome measure. In recent phase III studies, relapse rate and EDSS progression have been shown to be related, but the magnitude of the correlation between these variables has been weak. High-dose (8 mIU) interferon beta-1b (IFNβ-1b, Betaseron) administration reduced relapse rate and MRI worsening and there was a trend suggesting slowing of impairment progression (EDSS change) which approached but did not reach statistical significance for the first 4 years of observation [29]. Paradoxically, low-dose IFNβ-1b (1.6 mIU) was associated with a shorter time to EDSS worsening (e.g., earlier treatment failure) than occurred with placebo despite a trend to lower relapse rate and MRI activity [29]. In a later analysis of the IFNβ-1b study, patients who did not form neutralizing antibodies continued to experience a beneficial effect on relapse rate and MRI activity [48]. Surprisingly, however, these patients were more likely to show EDSS progression than were patients who became neutralizing antibody positive. Interferon beta-1a (IFNβ-1a, Avonex) appeared to delay EDSS progression despite an effect on relapse rate reduction [3] that was relatively more modest than the reduction associated with 8 mIU IFNβ-1b administration. Patients who formed neutralizing antibodies to IFNβ-1a were similarly less likely to show EDSS progression than were patients who were neutralizing antibody negative [49]. This surprising and, as yet, unexplained paradoxical observation that EDSS progression was less likely to occur in patients who were neutralizing antibody positive requires further attention. It is unclear whether this observation represents a statistical aberration or suggests

that different mechanisms of injury may be responsible for relapses (blood–brain barrier disruption and new MRI lesion formation) and EDSS progression (axon loss). If the latter is true, presumably different therapeutic strategies will be needed to address these two independent aspects of disease activity. Glatiramer acetate (Copolymer-1, Copaxone) reduced annualized relapse rate to a greater degree than was seen with IFNβ-1a yet did not show a statistically significant reduction of EDSS progression. Sulfasalazine (Salazopyrin EN-tabs) did not slow EDSS progression yet favorably affected all the clinical measures of relapse-related worsening to a comparable degree to that seen in the three current FDA-approved attack-prevention therapies including annualized relapse rate, time to first attack, proportion of relapse-free patients and relapse severity at 2 years [50]. These examples from recent clinical trials highlight some of the uncertainties in relying on any single conventional outcome measure for phase III clinical trials (relapse rate, EDSS progression, MRI behavior) in determining efficacy. MS trialists feel most assured that efficacy has been demonstrated when each of the primary and secondary outcome measures shows similar favorable trends, thereby establishing consistency of treatment effect.

Blinding

Evaluator and patient blinding is particularly important when the primary outcome is a subjective measure. Most clinical measures such as relapse rate and EDSS change are prone to some subjectivity and thus evaluator and, whenever possible, patient blinding is desirable. With the advent of partially effective parenteral therapies such as the beta interferons and glatiramer acetate, future clinical trials will be increasingly complex as combination parenteral therapies will almost certainly be evaluated. Patient blinding may become more difficult in future trials of previously studied, partially effective therapies as patients will become increasingly familiar with common drug side effects (injection site irritation, 'flu-like symptoms, the glatiramer acetate "systemic reaction", etc.). Currently, the accepted paradigm in MS trials is for patients to be evaluated by two clinicians – one a treating physician and the other an evaluating physician. Both physicians may be blinded, but particular care is taken to blind the evaluating physician, for example, by hiding injection sites (IFNβ-1b) [2], by headcovers (cyclophosphamide) [51] and by blocking access to both laboratory toxicity data and previous clinical assessments and impairment scores. The need to blind the evaluator was well shown in the Canadian Cyclophosphamide and Plasma Exchange trial [51]. In this study, a false positive (type I error) conclusion that oral cyclophosphamide and weekly plasma exchange was more effective than placebo treatment might have been reached if unblinded physicians' assessments had been used for the primary analysis in place of the blinded evaluators' scores for the primary analysis [52].

The two-physician model outlined above has now been used in the IFNβ-1b, IFNβ-1a and sulfasalazine trials. A similar model was used in the glatiramer acetate trial, although the adequacy of the blinding was not reported at the conclusion of the study. In the sulfasalazine study, a "forced" choice approach, wherein the physician was given only two options – "active treatment" or "placebo" – was used to assess blinding; this was done to reduce the likelihood that an unconscious awareness of the true assignment would go undetected. In addition, a novel approach to assess blinding was used in this trial. The EDSS scores assigned by the treating and evaluating neurologists were compared; if blinding had been compromised, it would have been more likely to occur among the treating neurologists. If this were the case, the difference between the treating and evaluating neurologists' evaluation of the change in the EDSS score from baseline would be negative for active-treated patients and positive for patients receiving placebo [50]. This approach could be used in future clinical trials to assess the success of blinding.

Duration of Follow-up

Three recent phase III clinical trials have been able to demonstrate a meaningful reduction in relapse rate with 2 years of follow-up. Two of these trials were unable to demonstrate an effect on EDSS progression at 2 years (or even at 4 years in the IFNβ-1b trial); however, the IFNβ-1a trial revealed slowing of EDSS progression within 2 years, even though only 57% of patients completed 24 months of follow-up. This result is somewhat surprising given that IFNβ-1a had the least robust impact on annualized relapse rates of the three agents. The IFNβ-1a trial highlights the importance of the behavior of the control group in assessing treatment outcome. In this trial, placebo-treated patients were twice as likely to "fail" at 1 year compared with the placebo group in the IFNβ-1b study. Although it is hazardous to compare outcomes across trials, particularly when eligibility criteria differ slightly as in this example, the proportion of patients showing evidence of EDSS progression was virtually identical in the patients receiving IFNβ-1a and high-dose IFNβ-1b. The major difference in patient response in these trials was the failure rate in the control group in the first year. Similar problems have been seen with other MS trials in which apparent treatment efficacy is perhaps better explained by unexpectedly poor performance of the control group, exaggerating the difference between the two treatment arms. This issue is discussed in greater detail in the next section.

The concept of "confirmed" treatment failure has been introduced to minimize the problems with EDSS reliability and transient, relapse-related EDSS worsening. Using this paradigm, EDSS progression must be recorded on two consecutive visits separated by a period of 3–6 months before criteria for failure are met. It is unclear whether 3 or 6 months is the appropriate interval for measurement of "confirmed worsening"; different trials have used different intervals. The optimal duration of a clinical trial will vary depending on the hypothesis to be tested and the type of MS patient being studied. It is crucial that clinical trials be carried on for a sufficient duration to reduce the likelihood of either of type I (false positive) or type II (false negative) error. The recently completed Mayo Clinic–Canadian Cooperative Study of Sulfasalazine in Active Multiple Sclerosis is an excellent example of this principle [50]. The primary outcome measure in this trial was delay or prevention of EDSS progression. The trial was designed for at least a 36 month period of follow-up on all enrolled patients. Sulfasalazine did not prevent EDSS progression. Within the first 18–24 months of enrollment, however, sulfasalazine-treated patients experienced a reduction in a number of clinical and MRI phenomena consistent with acute relapses. These trends were lost or reversed in the second half of the trial. The magnitude of the reduction of relapse-related phenomenon was such that it was conceivable that this agent might have been considered an inexpensive and safe reasonable alternative to the three parenteral, FDA-approved drugs for relapsing MS if relapse-related phenomenon had been considered the primary outcome measure and if the trial had been designed with only 2 years of follow-up. This same phenomenon was seen in the recently completed trial of riluzole in patients suffering from amyotrophic lateral sclerosis [53]. Treated patients had an early delay in progression to death or tracheotomy. This benefit was unfortunately lost by 15–18 months of follow-up. This agent was approved for use by the FDA because of this early benefit in this otherwise untreatable illness.

Control Group

The comparison in a trial is between the outcome in the treated and control groups. The behavior of the control group is the major determinant of the power of the study. Given the variability in the behavior of the control group, an adequate sample size is necessary to obtain sufficient precision about the untreated behavior of the disease. Problems induced by variations in the control group may be magnified by the recent practice to randomize only a third to a quarter of the patients to the placebo-treated control group in order to maximize the number of patients being offered active treatment and to assess multiple treatment limbs, often different doses of the same agent. It is generally assumed that if the inclusion and exclusion criteria are identical in two treatment trials, the placebo control groups should have a similar outcome. However, experience with several clinical trials has revealed that differences in behavior of the control groups often exceed the differences between the treated and control group in either study; for example, comparing the studies of IFNβ-1a and IFNβ-1b, a trend to favorable effect on sustained worsening of disability *at 3 years* was seen in favor of IFNβ-1b: 20% sustained worsening in the high dose 8 mIU group versus 28.0% in the placebo group [2]. The result was not statistically significant. However, in the IFNβ-1a study, 18.2% in the active treatment group were treatment failures *over 2 years* versus 35.5% in the placebo group [3]. The control group behaved significantly worse in the IFNβ-1a study, which enhanced the power of that study to detect a statistically significant difference. The difference in the behavior of the control groups could be due to differences in the application of the EDSS, differences in selection criteria, or to "drop-outs" in the IFNβ-1b study. This difference in the behavior of the control group complicates the examination of the relative efficacy of these two agents. The same argument could be made about the attack rate, which was significantly greater at baseline in the IFNβ-1b study. The decline in the attack rate at 2 years was significantly more impressive in the IFNβ-1b study (0.84 vs 1.27, $p = 0.0001$) than in the IFNβ-1a study (0.67 vs 0.82, $p = 0.04$). These statistical differences, while in the same direction, are trends in the one study and statistically significant differences in the other. These differences are of questionable clinical significance but are sufficient to result in approval or rejection of an indication for an agent and are, therefore, of significant interest to those with an interest in the evaluation of therapeutic agents in MS.

Major variations in the behavior of the control groups from that encountered in similar clinical trials or from expected norms from natural history data are predictors of poor reproducibility of the studies.

What generates the variations in the behavior of the control groups? Many of the outcome measures such as the EDSS are imprecise and have been subject to modifications and/or agreement by groups of investigators participating in clinical trials. Minor differences in the application of the function systems and EDSS likely constitute significant degrees of variation in clinical trials in which a 1.0 point EDSS change is sufficient to result in treatment failure. Furthermore, as previously mentioned, the probability of change in terms of the EDSS varies significantly according to baseline EDSS. Patients with baseline EDSS scores of 4 and 5 are much more likely to deteriorate by 1.0 point over the course of a 2 to 3 year trial [54]. The proportion of patients enrolled with a baseline EDSS score in the 4.0–5.5 range versus in the 6.0 or greater range in clinical trials of progressive MS can significantly affect the behavior of the control group.

The situation will be improved by the development of a more precise set of guidelines for rating EDSS and/or by adoption of continuous and quantitative outcome measures in MS, as suggested by the Task Force on Clinical Outcome Measures established by the National MS Society. Modifications have been instituted in most clinical trials to equate a 0.5 point change at baseline EDSS 6.0 or greater as equivalent to a 1.0 point worsening at lower levels.

Virtually all phase III MS trials in the "modern era" have been placebo-controlled. There are several reasons to require a placebo control group. MS is a highly unpredictable disease. Few clinically identifiable factors reliably predict short-term prognosis. Apparent "stabilization" after enrollement in terms of standardly applied outcome measures is common and may be accounted for by regression to the mean, a "placebo effect", and (in)sensitivity of the outcome measures. Differences in clinical behavior with time between patients and within individual patients have generally exceeded both the sensitivity and the reproducibility of the clinical measures and the magnitude of treatment effects expected from active agents.

The concept of "equipoise" is pertinent to the choice of the control group (e.g., placebo or "best current treatment"). Introduced in 1987 by Freedman [55], this concept states that there should be genuine uncertainty whether treatment A or treatment B is preferable. Investigators (and patients) should be "equally poised" with regard to their preference of which treatment is given. If two treatments are not felt to be equivalent, ethical practice dictates that the superior treatment be used. One survey of professionals and laypersons suggested that 50% of those surveyed felt it was unethical, in general, to proceed with a clinical trial if equipoise was disturbed beyond a ratio of 70:30. A greater level of equipoise (approximately 50:50) is warranted for clinical trials of illnesses involving either children or progressive, life-threatening diseases [56]. A greater disturbance of equipoise was acceptable for short-term symptomatic trials. It is important to emphasize that a clinical trial in progress must be reviewed and eligibility criteria and consent forms revised if other therapies have been demonstrated to be more effective than those under study during the course of the trial (e.g., the original equipoise has been disturbed). In some cases, trials must be terminated for this reason.

Widespread acceptance that there are now three partially effective therapies for patients with relapsing-remitting MS clearly complicates the choice of the control group for future treatment trials in this subgroup. Randomized, controlled clinical trials cannot be conducted ethically unless there is agreement among experts in the field that the experimental treatment to be studied has a high likelihood of being equally effective or more effective than the "standard treatment." It has been shown that IFNβ-1b, INFβ-1a and glatiramer acetate are more effective at reducing relapse rate, and possibly progression of impairment in the case of IFNβ-1a, than placebo. Although these three agents have not been uniformly accepted and licensed worldwide, it is no longer likely that placebo will be considered "standard therapy" in clinical trials in patients with relapsing-remitting MS in the USA. It is possible that future trials of therapy for relapsing-remitting MS may still include a placebo group but presumably only if a stipulation is included in the enrollment criteria that the trial is restricted to patients who have refused or who have failed one or more of these three parenteral agents.

There is currently less convincing evidence that any treatment significantly alters the progressive phase of secondary progressive and primary progressive MS. Similarly, no treatment has yet been shown to reverse long-standing neurological dysfunction (e.g., blindness, paralysis, dementia). No treatment has been proven to delay or prevent further episodes of inflammatory demyelination in patients with isolated neurological syndromes suggesting MS (e.g., optic neuritis, brainstem syndromes, partial transverse myelitis). A secondary analysis of the Optic Neuritis Treatment Trial initially suggested that the combination of intravenous methylprednisolone administered for 3 days and oral prednisone for 11 days might delay the onset of further relapses which would lead to a diagnosis of clinically definite MS [17]. Unfortunately, with prolonged follow-up of patients in this trial, the early beneficial response has not been sustained. Clinical trials designed to address these research questions should continue to be placebo-controlled.

The control group may play an important role in helping to recognize and anticipate potentially serious treatment-related adverse events, particularly when the adverse events are unanticipated and not readily attributed to the active treatment. In the recently terminated phase III trials of linomide (Roquinimex), serious ischemic heart disease complications occurred in linomide-treated patients and not in the placebo group. In this unfortunate example, it was exceedingly helpful that control patients were receiving a placebo (rather than a second active agent). Until a very large number of MS patients have been treated with any of the new "standard" treatments, we will be uncertain whether rare and unanticipated potentially serious events occurring in a clinical trial are related to one of the therapies under study.

Other Factors

It is important to measure and report compliance with the treatment protocol in any clinical trial. This need was highlighted in the Coronary Drug Research Group Study of cholesterol-lowering agents in which it was demonstrated that compliant patients did better than noncompliant patients with regard to survival, regardless of the treatment assignment (e.g., clofibrate or placebo) [57].

The "intent-to-treat" analysis is widely used. The problems of this analysis are discussed elsewhere (see Chapters 12 and 13).

Survival analysis techniques (e.g., time-to-event) take advantage of all clinical events, regardless of the duration of follow-up for the individual case in the trial. This approach enhances statistical power and reduces the effect of patients who discontinue treatment during the course of the trial. On the other hand, there is also an advantage to analyzing all available data at the end of a long clinical trial to capture clinical events that have occurred after the primary outcome has been reached (e.g., after "time to failure"). This technique permits a comparison of the magnitude of the treatment effect by analyzing the proportion of patients with larger and more convincing increments of disability progression, such as becoming wheelchair-dependent. This form of analysis is subject to multiple confounding influences, however, as failing patients may be receive different treatments on and off approved experimental protocols.

Results may be reported as either "absolute" or "relative" risk reduction. One study has shown that readers may be more influenced by the degree of "relative" risk reduction even for identical data [58]. The clinical relevance of these risk reductions is of greater significance than the statistical method used to highlight the observation, and one should recall that the absolute risk reduction may be very small despite a sizable benefit in terms of relative risk.

Trialists should report 95% confidence intervals. Readers should be wary of apparently positive results in which the confidence intervals include zero or 1 for relative risk. Trialists should report the alpha and beta used in the initial sample-sized calculations.

One problem inherent in all clinical trial research is the generalizability of the trial results. Most clinical trials are largely exclusive, rather than inclusive. There is a natural trend to expand the indications for the use of the putative agent after a positive result has been published. This behavior typically leads to unrealistic physician and patient expectations and competition for patient resources for clinical trials which assess expanded indications for an agent. One example of such difficulties encountered were those initially in recruiting patients for the IFNβ-1b SPMS trial because of widespread use of this drug in this group of patients even though unproven as a treatment for secondary progressive MS.

Conclusions

Most clinical trials in MS have been conducted to target attack frequency or change in disability. In phase I and II trials, which are generally 12 months in duration, the primary outcome measure is dynamic MR activity, generally numbers of gadolinium-enhancing and/or new or active T2-weighted lesions detected by monthly MR scanning. In phase III pivotal trials, which are generally 3 years in duration, the primary outcome measures are relapse rate for patients with relapsing-remitting MS and change in disability for patients with secondary progressive MS.

We have identified numerous pitfalls, some of which are specific to MS clinical trials and others which are not. A strategy to identify long-term benefit of agents found to have short-term efficacy in phase III clinical trials is currently lacking and should be an important focus of future MS clinical trial research.

Acknowledgments. Laura Irlbeck typed this manuscript.

References

1. Sriram S. Future of multiple sclerosis therapeutics: rational approaches targeting putative pathogenic mechanisms. In: Goodkin DE, Rudick RA, editors. Multiple sclerosis: advances in clinical trial design, treatment, and future perspectives. Berlin Heidelberg New York: Springer, 1996:47–62.
2. The IFNB Multiple Sclerosis Study Group. Interferon beta-1b is effective in relapsing-remitting multiple sclerosis. I. Clinical results of a multicenter, randomized, double-blind, placebo-controlled trial. Neurology 1993;43:655–661.
3. Jacobs LD, Cookfair DL, Rudick RA, et al. Intramuscular interferon beta-1a for disease progression in relapsing multiple sclerosis. The Multiple Sclerosis Collaborative Research Group (MSCRG). Ann Neurol 1996;39:285–294.
4. Johnson KP, Brooks BR, Cohen JA, et al. Copolymer 1 reduces relapse rate and improves disability in relapsing-remitting multiple sclerosis: results of a phase III multicenter, double-blind placebo-controlled trial. The Copolymer 1 Multiple Sclerosis Study Group [see comments]. Neurology 1995;45:1268–1276.
5. Miller DH, Albert PS, Barkhof F, et al. Guidelines for the use of magnetic resonance techniques in monitoring the treatment of multiple sclerosis. Ann Neurol 1996;39:6–16.
6. Weinshenker BG. The natural history of multiple sclerosis. Neurology 1995;13:119–146.
7. Lublin FD, Reingold SC, National Multiple Sclerosis Society (USA). Defining the clinical course of multiple sclerosis: results of an international survey. Neurology 1996;46:907–911.
8. Matthews PM, Francis G, Antel J, Arnold DL. Proton magnetic resonance spectroscopy for metabolic characterization of plaques in multiple sclerosis [published erratum appears in Neurology 1991;41:1828]. Neurology 1991;41:1251–1256.
9. Weiner HL, Mackin GA, Orav EJ, et al. Intermittent cyclophosphamide pulse therapy in progressive multiple sclerosis: final report of the Northeast Cooperative Multiple Sclerosis Treatment Group. Neurology 1993;43:910–918.
10. Abbruzzese G, Gandolfo C, Loeb C. Bolus methylprednisolone versus ACTH in the treatment of multiple sclerosis. Ital J Neurol Sci 1983;4:169–172.
11. Barnes MP, Bateman DE, Cleland PG, et al. Intravenous methylprednisolone for multiple sclerosis in relapse. J Neurol Neurosurg Psychiatry 1985;48:157–159.
12. Weiner HL, Dau PC, Khatri BO, et al. Double-blind study of true vs sham plasma exchange in patients treated with immunosuppression for acute attacks of multiple sclerosis. Neurology 1989;39:1143–1149.
13. Kurtzke JF, Beebe GW, Nagler B, Auth TL, Kurland LT, Nefzger MD. Studies on the natural history of multiple sclerosis. 7. Correlates of clinical change in an early bout. Acta Neurol Scand 1973;49:379–395.
14. Lucchinetti CF, Noseworthy JH, Rodriguez M. Promotion of endogeneous remyelination in multiple sclerosis. MS 1997;3:7–75.
15. Noseworthy JH, O'Brien PC, van Engelen BGM, Rodriguez M. Intravenous immunoglobulin therapy in multiple sclerosis: progress from the Theiler's virus model to a randomized, double-blind, placebo-controlled clinical trial. J Neurol Neurosurg Psychiatry 1994;57(Suppl):11–14.
16. van Engelen BG, Hommes OR, Pinckers A, Cruysberg JR. Barkhof F, Rodriguez M. Improved vision after intravenous immunoglobulin in stable demyelinating optic neuritis [letter]. Ann Neurol 1992;32:834–835.
17. Beck RW, Cleary PA, Trobe JD, et al. The effect of corticosteroid for acute optic neuritis on the subsequent development of multiple sclerosis. N Engl J Med 1993;329:1764–1769.
18. Jacobs LD, Beck RW, Simon JH, Kinkel RP, Brownscheidle CM, Murray TJ. Simonian NA, Slasor PJ, Sandrock AW. Intramuscular interferon beta-1a therapy initiated during a first demyelinating event in multiple sclerosis. N Engl J Med 2000;343:898–904.
19. Krupp LB, Larocca NG, Muir-Nash J, Steinberg AD. The fatigue severity scale: application to patients with multiple sclerosis and systemic lupus erythematosus. Arch Neurol 1989;46:1121–1123.
20. Fisk JD, Pontefract A, Ritvo PG, et al. The impact of fatigue on patients with multiple sclerosis. Can J Neurol Sci 1994;21:9–14.
21. Ashworth B. Preliminary trial of carisoprodol in multiple sclerosis. Practitioner 1964;192:540–542.

22. Keith RA, Granger CV, Hamilton BB, et al. The functional independence measure: a new tool for rehabilitation. In: Eisenber MG, Grzesiak RC, editors. Advances in clinical rehabilitation. Berlin Heidelberg New York: Springer, 1987:6–18.

23. Eisen A. Electromyography in disorders of muscle tone. Can J Neurol Sci 1987;14:501–505.

24. Bajd T, Vodovnick L. Pendulum testing of spasticity. J Biomed Eng 1984;6:9–16.

25. Vickrey BG, Hays RD, Harooni R, et al. A health-related quality-of-life measure for multiple sclerosis. Qual Life Res 1995;4:187–206.

26. Schiffer RB, Herndon RM, Rudick RA. Treatment of pathologic laughing and weeping with amitriptyline. N Engl J Med 1985;312:1480–1482.

27. Willoughby EW, Grochowski E, Li DK, Oger J, Kastrukoff LF, Paty DW. Serial magnetic resonance scanning in multiple sclerosis: a second prospective study in relapsing patients. Ann Neurol 1989;25:43–49.

28. Miller DH, Barkhof F, Nauta JJP. Gadolinium enhancement increases the sensitivity of MRI in detecting disease activity in multiple sclerosis. Brain 1993;116:1077–1094.

29. The IFNB Study Group University of British Columbia MS/MRI Analysis Group. Interferon beta-1b in the treatment of multiple sclerosis: final outcome of the randomized, controlled trial. Neurology 1995;45:1277–1285.

30. Filippi M, Horsfield MA, Morrissey SP, et al. Quantitative brain MRI lesion load predicts the course of clinically isolated syndromes suggestive of multiple sclerosis. Neurology 1994;44:635–641.

31. Stone LA, Smith ME, Albert PS, et al. Blood–brain barrier disruption on contrast-enhanced MRI in patients with mild relapsing-remitting multiple sclerosis: relationship to course, gender, and age. Neurology 1995;45:1122–1126.

32. Thompson AJ, Kermode AG, Wicks D, et al. Major differences in the dynamics of primary and secondary progressive multiple sclerosis. Ann Neurol 1991;29:53–62.

33. van Walderveen MAA, Barkhof F, Hommes OR, et al. Correlating MR imaging and clinical disease activity in multiple sclerosis: relevance of hypointense lesions on short TR/TE ("T1-weighted") spin-echo images. Neurology 1995;45: 1684–1690.

34. Petkau J. Statistical and design considerations for multiple sclerosis clinical trials. In: Goodkin DE, Rudick RA, editors. Multiple sclerosis: advances in clinical trial design, treatment, and future perspectives. Berlin Heidelberg New York: Springer, 1997:63–103.

35. Weinshenker BG, Bass B, Rice GPA, et al. The natural history of multiple sclerosis: a geographically based study. II. Predictive value of the early clinical course. Brain 1989;112:1419–1428.

36. Weinshenker BG, Bass B, Rice GP, et al. The natural history of multiple sclerosis: a geographically based study. I. Clinical course and disability. Brain 1989;112:133–146.

37. Weinshenker BG, Noseworthy JH, Rice GPA, et al. The natural history of multiple sclerosis: a geographically based study. IV. Applications to planning and interpretation of clinical therapeutic trials. Brain 1991;114:1057–1067.

38. Whitaker JN, McFarland HF, Rudge R, Reingold SC. Outcome assessment in multiple sclerosis clinical trials: a critical analysis. MS 1995;1:37–47.

39. Kidd D, Thorpe JW, Kendall BE, et al. MRI dynamics of brain and spinal cord in progressive multiple sclerosis. J Neurol Neurosurg Psychiatry 1996;60:15–19.

40. Noseworthy JH, Vandervoort MK, Wong CJ, Ebers GC. Inter-rater variability with the Expanded Disability Status Scale (EDSS) and Functional Systems (FS) in a multiple sclerosis

41. Amato MP, Fratiglioni L, Groppi C, Siracusa G, Amaducci L. Interrater reliability in assessing functional systems and disability on the Kurtzke scale in multiple sclerosis. Arch Neurol 1988;45:746–748.

42. Goodkin DE, Cookfair D, Wende K, et al. Inter- and intrarater scoring agreement using grades 1.0 to 3.5 of the Kurtzke Expanded Disability Status Scale (EDSS). Multiple Sclerosis Collaborative Research Group. Neurology 1992;42:859–863.

43. Goodkin DE, Bailly RC, Teetzen ML, Hertsgaard D, Beatty WW. The efficacy of azathioprine in relapsing-remitting multiple sclerosis. Neurology 1991;41:20–25.

44. Noseworthy JH, Vandervoort MK, Hopkins M, Ebers GC. A referendum on clinical trial research in multiple sclerosis: the opinion of the participants at the Jekyll Island workshop. Neurology 1989; 39:977–981.

45. Sipe JC, Knobler RL, Braheny SL, Rice GPA, Panitch HS, Oldstone MBA. A neurologic rating scale (NRS) for use in multiple sclerosis. Neurology 1984;34:1368–1372.

46. Goodkin DE, Rudick RA, VanderBrug MS, et al. Low-dose (7.5 mg) oral methotrexate reduces the rate of progression in chronic progressive multiple sclerosis. Ann Neurol 1995; 37:30–40.

47. Hauser SL, Dawson DM, Lehrich JR, et al. Intensive immunosuppression in progressive multiple sclerosis: a randomized, three-arm study of high-dose intravenous cyclophosphamide, plasma exchange, and ACTH. N Engl J Med 1983;308:173–180.

48. IFNB Multiple Sclerosis Study Group and the University of British Columbia MS/MRI Analysis Group. Neutralizing antibodies during treatment of multiple sclerosis with interferon β-1b: experience during the first three years. Neurology 1996;47:889–894.

49. Rudick RA, Jones W, Alam J, et al. Significance of serum neutralizing antibodies to Avonex (IFNβ-1a) in multiple sclerosis [abstract]. Neurology 1997;48:A80.

50. Noseworthy JH, O'Brien PC. Mayo Clinic–Canadian Cooperative MS Study Group. The Mayo Clinic–Canadian Cooperative Study of Sulfasalazine (Salazopyrin EN) in Active Multiple Sclerosis: preliminary report [abstract]. Neurology 1997;51: 1342–1352.

51. The Canadian Cooperative Multiple Sclerosis Study Group. The Canadian cooperative trial of cyclophosphamide and plasma exchange in progressive multiple sclerosis. Lancet 1991;337:441–446.

52. Noseworthy JH, Ebers GC, Vandervoort MK, Farquhar RE, Yetisir E, Roberts R. The impact of blinding on the results of a randomized, placebo-controlled multiple sclerosis clinical trial. Neurology 1994;44:16–20.

53. Bensimon G, Lacomblez L, Meininger V, et al. A controlled trial of riluzole in amyotrophic lateral sclerosis. N Engl J Med 1994;9:585–591.

54. Weinshenker BG, Issa M, Baskerville J. Meta-analysis of the placebo-treated groups in clinical trials of progressive MS. Neurology 1996;46:1613–1619.

55. Freedman B. Equipoise and the ethics of clinical research. N Engl J Med 1987:317:141–145.

56. Johnson N, Lilford RJ, Brazier W. At what level of collective equipoise does a clinical trial become ethical? J Med Ethics 1991;17:30–34.

57. Anonymous. Influence of adherence to treatment and response of cholesterol on mortality in the coronary drug project. N Engl J Med 1980;303:1038–1041.

58. Naylor D, Phil D, Chen E, Strauss B. Measured enthusiasm: does the method of reporting trial results alter perceptions of therapeutic effectiveness? Ann Intern Med 1992;117:916–921.

32. Multiple Sclerosis: Experience with Large Clinical Trials

D.L. Cookfair, B. Weinstock-Guttman and J.A. Cohen

Introduction

Until recently, multiple sclerosis (MS) was considered largely an untreatable disorder. Therapy was limited to the alleviation of symptoms, and corticosteroid or ACTH treatment of acute relapses. The last decade has been a period of great advances, culminating in the licensure of three agents demonstrated to be of benefit in relapsing MS. Presently, there are more than 100 potential therapies for MS at varying stages of testing.

Natural History

Potential clinical goals of disease-modifying therapies in MS are based on knowledge of the natural history of the disease. These goals include accelerating or improving recovery from acute relapses, reducing the frequency or severity of relapses, slowing or preventing the accumulation of permanent disability resulting from relapses or progression, and reversing fixed disability. The use of consistent terminology describing disease course is essential for investigators conducting clinical trials and for clinicians translating the results of trials into clinical practice. A standardized nomenclature for the clinical classification of MS disease stages was recently proposed [1].

Approximately 70–80% of MS patients initially develop neurological manifestations in the setting of acute relapses early in the disease course [2]. Typically, the neurological symptoms and signs of a relapse evolve over several days to weeks then improve or resolve over weeks to months. Approximately 25% of patients who experience an acute relapse recover completely, with partial or no recovery in the remainder. The relationship between the duration of manifestations and chance for subsequent recovery was examined by Muller [3]. Whereas symptoms of 2 months' duration or less had a 85%

chance of resolving completely, only 30% of symptoms present for 3 months resolved, and only 10% of symptoms present at 6 months resolved. Incomplete recovery from relapses leads to the accumulation of neurological deficits.

Considerable variability exists in relapse rate, both between patients and in individual patients over time. Some [2] but not all [4] investigators have found that increased relapse rate early in the course of MS predicts increased risk of disability later. A high proportion of patients previously with a relapsing course evolve into a gradually progressive course (secondary progressive) with a median time of approximately 11–15 years from the onset of symptoms [2]. However, a follow-up study of relapsing MS patients showed that while a substantial number (~30%) remained stable, 15% evolved into a progressive course during a 2 year observation period [5].

Studies of patients with progressive MS present additional challenges. The timing of transition from relapsing to secondary progressive MS usually can be made accurately only in retrospect. During the transition from relapsing to secondary progressive MS, there may be relapses superimposed on gradually worsening disability. Later, disability worsens without relapses. Typically, there is gradual worsening of pre-existing neurological deficits rather than the appearance of new deficits. Therefore, delaying the transition from a relapsing to a secondary progressive course is an extremely difficult endpoint to determine in practice.

It remains unclear whether there is a pathogenic difference between relapsing and secondary progressive MS. Approximately 15% of patients have a progressive course from onset without relapses (primary progressive MS). Several lines of evidence distinguish this form of MS: a distinct immunogenetic pattern, later onset, clinical features typical of a myelopathy, and reduced lesion activity and gadolinium enhancement on cranial magnetic resonance imaging (MRI). Because of clinical differences that would necessitate utilization of different endpoints and because of inferred biological difference, it has been customary in recent trials to distinguish those with the relapsing and progressive forms of the disease and, more recently, to distinguish those with relapsing/secondary progressive MS from those with primary progressive MS.

In the past, investigators assumed that patients with a progressive course were likely to have predictable continuous deterioration. Therefore, early trials in MS restricted enrollment to patients with chronic progressive disease [6,7]. Also, this assumption led to the lack of inclusion of a control group in some studies [6]. However, the rate of progression within a cohort of MS patients may be quite variable over a period of several years. Prospective clinic-based data indicated that up to 44% of patients with progressive MS may spontaneously stabilize during a 2 year follow-up period [5]. This phenomenon has been confirmed by analysis of the behavior of control groups in several experimental trials. Although inclusion criteria required confirmed progression prior to the trial, up to 50% of patients in the placebo groups remained stable during the trials [8,9]. Clearly, progression does not necessarily proceed inexorably in MS, emphasizing the need for appropriate parallel control groups.

General Considerations in the Design and Conduct of Large Clinical Trials in Multiple Sclerosis

Large Clinical Trials in Multiple Sclerosis: The Phase III Trial

Phase III trials are meant to provide definitive evidence of therapeutic efficacy and safety, and are the final studies conducted prior to application for licensure of a new therapeutic agent. As such, phase III studies must be rigorous in nature. A well-designed phase III trial is controlled, double-blind and randomized. Sample size requirements associated with definitive phase III trials in MS usually necessitate the participation of multiple centers. Objective endpoints must be clearly defined before the study begins, and a specific primary outcome must be explicitly identified. The various aspects of a well-designed trial are strongly interrelated. For example, the statistical analyses that are planned will depend in large part on the outcome measures that have been chosen, which in turn must reflect the objectives of

the study. However, there are three underlying considerations that drive the majority of decisions regarding specific aspects of trial design in a phase III trial: the target chosen for intervention, the ability of a particular design strategy to maximize power to detect therapeutic efficacy, and the feasibility of the proposed methodology.

Targets for Intervention

The four major targets for intervention in MS are symptoms, relapses, disease progression and neurological recovery. There have been many clinical trials that have focused on MS symptoms such as fatigue, spasticity and tremor. The heterogeneity in disease manifestations from patient to patient and in individual patients over time, together with the occurrence of multiple symptoms in varying combinations in individual patients, sometimes pose design problems for trials of symptomatic therapies in MS. However, the issues involved in the design and conduct of studies which target the disease process itself are even more complicated. As such, the statistical design of such studies is usually more sophisticated. There are two recent reports describing phase III trials in which the primary target for intervention was relapses: interferon beta-1b (IFNβ-1b) [10] and Copolymer-1 (glatiramer acetate, Cop-1) [11] and a recent phase III trial of IFNβ-1a in which disease progression was the primary target for intervention [12]. All three of these agents ultimately were licensed in the United States. To date, there have been no phase III trials that target neurological recovery for intervention. Trials to detect recovery of neurological function pose unique design problems. This review will focus on issues encountered in definitive trials to demonstrate beneficial effects on relapse rate and disease progression.

Maximizing Power to Detect Therapeutic Efficacy

The power of a clinical trial refers to the likelihood that the study will succeed in detecting a treatment effect if one genuinely exists. A powerful study is likely to find a difference in the treated versus control arms if a difference is truly there; a weak study may fail to detect a difference that truly exists. In the past, phase III trials targeting relapses and disease progression for intervention were placebo-controlled. However, with the recent approval of three partially effective disease-modifying agents as treatment for relapsing MS [10–12], future therapies may be required to demonstrate a treatment effect that is significantly greater than that seen in actively treated controls. The size of the treatment difference that must be detected is likely to be smaller, resulting in a substantial increase in the power needed to detect therapeutic efficacy. This has important implications for the design of future phase III trials for MS.

The power of a study to detect a genuine treatment effect can be increased by improving the precision of study outcome measures and increasing the number of primary outcome events observed during the trial [13]. Methods to enhance precision include developing standardized ways of measuring trial outcomes, including detailed written instructions, training the observers who determine the outcome, testing the performance of those observers, refining the measurement instruments themselves, and using repeated measures to determine outcome rather than a single observation. Ways to increase the number of primary outcome events observed during the trial include increasing trial duration or sample size, enrolling subjects who are at greatest risk of developing the outcome, expanding the definition of what constitutes an outcome measure, increasing the size of the treatment arm difference that is to be detected, and using more powerful statistical techniques.

Feasibility

Another important consideration when designing a phase III trial is the feasibility of the proposed methodology. Not only the study treatment, but also the type and frequency of outcome measurements must be acceptable to the patients and investigators who will participate in the study. Failure to consider these issues when designing a trial may reduce the number of patients willing to participate or the rate at which they can be accrued. It also could lead to accrual of patients who are not representative of the target population for which the treatment is intended. Furthermore, treatment noncompliance rates and loss to follow-up during the study might be increased, reducing the power of the study to detect a treatment effect of the size specified in the sample size calculations. Increasing sample size can dramatically increase a study's power to detect differences between treatment arms. However, in order for it to be feasible to carry out a study, sample size requirements must not exceed the number of patients meeting study eligibility criteria who are available at the study sites, or the professional and financial resources available to carry out the study. Therefore, design strategies must be chosen which maximize power while minimizing the sample size required to achieve that level of power.

Designing a Phase III Trial in Multiple Sclerosis

Certain design aspects of phase III trials require a greater depth of pre-trial planning than comparable aspects of studies at earlier stages of drug development. Methods for reducing bias and the statistical plan must be more sophisticated and described in more detail. A single primary outcome must be clearly identified, and the manner in which this outcome will be measured must be established before the trial begins. Detailed sample size calculations must be provided that clearly demonstrate that the sample size planned has sufficient power to detect therapeutic benefit as measured by the primary outcome measure if the anticipated therapeutic efficacy indeed exists. For these reasons, the sections which follow deal specifically with design issues associated with phase III trials for MS.

The Study Protocol

An important part of the pre-trial planning process is the preparation of a study protocol. The study protocol for a phase III trial is the written plan for the study and must include detailed information concerning every aspect of the trial [14], including the rationale for conducting the trial, the study objectives, trial design, procedures, and an outline of the planned statistical analyses. Patient selection criteria, the numbers of patients to be screened and enrolled, and the treatment groups must be described. The endpoints to be used in the study must be defined, and details concerning the manner in which each endpoint or outcome will be measured must be given. Procedures for accruing patients, administering treatment, and monitoring and ensuring patient safety must also be described, along with procedures for data collection, data management and quality control. The various resources needed to carry out the trial must be clearly identified in the protocol, and the feasibility of the trial must be demonstrated.

Defining Study Objectives

Testing multiple hypotheses in the same study increases the likelihood that at least one of the results will be statistically significant due to chance alone. The different outcomes measured in association with these multiple hypotheses may require a different schedule of examinations and different methods for ensuring adequate measurement precision. For these reasons, it is strongly recommended that phase III trials specify a single primary outcome that is used as the basis for all power and sample size calculations. When choices must be made regarding use of trial resources or specific aspects of trial design, strategies which emphasize precise measurement of this primary outcome should take precedence over considerations regarding secondary outcomes.

Selection of Study Subjects

The type of MS patient included in a trial has important implications for detecting efficacy. For example, a therapy that is strongly effective in patients with relapsing MS but not at all effective in patients with progressive MS may appear to be ineffective if the study population includes a mixture of the two types. The rate of occurrence of primary outcome events also may be increased by restricting the type of patients included in the study.

Comparison Groups

In designing a phase III trial in MS, it is important to remember that the disease manifestations and course may change significantly during the study period. Thus, for definitive trials, parallel control groups are required. For example, most prospective studies indicate that relapse rates in unselected clinic-based patient populations are in the range of 0.4 to 1 relapse per year [5]. During a 2 to 3 year observation period, the usual length of definitive clinical trials in MS, relapse rate remained relatively constant in a clinic population [5]. However, it has been observed in many trials that relapse rate in the control group decreases after initiation of the trial relative to the pre-trial period [10–12]. This phenomenon has been attributed to stricter definitions of relapse in trials, placebo effect and regression to the mean. In this case, regression to the mean refers to natural stochastic variability of relapse rate, so that if patients are selected based on active disease defined as a required number of relapses in the period immediately preceding the study, they may be less likely to experience a relapse during the study as their relapse rate regresses to the overall mean value.

The number of groups to be studied is also an important consideration. A controlled trial which divides a set number of patients into three treatment groups will have less power than a trial which is identically designed and executed in every other respect but divides the same number of patients into only two groups. Therefore, while including more than two treatment arms may provide useful information regarding efficacy (particularly if a dose-effect is seen), if the number of patients available or other

trial resources are limited, investigators should consider using a two-arm design.

Structuring the Trial to Protect Blinding

It is critical that the evaluations in a trial leading to determination of the endpoints are not biased by knowledge of treatment group. This is why a well-designed phase III trial is both double-blind and randomized. The importance of this issue was illustrated in the recent phase III trials of IFNβ-1b, IFNβ-1a and Cop-1, in which relatively modest treatment effects were seen and side-effects existed that could jeopardize blinding. For these reasons, the standard study structure in recent MS trials has included three blinded roles: a treating neurologist (who oversees therapy and makes treatment decisions), a study nurse (who serves as the contact person at the study site for study patients, monitors adverse effects and monitors compliance) and an evaluator (who performs the assessments on which the study outcome is based without access to historical data). In the case of the IFNβ-1b, IFNβ-1a and Cop-1 phase III trials the evaluator was a second neurologist. In future trials utilizing functional measures not based directly on the neurological examination, it should be possible to utilize nurses, physical or occupational therapists, or trained technicians to perform these outcome assessments.

Outcome Measures

The type of outcome measure chosen, the manner in which it is measured, and the frequency with which it is measured all affect the power of a study to detect a genuine treatment effect. As the precision (reproducibility) and accuracy of an outcome increase, so does its power to detect a genuine treatment effect. The ideal outcome measure is not only precise and accurate, but also easy to administer or observe, acceptable to patients, sensitive to change and clinically relevant [15]. Currently, the two most common targets for intervention in trials for MS are relapse rate and progression of neurological disability.

Relapses

Relapses are used as an outcome in studies where the goal of therapy is to reduce the severity or length of individual relapses, or as a clinical measure of disease activity in trials involving disease-modifying agents. An example of the first type of study is the double-blind placebo-controlled trial that showed that patients treated with ACTH had a more rapid resolution of the neurological deficits associated with acute relapses, although the extent of recovery was not improved [16]. Examples of the second type of study include phase III trials for three recently approved therapeutic agents IFNβ-1b [10], IFNβ-1a [12] and Cop-1 [11]. Design issues which should be considered when relapses are used as an outcome include the definition of a relapse for the purpose of the study, methodology for detecting relapses, methodology for determining the relapse length and severity, statistical analysis of relapse data, and appropriate comparison of relapse data across studies.

There are several published reports that provide the on-study definitions used to establish the occurrence of relapses [10–12]. Most require the appearance, following a period of neurological stability (usually 1 month), of new neurological deficits or worsening of pre-existing ones that lasts at least 24 h (to distinguish a true relapse from transient fluctuations in disease manifestations). It also is common to require the absence of fever or other intercurrent illness in order to distinguish a true relapse from worsening that often accompanies febrile illness. Trials in which relapse rate serves as the primary endpoint have specified objective changes in the examination or a rating scale derived from the examination necessary for an event to constitute a relapse. The definition of worsening, the minimum time requirements for symptom length and the length of the prior period of stability have varied from study to study. These differences have important ramifications for the outcome of the trial itself. Stricter definitions will reduce the number of "false positive" relapses detected (i.e., identifying as relapses clinical events that are not in reality relapses) but may result in a failure to detect milder relapses. Less strict definitions will lead to greater sensitivity with regard to mild relapses but will increase the number of "false positive" relapses detected.

Relapse data are likely to be more complete if detection of relapses is investigator-driven rather than patient-driven, and active "case-seeking" methods are used to detect relapses between scheduled visits (e.g., weekly telephone interviews by a study nurse who schedules a visit if a relapse is suspected on the basis of this interview). Determining the length and severity of a relapse is time-consuming for study personnel and, in the case of length, difficult to determine with a high degree of accuracy. Therefore, it may not always be feasible to measure these two parameters for studies in which relapses represent a secondary outcome. Finally, in patients in the transition period between relapsing and secondary progressive MS, it may be difficult to distinguish relapses from progression.

Disability

A number of scales have been developed as clinical measures of disease progression in clinical trials for MS [17]. The Kurtzke Expanded Disability Status Scale (EDSS) [18] is the most frequently used and the best validated. The EDSS utilizes data from the neurological examination to categorically rate severity in eight functional systems (FS scores). The FS scores, the distance the patient is able to walk and the assistance required, and for more severely disabled patients the ability to carry out activities of daily living, are used to determine a single score for disease severity. Scores range from 0 to 10 in 0.5 step increments, with higher scores indicating more severe disease. Advantages of the EDSS over other scales include its widespread use and familiarity to MS investigators, its assessment of a wide spectrum of neurological functions, and the fact that it allows simple comparison between patients and of individual patients over time.

The EDSS has certain disadvantages [17]. For example, the way in which the EDSS is scored varies depending on where on the scale a patient's score lies. In its lower range, the EDSS score is based on the FS scores. In its middle range, the EDSS score is based primarily on ambulatory ability, and, thus, becomes insensitive to changes in vision, cranial nerve function and upper extremity function. Also, like all scales based on the routine neurological examination, the EDSS is insensitive to cognitive dysfunction. Furthermore the EDSS is an ordinal scale, not an equal-interval scale. Therefore, the proportions of patients at EDSS steps and the time spent at each EDSS step varies along the scale [19,20]. These properties of the scale must be taken into account when planning the analysis of EDSS data.

The complexity and ambiguity in how the FS scores are defined and rated and how the EDSS score is calculated from the FS scores combined with other data contribute to high intra- and inter-rater variability [21–23], which is greatest in the lower range (i.e., EDSS score less than 4.0). There are several ways to improve the reliability of the EDSS as a measure of disability progression in the clinical trial setting [23]. Pre-study training of examining physicians and operationally redefining some of the FS scores can improve consistency in performing the examination and scoring the findings. Also, because inter-rater variability generally is higher than intra-rater variability, many study protocols stipulate that the EDSS determination should be performed by a single rater for an individual patient over the course of a trial. Assessment of intra- and inter-rater reliability on a study-by-study basis should be performed to determine the smallest change in EDSS that can be reliably detected in the context of that particular study. Finally, although using two sets of blinded physicians to follow patients during the trial is cumbersome, utilization of an examining doctor who determines the EDSS score without access to the history lessens the influence of disease symptoms or medication side-effects on scoring the more subjective aspects of the neurological examination.

The definition of treatment failure used during the analysis of EDSS data must also be chosen with care. Small differences in the EDSS score may not be detected reliably in the clinical trial setting due to increased intra- and inter-rater variability. Also, the clinical relevance of treatment failure based on small changes in EDSS score may not be evident. Conversely, definitions of treatment failure requiring a large change in EDSS score may be more clinically relevant and less subject to variability but will reduce sensitivity to change, running the risk of a type II error. Because of the different properties of the scale at different levels of disability, many trials have defined treatment failure to require less change (worsening) in EDSS score for patients with a baseline EDSS score at the high end of the scale (for example greater than 5.0) than for patients with lower a baseline EDSS score [19,20]. Finally, it is important that change in the EDSS score be confirmed at a later point (e.g., 3 months later) before it is considered to signify sustained progression in disability, to avoid transient increases in the score due to rater variability, day-to-day fluctuations in neurological status and acute relapse.

To address the perceived shortcomings of the EDSS, a number of timed functional tests have been proposed as alternative approaches to measuring neurological impairment and disability in MS trials. For example, measuring the actual time to walk 25 feet (8 m) rather than scoring ambulation using an ordinal scale as is done with the EDSS or Ambulation Index [6], provides a more sensitive measure of change in ambulation ability [24]. Similarly, the box-and-block test and 9-hole peg test are easy to perform, reproducible tests of upper extremity motor function. Both are more sensitive to detecting upper extremity motor dysfunction and in following change in function over time than the EDSS [25]. A composite measure (see below) combining the EDSS, the box-and-block test, the 9-hole Peg Test and Ambulation Index was more sensitive to neurological worsening than the EDSS alone in a phase II study of low-dose oral methotrexate in progressive MS [26]. In the cyclosporine phase III trial, a comprehensive battery of tests of neurological performance, including measures of cognitive function, upper extremity function, lower extremity function and gait, was shown to detect neurological progression in a more sensitive manner than the EDSS [27].

There are several potential advantages of functional testing methods. In general, the tests are easy to administer and reproducible. Many functional measures can be administered by trained technicians or nurses. In a phase III trial where disability data are collected on large numbers of patients over time, this attribute represents a significant practical advantage over the EDSS, which is based on the neurological examination. Functional measures yield quantitative results on a continuous scale. The findings on functional tests reflect the types of neurological dysfunction present and their severity more directly than relying on inference from findings on the neurological examination. Finally these tests assess functions that may be poorly reflected in the EDSS score, for example upper extremity function in patients with EDSS scores in the 4.0–7.0 range.

Functional testing has several potential disadvantages. Some of the tests require specialized equipment or expertise and, in general, these tests are unfamiliar to neurologists. More importantly, most have not been validated in the MS population. The amount of change that represents a meaningful clinical change is not always readily apparent. Finally, performance on these tests may be affected by a variety of neurological manifestations, making it difficult to equate test results to a patient's symptoms or findings on the neurological examination. For example, walking speed conceivably could be affected by abnormalities of vision, vestibular function, cerebellar function, muscle strength, muscle tone and sensation.

Neuropsychological Assessment

There are several reasons why neuropsychological assessment should be included as an outcome measure in MS clinical trials. Cognitive impairment is a common manifestation of MS, occurring in 50–60% of patients [28,29]. Cognitive impairment is related to cerebral lesion burden as quantified by MRI [30,31], and deterioration in cognitive function correlates with increasing lesion burden on MRI [31]. MS-related cognitive impairment occurs relatively independently of disease duration, disease course and physical impairment [32]. Therefore, measurement of cognitive function provides information concerning disease involvement that is different from and complementary to that provided by other clinical measures. Finally, cognitive dysfunction has important ramifications regarding functioning at home, quality of life and employment [33].

The results of neuropsychological testing in a number of small phase II trials have been reported, for example studies of interferon alpha [34], low-dose oral methotrexate [35] and 4-aminopyridine [36], and as an add-on study at a subset of sites in the IFNβ-1b phase III trial [37]. In general, the neuropsychological measures employed covered only a few cognitive domains. More comprehensive neuropsychological assessments were included in the phase III trials of IFNβ-1a and Cop-1. Analyses for the IFNβ-1a phase III study have been completed. Results indicate that relapsing MS patients treated with IFNβ-1a for 2 years performed significantly better than placebo patients on a composte battery of information processing and learning/recent memory, cognitive domains commonly disrupted by MS [38]. All these studies suggest that components of a comprehensive neuropsychological test battery, in particular measures of attention and concentration, may be useful as an outcome measure in MS trials.

Composite Outcome Measures

The variable course of MS makes the development of reliable, objective clinical outcome measures difficult. With the emergence of partially effective therapies, furture trials will have to compare two active treatment groups. In this setting the shortcomings of the EDSS discussed above become more prominent. Unless outcome measures are developed that have greater power to detect therapeutic efficacy than those currently available, the increased sample size necessary to conduct definitive phase III trials may become prohibitive.

A potential way to increase power without increasing sample size is to use a new outcome measure. There are two ways in which using a different outcome may reduce sample size. The first is if its use results in an increase in the number of primary outcome events which occur in the control population in a given period of time. The second is if its use results in more precise measurements (i.e., less measurement variability) than the outcome it replaces. In 1996, the National Multiple Sclerosis Society (NMSS) Clinical Outcomes Assessment Task Force published specific recommendations for the attributes of alternative measurement approaches in MS clinical trials [38]. Their recommendations support the development of a multidimensional composite outcome measure [39]. This committee and other investigators acquired contemporary clinical trial and historical multiple sclerosis data for meta-analyses of primary and secondary outcome assessments to provide a basis for recommending a new outcome measure. A composite measure encompassing the major clinical dimensions of arm, leg and cognitive function was identified and termed the Multiple Sclerosis Functional Composite (MSFC). Rating scales based on the standard neurological

examination (e.g., the EDSS) certainly could be included as a component of a composite outcome measure [26]. However, functional measures offer several advantages in terms of practicality and measurement properties. The phase III trial of IFNβ-1a in secondary progressive MS will employ the MS functional composite outcome measure comprising the timed 25-foot walk, 9-hole peg test and Paced Auditory Serial Addition Test. The EDSS and quantitative MRI are utilized as secondary outcome measures [40].

Surrogate Outcome Measures

Clinical trials in MS are made more difficult because MS is a heterogeneous disease both in how it manifests clinically and the severity of these manifestations. Also MS is a chronic disease with clinical changes developing over time periods that exceed those reasonably studied in a clinical trial. These aspects of MS make it important to utilize measurement tools capable of reliably detecting small changes in neurological status in as short a time as possible. A surrogate outcome is a laboratory test measurement that is used in place of a clinical measure [41]. The utility of a surrogate outcome is to confirm the validity of concurrent small changes in clinical measures or to predict future change in a clinical measure when the length of follow-up in the trial precludes observing major clinical changes. A surrogate measure may also be useful to subcategorize patients when a potential treatment is effective for only a subgroup and to look for a biological effect of a potential treatment, for example to help in determining dose. An important characteristic of a primary outcome measure for a definitive phase III trial is that it be clinically relevant. From a regulatory perspective, this means that for a surrogate marker to be used in place of a clinical outcome it must be highly predictive of that clinical outcome [41]. Ideally, the surrogate measure should also be more precise and accurate than the clinical outcome. A number of potential surrogate measures have been proposed for MS trials, including MRI, urine myelin basic protein-like material (UMBPLM) and evoked potentials (EP).

Participants in a 1995 workshop sponsored by the NMSS discussed the role of MRI in clinical trials for MS [42]. MRI was proposed as a potential surrogate outcome because it was perceived to be more objective, sensitive and reproducible than clinical rating scales such as the EDSS and to provide a more direct view of the pathological process [42]. Unlike the EDSS, MRI is not biased toward the detection of lesions affecting ambulation, since most brain lesions do not contribute to ambulatory disability.

The workshop noted that MRI has several attributes that make it an appropriate outcome for phase I/II MS trials. However, they concluded that the MRI does not currently meet the criteria necessary to replace a clinical outcome as the primary outcome measure in a definitive phase III trial for MS because of problems with reproducibility, biological variability, and the poor correlation between MRI and available clinical outcomes. Other authors have come to the same conclusion [43]. In phase III trials, quantitative MRI serves as an important secondary outcome measure, to support the primary clinical outcome.

The use of MRI in trials has been discussed more recently by another NMSS task force [44]. The best-evaluated role for MRI is as a measure of the current disease activity. The utility of this approach results from the observation that radiographic disease activity exceeds the clinical relapse rate by up to 10- to 20-fold [45,46]. In the IFNβ-1b phase III trial, 52 patients at one center underwent MRI studies every 6 weeks to assess radiographic disease activity, defined as the presence of new or enlarging lesions on T2-weighted scans [43]. There was a significant reduction in active scans, the number of active lesions per year and number of new lesions per year in the high-dose IFNβ-1b-treated group as compared with placebo-treated patients. A beneficial effect on disease activity as measured by MRI was also seen in the IFNβ-1a phase III trial. IFNβ-1a treatment resulted in a significant reduction in the number of new, enlarging, and new plus enlarging T2-hyperintense lesions accumulating over 2 years [46]. Patients in this trial also underwent yearly gadolinium-enhanced MRI. Baseline T1-weighted scans following administration of gadolinium were available from 132 placebo-treated patients and 141 IFNβ-1a-treated patients. At baseline, the mean number of gadolinium-enhancing lesions was 2.32 in the placebo-treated patients versus 3.17 in the IFNβ-1a-treated patients. This difference was not statistically significant. The mean number of lesions decreased in the placebo group to 1.59 at year one and 1.65 at year two but decreased further in the IFNβ-1a-treated patients to 1.04 and 0.80 respectively. These differences were significant at both years one and two. The beneficial effect seen on MRI-detected disease activity corroborated the clinical benefit seen in both trials.

Based on statistical modeling of data from monthly gadolinium-enhanced MRI scans, investigators have proposed potential approaches to utilizing frequent gadolinium-enhanced MRI scans in early screening studies of potential disease therapies [48,49]. The use of frequent gadolinium-enhanced scans would be anticipated to be most useful in the evaluation of agents expected to have a direct, rapid

effect on lesion formation. Also, utilization of MRI in this way probably will be more useful early in the disease course, as the rate of gadolinium enhancement appears to decrease when the disease evolves into a secondary progressive phase [50].

MRI has been used as a measure of disease severity, as reflected in total intracranial T-2 lesion burden. [43,51,47]. Both the IFNβ-1b and the IFNβ-1a phase III trials showed a greater increase in T2-lesion area for placebo patients than treated patients, although in the IFNβ-1a study this difference did not reach statistical significance [42,50,46].

Data from the IFNβ-1a study demonstrated prominent between-patient variability both in total T2-lesion burden at baseline and in change in burden over time, despite using a computer-assisted MRI image segmentation approach that minimized intra- and inter-rater variability in total T2-lesion volume determination. Other groups also have reported marked month-to-month variability in T2-lesion burden despite utilization of automated image analysis approaches [52]. This lability in T2-lesion volume suggests that much of the T2-signal abnormality represents edema in some patients and illustrates the need to subcategorize T2-lesions to distinguish the differing pathology that may contribute to the T2-lesion burden. Certain lesion subtypes have shown better correlation with progression of disability, for example hypointense lesions on T1-weighted images [53] and lesions demonstrating marked reduction in magnetization transfer [54]. Both these features are postulated to reflect tissue damage rather than inflammation and edema alone.

A number of biological markers have been described in MS, which have been postulated to reflect disease activity and in theory could be used to monitor putative treatments. These changes have included immunological abnormalities in cerebrospinal fluid (CSF), changes in peripheral blood lymphocyte populations, cytokine levels in blood or CSF, and changes in soluble forms of adhesion molecules. Unfortunately, none of these has been validated as a biological surrogate marker for use in MS trials. The closest has been myelin basic protein (MBP)-like material in CSF and urine.

Release of myelin components in body fluids (e.g., CSF, blood or urine) would be expected during active myelin damage. Proteolipid protein and MBP account for over 90% by weight of central nervous system (CNS) myelin proteins. MBP-like material (MBPLM) is not present normally in human CSF, but can be detected by radioimmunoassay in CSF in nanogram per milliliter concentrations following acute inflammatory, infectious, ischemic or traumatic CNS damage [55]. This MBPLM in CSF is a complex mixture of peptides of heterogeneous size postulated to result from the action of various enzymes in the CNS or CSF on MBP. An increase in MBPLM in CSF can be detected within 5 days of the onset of acute MS relapse, particularly involving the cervical spinal cord, and rapidly resolves over 2 weeks. No relationship between CSF MBPLM concentration and other CSF parameters, including immunoglobulin, has been seen. The level of CSF MBPLM is predictive of the clinical response to corticosteroid treatment of the relapse [56]. There is no relationship between CSF MBPLM concentration and progression.

MBPLM can be detected in the serum of patients with MS, but technical factors preclude it being a useful test. MBPLM also can be detected in concentrated urine (UMBPLM) from normal subjects, and is increased in selected patients with MS. There is no direct relationship between the presence or concentration of MBPLM in CSF and UMBPLM; it appears they represent distinct products [57]. Increased UMBPLM does not correlate with clinical relapses. Rather, UMBPLM concentration correlates with the T2-lesion burden on cranial MRI [58]. Increased levels appear to predict conversion to from a relapsing to a secondary progressive course [59].

Multi-modality sensory EP are useful in clinical practice to detect lesions in sensory pathways that are clinically silent. EP have been used in a number of clinical trials with variable utility. In general, visual evoked potentials (VEP) have been most useful due to their ease of performance and measurement relative to brainstem auditory evoked potentials (BAEP) or somatosensory evoked potentials (SEP). Careful attention must be paid to factors that can influence the reproducibility of EP, including technical factors in the recording, how latencies and amplitudes are determined, body temperature, degree of fatigue and time of day. EP appear to be more sensitive for detecting asymptomatic worsening or its lack. They are less useful for demonstrating improvements as they remain abnormal even after active inflammatory demyelination has resolved, reflecting persisting damage to tracts. Improvement in sensory pathways with rate- or temperature-dependent block and labile conduction has been demonstrated by EP for several agents thought to improve conduction in demyelinated tracts, including digoxin [60] and 4-aminopyridine [61–63]. In a 3 year, double-blind, placebo-controlled study of azathioprine with or without methylprednisolone in chronic progressive MS [64], treatment effects on VEP and upper extremity sensory evoked potential latencies progressively increased over the 3 years of the trial, and between-group differences became statistically significant at year two. A treatment effect favoring azathioprine was demonstrated with EP 1 year before between-group differences were seen in the standard neurological examination scores [65].

Quality of Life

Quality of life (QOL) refers to an individual's level of satisfaction with valued aspects of life, such as physical, emotional and social well-being. Health-related QOL refers more specifically to QOL as modified by illness and its treatment [66]. There are several reasons why MS has important consequences as regards QOL. MS typically presents during early adulthood and is a chronic disease. MS often impairs multiple systems, leading to a wide variety of functional difficulties. The heterogeneous manifestations of MS and the variable rate over which they develop lead to uncertain prognosis. Maintaining and improving QOL are important goals in the management of any chronic disease. However, improvements in clinical or laboratory outcomes do not always translate into improved QOL for the patient. In some instances, significant side-effects associated with an effective treatment may actually have a negative impact on QOL.

While clinical outcomes such as relapse rate and disability progression remain the primary outcomes for phase III MS trials, there is increasing recognition that patient-based assessment of QOL is an important secondary outcome. Unfortunately, the assessment of QOL is impeded by a number of factors which can have even greater impact in the setting of a large clinical trial. Quantitative assessment of QOL can be time-consuming, and measurement is dependent on language and cognitive abilities, which sometimes are impaired in patients with MS [67]. Also, QOL may be affected by factors unrelated to either disease or treatment, complicating the analysis and interpretation of results. Finally, instruments that have adequate metric properties to measure QOL in MS at a single point in time may not be sensitive to changes in QOL over time.

Several cross-sectional studies of patients with MS have found that increasing disability is associated with poorer QOL [66,68,69]. Results of a study comparing QOL in patients with MS, inflammatory bowel disease and rheumatoid arthritis suggested that QOL was poorest among patients with MS [70]. However, due in part to the difficulties described above, the number of large MS clinical trials reporting QOL results has been limited to date. In a controlled study involving 54 MS patients, exercise training resulted in improved fitness and a positive impact on QOL [71]. Initial results from the IFNβ-1a phase III trial indicated that patients with relapsing MS and mild disability often experience health-related physical and psychosocial dysfunction despite their low levels of disability [72]. Preliminary data have been presented which suggest that the delay in worsening in physical disability associated with treatment with IFNβ-1a [73] was associated with improved QOL [72].

In both these studies QOL was measured using the Sickness Impact Profile (SIP), a performance-oriented health status measure with documented validity and reliability that has been used to study QOL in a wide variety of chronic disease populations [74,75]. The SIP provides information on the impact of illness on a broad range of activities of daily living. Summary scores for physical and psychosocial functioning along with an overall SIP score are determined. Both a strength and a limitation of the SIP is that it is a generic rather than disease-specific health status measure. While this attribute makes it possible to compare QOL in MS patients with other chronic disease populations using the SIP, there may be certain problems specific to patients with MS that are not measured as well as they might be with a disease-specific measure. Also, the SIP provides a wealth of information, but it can be lengthy to administer. Another well-regarded generic measure of QOL is the SF-36 from the Medical Outcomes Study [76]. Because the SF-36 was developed more recently than the SIP, opportunities to evaluate its usefulness in studies involving MS patients have been more limited. The SF-36 has been shown to be both reliable and valid in studies of other disease populations, and is considerably shorter than the SIP [77].

One approach that has been suggested to improve the ability to detect QOL issues specific to patients with MS without sacrificing the strengths inherent in generic instruments such as the SIP and SF-36 is to use a short generic measure such as the SF-36 in combination with disease or symptom-specific measures [66,67]. Other measures are available or under development which may prove useful in the measurement of QOL in the setting of large phase III trials for MS [66,67]. Ultimately, when choosing QOL measures for use in a clinical trial for MS, investigators will need to evaluate the merits of the proposed QOL measure within the context of the planned trial. This assessment includes documenting the reliability and validity of the proposed measure as it applies specifically to the assessment of QOL in MS patients, and ensuring that the measure will be sensitive to change over time in the population to be studied.

Statistical Analysis Plan

Establishing a detailed statistical plan prior to the start of data collection is extremely important to the ultimate success of a phase III clinical trial. In addition to detailing a plan for efficacy analyses, investigators should also make plans for interim safety analyses. These aspects of the analysis and the other factors that should be considered during the development of the statistical analysis plan are described below.

Intent-to-Treat Analysis

Analyses should be conducted according to an intent-to-treat design, i.e., all study subjects should continue to be followed and analyzed according to their randomization assignments, even if they discontinue treatment while on-study. A discussion of the advantages and disadvantages of this analysis is given elsewhere (see Chapters 12 and 13).

Interim Safety Analyses

Interim analyses of outcome data should be conducted only in the context of safety monitoring. The endpoints to be analyzed and the number and timing of analyses should be specified in advance, as well as details regarding who will see interim results and under what conditions the results will be seen. p values derived from these analyses should be adjusted for multiple testing using appropriate methodology, such as that described by Fleming et al. [78], in order to avoid stopping the study prematurely as a result of a significant finding due solely to the large number of interim analyses conducted (i.e., a type I error).

Efficacy Analyses

The statistical approach used to analyze the data from a clinical trial depends mainly on the type of outcome variable that is utilized. Therefore, specific methods that commonly are used in the analysis of relapses and progression of disability are described below, along with other important issues to consider when developing the plan for efficacy analysis.

The most commonly used method for analyzing relapse data is to count the number of relapses and estimate an annualized relapse rate for each treatment arm. This often is accomplished by dividing the overall number of relapses by the total number of on-study person-years of follow-up contributed by patients in each treatment arm during the course of the study. The relapse rates for the different treatment arms are then compared, and a test of statistical significance is conducted to determine whether patients treated with the therapeutic agent have a lower relapse rate than patients in the control arm of the study. The annual relapse rate has been widely reported by many authors [10–12]. However, this approach is somewhat problematic in that it is dependent on the assumption that time to a patient's first relapse is independent of time to a patient's second relapse [12]. In other words, it assumes that there are no patients with inherently higher relapse rates than other patients. The validity of this underlying assumption is questionable. One analytic approach that may be taken when dealing with this problem is that used in the phase III trial of Cop-1 as a treatment for relapsing MS [11]. In this study, multivariate analysis of covariance was used to compare relapse rates for the two treatment arms that had been adjusted for duration of disease, sex, pre-study relapse rate and baseline EDSS by including these as covariates in the analysis. The proportions of relapse-free patients in the treatment arms were estimated from a logistic regression model after adjusting for the same set of covariates.

Cross-study comparisons of the magnitude of beneficial treatment effects on relapse rate are a common occurrence. However, caution should be exercised when comparing results from different studies. Differences in study entry criteria, pre-study relapse rates, definitions of relapses and methods to detect them, along with the differing analytical techniques used to determine relapse rate and proportion of relapse-free subjects, limit the utility of such comparisons.

A commonly used method to analyze EDSS data is the comparison of mean within-patient change in EDSS between two fixed points in time (e.g., baseline to end of study) in the treated and control arms using a *t*-test. There are several problems associated with this approach. The nonlinear nature of the EDSS suggests that nonparametric statistics would be more appropriate. Also, change in EDSS from one point to a second point does not necessarily indicate the occurrence of disease progression, since a temporary worsening in EDSS can occur during a relapse and may not be permanently sustained. Thus, an increase in EDSS from baseline to the end of study which is not reconfirmed at a later date may actually signify new disease activity rather than the accumulation of sustained disability. In most phase III trials for MS, patients are evaluated several times throughout the course of the study. The pre-post design described above uses data from only two of these evaluations, ignoring all the data collected in between. In general, statistical methods that make use of repeated measures result in more power than the simpler pre-post approach to data analysis. Finally, patients lost to follow-up while on study cannot be included in a pre-post analysis. When the loss to follow-up rate is high, it can introduce substantial bias into study results.

An alternative approach for analyzing disability data is to utilize life table methodology. Also referred to as survival analysis or time to failure analysis, this approach compares groups with regard to differences in time to reach a particular event, e.g., sustained disability [12,79]. Use of survival analysis is especially appropriate when it is expected that some patients may not complete the entire trial, a common phenomenon in trials involving large numbers of MS patients, lengthy follow-up periods, or therapeutic agents with significant side-effects. In this approach, the trial is deliberately designed such that patients entered into it will be followed for variable lengths of time. The advantages of survival analysis over a fixed point or pre-post type of design is that it allows one to incorporate information on individuals who are lost to follow-up during the trial up to the point that they are censored (i.e., "lost"). Thus, it is not necessary to eliminate patients from the analysis because they fail to complete the entire study or to ignore the large amount of data which is collected between the beginning and the end of the study for patients who complete the entire trial.

The most widely used approach to survival analysis in the context of clinical trials in general is the Kaplan–Meier method [80]. This method does not assume that data are normally distributed. It allows one to generate descriptive graphs that can be used to compare the two treatment groups visually. The Kaplan–Meier curve depicts the cumulative proportion of patients "surviving," i.e., not becoming treatment failures over time. Data can also be analyzed so as to indicate the cumulative proportion of patients "failing," e.g., sustaining a 1.0 step worsening in EDSS from baseline over time [81]. A *p* value is calculated using the log-rank test to determine whether observed differences are statistically significant [81]. Kaplan–Meier methodology has been routinely used in phase III trials for cancer and cardiovascular disease for over 20 years [83]. The use of survival analysis in the context of MS clinical trials is somewhat more complex than in the usual cancer trial, due to the nature of the endpoint, i.e., disease progression rather than death. Nevertheless, this methodology is being used with increasing frequency in MS trials to analyze both disease progression and relapse data [8,10–12,23,26,84,85]. In addition to the Kaplan–Meier technique, investigators also may wish to use Cox modeling (another form of survival analysis), when appropriate, to assess the effects of baseline disease characteristics or prognostic variables on treatment efficacy [86]. Assuming the data to be analyzed meet the underlying assumptions required by these techniques, statistical methods such as multivariate ANOVA or an overall test for time trend should be considered when one wishes to examine mean trends over time rather than time to a particular event [87].

Treatment Lag Time

Most studies are designed as though the effect of treatment will be seen as soon as patients begin their treatment. In some instances, there may be a lag between the time patients begin treatment and the time the treatment begins to show efficacy. Failing to account for the impact of lag time when estimating sample size and analyzing outcome data may result in negative findings even though a therapy is efficacious. The practical implications of this phenomenon may be seen when considering the design of a study in which the therapy to be tested is a disease-modifying agent thought to reduce likelihood of relapse. It is typical in studies involving relapsing patients to require that patients be free of relapses for 1–2 months prior to accrual but have a pre-study relapse rate that suggests active disease [10–12]. If a patient's pre-study relapse rate is high, that patient may be at higher risk than usual of suffering an exacerbation at the time they are accrued to the study because they have been required to be stable for at least 30–60 days in order to meet study eligibility criteria. If the therapeutic agent acts in such a manner that it will take 6 months before therapy begins to have effect on relapse frequency, a study in which relapses are analyzed by evaluating the proportion of subjects who are still relapse-free at the end of the study may show only a weak, nonsignificant effect on relapses. The same data, analyzed in a manner that takes treatment lag time into account, might yield highly significant results clearly demonstrating treatment efficacy.

Sample Size and Trial Duration

Sample Size

The statistical methodology used to establish sample size must reflect the primary outcome measure and the statistical methods that will be used to analyze it. Other factors also must be considered when making sample size calculations. The size of the minimum treatment effect to be detected must be specified. Since it requires less power to detect large differences between groups than small ones, studies seeking to detect a small treatment effect will require more patients than those that seek to detect large treatment effects.

To minimize the likelihood of making type I and type II errors, the investigator must set the maximum chance of making these errors in advance. In phase III clinical trials, the alpha level (the probability of making a type I error, also known as level of statistical significance) is typically set at 0.05. The beta level (the probability of making a type II error) is typically set at 0.20 (corresponding to a power of 80%) [13]. This means that there will be a 5% chance that an observed treatment effect is actually a false positive finding resulting from chance, and an 80% likelihood of finding a genuine treatment effect of the size specified during sample size calculations.

Assumptions must also be made concerning the rate at which primary outcome events are expected to occur in the control group. These assumptions should be based on observed data from similar patients in other clinical trials who received the same treatment (for trials with active controls) or lack of treatment (for placebo-controlled trials). An example of sample size calculations for an MS study in which this was done is provided in the phase III trial of IFNβ-1a [12]. Time to onset of sustained worsening in disability, defined as deterioration from baseline of at least 1.0 point on the EDSS persisting for at least 6 months, was the primary outcome and the treated and placebo arms were compared using a stratified log-rank test in a Kaplan–Meier time to failure analysis. The expected placebo progression rate used in sample size calculations for this study was based on the median time to progression in the placebo arm of a previous clinical trial of Cop-1 [88].

The expected rate of noncompliance among patients in the treatment arm of the study is another important factor to consider in determining sample size. For example, in an intent-to-treat design, patients who stop or miss treatments continue to be followed, if possible, and their outcome data are analyzed as though they were still receiving treatment. If a much larger than expected percentage of treated patients discontinue treatment before the end of the study, an apparently negative study could result when efficacy actually exists. For this reason, sample size calculations should assume a much larger rate of treatment discontinuation than is actually anticipated. Whenever feasible it is wise to make a "worst case scenario" type of assumption concerning the percentage of patients that will be lost to follow-up.

Altering the assumptions concerning any of the factors discussed above can change the sample size required for the trial. It is important to remember when making sample size calculations that a sample size that provides sufficient power to detect the primary outcome does not necessarily have sufficient power to detect secondary outcomes. For example, several studies have shown that T2-lesion volume on cranial MRI and the EDSS are only weakly correlated [42]. Therefore, it should not be assumed that a study designed to detect a sustained worsening in EDSS will have sufficient power to detect a change in T2-lesion volume.

Duration of the Trial

The duration of the trial is based in part on the amount of time it is expected to take for a certain number of primary outcome events to occur in the control population, the size of the treatment effect one hopes to detect and the rate at which eligible patients can be accrued to the study. Assuming that rates of treatment discontinuation and loss to follow-up do not increase as a result of increasing the duration of a trial, increasing trial duration will usually increase power since it allows time for additional primary outcome events to occur.

Study Procedures

There are a number of published works available that provide excellent descriptions of the day-to-day activities involved in conducting a successful trial, along with practical advice on how best to carry out these activities [13,15]. A recent work deals specifically with the various procedures, roles and responsibilities associated with the conduct of a phase III trial for MS [85].

Procedures for the actual conduct of the study should be planned thoroughly in advance, since the manner in which trial procedures are carried out may also affect the power of a study to detect efficacy. Key to the successful completion of a clinical trial is a strong and smoothly functioning administrative structure [85]. Most phase III trials for MS will be multicenter. Therefore, methods for ensuring uniformity in the performance of procedures across centers must be established before the trial begins. Case report forms and general procedures for data collection and data management should be fully developed and documented before the trial begins. The volume of data, quality of data, and need for double-blind in phase III trials generally necessitates the establishment of a separate data coordinating center (DCC). The DCC is responsible for coordination of all data collection and data management activities associated with the trial, ensuring the quality of the data that are entered into the database and analyzing the trial data. Ideally, the DCC should be both administratively and physically separate from the clinical centers involved in the trial. Another center that is a usual part of phase III trials is the treatment coordinating center (TCC). The TCC is responsible for coordinating treatment administration and monitoring clinical activities during the trial.

Conclusions

Large clinical trials in MS share many design features with trials in other diseases. However, several aspects of trials in MS pose special design problems. Trials of new agents in MS are complicated by our lack of knowledge of the underlying etiology of the disorder and incomplete understanding of its pathogenesis. There is tremendous heterogeneity in the disease, in terms of the range of clinical manifestations patients exhibit, the severity of these manifestations, and the course over which they develop. MS is a disease in which disability may accumulate over decades. Clinical trials of agents to alter the course of the disease, in contrast, are limited to several years in length. These characteristics place special demands on the outcome measures used and analysis methods. Increasing understanding of the nature of the disease process and recent successes in clinical trials have created new optimism that increasingly more effective treatments will be identified in the future.

References

1. Lublin FD, Reingold SC. Defining the clinical course of multiple sclerosis: results of an international survey. Neurology 1996;46:907–911.
2. Weinshenker BG, Bass B, Rice GPA, Noseworthy J, Carriere W, Baskerville J, et al. The natural history of multiple sclerosis: a geographically based study. 2. Predictive value of the early clinical course. Brain 1989;112:1419–1428.
3. Muller R. Studies in disseminated sclerosis. Acta Med Scand 1949;133(Suppl 222):1–214.
4. Kurtzke JF, Beebe GW, Nagler B, Kurland LT, Auth TL. Studies on the natural history of multiple sclerosis. 8. Early prognostic features of the later course of the illness. J Chron Dis 1977;30:819–830.
5. Goodkin DE, Hertsgaard D, Rudick RA. Exacerbation rates and adherence to disease type in a prospectively followed-up population with multiple sclerosis: implications for clinical trials. Arch Neurol 1989;46:1107–1112.
6. Hauser SL, Dawson DM, Lehrich JR, Beal MF, Kevy SV, Propper RD, et al. Intensive immunosuppression in progressive multiple sclerosis: a randomized, three-arm study of high-dose intravenous cyclophosphamide, plasma exchange, and ACTH. N Engl J Med 1983;308:173–180.
7. Myers LW, Fahey JL, Moody DJ, Mickey MR, Frane MV, Ellison GW. Cyclophosphamide "pulses" in chronic progressive multiple sclerosis: a preliminary clinical trial. Arch Neurol 1987;44:828–832.
8. The Multiple Sclerosis Study Group. Efficacy and toxicity of cyclosporine in chronic progressive multiple sclerosis: a randomized, double-blind, placebo-controlled clinical trial. Ann Neurol 1990;27:591–605.
9. The Canadian Cooperative Multiple Sclerosis Group. The Canadian cooperative trial of cyclophosphamide and plasma exchange in progressive multiple sclerosis. Lancet 1991;337: 441–446.
10. The IFNB Multiple Sclerosis Study Group. Interferon beta-1b is effective in relapsing-remitting multiple sclerosis. I.

Clinical results of a multicenter, randomized, double-blind, placebo-controlled trial. Neurology 1993;43:655–661.

11. Johnson KP, Brooks BR, Cohen JA, Ford CC, Goldstein J, Lisak RP, et al. Copolymer 1 reduces the relapse rate and improves disability in relapsing-remitting multiple sclerosis: results of a phase III multicenter, double-blind, placebo-controlled trial. Neurology 1995;45:1268–1276.

12. Jacobs LD, Cookfair DL, Rudick RA, Herndon RM, Richert JR, Salazar AM, et al. Intramuscular interferon beta-1a for disease progression in relapsing multiple sclerosis. Ann Neurol 1996; 39:285–294.

13. Hulley SR, Cummings SR. Designing clinical research: an epidemiological approach. Baltimore: Williams and Wilkins, 1988.

14. Clagett N. The biological IND. In: Mathieu M, editor. Biologics development: a regulatory overview. Waltham, MA: Paraxel International, 1993:53–75.

15. Meinert CL. Clinical trials: design, conduct and analysis. Oxford: Oxford University Press, 1986.

16. Rose AS, Namerow NS, Kuzma JW, Scheinberg LC, Brown AJ, Rumberg J, et al. Cooperative study in the evaluation of therapy in multiple sclerosis: ACTH vs placebo – final report. Neurology 1970;20:1–59.

17. Willoughby EW, Paty DW. Scales for rating impairment in multiple sclerosis: a critique. Neurology 1988;38:1793–1798.

18. Kurtzke JF. Rating neurologic impairment in multiple sclerosis: an expanded disability status scale (EDSS). Neurology 1983;33:1444–1452.

19. Ellison GW, Myers LW, Leake BD, Mickey MR, Ke D, Syndulko K, et al. Design strategies in multiple sclerosis clinical trials. Ann Neurol 1994;36:S108–S112.

20. Weinshenker BG, Issa M, Baskerville J. Long-term and short-term outcome of multiple sclerosis: a 3-year follow-up study. Arch Neurol 1996;53:353–358.

21. Amato MP, Fratiglioni L, Groppi C, Siracusa G, Amaducci L. Interrater reliability in assessing functional systems and disability on the Kurtzke scale in multiple sclerosis. Arch Neurol 1988;45:746–748.

22. Noseworthy JH, Vandervoort MK, Wong CJ, Ebers GC, the Canadian Cooperative MS Study Group. Interrater variability with the expanded disability status scale (EDSS) and functional systems (FS) in a multiple sclerosis clinical trial. Neurology 1990;40:971–975.

23. Goodkin DE, Cookfair D, Wende K, Bourdette D, Pullicino P, Scherokman B, et al. Inter- and intrarater scoring agreement using grades 1.0 to 3.5 of the Kurtzke Expanded Disability Status Scale (EDSS). Neurology 1992;42:859–863.

24. Schwid SR, Goodman AD, Mattson DH, Mihai C, Donohue KM, Petrie MD, et al. The measurement of ambulatory impairment in multiple sclerosis. Neurology 1997;49:1419–1424.

25. Goodkin DE, Hertsgaard D, Seminary J. Upper extremity function in multiple sclerosis: improving assessment sensitivity with box-and-block and nine-hole peg tests. Arch Phys Med Rehabil 1988;69:850–854.

26. Goodkin DE, Rudick RA, Medendorp SV, Daughtry MM, Schwetz KM, Fischer J, et al. Low-dose (7.5 mg) oral methotrexate reduces the rate of progression in chronic progressive multiple sclerosis. Ann Neurol 1995;37:30–41.

27. Syndulko K, Tourtellotte WW, Baumhefner RW, Ellison GW, Myers LW, Belendiuk G, et al. Neuroperformance evaluation of multiple sclerosis disease progression in a clinical trial: implications for neurological outcomes. J Neurol Rehabil 1993;7: 153–176.

28. Heaton RK, Nelson LM, Thompson DS, Burks JS, Franklin GM. Neuropsychological findings in relapsing-remitting and chronic-progressive multiple sclerosis. J Consult Clin Psychol 1985;53:103–110.

29. Rao SM, Leo GJ, Bernardin L, Unverzagt F. Cognitive dysfunction in multiple sclerosis. I. Frequency, patterns, and prediction. Neurology 1991;41:685–691.

30. Rao SM, Leo GJ, Haughton VM, St. Aubin-Faubert P, Bernadin L. Correlation of magnetic resonance imaging with neuropsychological testing in multiple sclerosis. Neurology 1989;39: 161–166.

31. Hohol MJ, Guttmann CRG, Orav J, Mackin GA, Kikinis R, Khoury SJ, et al. Serial neuropsychological assessment and magnetic resonance imaging analysis in multiple sclerosis. Arch Neurol 1997;54:1018–1025.

32. Fischer JS, Foley FW, Aikens JE, Ericson GD, Rao SM, Shindell S. What do we really know about cognitive dysfunction, affective disorders, and stress in multiple sclerosis? A practitioner's guide. J Neurol Rehabil 1994;8:151–164.

33. Rao SM, Leo GJ, Ellington L, Nauertz T, Bernardin L, Unverzagt F. Cognitive dysfunction in multiple sclerosis. II. Impact on employment and social functioning. Neurology 1991;41: 692–696.

34. Durelli L, Bongioanni MR, Cavallo R, Ferrero B, Ferri R, Ferrio MF, et al. Chronic systemic high-dose recombinant interferon alfa-2a reduces exacerbation rate, MRI signs of disease activity, and lymphocyte interferon gamma production in relapsing-remitting multiple sclerosis. Neurology 1994;44: 406–413.

35. Fischer JS. Use of neuropsychologic outcome measures in multiple sclerosis clinical trials: current status and strategies for improving multiple sclerosis clinical trial design. In: Goodkin DE, Rudick RA, editors. Multiple sclerosis: advances in clinical trial design, treatment and future perspectives. Berlin Heidelberg New York: Springer, 1996:123–144.

36. Smits RCF, Emmen HH, Bertelsmann FW, Kulig BM, van Loenen AC, Polman CH. The effects of 4-aminopyridine on cognitive function in patients with multiple sclerosis: a pilot study. Neurology 1994;44:1701–1705.

37. Pliskin NH, Hamer DP, Goldstein DS, Towle VL, Reder AT, Noronha A, et al. Improved delayed visual reproduction test performance in multiple sclerosis patients receiving interferon β-1b. Neurology 1996;47:1463–1486.

38. Flscher JS, Priore RL, Jacobs LD, Cookfair DL, Rudick RA, Herndon RM et al. Neuropsychological effects of Interferon Beta-1a in relapsing multiple sclerosis. Ann Neurol 2000, in press.

39. Rudick R, Antel J, Confavreux C, Cutter G, Ellison G, Fischer J, et al. Recommendations from the National Multiple Sclerosis Society Clinical Outcomes Assessment Task Force. Ann Neurol 1997;42:379–382.

40. Cutter GR, Baier ML, Rudick RA, Cookfair DL, Fischer JS, Petkau J et al. Development of a multiple sclerosis functional composite as a clinical trial outcome measure. Brain 1999;122:871–872.

41. Kirby N. The clinical testing of biologics. In: Mathieu M, editor. Biologics development: a regulatory overview. Waltham, MA: Paraxel International, 1993:53–75.

42. Evans AC, Frank JA, Antel J, Miller DH. The role of MRI in clinical trials of multiple sclerosis: comparison of image processing techniques. Ann Neurol 1997;41:125–132.

43. Paty DW, Li DKB, the UBC MS/MRI Study Group, the IFNB Multiple Sclerosis Study Group. Interferon beta-1b is effective in relapsing-remitting multiple sclerosis. II. MRI analysis results of a multicenter, randomized, double-blind, placebo-controlled trial. Neurology 1993;43:662–667.

44. Miller DH, Albert PS, Barkhof F, Francis G, Frank JA, Hodgkinson S, et al. Guidelines for the use of magnetic resonance techniques in monitoring the treatment of multiple sclerosis. Ann Neurol 1996;39:6–16.

45. Harris JO, Frank JA, Patronas N, McFarlin DE, McFarland HF. Serial gadolinium-enhanced magnetic resonance imaging

scans in patients with early, relapsing-remitting multiple sclerosis: implications for clinical trials and natural history. Ann Neurol 1991;29:548–555.

46. Thompson AJ, Miller D, Youl B, MacManus D, Moore S, Kingsley D, et al. Serial gadolinium-enhanced MRI in relapsing-remitting multiple sclerosis of varying disease duration. Neurology 1992;42:60–63.

47. Simon JH, Jacobs LD, Campion M, Wende K, Simonian N, Cookfair DL, et al. Magnetic resonance studies of intramuscular interferon β-1a for relapsing multiple sclerosis. Ann Neurol 1998;43:79–87.

48. McFarland HF, Frank JA, Albert PS, Smith ME, Martin R, Harris JO, et al. Using gadolinium-enhanced magnetic resonance imaging lesions to monitor disease activity in multiple sclerosis. Ann Neurol 1992;32:758–766.

49. Nauta JJP, Thompson AJ, Barkhof F, Miller DH. Magnetic resonance imaging in monitoring the treatment of multiple sclerosis patients: statistical power of parallel-groups and crossover designs. J Neurol Sci 1994;122:6–14.

50. Goodkin DE, Rudick RA, VanderBrug Medendorp S, et al. Low-dose oral methotrexate in chronic progressive multiple sclerosis: analyses of serial MRIs. Neurology 1996;47:1153–1157.

51. The IFNB Multiple Sclerosis Study Group, University of British Columbia MS/MRI Analysis Group. Interferon beta-1b in the treatment of multiple sclerosis: final outcome of the randomized, controlled trial. Neurology 1995;45:1277–1285.

52. Stone LA, Albert PS, Smith ME, DeCarli C, Armstrong MR, McFarlin DE, et al. Changes in the amount of diseased white matter over time in patients with relapsing-remitting multiple sclerosis. Neurology 1995;45:1808–1814.

53. Truyen L, van Waesberghe JHTM, van Walderveen MAA, van Osten BW, Polman CH, Hommes OR, et al. Accumulation of hypointense lesions ("black holes") on T1 spin-echo MRI correlates with disease progression in multiple sclerosis. Neurology 1996;47:1469–1476.

54. Gass A, Barker GJ, Kidd D, Thorpe JW, MacManus D, Brennan A, et al. Correlation of magnetization transfer ratio with clinical disability in multiple sclerosis. Ann Neurol 1994;36:62–67.

55. Cohen SR, Herndon RM, McKhann GM. Radioimmunoassay of myelin basic protein in spinal fluid: an index of active demyelination. N Engl J Med 1976;295:1455–1457.

56. Whitaker JN, Layton BA, Herman PK, Kachelhofer RD, Burgard S, Bartolucci AA. Correlation of myelin basic protein-like material in cerebrospinal fluid of multiple sclerosis patients with their response to glucocorticoid treatment. Ann Neurol 1993;33:10–17.

57. Whitaker JN. The presence of immunoreactive myelin basic protein peptide in urine of persons with multiple sclerosis. Ann Neurol 1987;22:648–655.

58. Whitaker JN, Kachelhofer RD, Bradley EL, Burgard S, Layton BA, Reder AT, et al. Urinary myelin basic protein-like material as a correlate of the progression of multiple sclerosis. Ann Neurol 1995;38:625–632.

59. Whitaker JN, Williams PH, Layton BA, McFarland HF, Stone LA, Smith ME, et al. Correlation of clinical features and findings on cranial magnetic resonance imaging with urinary myelin basic protein-like material in patients with multiple sclerosis. Ann Neurol 1994;35:577–585.

60. Kaji R, Happel L, Sumner AJ. Effects of digitalis on clinical symptoms and conduction variables in patients with multiple sclerosis. Ann Neurol 1990;28:582–584.

61. Davis FA, Stefoski D, Rush J. Orally administered 4-aminopyridine improves clinical signs in multiple sclerosis. Ann Neurol 1990;27:186–192.

62. van Diemen HAM, Polman CH, van Dongen TMMM, van Loenen AC, Nauta JJP, Taphoorn MJB, et al. The effect of 4-aminopyridine on clinical signs in multiple sclerosis: a ran-

domized, placebo-controlled, double-blind, cross-over study. Ann Neurol 1992;32:123–130.

63. van Diemen HAM, Polman CH, Koetsier JC, van Loenen AC, Nauta JJP, Bertelsmann FW. 4-Aminopyridine in patients with multiple sclerosis: dosage and serum level related to efficacy and safety. Clin Neuropharm 1993;16:195–204.

64. Ellison GW, Myers LW, Mickey MR, Graves MC, Tourtellotte WW, Syndulko K, et al. A placebo-controlled, randomized, double-blind, variable-dosage, clinical trial of azathioprine with and without methylprednisolone in multiple sclerosis. Neurology 1989;39:1018–1026.

65. Nuwer MR, Packwood JW, Myers LW, Ellison GW. Evoked potentials predict the clinical changes in multiple sclerosis drug study. Neurology 1987;37:1754–1761.

66. Vickrey BG, Hays RD, Harooni R, Myers LW, Ellison GW. A health-related quality of life measure for multiple sclerosis. Qual Life Res 1995;4:187–206.

67. LaRocca NG, Ritvo PG, Miller DM, Fischer JS, Andrews H, Paty D. Quality of life assessment in multiple sclerosis trials: current status and strategies for improving multiple sclerosis clinical trial design. In: Goodkin DE, Rudick RA, editors. Multiple sclerosis: advances in clinical trial design, treatment and future perspectives. Berlin Heidelberg New York: Springer, 1996:145–160.

68. Devins GM, Seland TP. Emotional impact of multiple sclerosis: recent findings and suggestions for future research. psychol Bull 1987;101:363–375.

69. Aronson KJ. Quality of life among persons with multiple sclerosis and their caregivers. Neurology 1997;48:74–80.

70. Rudick RA, Miller D, Clough JD, Gragg LA, Farmer RG. Quality of life in multiple sclerosis: comparison with inflammatory bowel disease and rheumatoid arthritis. Arch Neurol 1992;49:1237–1242.

71. Petajan JH, Gappmaier E, White AT, Spencer MK, et al. Impact of aerobic training on fitness and quality of life in multiple sclerosis. Ann Neurol 1996;39:432–441.

72. Cookfair DL, Fischer J, Rudick R, Bourdette D, O'Reilly K, Jacobs L, et al. Quality of life in low-disability multiple sclerosis patients participating in a phase III trial of interferon beta-1a for relapsing multiple sclerosis. Ann Neurol 1996;40:550.

73. Rudick RA, Goodkin DE, Jacobs LD, Cookfair DL, Herndon RM, Richert JR, et al. Impact of interferon beta-1a on neurologic disability in relapsing multiple sclerosis. Neurology 1997;49:358–363.

74. Bergner M, Bobbitt RA, Pollard WE, Martin DP, Gilson DS. The sickness impact profile: validation of a health status measure. Med Care 1976;14:57–67.

75. Bergner M, Bobbitt RA, Carter B, Gilson BS. The Sickness Impact Profile: development and final revision of a health status measure. Med Care 1981;19:787–805.

76. Ware JE, Sherbourne CD. The MOS 36-item Short Form Health Survey (SF-36). Med Care 1992;30:473–481.

77. Ware JE, Snow KK, Kosinski M, Gandek B. SF-36 Health Survey: manual and interpretation guide. Boston, MA: The Health Institute, New England Medical Center, 1993.

78. Fleming TR, Harrington DP, O'Brien PC. Designs for group sequential test. Control Clin Trials 1984;5:348–361.

79. Anderson S, Auquier A, Hauck WW. Statistical methods for comparative studies: techniques for bias reduction. New York: Wiley, 1980.

80. Kaplan EL, Meier P. Nonparametric estimation from incomplete observations. J Am Stat Assoc 1958;53:457–481.

81. Kalbfleish JD, Prentice RL. The statistical analysis of failure time data. New York: Wiley, 1980.

82. Mantel N. Evaluation of survival data and two new rank order statistics arising in its consideration. Cancer Chemoth Reports 1966;50:163–170.

83. Peto R, Pike MC, Armitage P, Breslow NE, Cox DR, Howard SV, et al. Design and analysis of randomized clinical trials requiring prolonged observation of each patient. Br J Cancer 1977; 35:1–39.

84. Bornstein MB, Miller A, Slagle S, Weitzman M, Drexler E, Keilson M, et al. A placebo-controlled, double-blind, randomized, two-center, pilot trial of Cop 1 in chronic progressive multiple sclerosis. Neurology 1991;41:533–539.

85. Rudick RA, Cookfair DL. Conduct of clinical trials in multiple sclerosis. In: Raine CS, McFarland HF, Tourtellotte WW, editors. Multiple sclerosis: clinical and pathogenetic basis. London: Chapman and Hall, 1997:341–353.

86. Cox DR. Regression models and life tables. J R Stat Soc 1972; 34:187–220.

87. Fleiss JL. The design and analysis of clinical experiments. New York: Wiley, 1986.

88. Bornstein MB, Miller A, Slagle S, Weitzman M, Crystal H, Drexler E, et al. A pilot trial of Cop 1 in exacerbating-remitting multiple sclerosis. N Engl J Med 1987;317:408–414.

33. Motor Neurone Disease: Ethics, Outcome Variables and Clinical Scales

R.J. Guiloff and A. Goonetilleke

Introduction

Clinical trials in motor neurone disease (MND; USA: amyotrophic lateral sclerosis, ALS) present challenging ethical and methodological problems and practical difficulties in their implementation. Some of these are shared with other neurological disorders and others are more disease-specific. The fatal progressive course over a median of 2–3 years and the patchy, incapacitating and variable clinical expression are major features of the disorder.

A number of ethical issues, some related to the nature of MND, will be considered first in this chapter. For example, due to the course of the disease, patients participating in clinical trials may not benefit from the drug even if it is shown to be effective. The use of historical controls (thus avoiding the use of placebo), the hidden benefits of participating in a clinical trial, and even the basic trial design chosen all have ethical implications. The disease is far less common than other neurological conditions so that funding for clinical trials from all sources is much less than for a number of other diseases. Thus, the question of screening as many drugs as possible, appropriately and efficiently, to make the most of available resources, also becomes an ethical matter.

The outcome variables selected for a clinical trial will be presented in relation to the basic trial designs in which they are used. Time to death seems an obvious outcome variable for a fatal disease, but increase in survival without a reduction in the rate of progression of disability is not acceptable to many MND patients. Studies addressing survival are costly and the rate of dropouts in clinical trials in this disease is consistently high (20–25% or more), often posing unresolved problems for the interpretation of statistical results. A number of other outcome variables may be required for both phase II and III studies. This has led to the development of quantitative measurements of muscle force, respiration, bulbar function and activities of daily living and to the description of qualitative and quantitative clinical scales for use in MND. These measurements and scales will also be reviewed and critically discussed in this chapter. Qualities of life measures are mentioned in Chapter 34.

Ethics

Many of the ethical issues in MND clinical trials are shared with other neurological diseases. The severity and poor prognosis of MND, along with the heterogeneous clinical picture, pose more specific ethical issues.

General Aspects

The requirements for human clinical therapeutic trials outlined in the Declaration of Helsinki by the World Medical Association have been accepted internationally as the basis for ethical clinical research. Individual countries have developed their own approach to the implementation of such guidelines. In the United Kingdom the British Medical Association provide their own guidelines on medical research on human subjects. In addition, a system of local ethics committees have to approve the protocols for all proposed trials within individual hospitals and regions.

It can be argued that a properly conducted study is most likely to answer the question as to the efficacy of the drug being tested. A randomised double-blind placebo-controlled trial is considered the gold standard in trial design. There has been debate about the use of placebos in clinical trials generally

[1], particularly in disorders with significant mortality such as MND. The use of a placebo can be justified if there is no standard intervention that has already been shown to be superior to placebo, and the trial patients are aware of the chances of receiving either the placebo or the study drug [2].

Investigators must ensure that results are being monitored during the trial, allowing early termination of the trial if significant beneficial or harmful effects of the study drug appear [3]. Conversely, trials may need extension beyond the original sample size or planned period of follow-up [4]. For example, if the actual event rates observed during the trial were less than the figures used to estimate sample sizes at the beginning of the study the trial would lack the statistical power to detect, or exclude, any significant drug effects, unless recruitment and/or follow-up were extended.

The time intervals at which the data are to be monitored during a trial should be determined before the trial begins. The number of checks should be sufficient to detect rapidly any serious adverse effects of the study drug. Excessive checks need to be avoided, as repeated testing at the same level of significance increases the chance of incorrectly rejecting the null hypothesis (Ho) of there being no difference between treatment groups. For example, if using a significance level of 5% the chances of incorrectly rejecting Ho after only one test is only 5%. If Ho is tested twice during the study the probability of incorrectly rejecting Ho chances increases to 8%, and up to 14% and 20% after testing five or ten times respectively [5].

Specific Considerations

In any clinical trial there is a possible conflict between the ethics of benefit to individual patients and benefit to all patients with the disorder [6]. *Individual ethics* refers to the fact that each patient should receive the treatment that is likely to be most

beneficial to them, whereas *collective ethics* relates to achieving medical progress as quickly as possible so that all patients with the disorder can benefit. Most trials in MND monitor the effects of potential therapeutic agents on individual patients over a period of 12 months or more, a relatively long period compared with the overall median survival of 2–3 years. Approximately 20–30% of patients may therefore die during a 12 month study. It follows that many patients entering MND trials are unlikely to benefit themselves, even if the drug is eventually shown to be effective.

There are hidden benefits in participating in a trial, even in patients randomised to the placebo group. The regular medical supervision of patients during trials often results in earlier assessment of potential consequences of the disease process (e.g. dysphagia or respiratory failure) and appropriate medical intervention (e.g. gastrostomy, respiratory assistance) may also be instituted earlier. Regular clinical and laboratory monitoring may also detect other unrelated disorders (e.g. hypertension, diabetes mellitus) which may otherwise have remained latent.

The use of historical controls in MND has been advocated by some groups in the past [7] in order to give all patients the chance to receive the putative active drug and avoid placebo. The changes and improvements in clinical practice over the years (e.g. gastrostomy, assisted ventilation) make this approach prone to error. The median survival of the historical and current populations may be quite different. Control populations in published clinical trials in MND show substantial differences in mortality (see Table 33.1). For example, a particularly high mortality in the control group was seen in the riluzole trials [8,9]. Further, the effect of close monitoring during a trial is not properly controlled for if historical controls are used. Putative beneficial effects related to such monitoring could be attributed to the tested drug.

Table 33.1. Comparison of 12 month mortality rates in the control groups of some ALS trials

Study	Drug	Entry criteria	n	FVC (% normal)	Age (years)	Deaths (%)
Plaitakis et al. [11]	BCAA	Ambulant	11	?	53.7 ± 11.5	18
Smith et al. [12]	hGH	Ambulant	37	?	58.5 ± 10.3	16
Bensimon et al. [8]	Riluzole	<60 months disease, 20–75 years old, FVC > 60% normal	78	86 ± 18	58.1 ± 11.0	42
Goonetilleke and Guiloff [13]	RX77368	<36 months disease, 18–80 years old, FVC > 1.0 litre	15	79.7 ± 40	55.1 ± 11.1	20

FVC and age are expressed as mean ± SD.

n, number in control group; FVC, forced vital capacity; BCAA, branched chain amino acids; hGH, human growth hormone; RX77368 is the name of a TRH analogue.

Crossover studies ensure exposure of all patients to the study medication at some stage. The relentless progression of the disease in many cases means that the study periods may not represent comparable stages of the disease process. Further, in view of the comparatively long follow-up and washout periods required to assess the effect of a drug relative to median survival in MND, the consensus is that the use of a crossover study design is inappropriate for phase III trials in this disease [10]. These current consensus guidelines, surprisingly, still accept historical controls and crossover design for phase II trials.

No therapeutic agents to date (some may argue that riluzole is a possible exception) have been shown to have a definite and significant clinical effect on the disease process or on the manifestations of the disease. The authors argue that the use of placebo-controlled, parallel groups, randomised and double-blind designs is currently ethically justified in MND. A double-blind study minimises the risk of bias, and corrects for external factors.

Outcome Variables

The selection of the outcome variables in a given trial is of paramount importance. The ones chosen need to be appropriate to the questions asked and to the study design (event rate, hazard rate or continuous variable, see below). They also need to be clinically meaningful and easy to implement in a clinical trial setting. The number of outcome variables also influences the level of statistical significance required. Usually one outcome variable is chosen, or at the most two, to decide on the efficacy of a drug. A number of secondary outcome measures may also be used.

Event Rate Studies

An important effect of a potential therapeutic agent would be the demonstration of a significant reduction in a relevant event. Relevant events in MND include the number of deaths or of major disability (e.g. respiratory failure, gastrostomy, inability to use an upper limb or to walk). Event rate studies measure the *proportion of patients experiencing an event* during a period of time. Advantages of this design over hazard rate studies (see below) include the following: it is easier to plan a termination date for the trial, a shorter time is required to complete the trial and smaller sample sizes are required. However, there is no overall consensus as to the *degree* by which the proportion of such events would need to

be improved by a drug to be considered clinically "significant".

Hazard Rate Studies

Hazard rate studies entail the analysis of the *time to a relevant event*. Such events in MND have included time to death, requirement of gastrostomy or respiratory failure. These trials generally continue until both drug and control groups reach the appropriate end-points specified in the protocol. The methodology for hazard rate studies, in particular survival, has been developed mainly in relation to cancer therapy trials and will not be discussed further here. Time to death or respiratory failure was used in the recent riluzole trials [8,9]. A conventional phase II trial to establish biological efficacy does not appear to have been undertaken for this drug. Instead it was attempted to prove efficacy in phase III studies with an intention-to-treat analysis comparing the drug with placebo. There was a high a relatively high death rate in the control group compared with a number of recent previous MND clinical trials [11–13] (Table 33.1). There was also a high rate of dropouts (about 25%). The problems related to the use of the intention-to-treat analysis to prove efficacy, particularly when the dropout rate is high are discussed in the general section of this book (see Chapters 12 and 13).

Continuous Response Variables

Disadvantages of both event rate and hazard rate trial designs in MND are the relatively large numbers of patients required compared with the number actually available for such studies. Trials requiring large sample sizes limit the number of drugs that can be tested at any one time, and therefore have high human, in addition to economic, costs.

A methodology that requires relatively small numbers of patients and yet retains sufficient statistical power is required to screen a number of potential therapeutic agents at the same time. The continuous response variable design, by employing interval data, requires smaller sample sizes. This is one reason for the development of the quantitative clinical scales discussed in detail below.

This trial design has been used advantageously to screen new drugs for significant biological effects (phase II studies) using as few as 30 patients [13]. A large number of drugs could potentially be assessed simultaneously in small groups of patients and controls throughout many centres for biological efficacy with a similar design. In a disease as devastating as MND, and without known cure, such intensive screening should be a priority for the clinical scientific community and the funding agencies. If an effect is demonstrated, the drug may then be assessed in trials using an event rate or hazard rate trial design (see above), which require larger patient numbers and are far more expensive.

Each of these types of studies has been used in clinical trials in MND.

Clinical Neurophysiology Variables

Electromyographic variables are not currently widely accepted as useful outcome measures in MND clinical trials in spite of having the appeal of objectivity. A variety of variables have been used including compound muscle action potential, motor unit potential analysis (macro EMG and concentric needle), single-fibre EMG (fibre density and jitter) and motor unit number estimates (MUNE). The clinical relevance of these measurements is less obvious than their biological significance. A number of issues related to standardisation of the techniques, accuracy, sensitivity and reliability need to be addressed before their use can become widespread. Of the available methods MUNE seems the most promising [14,15]. If MUNE reflects accurately the number of motor neurones present in a segment of the ventral horn, then a biological effect of a drug that reduces the rate of motor neurone loss may be demonstrable with this technique.

Clinical Scales

The rest of this chapter will focus on a critical discussion on the development of clinical scales for MND, both qualitative and quantitative. They are used in clinical practice to follow up the progression of the condition in several centres [16] and in natural history studies [17,18]. They have also been used for phase II and in some phase III clinical trials. The challenge has been to produce scales that are sensi-

tive, accurate and reliable while also being transparent enough to reflect the patchy involvement by the disease process. In the design of such scales much attention has therefore been paid recently to topographical subscores (bulbar, respiration, cervical enlargement, lumbar-sacral enlargement) in order to describe the differential involvement of such regions in individuals and in groups of patients. Such four subscores describe accurately the evolution of the disease in individuals and in groups of patients [13,16].

Qualitative Scales

The Norris Scale (Appendix A)

The Norris Scale was the first widely used MND scale, and has evolved since its original description [19] to its current form (Appendix A). The scale is simple to administer, and has been used in a number of clinical situations during the last 20 years. The scale comprises 34 items that measure involvement in Bulbar, Respiratory, Arm, Trunk, Leg and General domains, the relative weights for each subdomain being 15, 6, 26, 9, 26 and 18 respectively (Table 33.2). Bulbar and respiratory function, which many would consider to be functions of critical importance in MND, are therefore given a relative weight of only 21% of the total score. Bowel and bladder function is also assessed, though these functions are rarely involved in MND. The validity of combining items that reflect self-reported function (65%) and symptoms (6%) as well as clinical signs (29%) can also be questioned. Other methodological difficulties with the Norris Scale include the mixing of impairments and disabilities in the same scale.

Appel ALS Scale (Appendix B)

The Appel ALS scale was developed using an analysis of a data set accrued from 74 MND patients

Table 33.2. The relative weights assigned to six domain subscores of some qualitative ALS scales

	Bulbar	Respiratory	Upper limb	Trunk	Lower limb	General
Norris, 1974	15	6	26	9	26	18
Appel, 1987	18	18	34	0	30	0
Hillel, 1989	50[a]	0[b]	25	0	25	0
ALSFRS, 1995[c]	30	10	20 (20–30)	10 (0–10)	20	0
CXALS, 1995[c]	25%	25%	25%	—	25%	—

ALSFRS, ALS Functional Rating Scale; CXALS, Charing Cross Qualitative ALS Rating Scale.
[a] Speech and swallowing scores combined.
[b] A measure of vital capacity has been suggested as an additional score of the ALSSS.
[c] The use of a total score has been discouraged by the authors of these scales (see text).

involved in a study over 4 years [20]. All had upper and lower motor neurone signs with minimal bulbar compromise at the beginning of the study. A number of items were used to create five separate domain subscores (bulbar, respiratory, muscle strength, lower extremity function and upper extremity function). Each domain had a score of 6 for normal function and 30–36 for maximal dysfunction. The total score was a sum of the scores for the five groups, with scores therefore ranging from 30 points for normal function to 164 for maximal dysfunction.

Methodological considerations for this rating scale include the fact that the patients studied appeared selective, with all having initial scores <80, which is approximately 50% of the total score. The performance of the scale on more severe patients is unknown. A number of the timed tests present in the upper and lower extremity function scores may be prone to learning effects [21]. Such a learning effects may explain some of the initial improvements in scores seen in two of the three individual patient progression rates shown in the original publication (figure 1 in [20]).

Reproducibility rates quoted for the Appel ALS Scale include an intra-class correlation coefficient for a single examination of 51 patients by four raters of 0.757, and a test–retest correlation coefficient (patients retested within a 3 week period) of 0.99. The mean difference in scores between assessments was less than one point for each domain and 1.65 points for the overall score, the latter being equivalent to 1.0% of the maximum possible score [20].

The reproducibility rates quoted may not be widely applicable, because (a) all the raters had a minimum of 1 year's experience, (b) some of the items in the scale (e.g. regarding diet, need for assistive devices) are dependent on patient responses to specific questions, which may be remembered by the patient in the second assessment, and (c) the use of an intra-class correlation coefficient is only appropriate for interval data, with no evidence provided to validate the assumption that this scale may be considered an interval one. The relative weights assigned to bulbar, respiratory, arm, trunk and leg domain subscores of 18:18:34:0:30 appear somewhat arbitrary (Table 33.2), as do the weights for individual items within the subscores. The validity of these weights can also be questioned, with only 36% of the total scale represented by bulbar and respiratory function. There was evidence for a certain degree of concurrent validity for the scale. When two nurse-clinicians independently placed 74 patients into five clinical stages of severity, there appeared to be a correlation between this independent means of assessment of severity and the Appel ALS scores for the patients (table 2 in [20]).

Longitudinal assessments over 2 years using this scale suggest linear changes in group scores. Marked differences in progression rates were noted between subjects, with a greater than 20-fold difference in the progression rates of the slowest and most rapid declines. The scale appeared to contain some prognostic capabilities [18,20]. If there was a change of >22 points in 6 months, the patient would usually be totally dependent and wheelchair-bound or terminally ill by 1 year. The average overall total scores for various levels of functions were as follows: independent function 52, able to work but needing some assistance 75, unable to work 119, and being completely bed-bound 135. However, the standard deviations or ranges to these readings were not provided so that the true correlative nature of the scores to function cannot be accurately ascertained.

The Hillel ALS Severity Scale (Appendix C)

The Hillel ALS severity scale (ALSSS) was developed as an ordinal scale that assesses speech, swallowing, upper and lower limb functions using a 0–10 ordinal scale. The scores for speech and swallowing could be summated to form a Bulbar score, and upper and lower limb function summated to form a Spinal score. The ALSS requires an interview and a limited physical examination, and takes 5–10 minutes to administer. Its main advantage is that it can be easily and rapidly administered by a variety of health workers. A study on reliability was performed by analysing the scores obtained by three raters on 19 MND patients over a period of 2 days, and obtained a mean inter-rater reliability coefficient of 0.95 (range of 0.93–0.99) for the four components of the scale [22]. Overall, the three raters were within 1 point in 91% of evaluations. The three raters were within one point on the scale for 100% (48/48) of evaluations for speech; results of 91% (52/57), 84% (48/57) and 91% (52/57) were obtained for swallowing, upper and lower limb functions respectively. Seventeen of these patients also underwent a more thorough speech analysis, and resultant scores for speech intelligibility, oral diadochokinetic rates and words per minute had correlation coefficients of 0.88, 0.86 and 0.81 with the ALSSS speech scores.

The ALSSS scores for 138 patients were then studied during a prospective study, during which 32 patients died. When the mean scores from the last visit where analysed for the 106 patients who remained alive in comparison with the mean scores for the 32 patients who died, no significant differences could be detected. As 80% of the deaths (in which the cause of death could be identified) were due to respiratory failure, it was suggested that a measure of vital capacity should also be included as an additional score of the ALSSS.

The ALS Functional Rating Scale (Appendix D)

The ALS Functional Rating scale was devised on similar principles to those used in the construction of the Unified Parkinson's Disease Rating Scale (UPDRS), and is primarily a measure of *disability* in MND patients. The patient or companion rates the patient's function for each of 10 items of the scale from 4 (normal) to 0 (unable to attempt the task). Although a summated total score (0–40) may be used, greater validity is to be obtained by considering individual items of the scale separately. In this way one may consider the time taken for an individual MND patient, or an MND population, to obtain a 1 point drop in score for each item. For example, nearly all patients drop one point from normal in the Dressing and Hygiene subscore by 12 months, whereas Handwriting and Feeding subscores may take 12–24 months to drop by 1 point.

A study of the ALSFRS [23] compared with quantitative dynamometry and other measures of daily function in 75 MND patients concluded that the ALSFRS (i) showed considerable internal consistency, with values of Cronbach's of greater than 0.6 for all individual items of the scale; and (ii) showed good test–retest reliability (for readings obtained from patients on two separate occasions) with Pearson correlation coefficients of greater than 0.88 for all test items, kappa coefficients of 0.59–0.82, and mean absolute differences ($\pm$ SDs) of 0.46 $\pm$ 0.46 for upper extremity functions, 0.59 $\pm$ 0.72 for lower extremity functions and 1.34 $\pm$ 1.37 for the total ALSFRS score.

The following methodological points need to be considered regarding the validation data for the ALSFRS:

(1) Cronbach's is rarely used in evaluating clinimetric scales as (i) high values may be obtained by scales consisting of items showing high levels of inter-correlation but lacking biological significance, and (ii) certain items may be included in the scale that showed a high interdependent correlation but were essentially redundant as they measured the same function [24].
(2) The use of correlation coefficients as indices of repeatability has been criticised [25], as it reflects the closeness to any straight-line relation between two sets of readings, irrespective of the differences between them. The percentage dif-

ference is an index that immediately conveys the degree of closeness between two sets of readings. The mean ($\pm$ SDs) absolute differences for the ALSFRS expressed as percentages were 11.5 $\pm$ 11.5% for upper extremity functions, 14.8 $\pm$ 18.0% for lower extremity functions and 33.5 $\pm$ 34.3% for the total ALSFRS score. The two sets of readings for each patient using the ALSFRS were apparently obtained by the same nurse-coordinator or physical therapist at the study site. These findings suggest a reasonable degree of intra-rater repeatability. Information on inter-rater repeatability was not given.

(3) A factor analysis revealed four factors, corresponding to (i) coordinated mostly upper limb function (writing, feeding, turning, dressing), (ii) bulbar function (speech, swallowing, salivation), (iii) respiration (breathing) and (iv) gross, less finely controlled activities (dressing, turning, walking, climbing, breathing). As can be seen the item cutting did not appear in any of the four factors identified in the analysis, whereas some items (i.e. turning, dressing, breathing) appeared in more than one factor. Although only writing, cutting and dressing were considered together in the subjective upper limb ALSFRS, writing and dressing appeared with feeding and turning, but without cutting, in the factor analysis. Similarly, walking and climbing stairs were considered together as representing subjective lower limb ALSFRS whereas these two functions appeared together with dressing, turning and breathing in the factor analysis.
(4) Bulbar and respiratory function are represented by 40% of the total score.
(5) Transparency of the scale is lost if the total ALSFRS is used.

This scale is also considered in Chapter 34.

Charing Cross Qualitative ALS Rating Scale (Appendices E, F) [13,16]

The Charing Cross Qualitative ALS Rating Scale was designed to assess important qualitative changes in severity of involvement in the bulbar, respiratory, upper limb and lower limb regions. A number of rating scales used in MND possess face validity but their various grades may be judged to be somewhat arbitrarily assigned. This methodological difficulty was specifically addressed during the construction of the Charing Cross Qualitative ALS Rating Scale. In a longitudinal study of 16 MND patients (mean follow-up of 13.5 months, range 1–31 months) all patients were assessed on a monthly basis. Patients were each assigned one of six qualitative grades for respiratory, upper limb, lower limb, and activities of daily living function. The grades were chosen on the basis of face validity, and covered all deficits ranging from complete absence to normal function. Patients were also assessed using the Charing Cross Quantitative ALS Rating Scale (see below), thereby obtaining interval scores (as % normal values) of these functions. This data-set was then used to calculate the means and standard deviations of the interval scores that corresponded to each of the six qualitative grades. If some qualitative grades had similar % normal scores they were merged as a single grade. In this manner, four grades representing distinctly different mean interval scores were found for respiration, upper limbs and lower limbs.

Assigning qualitative grades for bulbar function is more difficult, as there are a number of important different combinations of speech and swallowing abnormalities observed in clinical practice. Six different grades of speech and swallowing impairment were initially used. During a longitudinal study of 20 MND patients, each was patient assessed on 10 separate monthly visits. Such grades were assigned to each patient in addition to obtaining interval data for these functions using the bulbar tests (e.g. tongue protrusion, word repetition, jaw movement and swallowing) of the Charing Cross Quantitative ALS Rating Scale (see below). The readings obtained by the quantitative tests, expressed as percentages of normal readings, were then used as variables for a cluster analysis, which consistently revealed a five-cluster solution by 10 different clustering methods.

The different steps in obtaining the qualitative grades of function for the Charing Cross Qualitative ALS Rating Scale fulfil a number of criteria for a valid clinical scale. The different grades describe all the different types of deficit seen in MND, are mutually exclusive, transparent, have suitable discrimination, and are clinically plausible.

It has been recommended that the grades assigned for different functions should be kept separate, and not be combined into a single overall score. Although a single global score has certain advantages (e.g. simplicity of use, data reduction), the validity of such a score must be questioned. For this reason the authors of the Charing Cross Qualitative ALS Rating Score suggest the use of a tandem profile of functional grades to describe patients. For example a tandem profile of B4R4U1L1A1 would be used to describe a patient with normal bulbar and respiratory function, loss of function in one or both arms, unable to walk, and who is totally dependent in activities of daily living.

Quantitative Assessments

In the 1980s many research groups realised that existing methods of evaluating MND patients (e.g. neurological examination, manual muscle testing, rating scales) were inadequate for meaningful longitudinal assessments of function. The disadvantages of their use included:

1. Basis on ordinal scales, with attributes classified according to rank (e.g. MRC grades, "mild/moderate/severe" deficits) thereby limiting statistical procedures to non-parametric methods.
2. The differences in ranks were often known to be unequal. For example, using the MRC scales it was shown that 3% of the total force of biceps brachii was represented by the grades 0–3, whilst 97% was represented by grades 4–5 [26]. Similarly, a change in Norris ALS score from 37 to 30 is not the same as from 77 to 70 to either patient or examiner, though both represented a 7 point decline [27].
3. The validity and reliability of many existing scales had yet to be ascertained.
4. Lack of sensitivity led to an inability to detect small but significant changes in function.
5. Allocated grades were dependent on the judgement of the rater.

Quantification of neurological deficit overcame many of these difficulties, and had already been introduced by Tourtellotte in the evaluation of multiple sclerosis [28]. Quantification has centred on the development of measurements of muscle strength, respiration, bulbar function and a number of timed activities.

Muscle Strength Function

The need for a more objective and accurate means of testing muscle strength than by qualitative grading scales (e.g. MRC scale) was met by a proliferation of dynamometers. Quantitative strength measurements can be performed under isokinetic or isometric conditions. Under isokinetic conditions the torque produced by a muscle group is recorded as the limb moves through the entire range of movement with a pre-set speed. Disadvantages of this technique include the fact that variables such as muscle length, velocity of movement and limb weight can affect the movement, and the relative expense of the equipment and time required for such measurements. Therefore isometric measurements have become more commonplace, whereby the examiner holds the patient's limb immobile as individual muscle groups are examined. Different types of dynamometers may be used, including spring balances, cable tensiometers, strain gauges and hand-held dynamometers. Fixed dynamometers have been shown to produce highly reproducible readings, though the equipment required can be expensive and difficult to use on disabled patients. Hand-held devices overcome these problems, and the reproducibility and variability of readings obtained by a single rater compare well with those obtained by fixed devices [25].

The readings are expressed in units of force, typically as newtons or kg-force. The data may be further transposed to *percentage of normal* (% normal) by comparing patients' values with matched control values. Sex and age matching is the minimal requirement in obtaining valid % normal readings. Suitable control values have been published for both strain gauge [29] and hand-held dynamometers [30]. When expressed as % normal, muscle groups may be combined to form composite scores (e.g. upper limb, lower limb and global scores), which provides a means of data reduction but also further improves reproducibility and variability of muscle strength measurements [19]. A further discussion on this topic can be found in Chapter 34.

Bulbar Function

The methodology for the quantitative measurement of bulbar function in MND is less advanced than for the assessment of muscle strength in the limbs. Although measurements of the maximal voluntary contraction of some bulbar muscles (e.g. jaw, lips, tongue) can be made [31], quantifying the strength of other more functionally important muscles (e.g. pharyngeal and laryngeal muscles) is more difficult. Timed tests of jaw movements, tongue protrusion, speech and swallowing can produce highly reproducible readings. However, there are "learning effects" in MND patients in some of the tests and these need to be considered (see Charing Cross Quantitative ALS Rating scale).

Respiratory Function

The majority of MND patients die from respiratory failure, and measures of respiratory function have been consistently shown to be one of the best predictors of survival in this disease. Although various other indices of respiratory function (e.g. maximal voluntary ventilation [32], maximal inspiratory and expiratory pressures [33,34]) have been suggested as the most sensitive tests, the use of vital capacity remains the most popular. All tests of respiratory function should be expressed as % normal values after comparison with readings from sex-, age- and height-matched control values.

Activities of Daily Living (ADL)

A number of quantitative tests of ADL function have been used in a variety of neurological disorders [35]. Many employ timed tests of various day-to-day tasks (e.g. rising from a chair, walking a set distance, use of pegboard, placing coins etc.) that may be affected by the disease process. Such activities depend on critical levels of function (e.g. rising from a chair and walking require muscles that are sufficiently strong to act against gravity), and they therefore often show a non-linear relationship with muscle strength measurements [36]. As tests of ADL function reflect performance of day-to-day activities the interpretation of their results are immediately apparent, and thereby possess face validity for both clinicians and patients.

Quantitative Clinical Scales

Tufts Quantitative Neuromuscular Examination (Appendix G). The Neuromuscular Research Unit at Tufts New England Medical Center was one of the first groups to adopt a quantitative approach in developing a rating scale for detecting involvement of relevant functions in MND. The stages involved in the formation of the current Tufts Quantitative Neuromuscular Examination (TQNE) test protocol included:

(a) *Quantification of relevant functions.* Seventy quantitative test items were initially selected to represent functions affected in MND. These included pulmonary, bulbar and muscle force function, as well as various ADL.

(b) *Data collection.* The aforementioned items were tested on 35 normal controls and 10 MND patients using the same rater (a physical therapist) throughout. Intra-rater reliability was ascertained by the same rater retesting all subjects 3–5 hours later. Inter-rater reliability was ascertained by testing 10 normal controls and 10 MND subjects by two raters (both physical therapists) 3–5 hours apart [37]. For pulmonary function and timed activities the mean intra-rater test–retest correlation coefficient (r) was 0.88 for normal controls and 0.96 for MND patients, and the mean per cent differences of readings on retesting of were 6.1% and 8.5% respectively; for isometric strength $r = 0.96$ (controls) and 0.98 (MND), with mean per cent differences of 6.5% and 8.9% respectively; for inter-rater reliability of timed tests, $r = 0.84$ (controls) and 0.98 (MND), with mean per cent differences of 5.2% and 5.5% respectively; for isometric strength, $r = 0.95$ (controls) and 0.98

(MND), corresponding to per cent differences of 7.6% and 8.2%. Based on these results the test items were said to have "excellent test–retest reliability" by the authors.

(c) *Selection of test items.* The aforementioned data were then analysed for "reliability and redundancy". This involved using data from 35 normal controls to eliminate items with test–retest correlation coefficients <0.70, and performing a cluster analysis on data from 176 MND patients to eliminate items with a high degree of redundancy.

(d) *Data reduction.* The need for data reduction had become immediately apparent after the use of a number of test items in several clinical trials [38–40]. This was achieved by the formation of composite scores [41]. The steps involved in the formation of such scores required standardising items in the TQNE which were measured in different units. The procedure selected was the *Z*-score transformation, where:

$$Z = \frac{\text{raw value from test} - \text{MND population mean for that test}}{\text{MND standard deviation for that test}}$$

e.g. a *Z*-score of +1 represents 1 standard deviation above the MND population mean for that test.

These scores are expressed in comparison with an MND population's mean and standard deviation for each test, using an MND population attending the Tufts New England Medical Centre. *Megascores* for bulbar, respiratory, upper limb, lower limb and timed hand function were then calculated by averaging the *Z*-transformed items within each category.

The TQNE protocol is estimated to take 60 min to perform, which can be rather onerous for both patients and raters. Also, testing severely disabled patients with a fixed dynamometer (strain-gauge device) can be impractical. Relevant methodological considerations when using the TQNE include:

(a) Significant "learning effects" are to be expected in some timed activities (e.g. speech tests, pegboard tests) used in the TQNE (see also Charing Cross Quantitative ALS Rating Scale), which have not been accounted for during the process of data gathering. Ignoring such effects during baseline assessments may lead to spurious "improvements" during a longitudinal study.

(b) The main index used in assessing reliability of TQNE test items was the correlation coefficient, with elimination of items with test–retest *r* < 0.70. This may have resulted in the retention of some test items with poor retest reliability (e.g. pegboard, grip). Conversely items with poor correlation coefficients (due to homogeneity for

that function within the tested MND population) but with good reliability, as evidenced by low per cent differences, may have been eliminated. Correlation coefficients indicate the closeness of readings to any straight-line relationship, irrespective of the differences between them. Their use as indices of reliability in test–retest situations has therefore been criticised [25]. Also, due to the degree of functional heterogeneity present in disease populations, there is an increased likelihood of patients maintaining their relative ranks in test–retest studies compared with normal control populations. Therefore, resultant high correlation coefficients may be reflecting the greater degree of heterogeneity for the function tested in a population rather than the true reliability of that test. The use of per cent difference between readings on retesting may better reflect the degree of closeness between two sets of readings irrespective of their absolute values. Examples of this point in relationship to the test items considered in the development of the TQNE are illustrated in the original publications. The isometric strength test *gripL* (i.e. grip with left hand) has an excellent intra-rater correlation coefficient of 0.99 in MND patients, but the degree of difference on retesting is 17.2% (see table 4 in [27]). In contrast, *FVC* in normals has a relatively low correlation ($r = 0.88$), whereas there is only a 5.7% difference on retesting (see table 4 in [37]).

(c) Cluster analysis was another method employed in selecting test items for the TQNE but scant details are available on this step of item selection (e.g. type of cluster analysis performed). The following points regarding the use of cluster analyses must be considered. (i) Their use in finding clusters of variables that measure closely related functions is similar to a principal component analysis. Indeed, when the variables are measured on a continuous scale (as all 70 original test items considered for the TQNE were), most would consider a principal component analysis more appropriate [42]. (ii) It is well recognised that the results obtained by cluster analysis depend on a number of considerations (e.g. type of clustering used, which variables are thought to be important). (iii) Although popular in the 1960s, cluster analysis has found less favour in recent years [43,44].

(d) The aforementioned steps resulted in the reduction of test items from 70 to 29, which came to comprise the TQNE protocol in 1986. By 1988 the number of test items had been reduced to 28. Timed walking was eliminated but the reasons are not stated in the literature; the final TQNE therefore contains no timed lower limb activities.

(e) The use of Z-scores (see above) by comparison with an MND population based at Tufts New England Medical Centre may not be valid for populations based elsewhere in the world. A major disadvantage of the use of Z-scores is that a patient's deficit expressed in this way is difficult to visualise – for example how severely affected is a patient 1 standard deviation below an MND population mean for that test? In addition, the unit of decline in terms of function is different for each test since the mean for each test is peculiar to the base MND population.

(f) The degree of bulbar involvement is an important feature in MND, both for natural history studies and in clinical trials. A composite score for bulbar function should attempt to assess the degree of involvement of jaw, face, pharynx/palate and tongue. In the TQNE megascore "oro-pharyngeal function" consists only of two word-repetition tasks. Jaw function is not represented, and pharyngeal function is only partially assessed. The TQNE megascore assesses function in the upper limbs (i.e. "timed hand activities"), but an equivalent for lower limb function is not present in the protocol (such as. standing, walking, running).

(g) A factor analysis of TQNE items has been published (Table 33.3) [45]. It is unclear what data this analysis was performed on. In particular, it is not clear (i) the number of MND subjects considered, (ii) the number of assessments made on individual subjects, (iii) whether the same number of assessments were made on all subjects, (iv) whether analysis was performed on raw or standardised data, (v) what criteria were used for the number of factors extracted in the analysis. All these factors could potentially have significant effects on the results obtained from a factor analytic procedure. It can be seen from the results of this analysis (Table 33.3) that certain test items subsequently grouped together in the same megascore violate, in a statistical sense, the assumption that they represent the same underlying factor. In particular, (i) phone dialling – *phoneR* loads most heavily on factor 3, whilst *phoneL* does so on factor 5 (the latter only having a loading of 0.136 on factor 3), (ii) pegboard – similarly, *pegbdR* and *pegbdL* load on factors 3 and 5 respectively, (iii) arm strength – *gripR* and *gripL* load more heavily on factors 3 and 5, (iv) leg strength – *hipextL* and *hipflexR* load more heavily on factor 2, the latter stated as representing arm strength.

Charing Cross Quantitative ALS Rating Scale (Appendices H, I). Various items of function, assessed by quantitative methods and expressed as % normal by comparison with age- and/or sex-matched controls as appropriate, have been combined to form composite scores of bulbar, respiratory, upper limb muscle force, lower limb muscle score and ADL [13]. The methods of obtaining measurements for the individual items for each type of score have been previously described and validated [13,16,25,35,46]. Normal mean values in controls used to express readings in patients as percentage of normal for bulbar and activities of daily living tests are given in Appendix I.

A factor analysis of these various quantitative tests (see Table 33.4), expressed as % normal values, has shown that grouping the individual items to form composite scores is appropriate [13,16]. Such factors are consistent with the research (and clinical) criteria used to diagnose MND which consider the upper and lower motor neurone involvement by topographical regions (bulbar, cervical, thoracic, lumbosacral) [47].

Bulbar function is assessed by performing timed tests for tongue protrusion, word repetition, jaw movements and swallowing. As the speed at which these repetitions are performed by the patients increases with the number of sessions performed [21,48,49], about 10 sessions are required to eliminate the effects of this "learning curve". Respiratory function is assessed by measuring forced vital capacity (FVC). Initially, the degree of chest expansion (inspiratory–expiratory chest circumference difference) was also measured. Interestingly, there also appears to be a learning curve for FVC in bulbar MND patients [16] so that it is important to check this when establishing baseline values for this group of patients.

The quantitative measurements of muscle strength are obtained using a hand-held dynamometer. Care was taken to take a representative sample of four muscles muscle groups in each limb. Thus all segments of a limb, and all limbs, are equally represented in the final composite score for muscle force. There is one shoulder muscle group (shoulder abduction), one arm muscle (biceps), one forearm muscle (finger extensors) and one small hand muscle (first dorsal interosseous). In the lower limbs there is one hip muscle (hip flexion), one thigh muscle (quadriceps), one leg muscle (tibialis anterior) and one small foot muscle (extensor digitorum brevis). Thus, the face validity of the muscle score is self-evident.

The overall accuracy of readings obtained by hand-held dynamometry has been shown to be 3%,

Table 33.3. Rotated factor loadings from a factor analysis of 47 TQNE test items

Item	Factor1	Factor2	Factor3	Factor4	Factor5	Factor6
FVC	0.215	0.763	0.003	0.199	−0.008	−0.039
MVV	0.105	0.728	−0.114	0.339	0.020	0.138
Pa	0.114	−0.056	0.141	−0.904	−0.016	0.083
Pata	0.043	0.013	0.182	−0.907	−0.072	0.089
Blow	−0.013	0.238	−0.233	0.804	−0.144	0.116
Speech	−0.151	0.056	−0.066	0.930	0.101	−0.058
Swallow	−0.212	0.189	−0.051	0.810	−0.080	0.127
Distance	0.769	0.106	0.185	−0.125	0.047	0.425
Gait	0.859	−0.024	0.086	−0.225	0.156	0.299
Stairs	0.862	0.060	0.188	−0.173	0.123	0.272
Curbs	0.874	0.060	0.184	−0.141	0.142	0.282
Floor	0.595	0.245	0.289	−0.224	0.218	0.359
Toilet	0.803	0.085	0.227	−0.111	0.360	0.095
Bed	0.729	0.055	0.136	−0.129	0.373	0.172
Chair	0.790	0.155	0.203	−0.073	0.297	0.188
Tlegstan	0.311	0.107	0.039	0.074	−0.170	0.645
Comb	0.108	0.179	0.825	−0.155	0.108	0.271
Teeth	0.052	0.176	0.869	−0.162	−0.108	0.156
Faucet	0.108	−0.026	0.806	−0.143	−0.012	0.124
Wash	0.149	0.281	0.712	−0.235	0.346	0.162
Feed	0.003	0.118	0.910	−0.205	−0.054	−0.054
Cut	0.038	0.185	0.695	−0.124	0.498	−0.018
DressUE	0.156	0.172	0.773	−0.250	0.290	−0.022
DressLE	0.314	0.020	0.387	−0.289	0.555	0.198
Write	−0.034	0.088	0.720	−0.023	0.269	−0.061
PhoneR	−0.045	−0.056	−0.637	−0.265	−0.454	0.158
PhoneL	−0.210	−0.137	−0.136	−0.187	−0.709	0.070
PegbdR	0.119	0.044	0.710	−0.007	0.486	−0.253
PegbdL	0.135	0.023	0.296	−0.025	0.812	−0.087
ShdflexR	0.142	0.804	0.464	0.070	−0.009	0.086
ShdflexL	0.130	0.882	0.219	−0.056	0.171	0.131
ShdextR	0.234	0.829	0.361	0.140	−0.019	0.010
ElbflexR	0.165	0.698	0.612	0.108	−0.003	0.038
ElbflexL	0.114	0.795	0.241	−0.015	0.282	0.137
ElbextR	0.121	0.745	0.512	0.131	−0.012	0.049
ElbextL	0.259	0.791	0.223	0.004	0.195	−0.004
GripR	0.150	0.510	0.707	0.056	0.133	−0.129
GripL	0.140	0.479	0.250	−0.107	0.496	−0.010
HipextR	0.650	0.570	−0.124	0.086	0.090	−0.177
HipextL	0.572	0.679	−0.095	0.027	0.045	−0.099
HipflexR	0.640	0.643	−0.043	0.106	−0.170	−0.220
KneextR	0.709	0.539	0.069	0.078	−0.113	−0.181
KneextL	0.717	0.498	−0.018	−0.076	−0.001	−0.174
KneflexR	0.773	0.378	−0.100	0.099	−0.035	−0.189
KneflexL	0.812	0.362	−0.154	0.064	0.047	−0.112
DorsiR	0.841	0.162	0.132	−0.035	−0.078	−0.114
DorsiL	0.807	0.063	0.064	−0.101	0.030	0.004

Adapted from Figure 10.2 of Munsat et al. [45].
Number of subjects used in this factor analysis is unstated.

Table 33.4. Rotated factor loadings from a factor analysis of 30 quantitative test items used in the Charing Cross Quantitative ALS Rating Scale [16]

Item	Factor1	Factor2	Factor3	Factor4	Factor5
FVC	0.12	0.21	0.07	−0.59	0.60
IED	0.39	0.09	−0.10	−0.29	0.72
Ticker	−0.03	−0.09	−0.04	0.55	0.12
Tongue	0.05	0.09	−0.03	0.22	−0.08
Jaw	0.10	0.21	−0.03	0.77	−0.23
Swallow	0.03	0.01	−0.07	0.84	−0.02
Buttons	−0.13	−0.05	0.62	−0.17	−0.20
Writing	0.00	0.12	0.84	−0.10	−0.04
CoinsR	−0.07	0.03	0.77	−0.14	−0.14
CoinsL	−0.12	0.04	0.87	−0.13	−0.05
Stand	−0.02	0.01	0.76	0.11	0.21
Walk	−0.06	−0.03	0.77	0.16	0.22
ShabdR	0.91	0.05	−0.11	0.11	0.03
ShabdL	0.85	0.10	−0.12	0.09	0.09
ElbflexR	0.93	−0.01	−0.06	0.02	0.04
ElbflexL	0.92	0.04	−0.08	−0.04	0.17
ElbextR	0.85	0.04	−0.02	−0.08	0.10
ElbextL	0.87	0.18	−0.04	−0.03	0.20
FingextR	0.87	−0.15	0.00	0.07	−0.10
FingextL	0.92	−0.16	−0.02	−0.06	−0.04
DIOR	0.75	−0.22	−0.04	0.20	−0.21
DIOL	0.82	−0.17	−0.07	0.01	0.00
HipflexR	−0.06	0.86	0.03	0.04	0.36
HipflexL	−0.05	0.85	0.03	0.03	0.41
KneextR	−0.15	0.86	0.07	0.02	0.25
KneextL	−0.22	0.84	0.09	0.04	0.34
DorsiR	0.11	0.91	−0.11	0.07	−0.20
DorsiL	0.08	0.92	−0.06	0.09	−0.17
EDBR	0.04	0.89	0.01	−0.04	−0.21
EDBL	−0.01	0.91	0.11	0.00	−0.12

Data from 27 MND patients assessed on six consecutive months each.
Five factors extracted, according to eigenvalue >1.0 criterion.
IED, inspiratory–expiratory chest circumference difference; ticker, repetition of "ticker"×10; tongue, tongue protrusion ×10; jaw, jaw open/close ×10; swallow, swallow 100 ml of water through a straw; buttons, unfasten/fasten button; write, writing standard sentence; coins, placing four coins in slots; stand, rise from chair; walk, walking 25 feet (7.7 m).
The last 18 factors are individual muscle force dynamometry readings: e.g. DIO, index finger abduction; EDB, greater hallux extension.

and to be improved by greater experience of the rater [25]. Overall reproducibility was also shown to be good, with a mean % difference (difference between readings × 100/mean of 2 readings) of 13.2%, repeatability coefficient (2 × standard deviation of differences between repeated readings) of 2.17 kg-force, and overall Pearson correlation coefficient of 0.98 [25]. The use of upper limb and lower limb composite scores resulted in a mean coefficient of variation (CV) of ten readings of 5.8%, and compared well with those obtained by fixed devices [25].

The individual test items of the Charing Cross Quantitative ALS Rating Scale are obtained using methods that have been shown to produce accurate and reproducible measurements, with acceptable levels of variability. The grouping of individual test items to form composite scores was first checked for face validity, and then more formally investigated using a factor analysis. The scale has been used successfully to screen potential therapeutic agents; by employing a matched-pairs design only 30 patients were required to exclude a significant biological effect from a TRH analogue (RX77368) in MND [13]. Quality of life measures are mentioned in Chapter 34.

Conclusions

This chapter has discussed some ethical issues in clinical trials in MND. The methodological difficulties of using historical controls were highlighted. Using parallel placebo-controlled, randomised, double-blind designs currently remains ethical and the soundest approach to clinical trials in this disease. Outcome variables in event and hazard rate designs are considered for phase III trials. The reliance on the effect of drugs on survival alone may disregard significant biological effects on functions essential to the patient's well-being. A variety of techniques to quantify bulbar function, respiration, muscle force and activities of daily living have been developed. A number of qualitative and quantitative clinical scales have also been developed to address the need to assess such functions in MND. They include the Norris Scale, the Hillel Scale, the Appel Scale, the ALS Functional Rating Scale, the Charing Cross Qualitative and Quantitative Rating Scales and the Tuft Quantitative Neuromuscular Examination (TQNE). A critical review of such quantitative measurements and scales is presented. With the development of these measurement tools for MND it is now feasible to screen drugs for biological efficacy in small numbers of patients in phase II controlled trials. Large-scale screening in this manner, of many potential treatments for this devastating disease, in many centres throughout the world, is efficient in time and resources needed. Large, expensive and slow phase III trials should focus on drugs with significant or promising biological effects in phase II trials.

Appendices

Appendix A. The Norris ALS Scale

	3 *Normal*	2 *Impaired*	1 *Trace*	0 *No use*
1. Hold up head				
2. Chew food				
3. Swallowing				
4. Speech				
5. Roll over in bed				
6. Sit up				
7. Empty bowel/bladder				
8. Breathing				
9. Coughing				
10. Write name				
11. Work buttons, zippers				
12. Feed self				
13. Grip/lift self				
14. Grip/lift book/tray				
15. Grip/lift fork/pencil				
16. Change arm position				
17. Climb one flight of stairs				
18. Walk one block				
19. Walk across a room				
20. Walk with assistance				
21. Stand up from a chair				
22. Change leg position				
	Normal	*Hyper/Hypo*	*Absent*	*Clonic*
23. Stretch reflexes – arms				
24. Stretch reflexes – legs				
	Absent	*Present*	*Hyperactive*	*Clonic*
25. Jaw jerk				
	Flexor	*Mute*	*Equivocal*	*Extensor*
26. Plantar response – right				
27. Plantar response – left				
	None/rare	*Slight*	*Moderate*	*Severe*
28. Fasciculation				
29. Atrophy – face, tongue				
30. Atrophy – arms, shoulders				
31. Atrophy – legs, hips				
32. Labile emotions				
		0 to mild		*Moderate to severe*
33. Fatigability				
34. Leg rigidity				
Patient Subtotals				**PATIENT TOTAL SCORE**
Normal Subtotals	96	4		

Appendix B. The Appel ALS Scale

Bulbar (6–30 points)
Swallowing
- 3   General diet
- 6   Soft diet (soft, cooked; eliminates popcorn, nuts, cornbread etc.)
- 9   Mechanical soft diet (finely chopped or ground and thick liquids)
- 12   Pudding consistency diet (strained, pureed, blended and thick liquids)
- 15   Tube feedings

Speech
- 3   Clear
- 6   Slightly slurred on enunciation of pa/ta/ka
- 9   Slurred
- 12   Unintelligible
- 15   None

Respiratory (6–30 points)
- 6   Vital capacity (VC) less than 500 ml from highest previous recording or within 500 ml of predicted value
- 12   Change in VC of more than 500 ml from highest previous recording or from predicted VC, or need for incentive spirometry, medication or chest physiotherapy
- 18   Change in VC of more than 1000 ml from highest previous recording or from predicted VC, or need for intermittent positive-pressure breathing or suctioning
- 24   VC below 1800 ml or only able to record TV due to weakness
- 30   Endotracheal intubation or tracheostomy

Muscle strength (6–36 points)
Muscles of upper extremities (sum of MRC grades for deltoid, biceps, triceps, wrist extensor, wrist flexor, finger extensor and finger flexor on R and L side)
- 2   70
- 4   62–69
- 6   54–61
- 8   46–53
- 10   32–45
- 12   18–31
- 14   17

Muscles of lower extremities (sum of MRC grades for iliopsoas, quadriceps, hamstrings, ankle dorsiflexion, plantar flexion, toe extension, toe flexion on R and L side)
- 2   70
- 4   62–69
- 6   54–61
- 8   46–53
- 10   32–45
- 12   18–31
- 14   17

Grip (lb R grip + lb L grip)/2
- 1   60
- 2   46–59
- 3   20–45
- 4   <20

Lateral pinch (lb R pinch + lb L pinch)/2
- 1   14
- 2   10–13
- 3   5–9
- 4   <5

Muscle function – lower extremities (6–35 points)
Standing from chair (seconds)
- 1   0–1
- 2   1.5–3
- 3   3.5–5
- 4   >5
- 5   Unable

Standing from lying supine (seconds)
- 1   2
- 2   2.5–4
- 3   4.5–6
- 4   6.5–10
- 5   >10
- 6   Unable

Walking 20 feet/6 metres (seconds)
- 1   8
- 2   8.5–12
- 3   12.5–16
- 4   >16
- 5   Unable

Need for assistive devices
- 1   None
- 2   Ankle-foot orthosis/cane/boots
- 3   Walker, crutches, and/or occasional wheelchair (for long trips etc.)
- 4   Confined mostly or always to wheelchair
- 5   Confined to bed

Climbing and descending 4 standard steps (seconds)
- 1   5
- 2   5.5–8
- 3   8.5–12
- 4   12.5–18
- 5   >18
- 6   Unable

Appendix B. (*Continued*)

Hips and legs
1   Walks and climbs stairs without assistance
2   Walks and climbs stairs with aid of railing
3   Cannot climb stairs but walks unassisted and rises from chair
4   Cannot climb stairs but walks unassisted with either ankle–foot orthosis or cane
5   Cannot climb stairs but walks with minimal assistance or walks unassisted with crutches or walker
6   Cannot climb stairs but walks with crutches or walker with assistance or walks with total support
7   Confined to wheelchair
8   Confined to bed

Muscle function – upper extremities (6–33 points)
Dress and feed
1   Independent
2   Independent with aids (button hooks, zipper pull, padded utensils, plate holder: but no assistance)
3   Mini assistance (needs assistance cutting meat, buttons, shifting clothing)
4   Major assistance (caretaker does most of dressing and/or feeding)
5   Dependent

Propelling wheelchair 20 feet/6 metres (seconds)
1   11
2   11.5–20
3   20.5–30
4   30.5–40
5   >40
6   Unable

Arms and shoulders (grade the most affected side)
1   Starting with arms at the sides, abducts the arms in a full circle until they touch above the head

2   Raises arms above the head only by flexing the elbow or using the accessory muscles
3   Cannot raise hands above the head but raises glass of water to mouth
4   Raises hands to mouth but cannot raise glass of water to mouth
5   Cannot raise hands to mouth but can use hands to hold articles
6   Cannot raise hands to mouth and has no useful function of hands

Cutting Theraplast – dominant hand (seconds)
1   5
2   5.5–10
3   10.5–15
4   15.5–20
5   >20
6   Unable

Purdue pegboard (60 seconds): (no. of pegs R side + no. of pegs L side)/2
1   27–36
2   22–26
3   18–21
4   1–17
5   Unable

Blocks (60 seconds): (no. of blocks R side + no. of blocks L side)/2
1   75–95
2   62–74
3   43–61
4   1–42
5   Unable

Appendix C. The Hillel ALS Severity Scale

Speech

Normal Speech Processes

10	Normal	Patient denies any difficulty speaking, examination demonstrates no abnormality
9	Nominal abnormalities	Only the patient or partner notices speech has changed; maintains normal rate and volume

Detectable speech disturbance

8	Perceived changes	Speech changes are noted by others, especially during fatigue or stress; rate of speech remains essentially normal

Appendix C. (*Continued*)

7	Obvious abnormalities	Speech is consistently impaired; rate, articulation and resonance are affected; remains easily understood

Intelligible with repeating

6	Repeats occasionally	Rate is much slower; repeats specific words in adverse listening situations; does not limit complexity or length of messages
5	Repeats frequently	Speech slow and laboured; extensive repetition or a "translator" is often used; patient probably limits complexity or length of messages

Speech combined with non-vocal communication

4	Speech plus non-verbal	Speech is used in response to questions; intelligibility problems need to be resolved by writing or using a spokesperson
3	Limits speech to one word	Vocalises one word responses beyond yes/no; otherwise writes or uses a spokesperson; initiates communication non-vocally

Loss of useful speech

2	Speech to express motion	Uses vocal inflection to express emotion, affirmation and negation
1	Non-vocal	Vocalisation is effortful, limited in duration, and rarely attempted; may vocalise for crying or pain

Swallowing

Normal eating habits

10	Normal	Patient denies any difficulty chewing or swallowing; examination demonstrates no abnormality
9	Nominal abnormality	Only patient notices slight indicators such as food lodging in the recesses of the mouth or sticking in the throat

Early eating problems

8	Minor abnormality	Complains of some swallowing difficulties; maintains essentially a regular diet; isolated choking episodes
7	Prolonged time/smaller	Mealtime has significantly increased and smaller bite sizes are bite size necessary; must concentrate on swallowing thin liquids

Dietary consistency changes

6	Soft diet	Diet limited primarily to soft foods; requires special meal preparation
5	Liquified diet	Oral intake adequate; nutrition limited primarily to liquefied diet; adequate thin liquid intake usually a problem; may force self to eat

Needs tube feedings

4	Supplemental tube feedings	Oral intake alone no longer adequate; patient uses or needs a tube to supplement intake; patient continues to take significant (greater than 50%) nutrition orally
3	Tube feeding with occasional oral nutrition	Primary nutrition and hydration accomplished by tube; receives less than 50% nutrition orally

No oral feeding

2	Secretions managed with aspirator and/or medication	Cannot safely manage any oral intake; secretions managed with aspiration and/or medications; swallows reflexively
1	Aspiration of secretions	Secretions cannot be managed non-invasively; rarely swallows

Upper extremities (dressing and hygiene)

Normal function

10	Normal	Patient denies any weakness or unusual fatigue of upper extremities; examination demonstrates no abnormality

Appendix C. (*Continued*)

9	Suspected fatigue	Patient suspects fatigue in upper extremities during exertion; cannot sustain work as long as normal; atrophy not evident on examination

Independent and complete self-care

8	Slow self-care	Dressing and hygiene performed more slowly than usual
7	Effortful self-care	Requires significantly more time (usually double or more) and effort to accomplish self-care; weakness is apparent on examination

Intermittent assistance

6	Mostly independent	Handles most aspects of dressing and hygiene alone; adapts by resting, modifying (electric razor) or avoiding some tasks; requires assistance for fine motor tasks (e.g. buttons, tie)
5	Partial independence	Handles some aspects of dressing and hygiene alone; however, routinely requires assistance for many tasks such as make-up, combing hair, shaving

Needs attendant for self-care

4	Attendant assists patient	Attendant must be present for dressing and hygiene; patient performs the majority of each task with the assistance of the attendant
3	Patient assists attendant	Attendant directs the patient for almost all tasks; patient moves in a purposeful manner to assist the attendant; does not initiate self-care

Total dependence

2	Minimal movement	Minimal movement of one or both arms; cannot reposition arms
1	Paralysis	Flaccid paralysis; unable to move upper extremities (except, perhaps, to close inspection)

Lower extremities (walking)

Normal

10	Normal	Patient denies weakness or fatigue; no abnormality on examination
9	Fatigue suspected	Patient suspects weakness or fatigue in legs during exertion

Early ambulation difficulties

8	Difficulty on uneven terrain	Difficulty and fatigue when walking long distances, climbing stairs, and walking over uneven ground (even thick carpet)
7	Observed changes in gait	Noticeable change in gait; pulls on railings when climbing stairs; may use leg brace

Walks with assistance

6	Walks with mechanical device	Needs or uses cane, walker or assistant to walk; probably uses wheelchair away from home
5	Walks with mechanical device and assistant	Does not attempt to walk without attendant; ambulation limited to less than 50 feet (15 m); avoids stairs

Functional movement only

4	Able to support weight	At best, can shuffle a few steps with the help of attendant for transfers
3	Purposeful leg movements	Unable to take steps, but can position legs to assist attendant in transfers; moves legs purposely to maintain mobility in bed

No purposeful leg movement

2	Minimal movement	Minimal movement of one or both legs; cannot reposition legs independently
1	Paralysis	Flaccid paralysis; cannot move lower extremities (except, perhaps, to close inspection)

Appendix D. The ALS Functional Rating Scale

1. **Speech**
    4   Normal speech processes
    3   Detectable speech disturbance
    2   Intelligible with repeating
    1   Speech combined with non-vocal communication
    0   Loss of useful speech
2. **Salivation**
    4   Normal
    3   Slight but definite excess of saliva; may have night-time drooling
    2   Moderately excessive saliva; may have minimal drooling
    1   Marked excess of saliva with some drooling
    0   Marked drooling; requires constant use of tissue or handkerchief
3. **Swallowing**
    4   Normal eating habits
    3   Early eating problems – occasional choking
    2   Dietary consistency changes
    1   Needs supplemental tube feeding
    0   NPO (exclusively parenteral or enteral feeding)
4. **Handwriting**
    4   Normal
    3   Slow or sloppy; all words are legible
    2   Not all words are legible
    1   Able to grip pen but unable to write
    0   Unable to grip pen
5a. **Cutting food and handling utensils (without gastrostomy)**
    4   Normal
    3   Somewhat slow and clumsy, but no help needed
    2   Can cut most foods, although clumsy and slow; no help needed
    1   Food must be cut by someone, but can still feed self slowly
    0   Needs to be fed
5b. **Cutting food and handling utensils (with gastrostomy)**
    4   Normal
    3   Clumsy but able to perform all manipulations independently
    2   Some help needed with closures and fasteners
    1   Provides minimal assistance to caregiver
    0   Unable to perform any aspect of task
6. **Dressing and hygiene**
    4   Normal   function
    3   Independent and complete self-care with effort or decreased efficiency
    2   Intermittent assistance or substitute methods
    1   Needs attendant for self-care
    0   Total dependence
7. **Turning in bed and adjusting bed clothes**
    4   Normal
    3   Somewhat slow and clumsy, but no help needed
    2   Can turn alone or adjust sheets, but with great difficulty
    1   Can initiate, but not turn or adjust sheets alone
    0   Helpless
8. **Walking**
    4   Normal
    3   Early ambulation difficulties
    2   Walks with assistance (any assistive device including ankle foot orthosis)
    1   Non-ambulatory functional movement only
    0   No purposeful leg movement
9. **Climbing stairs**
    4   Normal
    3   Slow
    2   Mild unsteadiness or fatigue
    1   Needs assistance (including handrail)
    0   Cannot do
10. **Breathing**
    4   Normal
    3   Shortness of breath with minimal exertion (e.g. walking, talking)
    2   Shortness of breath at rest
    1   Intermittent (e.g. nocturnal) ventilator dependence
    0   Ventilator-dependent

Appendix E. The Charing Cross Qualitative ALS Rating Scale.

Grade	Description		
Bulbar	*Speech abnormality*		*Swallowing abnormality*
4	Normal	+	Normal
3b	Normal	+	Minimal to moderate
or	Minimal	+	Mild or moderate
3a	Minimal	+	Minimal
or	Minimal to moderate	+	Normal
2	Normal to minimal	+	Severe
or	Mild	+	Minimal to severe
or	Moderate or severe	+	Minimal or mild
or	Severe	+	Normal
1	Moderate or severe	+	Moderate or severe

Respiration

4	Normal
3	Dyspnoea on moderate exertion
2	Dyspnoea on mild exertion or at rest
1	Ventilator some/all of the time

Upper limb

4	Normal
3	Both arms functional, but some activities[a] take longer to perform
2	One or both arms lost some function (needs help in some activities[a])
1	One or both arms lost all function (needs help in all activities[a])

Lower limb

4	Normal
3	Abnormal gait, can walk the same distance as before (without device or helper)
2	Cannot walk the same distance as before or needs a device or helper(s)
1	Unable to walk

Activities of daily living

4	Normal
3	One or more activities take longer or occasional help heeded[b]
2	Totally dependent in one or more activities[b]
1	Totally dependent in all activities[b]

Speech abnormalities: minimal = always intelligible; mild = occasionally unintelligible (<50% of the time); moderate = mostly unintelligible (>50% of the time); severe = always unintelligible/anarthric.
Swallowing abnormalities: minimal = dysphagia with normal diet; mild = avoids some foods; moderate = modified diet (liquidised, pureed, liquid supplements); severe = gastrostomy/nasogastric tube.
Mild exertion = routine activities (wash, dress, walk 1 mile (1.5 km), two flights of stairs).
Moderate exertion = more than routine activities.

[a] Write, self-feed, dress (buttons and laces); [b] self-feed, dress, wash, toilet, stand, walk.

Appendix F. Charing Cross Qualitative ALS Rating Scale

Validation and equivalence of grades to percentage of normal function scores obtained with the Quantitative Charing Cross ALS Rating Scale.

Function and Grade	% Normal	SD
Bulbar		
4	90	16.2
3b	67.3	9.9
3a	58.4	17.5
2	42.2	11.0
1	28.0	9.9
Respiration		
4	96.7	35.9
3	76.4	33.4
2	41.6	15.4
1	17.6	13.3
Upper limb		
4	72.4	22.6
3	56.8	12.5
2	26.7	26.1
1	1.1	2.0
Lower limb		
4	95.1	12.1
3	42.6	22.0
2	20.8	13.0
1	11.8	10.5
Activities of daily living		
4	98.3	14.6
3	79.9	17.3
2	37.1	23.3
1	1.8	2.8

% Normal: For each grade the equivalent mean percentage of normal function as calculated with the quantitative Charing Cross ALS rating scale in the same patients is given.

SD is the standard deviation of the mean %Normal given for each function and reflects the dispersion of values for each qualitative grade in the population of MND patients that was studied.

Appendix G. The Tufts Quantitative Neuromuscular Examination (TQNE)

		Abbreviation	
A.	**Pulmonary function**		
	Forced vital capacity	FVC	1
	Maximal voluntary ventilation	MVV	1
B.	**Oropharyngeal.**		
	Time to repeat "pa" 20 times	pa	1
	Time to repeat "pata" 15 times	pata	1

Appendix G. (*Continued*)

C.	**Timed hand activities.**		
	Time dialling telephone number	phone R/L	2
	Number of pegs placed in a Purdue		
	pegboard in 30 seconds	pegbd R/L	2
D.	**Isometric arm strength.**		
	Shoulder extension	Shdext R/L	2
	Shoulder flexion	Shdflex R/L	2
	Elbow extension	Elbext R/L	2
	Elbow flexion	Elbflex R/L	2
	Grip strength	Grip R/L	2
E.	**Isometric leg strength.**		
	Hip flexion	Hipflex R/L	2
	Hip extension	Hipext R/L	2
	Knee extension	Kneext R/L	2
	Knee flexion	Kneeflex R/L	2
	Ankle dorsiflexion	Dorsi R/L	2

Total: 28

Both sides of the body are tested.

"Best of 2 trials" was used in all tests for data analysis.

An electronic strain-gauge tensiometer was used to assess strength. Grip strength was assessed by a Jamar dynamometer.

Appendix H. The Charing Cross Quantitative ALS Rating Scale

See also Appendix I.

Bulbar score

Tongue protrusion	Timed 10 repetitions of tongue protrusion
Word repetition	Timed 10 repetitions of the word "ticker"
Jaw movements	Timed 10 repetitions of opening/closing jaw
Swallowing	Timed swallow of 100 ml water using standard beakers and straws.

Respiratory score

Forced vital capacity	Forced vital capacity (ml)

Upper limbs

Shoulder abduction	}Readings obtained using hand-held dynamometrey, and then expressed
Elbow flexion	}as % normal values after matching to sex and age matched controls.
Finger extension	}Such % normal values from the eight muscle groups from both right and
Index finger abduction	}left sides would then be combined in a composite upper limb score.

Lower limbs

Hip flexion	}As for upper limbs
Knee extension	}
Ankle dorsiflexion	}
Greater hallux extension	}

Appendix H. (*Continued*)

Activities of daily living

Unfastening/fastening a button	Timed test, patient using both hands for test
Placing four coins, right	Timed test, patient using only right hand for test
Placing four coins, left	Timed test, patient using only left hand for test
Handwriting	Timed test, patient writing a standard sentence using dominant hand "John Brown walked a big dog"
Rising from a chair	Timed test to stand upright from a standard chair
Walking	Timed test, patient walks forward 25 feet (7.5 m), turns, and walks back 25 feet

Appendix I. The Charing Cross Quantitative ALS Rating Scale: Means and Standard Deviations for Timed Tests of Bulbar Function and Activities of Daily Living (ADL) in Normal Controls

Test	Mean	SD	Range
Bulbar			
Tongue protrusion	3.06	0.85	1.8–4.9
Word repetition "ticker"	2.45	0.33	1.7–3.0
Jaw movement	2.86	0.92	1.8–6.5
Swallowing	7.72	3.10	4.4–16.4
ADL			
Buttons	3.08	0.60	2.2–4.8
Coins, right hand	5.58	0.85	4.2–7.8
Coins, left hand	5.77	0.87	4.1–7.4
Handwriting	9.86	2.60	6.1–19.8
Rising from chair	1.10	0.25	0.7–1.5
Walking	9.05	1.45	6.8–11.9

Learning effects have been eliminated [46]. All times in seconds.
Bulbar: Values from 30 normal controls (13 men and 17 women). Mean age 51.1 years (SD 16.3), mean height 1.67 m, mean weight 64.3 kg.
ADL. Values from 30 normal controls (15 men and 15 women). Mean age 48 years (SD 14.6), mean height 1.67 m, mean weight 64.9 kg.

References

1. Bok S. The ethics of giving placebos. Sci Am 1974;231:17–23.
2. Friedman LM, Furberg CD, DeMets DL. Blindness. In: Fundamentals of clinical trials, 2nd ed. St Louis: Mosby-Year Book, 1985:71–81.
3. Friedman LM, Furberg CD, DeMets DL. Monitoring response variables. In: Fundamentals of clinical trials, 2nd edn. St Louis: Mosby-Year Book 1985:213–239.
4. Stamler J. Invited remarks. Clin Pharmacol Ther 1979;25:641–646.
5. Armitage P, McPherson CK, Rowe BC. Repeated significance tests on accumulating data. J R Stat Soc Ser A 1969;132:235–244.
6. Lellouch J, Schwartz D. L'essai therapeutique: ethique individuelle ou ethique collective? Rev Inst Int Statist 1971;39:127–136.
7. Pradas J, Finison L, Andres PL, Thornell B, Hollander D, Munsat TL. The natural history of amyotrophic lateral sclerosis and the use of natural history controls in therapeutic trials. Neurology 1993;43:751–755.
8. The Riluzole Study Group, Bensimon G, Lacomblez L, Meininger V. A controlled trial of riluzole in amyotrophic lateral sclerosis. N Engl J Med 1994;330:385–591.
9. Lacomblez L, Bensimon G, Leigh PN, et al. A dose ranging study of Riluzole in amyotrophic lateral sclerosis. Lancet 1996;347:1425–1431.
10. Miller RJ, Munsat TL, Swash M, Brooks BR. Consensus guidelines for the design and implementation of clinical trials in ALS. J Neurol Sci 1999;169:2–12.
11. Plaitakis A, Smith J, Mandeli J, Yahr MD. Pilot trial of branched-chain aminoacids in amyotrophic lateral sclerosis. Lancet 1988;I:1015–1018.
12. Smith RA, Melmed S, Sherman B, et al. Recombinant growth hormone treatment of amyotrophic lateral sclerosis. Muscle Nerve 1993;16:624–663.

13. Goonetilleke A, Guiloff RJ. Continuous response variable trial design in motor neuron disease: long term treatment with a TRH analogue (RX77368). J Neurol Neurosurg Psychiatry 1995;58:201–208.

14. Daube J. Motor Unit Number Estimate: Has its time arrived?. Amyotrophic Lateral Sclerosis 2000;1:68.

15. Gooch CL, Harati Y. Motor Unit Number Estimation, ALS and clinical trials. Amyotrophic Lateral Sclerosis 2000;1:71–82.

16. Guiloff RJ, Goonetilleke A. Natural history of amyotrophic lateral sclerosis. Observations with the Charing Cross amyotrophic lateral sclerosis scales. In: Serratrice G, Munsat T, editors. Pathogenesis and therapy of amyotrophic lateral sclerosis. Adv Neurol. 1995;68:185–198.

17. Ringel SP, Murphy JR, Alderson MK, et al. The natural history of amyotrophic lateral sclerosis. Neurology 1996;43:1316–1322.

18. Haverkamp LJ, Appel V, Appel SH. Natural history of amyotrophic lateral sclerosis. I. A database population. Validation of a scoring system and a model for survival prediction. Brain 1995;118:707–719.

19. Norris FH, Calanchini PR, Fallat RJ, et al. The administration of guanidine in amyotrophic lateral sclerosis. Neurology 1974;24:721–728.

20. Appel V, Stewart SS, Smith G, Appel SH. A rating scale for amyotrophic lateral sclerosis: description and preliminary experience. Ann Neurol 1987;22:328–333.

21. Guiloff RJ, Goonetilleke A. Longitudinal clinical assessments in motor neurone disease- relevance to clinical trials. In: Clifford Rose F, editor. ALS: from Charcot to the present and into the future. London: Smith-Gordon, 1993:73–82.

22. Hillel AD, Miller RM, Yorkston K, McDonald E, Norris FH, Konikow N. Amyotrophic lateral sclerosis severity scale. Neuroepidemiology 1989;8:142–150.

23. The ALS CNTF Treatment Study (ACTS) Phase I-II Study Group. The amyotrophic lateral sclerosis functional rating scale: assessment of activities of daily living in patients with amyotrophic lateral sclerosis. Arch Neurol 1996;53:141–147.

24. Feinstein AR. Organisation of the output scale. In: Clinimetrics. New Haven: Yale University Press, 1987:60–76.

25. Goonetilleke A, Modarres-Sadeghi H, Guiloff RJ. Accuracy, reproducibility and variability of hand-held dynamometry in motor neuron disease. J Neurol Neurosurg Psychiatry 1994;57:326–332.

26. van der Ploeg RJO, Oosterhuis HJGH, Reuvekamp J. Measuring muscle strength. J Neurol 1984;231:200–203.

27. Shafer SQ, Olarte MR. Methodological considerations for clinical trials in motor neurone disease. In: Rowland LP, editor. Human motor neuron diseases. New York: Raven Press, 1982:559–566.

28. Tourtellotte WW, Haerer AF, Simpson JF, Kuzma JW, Sikorski J. Quantitative clinical neurological testing. I. A study of a battery of tests designed to evaluate in part the neurological function of patients with multiple sclerosis and its use in a therapeutic trial. Ann NY Acad Sci 1965;122:480–505.

29. The National Isometric Muscle Strength (NIMS) Database Consortium. Muscular weakness assessment: use of normal isometric strength data. Arch Phys Med Rehabil 1996;77:1251–1255.

30. Bohannon RW. Reference values for extremity muscle strength obtained by hand-held dynamometry from adults aged 20 to 79 years. Arch Phys Med Rehabil 1997;78:26–32.

31. Barlow SM, Abbs JH. Orofacial fine motor control impairment in congenital spastics: evidence against muscle spindle related performance deficits. Neurology 1984;34:145–150.

32. Fallat RJ, Jewitt, Bass M, Kamm B, Norris FH. Spirometry in amyotrophic lateral sclerosis. Arch Neurol 1979;36:74–80.

33. Griggs RC, Donahue KM, Utell MJ, et al. Evaluation of pulmonary function in neuromuscular disease. Neurol Clin 1981;38:9–12.

34. Cohen JA, Gundesblatt M, Miller RM, et al. Predictive value of pulmonary function testing in ALS. Neurology 1985;35:72.

35. Potvin AR, Tourtellotte WW. Instrumented examination of activities of daily living. In: Quantitative examination of neurologic functions. Boca Raton, FL: CRC Press, 1985;1:167–180.

36. Andres PL, Thibodeau LM, Finison LJ, Munsat TL. Quantitative assessment of neuromuscular deficit in ALS. Neurol Clin 1987;5:125–141.

37. Andres PL, Hedlund W, Finison L, Conlon T, Felmus M, Munsat TL. Quantitative motor assessment in amyotrophic lateral sclerosis. Neurology 1986;36:937–941.

38. Bradley WG, Hedlund W, Cooper C, et al. A double-blind controlled trial of bovine brain gangliosides (cronassial) in amyotrophic lateral sclerosis. Neurology 1984;34:1079–1082.

39. Keleman J, Hedlund W, Murray-Douglas P, Munsat TL. Lecithin is not effective in amyotrophic lateral sclerosis. Neurology 1982;32:315–316.

40. Munsat TL, Easterday CS, Levy S, Wolff SM, Hiatt P. Amantadine and guanidine are ineffective in ALS. Neurology 1980;31:1054–1055.

41. Andres PL, Finison LJ, Conlon MPH, Thibodeau PTA, Munsat TL. Use of composite scores (megascores) to measure deficit in amyotrophic lateral sclerosis. Neurology 1988;38:405–408.

42. Armstrong P, Berry G. Statistical methods in medical research, 2nd ed. Oxford: Blackwell Scientific, 1987:344–346.

43. Cormack RM. A review of classification. J R Stat Soc 1971;134:321–367.

44. Everitt BS. Unresolved problems in cluster analysis. Biometrics 1979;35:169–182.

45. Munsat TL, Andres PL, Skerry LM. The use of quantitative techniques to define amyotrophic lateral sclerosis. In: Munsat TL, editor. Quantification of neurologic deficit. Boston, MA: Butterworth, 1989:129–139.

46. Goonetilleke A, Guiloff RJ. Accuracy, reproducibility and variability of quantitative assessments of bulbar and respiratory function in motor neuron disease. J Neurol Sci 1994:123 (Suppl):64–66.

47. Brooks BR. El Escorial World Federation criteria for the diagnosis of amyotrophic lateral sclerosis. Subcommittee on Motor Neuron Diseases/Amyotrophic Lateral Sclerosis of the World Federation of Neurology Research group on Neuromuscular Diseases and the El Escorial "Clinical limits of amyotrophic lateral sclerosis" workshop contributors. J Neurol Sci 1994;124(Suppl):96–107.

48. Modarres-Sadeghi H, Rogers H, Emami J, Guiloff RJ. Subacute adminstration of a TRH analogue (RX77368) in motorneuron disease: an open study. J Neurol Neurosurg Psychiatry 1988;51:1146–1157.

49. Guiloff RJ, Modarres-Sadeghi H, Rogers H. Motor neuron disease: aims and assessment methods in trial design. In: Clifford Rose F, editor. Amyotrophic lateral sclerosis. New York: Demos, 1990:19–31.

34. Motor Neurone Disease: Basic Designs, Sample Sizes and Pitfalls

B. Rix Brooks, M. Sanjak, D. Belden and A. Waclawik

Introduction

In the last quarter-century the assault on motor neurone disease (MND)/amyotrophic lateral sclerosis (ALS) was initiated by single-center small clinical trials with technically complex, not widely validated outcome measurements as multiple endpoints. Over time there was a steady escalation to multicenter large, sometimes international, clinical trials with one simple, easily and precisely determined outcome measurement as the primary endpoint. During this evolution, it became apparent that there was an imbalance in our understanding of the outcome measures employed in determining the potential treatment effects of interventions for MND/ALS. Foremost was the unclear relationship between standard clinical measures of muscle strength by manual muscle testing and computerized isometric muscle strength in MND/ALS patients. Furthermore, despite reproducibiity and accuracy testing of disease-specific clinimetric scales in MND/ALS patients with validity testing against standard general purpose disability scales, few studies compared different scales in the same MND/ALS patient population or appraised the properties of these clinimetric scales over time [1–14]. Both large and small clinical trials have employed analytic methods including simple descriptive statistics of the outcome measure with repeated measures, change from baseline or slope measurements. The controversial evaluation of the anti-glutamate drug, riluzole, employed a simple trial design with survival as the clinical endpoint [15–19]. This clinical trial design and analysis with event history (time-to-failure or survival) statistics highlighted the potential importance of study design.

In this chapter we will attempt to provide a fundamental understanding of the development of clinimetrics in MND/ALS. The evolution of techniques for clinical assessment and analysis of treatment effects in MND/ALS has been incremental. Single-center studies with small homogeneous groups of patients have been supplanted by large multicenter studies with multinational groups of MND/ALS patients assessed by a variety of clinimetrics. Initially, these clinimetrics were adopted from historically validated clinical studies of non-MND/ALS neuromuscular diseases and poliomyelitis, but more experience in a larger number of MND/ALS patients has provided extensive experience with a number of clinimetrics specifically designed for use in MND/ALS.

The assault on MND/ALS has been based on fundamental assumptions concerning the pathogenesis of motor neurone degeneration. In the last quarter-century, variously sized clinical trials have been conducted to evaluate therapies with:

- potentially ergotropic peptides (TRH, RX77368, DN1417) [20–28]
- potentially clinically active neurotrophic factors (GH, CNTF, BDNF, IGF-I) [29–34]
- potentially anti-glutamatergic/anti-oxidant drugs (riluzole, BCAA, N-acetyl-cysteine) [16–19,35–43]
- immunosuppressive therapies (cyclophosphamide, cyclosporine, total lymphoid irradiation) [44–48].

During this period, the natural history of MND/ALS has been analyzed in increasingly larger cohorts with respect to survival, manual muscle testing, quantitative measures of isometric and isokinetic strength, pulmonary function, and timed functional tests [1–4,6–14,49–55]. Clinical endpoints have been evaluated by event history (time to failure, survival) analysis, analysis of change in slopes or change from baseline with repeated measures of clinimetric scales, timed functional tests or continuous measurement of isometric strength [56].

The advances in the last decade have been consolidated with event history analysis of survival in the clinical trial of riluzole versus placebo over 18 months. Studies of larger size but shorter study periods did not demonstrate efficacy of neurotrophic factors (CNTF, BDNF) in limiting loss of isometric strength or forced vital capacity. Smaller studies selecting patient groups with different inclusion criteria (TRH analogue RX77368, rhGH, cyclophosphamide, cyclosporine) have not shown treatment effects in randomized controlled clinical trials. Selection of MND/ALS patients with progressive disease (rhIGF-I) on the Appel ALS Scale [32,33] led to conflicting results in two clinical trials.

Our experience in the recent decades has highlighted both the strengths and weaknesses of basic research, clinical science, clinical practice and organizational structures to focus on developing a cure for MND/ALS. As our ability to marshal resources to achieve this goal increased during the Decade of the Brain, the paucity of substantial information on the quantitative natural history of MND/ALS and other motor neurone diseases became apparent. The development of specific consortia – academic, regional, and international – provided new insights into several features of the clinical course of MND/ALS, but the practical marriage of industry and academia ushered in a new set of problems in terms of nomenclature and clinical style. At the end of this blush of clinical activity in appraising the effect of different treatments in MND/ALS, we are beset with a sense of scale that bewitches us into thinking that no treatment may be effectively evaluated in studies with fewer than 500–1000 patients.

Crucial to an evaluation of a treatment in MND/ALS is a determination of what is a clinically significant change, a discernment of what changes occur with high frequency in the first 12 months after MND/ALS patients are referred for treatment to a specialized MND/ALS Clinic, an insight into which study designs to employ in phase I, II and III clinical trials and an understanding of which statistical analytic methods will permit efficient utilization of MND/ALS patients in meaningful timely clinical trials.

Clinical Outcome Measures

The development of clinical outcome measures in MND/ALS has been reviewed previously [1–4,6–14,54–57, see also Chapter 33]. Reliability, accuracy and validity studies have been published

[10,11,57,58]. The outcome measures employed in clinical trials gauge pathology caused by the disease process, impairment caused by the pathology, disability caused by the impairment and handicap caused by the disability (Table 34.1) [59].

The measures to be employed are determined by the questions being asked. Survival analysis, employed in the riluzole clinical trials, measures the ultimate handicap – death – as the primary endpoint [15,16,18]. Change in the slope (rate of change) of the Appel ALS Rating Scale was employed as the primary endpoint in the USA rhIGF-I (Myotrophin) clinical trial [32]. Change in the slope of the forced vital capacity was the primary endpoint assessed in the BDNF clinical trials [34]. Change in the slope of the combined arm and leg isometric muscle strength megascore was the primary endpoint assessed in the Synergen-CNTF clinical trials [31]. Change from baseline in the Appel ALS Rating Scale was employed as the primary endpoint in the European rhIGF-I (Myotrophin) clinical trial [33]. Change from baseline in the combined arm and leg isometric muscle strength megascore was employed as the primary endpoint in the ACTS – CNTF clinical trial [30].

While the World Federation of Neurology Subcommittee on Motor Neuron Diseases of the Research Group on Neuromuscular Diseases formulated Consensus Guidelines for the Design and Execution of Clinical Trials in MND/ALS at Airlie House in 1994 [59] which were modified and amended by the World Federation of Neurology Committee on Motor Neuron Diseases at Airlie House in 1998 [242], no one clinical endpoint is required and many potential clinical endpoints are recommended. Much work is needed to sift and winnow the potential clinical outcome measures in MND/ALS to determine those measures that will provide information on clinical change early in the course of MND/ALS permitting efficient phase I, II and III clinical trials of treatments. A tactical approach to this problem is to evaluate the current clinimetrics with different statistical techniques to determine which analytic techniques may potentially increase the efficiency of MND/ALS clinical trials.

Pulmonary Function: FVC and VC

Forced vital capacity (FVC) has been studied in a large number of ALS patients and is a significant prognosticator for survival [34,53]. FVC was studied in our ALS patients as percent predicted relative to normal control subjects. Evaluation over time by repeated measures with last value carried forward

Table 34.1. Disease outcome measures in ALS

Pathology	
Motor neurone pathologic change	Ubiquitin (+) motor neurones
Motor neurone loss	Neurofilament (+) motor neurones
Corticospinal tract degeneration	Glial Fibrillary Acidic Protein (+) Corticospinal Tract Staining
Impairment	
Strength loss	
Lip, tongue, jaw	Maximal voluntary isometric contraction (MVIC)
	Timed tests
Arm	Medical Research Council manual muscle testing
Hand grip, index finger pinch	Maximal voluntary isometric contraction (MVIC)
Leg	Fixed:
	Tufts Quantitative Neurological Examination (TQNE)
	ACTS/WALS isometric muscle strength examination
	Hand-held:
	Charing Cross Quantitative ALS Rating Scale (ALS Quant)
Diaphragm	Inspiratory/expiratory force
	Respiratory rate
Breathing	Vital capacity (forced, slow)
	Peak inspiratory flow rate
Spasticity	Ashworth Spasticity Scale
	Rate of force generation
	Standing, turning and walking velocity
	Alternate motion rate
Fine Coordination Loss	Finger kinematics
	Pegboard
Disability	
Function Loss	
Speech	Intelligibility, Frenchay Scale
	ALS Functional Rating Scale (ALS FRS)
	Charing Cross Qualitative ALS Rating Scale (ALS Qual)
	Salpétrière ALS Rating Scale
	Hillel ALS Severity Scale
	Norris ALS Rating Scale
	Appel ALS Rating Scale
Swallow	Deglutition, ALS FRS, Charing Cross ALS Qual,
	Salpétrière, Hillel, Norris
Breathing	ALS FRS, Charing Cross ALS Qual,
	Salpétrière, Hillel, Norris
Arm	ALS FRS, Charing Cross ALS Qual,
	Salpétrière, Hillel, Norris, Appel
Leg	ALS FRS, Charing Cross ALS Qual,
	Salpétrière, Hillel, Norris, Appel
Handicap	
Independence loss	Quality of life scales
Work	Sickness Impact Profile (SIP), ALS Quality of Life (ASLQoL)
Social integration	
Self-care	Short-Form 36 (SF-36), ALS Quality of Life (ALSQoL)
Gastrostomy	ALS FRS, Salpétrière, Hillel, Norris, Appel
Respiratory support	ALS FRS, Charing Cross ALS Qual,
BiPAP, CPAP	Salpétrière, Hillel, Norris, Appel
Death	Survival

Pulmonary — Forced Vital Capacity

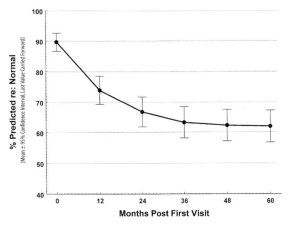

Fig. 34.1. Repeated measures analysis of forced vital capacity — mean ± 95% confidence limits [last value carried forward (LVCF)] — over 60 months after the first clinic visit in 305 MND/ALS patients.

Forced Vital Capacity — Sustained Drop from Baseline

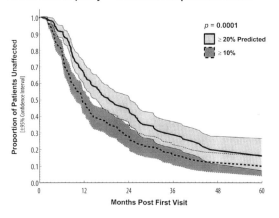

Forced Vital Capacity — Sustained Drop below Threshold

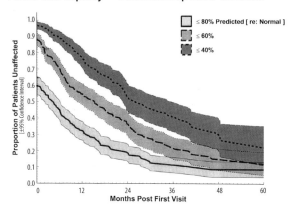

Fig. 34.2. Event history analysis (proportion of patients unaffected ± 95% confidence interval) of sustained drop in forced vital capacity by ≥10% or ≥20% predicted (relative to normal) (*top*) and event history analysis of a sustained drop below a fixed threshold of 80%, 60% or 40% predicted in forced vital capacity (*bottom*) over 60 months after the first clinic visit in 305 MND/ALS patients.

(LVCF) for missing data indicates that the mean FVC for 305 patients at entry was 90% predicted (Fig. 34.1). When FVC data for this population are presented using as an endpoint a sustained (present at ≥ two follow-up visits) specific drop by 10% predicted or 20% predicted evaluated by event history analysis, 55 of 100 patients will drop by 10% predicted or more in the first 12 months after first clinic attendance. During this period, 37 of 100 patients will drop by 20% predicted or more (Fig. 34.2, top). Because patients with any entry FVC may contribute to this endpoint, there may be an enrichment in the number of events that may occur during the first 12 months of attendance at an MND/ALS clinic. When using an endpoint defined as a fall below a defined threshold (80% predicted, 60% predicted, 40% predicted), a large proportion (40%) of patients was already below 80% predicted when first seen in the MND/ALS clinic and the change over time differed with the defined threshold (Fig. 34.2, bottom). In the first 12 months following attendance at clinic, 30 of 100 patients will fall below 80% predicted, 33 of 100 patients will fall below 60% predicted and 19 of 100 patients will fall below 40% predicted. Therefore more events will occur when the endpoint is defined as a specific sustained ≥10% predicted or ≥20% predicted drop.

FVC or slow vital capacity (VC) are reproducibly measured with excellent quality control and small intra-rater or inter-rater variability [60,61]. FVC and VC have been employed in several phase I–II and several phase III multicenter clinical trials in North America and Europe. In two completed (BDNFsc, BDNFit), one just completed (SR57746A-Xaliproden)

and two planned (BDNFsc, BDNFit) clinical trials FVC or VC are the primary endpoints. These endpoints are prognostic indicators of survival in MND/ALS [53]. Therefore, employment of these clinical outcome measures in ALS clinical trials might provide a surrogate indicator of the treatment effect on survival.

FVC is an excellent surrogate measure for MND/ALS clinical trials because there is a specific prognostic relationship between FVC and survival. The mean survival time for MND/ALS patients with FVC below a defined threshold is 19 months (80% predicted), 13 months (60% predicted) or 8.5 months (40% predicted) (Fig. 34.3). The mean survival time after falling below a specific threshold progressively decreases with decreasing percent predicted vital capacity with variable 95% confidence limits (Fig. 34.4).

FVC changes over the first 12 months following the initial clinic visit when measured as either endpoint analysis (change from baseline with LVCF), slope analysis (change in individual slopes with LVCF), sustained drop below a specific threshold (80% predicted, 60% predicted, 40% predicted) or a specific sustained drop from baseline (10% predicted, 20% predicted) demonstrate different sample size requirements. The sample sizes were determined based on a 90 percent power $(1 - \beta = 0.90)$ for deter-

mining a treatment effect with a two-sided significance $(\alpha = 0.05)$ [126]. When treatment effect sizes resulting in complete cessation of progression (100% arrest) or varying degrees of slowing of progression (75%, 50% and 25% arrest) were simulated, the sample sizes required in each treatment group as a function of the endpoint analysis employed were significantly different (Fig. 34.5). Event history analysis of FVC is particularly more efficient with respect to sample size requirements at smaller treatment effect

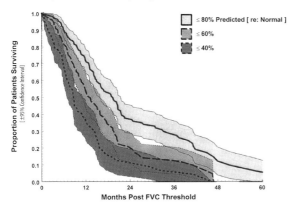

Fig. 34.3. Event history analysis (proportion of patients unaffected ± 95% confidence interval) of survival versus months after forced vital capacity threshold in 305 MND/ALS Patients.

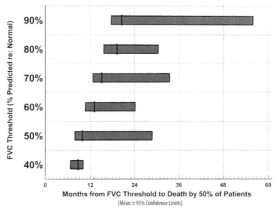

Fig. 34.4. Months from forced vital capacity threshold (% predicted relative to normal) to death of 50% of patients (mean ± 95% confidence interval) in 305 MND/ALS patients.

Fig. 34.5. Sample size required in each treatment arm (1 N) to demonstrate 25%, 50%, 75% or 100% arrest over 12 months follow-up to give two-sided confidence $(Z\alpha = 0.05)$ for type I error and power of 0.90 $(Z\beta = 0.05)$ to prevent type II error in forced vital capacity: endpoint analysis (change from baseline) [last value carried forward (LVCF)]; slope analysis (initial slope) (LVCF), event history analysis of a sustained drop below fixed threshold of 80%, 60% or 40% predicted, event history analysis of a sustained drop by ≥10% or ≥20% predicted from baseline based on 305 MND/ALS patients.

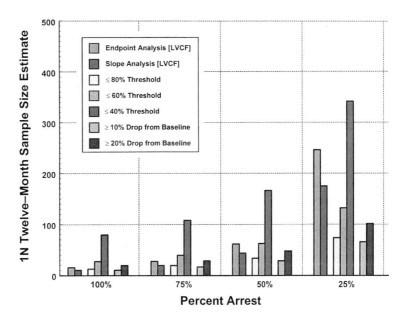

Coefficient of Variation of Vital Capacity

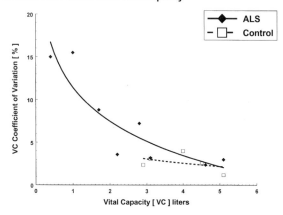

Fig. 34.6. Coefficient of variation of vital capacity in 8 MND/ALS patients and 4 control subjects versus vital capacity: Salpêtrière analysis.

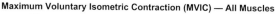

Maximum Voluntary Isometric Contraction (MVIC) — All Muscles

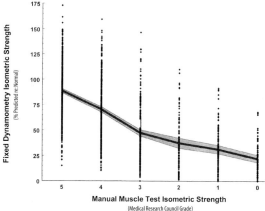

Fig. 34.7. Maximum voluntary isometric contraction (MVIC) – correlation of fixed dynamometry isometric strength (% predicted relative to normal) with manual muscle test isometric strength (Medical Research Council grade) – all muscles in 132 MND/ALS patients.

size than repeated measure techniques such as a change in slopes.

FVC and VC have excellent test–retest reliability and reproducibility in ALS patients [10–14,29–34, 60–67]. The variability in the test–retest FVC or VC measurements has been studied in large multicenter clinical trials of BDNF and SR57746A-Xaliproden. In multicen-ter trials, maintaining test–retest reproducibility throughout the course of the clinical trial requires frequent validation sessions to maintain the level of evaluator training. The test-retest reproducibility is identical in control subjects and MND/ALS patients with VC above 60% predicted but the coefficient of variation increases as the measured VC decreases (Fig. 34.6). This variability at low FVC or VC favors employing event history analysis of FVC or VC changes with threshold endpoints or specific drop endpoints at FVC or VC above 60% predicted.

Muscle Strength: MVIC and MMT

Throughout the last 15 years there has been a recurring polemic, grounded partially in perception and partially in fact, concerning the sensitivity and specificity of maximum voluntary isometric contraction (MVIC) [1–4,10–14,68–71]. MVIC, measured either by fixed or hand-held dynamometry, demonstrates change in isometric muscle strength, but its efficiency in providing clinical information over time has only recently been studied in MND/ALS. In other neuromuscular diseases, such as Duchenne muscular dystrophy and facioscapulohumeral muscular dystrophy, manual muscle testing provides similar and adequate information for discerning clinical change over time in long-term clinical studies [72–80].

To determine the relationship between MVIC and manual muscle test (MMT) strength in MND/ALS, MVIC and MMT assessments were performed in muscles measured independently cross-sectionally and longitudinally in 132 MND/ALS patients (M:F, 95:37; B:A:L, 26:59:47] by two raters with no review or discussion of measured values. MMT ratings were determined according to the Medical Research Council protocol [81] by one examiner and MVIC in the same muscles was measured by three examiners according to established protocol [57,82,83]. MVIC raw data were transformed into a muscle-specific percent predicted value determined by the age, gender, height and weight of each patient according to regression equations developed by the National Isometric Muscle Strength Database Consortium [82]. Previous regression equations had been based on smaller control samples and different baseline determinants [76–79].

Shoulder extensor, shoulder flexor, elbow extensor, elbow flexor, wrist extensor, wrist flexor, hip extensor, hip flexor, leg extensor, leg flexor and ankle dorsiflexor MVIC and MMT were studied individually (right/left) and analyzed separately or with both right and left muscles pooled. Results for individual muscles are presented on the University of Wisconsin (UW) ALS Clinical Research Center website (http://www.neurology.wisc.edu/alscrc/clintrialdata1). Employing a composite of all limb muscles measured cross-sectionally, the comparison of MVIC with MMT indicates that the mean MVIC is proportionate at each MMT ordinal rating (MMT-5, 94% predicted; MMT-4, 75% predicted; MMT-3, 55% predicted) (Fig. 34.7). The mean difference in MVIC between MMT-5 and MMT-4 or MMT-4 and MMT-3 at first visit is 20% ± 4% (standard deviation) predicted. This relationship does not exist below MMT-3. Similar results were noted in a smaller group of 12 MND/ALS patients studied in Germany before the development of the percent predicted regression equations. In this study [84] there was a proportional decrease in MVC measured by hand-held dynamometry with decreasing ordinal manual muscle test rating from normal (5) to good (4) to fair (3) strength, but a floor effect was suggested below fair (3) strength. A recent study comparing MMT with MVIC measured by fixed dynamometry and a disability scale, the ALS Functional Rating Scale (ALS FRS), in 20 MND/ALS patients indicated that MMT changed over time but MVIC was more sensitive to change and paralleled changes in the ALS FRS total score [6]. A more creative clinical analysis in 43 MND/ALS patients compared with 75 control subjects indicated that a similar relationship exists between MMT and hand-held dynamometry and that MVIC measured by hand-held dynamometry was more sensitive to change over time [9].

Our cross-sectional study was extended prospectively and longitudinally by looking at the sensitivity of muscle strength change over time in MND/ALS patients measured by repeated measures [mean MMT (ordinal units); mean MVIC (Z units), mean MVIC (percent predicted)], by a sustained fall of the muscle strength below a specific threshold (i.e., MMT ≤4, ≤3; MVIC ≤80%, ≤60%, ≤40% predicted), or by a sustained specific drop from baseline (i.e., MMT ≥1

ordinal unit; MVIC ≥1 Z unit; ≥10%, ≥20% predicted). The findings are similar for all muscles individually and can be reviewed on the website (see URL above). The composite MVIC for the arm muscles shows unique properties (Fig. 34.8). The event history analysis for a sustained drop in the composite isometric arm strength by ≥1 ordinal unit by MMT testing overlaps the drop in the composite isometric arm strength by ≥20% predicted by MVIC testing. The sustained drop by ≥10% predicted in arm isometric strength measured by fixed dynamometry antecedes the drop by ≥20% predicted and may be a surrogate measurement of change in arm strength in the first 12 months following attendance at a MND/ALS clinic. This clinimetric evaluated by event history analysis meets the need to have frequent events that may be measured in the study interval and may be relatively unaffected by loss to follow-up, which is minimal in the first 12 months following attendance at a MND/ALS clinic but increases dramatically between 12 and 24 months after the first visit.

Event history analysis also permits comparison of age, sex, site of onset and time after onset in matched case-historical control exploratory trials of therapies on isometric muscle strength in MND/ALS patients. Such quasi-experiments will allow evaluation, in some groups of patients, of therapeutic interventions such as drugs or medical devices that might be chosen for further study in appropriately controlled phase III clinical trials. One such drug is albuterol, which in 28 MND/ALS patients demonstrated a

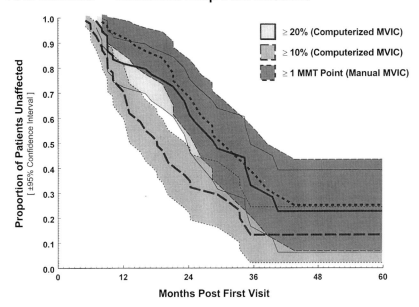

Fig. 34.8. Event history analysis (proportion of patients unaffected ± 95% confidence interval) of a sustained drop from baseline of computerized maximum voluntary isometric contraction (MVIC) by ≥10% predicted (relative to normal) or ≥20% predicted (relative to normal), or ≥1 MMT point drop in composite arm muscles (shoulder extensors, elbow extensors and elbow flexors) over 60 months after the first clinic visit in 132 MND/ALS patients.

Arm Muscles — Sustained Drop from Baseline

Legend:
- ≥ 20% (Computerized MVIC)
- ≥ 10% (Computerized MVIC)
- ≥ 1 MMT Point (Manual MVIC)

Y-axis: Proportion of Patients Unaffected [±95% Confidence Interval]

X-axis: Months Post First Visit

significant sparing effect on knee extensor and knee flexor strength compared with case-matched historical controls (Fig. 34.9).

In comparison with event history analysis of MVIC change in MND/ALS patients, the change over time of MVIC determined by repeated measures is associated with a large population standard deviation and requires correction for censuring due to loss to follow-up (Fig. 34.10). The change over time in the mean composite score based on MMT units, MVIC Z units or MVIC percent predicted shows comparable change over time but the different population standard deviations lead to different sample sizes depending on the method of analysis (Fig. 34.11). Mean MMT scores are least sensitive and require extraordinary sample sizes, even for large treatment

Manual MVIC — All Muscles

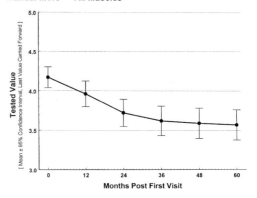

Knee Extensors — ≥ 10% Sustained Drop from Baseline

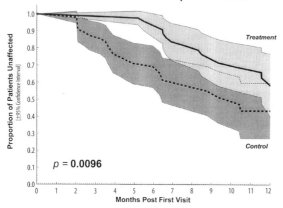

Knee Flexors — ≥ 10% Sustained Drop from Baseline

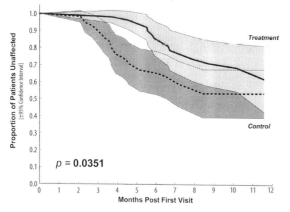

Computerized MVIC — All Muscles

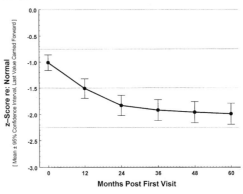

Computerized MVIC — All Muscles

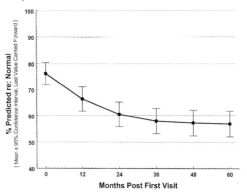

Fig. 34.9. Event history analysis (proportion of patients unaffected ± 95% confidence interval) of a sustained drop by ≥10% predicted (relative to normal) from baseline of computerized maximum voluntary isometric contraction (MVIC) in knee extensors (*top*) and knee flexors (*bottom*) in 28 MND/ALS patients treated with albuterol sulfate extended release tablets compared with 28 historical control MND/ALS patients matched for age, sex, site of disease onset and time after onset to first test.

Fig. 34.10. Repeated measures analysis of manual test (MMT) maximum voluntary isometric contraction (MVIC) — mean ± 95% confidence limits [last value carried forward (LVCF)] over 60 months after the first clinic visit in xx MND/ALS patients (*top*); computerized MVIC (Z-Score relative to Normal) — mean ± 95% confidence limits (LVCF) over 60 months after the first clinic visit in xx MND/ALS patients (*middle*); computerized MVIC (% predicted relative to normal) — mean ± 95% confidence limits (LVCF) over 60 months after the first clinic visit in 132 MND/ALS patients (*bottom*).

effects. *Z* unit and percent predicted measurements of MVIC are equally efficient with respect to sample sizes required to demonstrate complete arrest of disease progression. The MVIC percent predicted is more easily grasped clinically and the event history analysis of a sustained drop in strength by ≥10% predicted or ≥20% predicted requires fewer patients than endpoint analysis change from baseline or slope

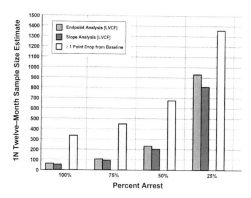

Manual MVIC — All Muscles

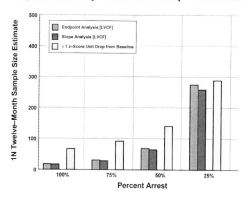

Computerized MVIC [z–Score re: Normal] — All Muscles

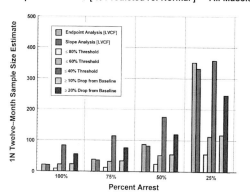

Computerized MVIC [% Predicted re: Normal] — All Muscles

analysis. The evaluation of muscle strength loss by a sustained drop below a threshold level is complicated by the fact that many patients may enter below the designated threshold level and the subsequent range of potential change is smaller, dependent upon the distribution of strength at baseline. Event analysis of sustained drops in MVIC below a specific threshold as percent predicted is comparably efficient to event analysis of sustained drops in MVIC by ≥10% predicted or ≥20% predicted; however, the latter method requires the event to occur during the study period whereas the threshold method is subject to the distribution of isometric strength at the beginning of the study period.

Analysis of the properties of ≥10% predicted, ≥20% predicted or a 1 MMT unit sustained drop, shows no statistically significant difference among ALS patients with bulbar, arm or leg onset as well as no statistical difference between males and females. No statistically significant difference for ALS patients above or below age 45 years is present (see URL above).

Event history analysis of single muscles or muscle groups is present for the UW ALS clinic on the website (see URL above). In previous analyses of limb muscle strength change over time in ALS patients, repeated measures techniques, rate of change by mean slope techniques and change from baseline have been presented for smaller groups of ALS patients [1–4,10–14,29–31,43]. Index finger pinch, wrist extension, jaw (masseter), and tongue (protrusion) strength changes only studied in limited group of patients previously are presented by the new event history analysis of sustained drop by ≥10% predicted or ≥20% predicted strength change for a large longitudinal study of UW ALS clinic patients (see URL above).

Both MMT and MVIC strength measurements have been employed in a large number of phase I–II clinical trials and in large multicenter phase III clin-

Fig. 34.11. Sample size required in each treatment arm (1 N) to demonstrate 25%, 50%, 75% or 100% arrest over 12 months follow-up to give two-sided confidence ($Z\alpha = 0.05$) for type I error and power of 0.90 ($Z\beta = 0.05$) to prevent type II error in manual muscle test (MMT) maximum voluntary isometric contraction (MVIC): endpoint analysis (change from baseline) (LVCF); slope analysis (initial slope) (LVCF), event history analysis of a sustained ≥1 MMT point drop from baseline (*top*); computerized MVIC (Z-score relative to normal): endpoint analysis (change from baseline) (LVCF); slope analysis (initial slope) (LVCF), event history analysis of a sustained ≥1 Z-score unit drop from baseline (*middle*); computerized MVIC (% predicted relative to normal): endpoint analysis (change from baseline) (LVCF); slope analysis (initial slope) (LVCF), event history analysis of a sustained drop below fixed threshold of 80%, 60% or 40% predicted, event history analysis of a sustained drop by ≥10% or ≥20% predicted from baseline (*bottom*). Based on a historical control sample of 132 MND/ALS patients.

ical trials. Intra- and inter-rater reliability have been assessed in a number of such clinical trials [56–58,68–70,75–80,83–86]. Test–retest reproducibility of MVIC across many centers was audited and quantified in two large phase III clinical trials that employed MVIC as the primary clinical endpoint [57,58]. Test–retest reliability across centers demonstrated a systematic decline in strength across centers, but, in addition, there was a significant systematic difference in variance across centers (Fig. 34.12). Within-center variance, though significant, did not affect the change in MVIC over time by center [30]. Similar results were obtained in other studies [29,31].

ALS Functional Rating Scale: ALS FRS Subscales

The ALS FRS is an outgrowth of the ALS CNTF Treatment Study (ACTS) and was a logical extension of the Hillel ALS Severity Scale [62–65]. The ALS FRS differs from the Norris ALS Scale and the Appel ALS Scale [87–89] in not mixing impairment and disability measures but just representing disability measures. It has been validated in a large number of ALS patients and has features which overlap the Charing Cross Qualitative and Quantitative ALS Rating Scale [1,3,12,51,53].

The ALS FRS has been employed in several small phase I–II and several large phase III multicenter trials in North America and Europe with excellent reproducibility, intra- and inter-rater reliability as well as content validity [51].

The total ALS FRS score has many interesting properties well described in the literature [1,51]. The mean ALS FRS total score changes over time comparably to the change in MVIC by percent predicted (Fig. 34.13). Similar findings occurred in the placebo group of patients in the ACTS clinical trial [89]. When the total ALS FRS score is presented as a ≥4-point drop (≥10% predicted) or as an ≥8-point drop (≥20% predicted), it is clear that 73 events per 100 patients occur by 12 months after the first visit for a sustained drop by ≥4 points and 40 events per 100 patients occur by 12 months for a sustained drop by ≥8 points (Fig. 34.14). When the total ALS FRS score is presented as a sustained drop below 80% predicted, 60% predicted, 40% predicted, it is clear that

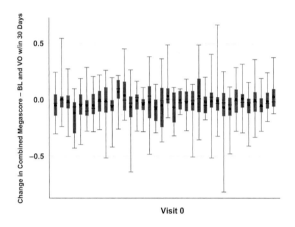

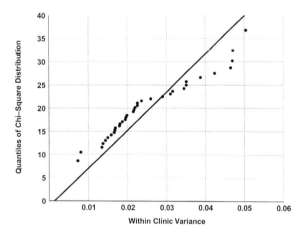

Fig. 34.12. Test–retest reliability of maximum voluntary isometric contraction muscle strength measured as combined arm–leg megascore at 36 clinic sites in the ALS CNTF Treatment Study (ACTS) [30,57]. Change in combined megascore between baseline and visit 0 ± standard deviation in 973 MND/ALS patients (*top*). Quantiles of chi-square distribution versus within-clinic variance at 35 clinic sites (*bottom*).

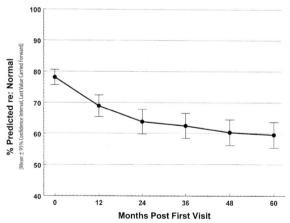

Fig. 34.13. Repeated measures analysis of ALS Functional Rating Scale total score – mean ± 95% confidence interval [last value carried forward (LVCF)] over 60 months after the first clinic visit in 132 MND/ALS patients.

ALS FRS Total Score — Sustained Drop from Baseline

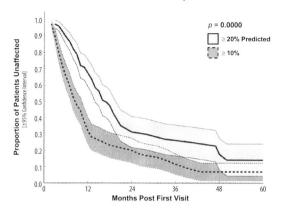

ALS FRS Total Score — Drop Below Threshold

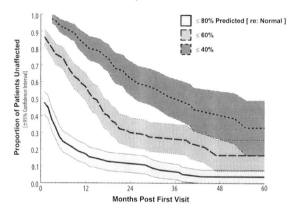

Fig. 34.14. Event history analysis (proportion of patients unaffected ± 95% confidence interval) of ALS functional rating scale total score – sustained drop in ALS FRS total score by ≥10% or ≥20% predicted (*top*); sustained drop below fixed threshold of 80%, 60% or 40% Predicted ALS FRS total score (*bottom*) over 60 months after the first clinic visit in 132 MND/ALS patients.

half of the patients were below 80% predicted at the first visit.

The subscales of the ALS FRS, when subject to analysis of a sustained drop below threshold after the first visit show clear, statistically significant, stepwise differentiation for the Speech, Feeding Self, Turning in Bed, Climbing Stairs and Walking subscales, defined by the individual steps in each subscale (see URL above). For the Swallowing and Breathing subscales, step 3 is clearly different from the other steps but steps 2, 1 and 0 are not statistically different (see URL above).

For the specific first point drop on the ALS FRS subscales from 4 to >3, only 35–50 events per 100 patients occur for Speech, Swallowing and Breathing in the first 12 months following attendance at the UW ALS Clinic. However, between 63 and 75 events per 100 patients occur during this period for Turning in Bed, Climbing Stairs and Walking. This finding is similar to the slow change in bulbar timed functional tests of alternate motion rates compared with lower extremity functional tests presented above (see URL above).

The ALS FRS is very efficient with respect to sample size for large treatment effect size but is less efficient for small treatment effect sizes (Fig. 34.15). For studies of 12 months duration, the ALS FRS is not as efficient as the FVC or VC percent predicted but is slightly more efficient than MVIC percent predicted.

Timed Functional Tests: Bulbar, Arms, Legs

Timed functional tests are components of the Tufts Quantitative Neurological Examination, Appel ALS Rating Scale, Charing Cross ALS Quantitative Rating Scale and ACTS Evaluation protocols [1–4,10–14]. In the Tufts Quantitative Neurological Examination the final clinimetric is a Z-score relative to other ALS patients, and in the ACTS Evaluation, the final clinimetric is a percent predicted score relative to normal [1]. In the Appel ALS Rating Scale, observed data are assigned an ordinal rank and incorporated into the final scale [1,87].

Standing, 360° axial turning and walking velocity measurements were dichotomized. For walking velocity, only 12% of UW ALS patients were below the 80% predicted threshold at the first visit (Fig. 34.16; see URL above). Over the next 12 months, 65 per 100 UW ALS patients show a sustained ≥10% predicted decine in walking velocity measured over 9 months (Fig. 34.16).

Rapid alternating movements of the hands defined as the rate of pronation followed by supination evaluated over 10 s showed 30% of patients below 80% predicted at the first visit (Fig. 34.17) and 40 of 100 patients showed a sustained drop by ≥10% predicted in the first 12 months following attendance at the UW ALS Clinic (Fig. 34.17).

The parallel rapid alternating motion rate for the tibialis anterior muscles is the foot tapping rate, defined as the rate evaluated over 10 s. At the first visit, 40% of patients are below 80% predicted and fewer than 35 of 100 patients showed a sustained drop by ≥10% predicted over the first 12 months following their first visit to the UW ALS Clinic (see URL above).

Bulbar alternate motion rates for the facial muscles are assessed by timed 10 repetitions of the word "pepper" and alternate motion rates for the

ALS Functional Rating Scale — Total

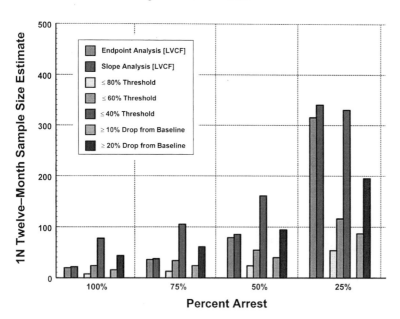

Fig. 34.15. Sample size required in each treatment arm (1 N) to demonstrate 25%, 50%, 75% or 100% arrest over 12 months follow-up in ALS Functional Rating Scale total score to give two-sided confidence ($Z\alpha = 0.10$) for type I error and power of 0.90 ($Z\beta = 0.05$) to prevent type II error: endpoint analysis (change from baseline) [last value carried forward (LVCF)]; slope analysis (initial slope) (LVCF), event history analysis of a sustained drop below fixed threshold of 80%, 60% or 40% predicted, event history analysis of a sustained drop by ≥10% or ≥20% predicted from baseline. Based on a historical control sample of 132 MND/ALS patients.

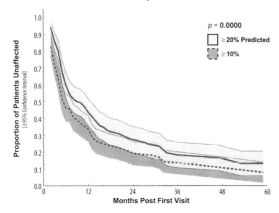

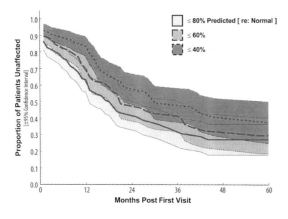

tongue muscles are assessed by timed 10 repetitions of the word "ticker". In both tests, 50–60% of patients were below 80% predicted at the first visit and little change occurred in the first 12 months (Fig. 34.18). By comparison with the above functional tests only 25–35 per 100 of patients demonstrated a sustained ≥10% predicted drop in the first 12 months after the first visit (Fig. 34.18).

The hierarchy of the percent of UW ALS patients demonstrating a ≥10% predicted sustained decline over the first 12 months following attendance at the UW ALS Clinic is leg (75–80%), arm (35–40%) and bulbar (20–25%) (see URL above).

Time to Specific Sustained Clinimetric Loss by 50% of Patients

The choice of clinimetrics for clinical trials is driven by the number of events which occur in the first 12 months following attendance at the MND/ALS clinic. The best clinimetrics will demonstrate a defined change in 50% of patients over a short period of time

Fig. 34.16. Event history analysis (proportion of patients unaffected ± 95% confidence interval) of walking velocity (speed of walking 30 feet in 10 s) – sustained drop in walking velocity by ≥10% or ≥20% predicted (*top*); sustained drop below fixed threshold of 80%, 60% or 40% predicted walking velocity (*bottom*) over 60 months after the first clinic visit in 198 MND/ALS patients.

Rapid Alternating Movement — Sustained Drop from Baseline

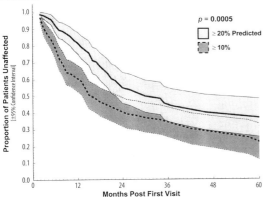

"Pepper" — Sustained Drop from Baseline

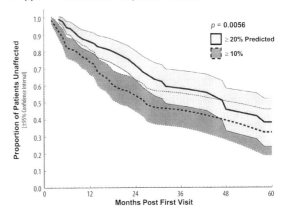

Rapid Alternating Movement — Drop Below Threshold

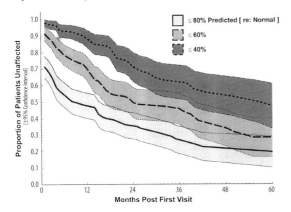

"Pepper" — Drop Below Threshold

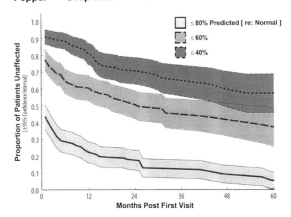

Fig. 34.17. Event history analysis (proportion of patients unaffected ± 95% confidence interval) of rapid alternating motion rate for hands (alternating pronation–supination in 10 s) – sustained drop in rapid alternating motion rate by ≥10% or ≥20% predicted (*top*); sustained drop below fixed threshold of 80%, 60% or 40% predicted rapid alternating motion rate (*bottom*) over 60 months after the first clinic visit in 198 MND/ALS patients.

Fig. 34.18. Event history analysis (proportion of patients unaffected ± 95% confidence interval) of alternative motion rate for facial muscles (10 repetitions of "pepper") – sustained drop in repetition rate by ≥10% or ≥20% predicted (*top*); sustained drop below fixed threshold of 80%, 60% or 40% predicted repetition rate (*bottom*) over 60 months after the first clinic visit in 198 MND/ALS patients.

prior to loss of follow-up. Event history analysis has been shown under certain circumstances to be more sensitive to clinical change [90–99]. A careful study of potential clinimetrics was conducted in MND/ALS patients with the result that a sustained drop by ≥10% predicted in vital capacity and walking velocity occurred in 50% of patients during the 8–14 months following initial evaluation at the MND/ALS clinic. Nearly half the patients showed a similar change in standing and turning velocity over 9–21 months following attendance at the clinic. MVIC measured by fixed dynamometry showed a similar change from 13 to 23 months after the first visit. MVIC measured by MMT yielded a ≥1 unit drop in 50% of patients over 26–60 months after first attendance at the MND/ALS clinic. Functional changes

occurred earlier, with changes in rapid alternating arm and leg movements in 50% of patients between 14 and 30 months after the first visit. Brainstem functional changes occurred in 50% of patients between 23 and 60 months after the initial evaluation. (Fig. 34.19).

Quality of Life Scales: SIP and SF-36

The Sickness Impact Profile (SIP) has been employed in the rhIGF-I (Myotrophin) clinical trials, the BDNF phase II–III clinical trial and the ALS Synergen CNTF clinical trial [31–34,102–103]. It is validated with a number of measures of disability in ALS patients [102]. The Short Form-36 (SF-36) derived from the Medical Outcomes Study has been validated in ALS patients [104]. Shortened versions are constitutive components of the ALS CARE Study ALS Patient Care Database forms used in the longitudinal North American ALS Registry [103]. At the first visit only 3% of UW ALS patients are below 80% predicted for the SIP quality of life scale while 8% of patients are below 80% predicted for the SF-36. During the next 18 months, 50% of patients fall below 80% predicted on the SIP but 70% of patients fall below 80% predicted on the SF-36 (Fig. 34.20). Moreover, 35% of patients fall below 60% predicted and 4% of patients fall below 40% predicted at 18 months post entry. Overall, there appears to be more change over time in the SF-36 scale than the SIP scale using event history analysis. A larger number of patients in the BDNF phase II–III clinical trial were studied longitudinally by both quality of life measures and will be reported shortly [105].

Survival

Survival of MND/ALS patients seen at MND/ALS clinics differs significantly from survival of MND/ALS patients in population-based studies [106,107]. Survival studies in the MND/ALS clinic

setting can add information with respect to survival following specific disease milestones. Percutaneous endoscopic gastrostomy is recommended commonly in MND/ALS patients with severe dysphagia leading to inanition. Quasi-experimental analysis of convenience samples of patients who do and do not follow the recommendation have shown conflicting outcomes including improved survival following gastrostomy tube placement [108,109]. In a similar group of UW MND/ALS patients, survival was studied following the onset of swallowing difficulties and no significant difference in survival was noted between the group of ALS patients receiving gastrostomy and those not receiving gastrostomy (Fig. 34.21).

Experimental and Quasi-experimental Designs for phase I, II and III Clinical Trials

The development of clinimetrics which provide a large number of events over the potential period for follow-up following first attendance at a referral MND/ALS clinic increases the potential for assess-ing treatment effects of different agents in these patients.

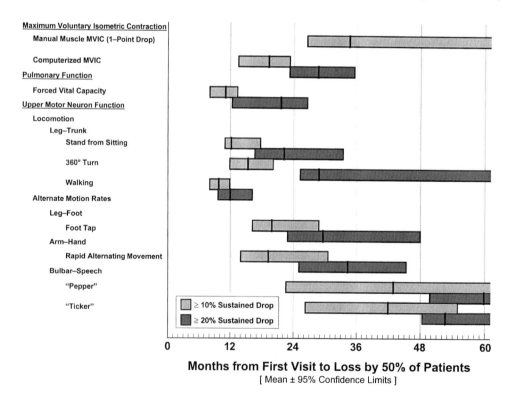

Fig. 34.19. Months from first visit to sustained drop in outcome measure by ≥10% or ≥20% predicted in 50% of MND/ALS patients. Open-ended right sided 95% confidence limit indicates <50% of ALS patients achieved the respective endpoint.

SF–36 Total Score — Drop Below Threshold

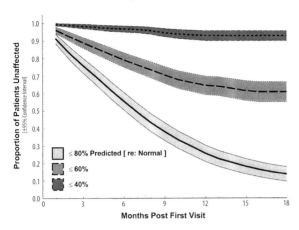

SIP Total Score — Drop Below Threshold

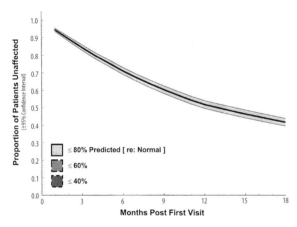

Fig. 34.20. Event history analysis (proportion of patients unaffected ± 95% confidence interval) of the end-point sustained drop below 80%, 60% or 40% predicted total score for Short Form-36 (SF-36) (n SF-36 = 62) or Sickness Impact Profile (SIP) (n SIP = 147) over 18 months in MND/ALS patients.

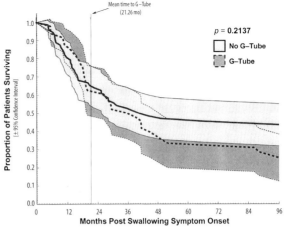

Fig. 34.21. Event history analysis (proportion of patients unaffected ± 95% confidence interval) of survival following onset of swallowing symptoms in 121 MND/ALS patients. Percutaneous endoscopic gastrostomy (PEG) tube placement was recommended at various times following onset of swallowing difficulties. In patients who accepted PEG tubes the mean time to insertion was 21.26 months. Survival in patients who did (n PEG = 49) and not (n no PEG = 72) receive PEG tubes was identical ($p = 0.2137$).

The goal of therapeutic research in MND/ALS is to measure treatment efficacy. The clinical domains in which to evaluate treatment efficacy are defined by the regional impact of impairment caused by MND/ALS (Table 34.1). The clinical trial calculus that is employed to evaluate therapeutic efficacy depends on the endpoint used to measure the clinical outcome [110–128], the hypothesis to be tested, the availability of MND/ALS patients with specific types of disease onset and involvement, the availability of competing treatments and the step in the drug development process (exploratory phase I, II; definitive phase II; definitive phase III and open-label phase IV). Both randomized clinical trials and non-randomized clinical trials constitute elements of this clinical trial calculus.

Randomized clinical trials (RCTs) include:

1. Clinical series with contemporaneous control subjects: each study patient is randomly assigned to treatment or control (subject-specific RCT) [29–34,35,36,39–45,99–101,114–128];
2. Clinical series with contemporaneous control subjects: each group of which is randomly assigned to treatment or control (group-specific RCT) [129];
3. Clinical series with randomized first treatment crossover control (crossover RCT) [20,23,74,130–135];
4. Individual with randomized first or multiple crossover treatment – control exposures (N-of-1 crossover RCT) [136–144].

Nonrandomized clinical trials include:

1. Clinical series with historical controls (observational study-historical controls) [145–154];
2. Clinical series with contemporaneous controls not randomly assigned to treatment (observational study – nonrandomized controls) [155–158];
3. Clinical series with different treatment dose-rates (observational studies comparing different treatment groups with nonrandom pre-assigned treatment – prospective or retrospective cohort studies) [159–169];
4. Clinical series with matched individual control subjects (prospective or retrospective case-control studies) [13,14,159];

5. Clinical series without case–control subjects (prospective or retrospective cross-sectional studies) [80,170–184];
6. Individual with nonrandomized first or multiple crossover treatment – control exposures (*N*-of-1 nonrandomized crossover) [185–190].

Nonrandomized clinical trials are a fundamental feature of quasi-experimental design which is quite commonly employed in MND/ALS research. Quasi-experiments lack random assignment to identify the treated and comparative groups. The most common version of this design is the non-equivalent groups design, which has been used to provide important information concerning BiPAP and PEG in ALS patients [108,190,191]. In each example there was a post-test survival but the groups were determined by criteria other than randomization. Other quasi-experimental designs include a double pre-test with a single post-test that is used to determine whether there is symptomatic improvement in swallowing or breathing following interventions [193]. Symptomatic treatments may be evaluated by crossover trial design when there is short-term onset and offset of the treatment, such as glycopyrrollate or atenolol in sialorrhea or ephedrine or pyridostigmine bromide in neuromuscular junction fatigue [136–144]. When there is delayed onset and offset, such as nortriptylline for lability then a pre-test/post-test quasi-experimental design may precede a parallel placebo-controlled clinical trial to evaluate treatment effect size. As seen above, quasi-experimental design may use concurrent convenience control groups and event history analysis [98,180,181]. Concurrent nonrandomized control groups may be studied prospectively as presented above for the potentially ergotropic drug, albuterol sulfate (Fig. 34.9).

The need for innovative tactics to assess treatment effects is increasing as we have a number of potential therapies, addressing various pathogenetic aspects of MND/ALS. Symptomatic features of MND/ALS may be addressed by *N*-of-1 crossover RCTs or crossover RCTs. Fundamental characteristics of the pathogenesis of MND/ALS resulting in progression of weakness must be addressed by other clinical trial designs outlined above. Different clinical trial designs may be required for each clinical trial depending upon the hypothesis to be tested [194–211].

Spread of disease from involved to uninvolved regions may be assessed in specific muscles by event history analysis of loss of strength by a sustained specific drop or a sustained drop below as specific threshold. Delay of progression in clinically affected muscles may be assessed by similar methods. Sample size requirements for event history analysis of muscle strength in individual muscles, pulmonary function, and timed functional activities are more efficient than sample sizes requirements for other analytic techniques of these same endpoints [90,91,212–241]. Repeated measures design assessing improvement of the clinical endpoint employed as the outcome measure may be applied to individual muscles, pulmonary function or timed functional activities. As formulated in the Airlie House Guidelines [59,242], phase I clinical trials should incorporate concurrent placebo-controlled patients and should be conducted for at least 6 months if clinical improvement is anticipated. Longer trials may be required if delayed onset of treatment effect will require prolonged treatment to assess potential toxicity.

Phase II clinical trials may utilize concurrent placebo controls, historical controls or a cross–over design. Phase II clinical trials are employed to screen agents with potential positive therapeutic value and to define therapeutic effect size to aid in planning phase III clinical trials. If improvement in strength or function is the endpoint, the trial should last at least 6 months. The first 3 months and repeated testing may identify learning and placebo effects. The second 3 months may substantiate treatment effect size and persistence. If stabilization or slowing of deterioration is the end point, the trial should last a minimum of 12 months depending on the nature of the drug or intervention. The number of events that occurs in the first 12 months following initial attendance at a MND/ALS clinic depends on the clinical endpont and how it is analyzed. Loss to follow-up is less than 10–15% in this first year depending on the MND/ALS clinic, but increases significantly in the second and third years after first attendance.

Phase III clinical trials should be controlled with the MND/ALS patient receiving the best available treatment for this disease. The patient may receive a placebo in comparison with the new treatment that is being tested or a dose-ranging study with the minimally effective dose compared with the maximum effective or tolerated dose as defined by phase II clinical trials. However, persistent ethical concerns have led to recommendations that dose-ranging from the minimally effective dose to the maximum effected dose be considered rather than placebo. Phase III clinical trials should include event history analysis of time to death, assessment of strength measured by maximum voluntary isometric contraction, pulmonary function, functional performance by the ALS rating scale and measurement of bulbar function.

The availability of computer software for clinical trial design, clinical trial execution and clinical trial analysis has permitted advances in the assault on MND/ALS [243–265]. Many standardized and validated software programs are also available on the Internet [266,267]. Both published and electronic resources may be used to enhance clinical trial design and minimize pitfalls in the evolution to factorial designs in the assessment of combination therapies in MND/ALS [268–271].

The strength of enhanced computer support for clinical trials in MND/ALS permits easy implementation of a standardized report format for patient-oriented clinical research [272–274]. The templates serve as a reminder of the crucial elements which must be provided to initiate, conduct and complete a valid clinical trial (Table 34.2).

Acknowledgements. The role of the World Federation of Neurology Subcommittee on Motor Neuron Diseases under leadership of Theodore Munsat, Micheal Swash, Nigel Leigh, Vincent Meininger, Robert Miller and Vianney de Jong in criticizing many of these concepts is greatly appreciated. The early and enduring excitement in assessing clinimetrics in MND/ALS was nurtured by my close friend Roberto Guiloff and his colleagues, who have led the way in careful assessment of repeated measures designs in MND/ALS. The studies reported in this chapter were supported in part by the Muscular Dystrophy Association, the Department of Veterans Affairs, Veterans Health Administration, VISN 12 and the University of Wisconsin General Clinical Research Center, National Institutes of Health (MR 344-555-6677). None of these studies would be possible without the continuing dedication of Kathryn Roelke, RN, ALS Clinical Nurse Specialist, and ALS Clinical Research Center Research Specialists Jennifer Parnell, Christy Dewitt and Crystal Halvorson. I am extremely grateful for their professional approach to the care of our MND/ALS patients.

Table 34.2. Checklist for reporting clinical trials

Title	1.	Identify the study as a randomized/nonrandomized clinical trial
Abstract	2.	Use a structured format: Context, Objective, Design, Setting, Patients, Intervention, Main outcome measures, Results, Conclusions
Introduction	3.	State prospectively defined hypothesis, clinical objectives and planned subgroup or covariate analysis
Methods		
Protocol	4.	Planned study population, together with inclusion/exclusion criteria
	5.	Planned interventions and their timing
	6.	Primary and secondary outcome measure(s) and the minimum important difference(s), and how the target sample size was projected
	7.	Rationale and methods for statistical analyses detailing main comparative analyses and whether they were completed on an intention-to-treat basis
	8.	Prospectively defined stopping rules (if warranted)
Assignment	9.	Randomization unit (e.g., individual, cluster, geographic) or method of treatment assignment
	10.	Method used to generate the allocation
	11.	Method of allocation concealment and timing assignment
	12.	Method to separate the generator from the executor of assignment
Blinding	13.	Describe mechanism (e.g., capsules, tablets); similarity of treatment characteristics (e.g., appearance, taste); allocations schedule control (location of code during trial and when broken); and evidence for successful blinding (blinding) among participants, person doing intervention, outcome assessors, and data analysts
Results		
Participants	14.	Provide a trial profile summarizing participant flow, numbers and flow and timing of randomized assignment, interventions, and follow-up measurements for each randomized group
Analysis	15.	State estimated effect of intervention on primary and secondary outcome measures, including a point estimate and measure of precision (confidence interval)
	16.	State results in absolute numbers when feasible (e.g., 10/20, not 50%)
	17.	Present summary data and appropriate descriptive and inferential statistics in sufficient detail to permit alternative analyses and replication
	18.	Describe prognostic variables by treatment group and any attempt to adjust for them
	19.	Describe protocol deviations from the study as planned, together with the reasons
Comment	20.	State specific interpretation of study findings, including sources of bias and imprecision (internal validity) and discussion of external validity, including appropriate quantitative measures when posssible
	21.	State general interpretation of the data in light of the totality of the available evidence

References

1. Brooks BR. Amyotrophic lateral sclerosis clinimetric scales: guidelines for administration and scoring. In: Herndon RM, editor. Handbook of clinical neurologic scales. New York: Demos Vermande, 1997:27–79.

2. Brooks BR, Lewis D, Rawling J, Sanjak M, Belden D, Hakim H, et al. The natural history of ALS. In: Williams AC, editor. Motor neuron disease. London: Chapman & Hall, 1994:131–170.

3. Brooks BR, Shodis KA, Lewis DH, Rawling JD, Sanak M, Belden DS, et al. Natural history of amyotrophic lateral sclerosis – quantification of symptoms, signs, strength and function. In: Serratrice G, Munsat T, editors. Pathogenesis and therapy of amyotrophic lateral sclerosis. Adv Neurol 1995;68:163–184.

4. Brooks BR, Sufit RL, DePaul R, Tan YD, Sanjak M, Robbins J. Design of clinical therapeutic trials in amyotrophic lateral sclerosis. In: Rowland LP, editor. Amyotrophic lateral sclerosis and other motor neuron diseases. Adv Neurol 1991;56:521–546.

5. Brooks BR. Emerging directions in ALS therapeutics – palliative therapies at the advent of the twenty-first century. Clin Neurosci 1996;3:386–392.

6. Andres PL, Skerry LM, Thornell B, Portney LG, Finison LJ, Munsat TL. A comparison of three measures of disease progression in ALS. J Neurol Sci 1996;139:64–70.

7. Andres PL, Finison LJ, Conlon T, Thibodeau LM, Munsat TL. Use of composite scores (megascores) to measure deficit in amyotrophic lateral sclerosis. Neurology 1988;38:405–408.

8. Andres PL, Skerry LM, Munsat TL. Measurement of strength in neuromuscular diseases. Boston: Butterworth, 1989:87–99.

9. Goonetileke A, Guiloff RJ, Nikhar N, Orrell RW, Tan SV. The clinical assessment of muscle force [abstract 1-02-04]. J Neurol Sci 1997;150(Suppl):S4.

10. Goonetilleke A, Guiloff RJ. Accuracy, reproducibility and variability of quantitative assessments of bulbar and repsiratory function in motor neurone disease. J Neurol Sci 1994;123:64–66.

11. Goonetilleke A, Modarres-Sadeghi H, Guiloff RJ. Accuracy, reproducibility, and variability of handheld dynamometry in motor neuron disease. J Neurol Neurosurg Psychiatry 1994;57:326–332.

12. Guiloff RJ, Goonetilleke A. Natural history of amyotrophic lateral sclerosis. Observations with Charing Cross Amyotrophic Lateral Sclerosis Rating Scales. In: Serratrice G, Munsat T, editors. Pathogenesis and therapy of amyotrophic lateral sclerosis. Adv Neurol 1995;68:185–198.

13. Guiloff RJ, Goonetilleke A. Longitudinal clinical assessments in motor neurone disease – relevance to clinical trials. In: Rose FC, editor. ALS – Charcot to the present and into the future. London: Smith-Gordon, 1994:73–82.

14. Guiloff RJ, Modarres-Sadeghi H, Rodgers H. Motor neuron disease: aims and assessment methods in trial design. In: Rose FC, editor. Amyotrophic lateral sclerosis: progress in clinical neurologic trials. New York: Demos, 1990:19–31.

15. Bensimon G, Lacomblez L, Meininger V, ALS Riluzole Study Group. A controlled trial of riluzole in amyotrophic lateral sclerosis. N Engl J Med 1994;330:585–591.

16. Lacomblez L, Bensimon G, Leigh PN, Gillet P, Meininger V, ALS/Riluzole Study Group II. Dose-ranging study of riluzole in amyotrophic lateral sclerosis, Lancet 1996;347:1425–1431.

17. Guiloff RJ, Goonetilleke A, Emani J. Riluzole and amyotrophic lateral sclerosis, Lancet 1996;348:336–337.

18. Lacomblez L, Bensimon G, Leigh PN, Gillet P, Meininger V. Riluzole and amyotrophic lateral sclerosis [Reply]. Lancet 1996;348:337.

19. Riviere M, Meininger V, Zeisser P, Munsat T. An analysis of extended survival in patients with amyotrophic lateral sclerosis treated with riluzole. Arch Neurol 1998;55:526–528.

20. Mitsumoto H, Salgado ED, Negroski D, Hanson MR, Salanga VD, Wilber JF, et al. Amyotrophic lateral sclerosis: effects of acute intravenous and chronic subcutaneous administration of thyrotropin-releasing hormone in controlled trials. Neurology 1986;36:152–159.

21. Brooks BR, Sufit RL, Montgomery GK, Beaulieu DA, Erickson LM. Intravenous thyrotropin-releasing hormone in patients with amyotrophic lateral sclerosis. Dose-response and randomized concurrent placebo-controlled pilot studies. Neurol Clin 1987;5:143–158.

22. Brooks BR. A summary of the current position of TRH in ALS therapy. Ann NY Acad Sci 1989;553:431–461.

23. Brooke MH. Thyrotropin-releasing hormone in ALS. Are the results of clinical studies inconsistent? Ann NY Acad Sci 1989;553:422–430.

24. Modarres-Sadeghi H, Rogers H, Emami J, Guiloff RJ. Subacute administration of a TRH analogue (RX77368) in motorneuron disease: an open study. J Neurol Neurosurg Psychiatry 1988;51:1146–1157.

25. Modarres-Sadeghi H, Guiloff RJ. Comparative efficacy and safety of intravenous and oral administration of a TRH analogue (RX77368) in motor neuron disease. J Neurol Neurosurg Psychiatry 1990;53:944–947.

26. Guiloff RJ. Use of TRH analogues in motorneurone disease. Ann NY Acad Sci 1989;553:399–421.

27. Goonetilleke A, Guiloff RJ. Continuous response variable trial design in motor neuron disease: long term treatment with a TRH analogue (RX77368). J Neurol Neurosurg Psychiatry 1995;58:201–208.

28. Hawley RJ, Kratz R, Goodman RR, McCutchen CB, Sirdofsky M, Hanson PA. Treatment of amyotrophic lateral sclerosis with the TRH analog DN-1417. Neurology 1987;37:715–717.

29. Smith RA, Melmed S, Sherman B, Frane J, Munsat TL, Festoff BW. Recombinant growth hormone treatment of amyotrophic lateral sclerosis. Muscle Nerve 1993;16:624–633.

30. Lotz B, Brooks B, Sanjak M, Weasler C, Roelke K, Parnell J, et al. A double-blind placebo-controllled clinical trial of subcutaneous recombinant human ciliary neurotrophic factor (rhCNTF) in amyotrophic lateral sclerosis, Neurology 1996;46:1244–1249.

31. Miller RG, Petajan JH, Bryan WW, Armon C, Barohn RJ, Goodpasture JC, et al. A placebo-controlled trial of recombinant human ciliary neurotrophic factor (rhCNTF) in amyotrophic lateral sclerosis. Ann Neurol 1996;39:256–260.

32. Lai EC, Felice KJ, Festoff BW, Gawel MJ, Gelinas DF, Kratz R, et al. Effect of recombinant human insulin-like growth factor-I on progression of ALS: a placebo-controlled study, Neurology 1997;49:1621–1630.

33. Borasio GD, Robberrecht W, Leigh PN, Emile J, Guiloff RJ, Jerusalem F, et al. A placebo-controlled trial of insulin-like growth factor-I in amyotrophic latearl sclerosis. Neurology 1998;51:583–586.

34. Cedarbaum JM, Stambler N, Brooks BR, Bradley W. Brain-derived neurotrophic factor in amyotrophic lateral sclerosis: a failed drug or a failed trial? Ann Neurol 1998;44:506–507.

35. Plaitakis A, Smith J, Mandeli J, Yahr MD. Pilot trial of branched-chain aminoacids in amyotrophic lateral sclerosis. Lancet 1988;I:1015–1018.

36. The Italian ALS Study Group. Branched-chain amino acids and amyotrophic lateral sclerosis: a treatment failure? Neurology 1993;43:2466–2470.

37. Rowland L. Branched-chain amino acids and amyotrophic lateral sclerosis. Neurology 1993;43:2437–2438.

38. Plaitakis A. Branched-chain amino acids and ALS. Neurology 1994;44:1982–1983.

39. Steiner TJ, SPECIALS Group. Multinational trial of branched-chain amino acids in amyotrophic lateal sclerosis [abstract]. Muscle Nerve 1994(Suppl);166.

40. Steiner TJ. Clinical trials. In: Williams AC, editor. Motor neuron disease. London: Chapman & Hall, 1994:701–724.

41. Tandan R, Bromberg MB, Forshew D, Fries TJ, Badger GJ, Carpenter J, et al. A controlled trial of amino acid therapy in amyotrophic lateral sclerosis. 1. Clinical, functional, and maximum isometric torque data. Neurology 1996;47:1220–1226.

42. Blin O, Pouget J, Aubresp G, Guelton C, Crevat A, Serratrice G. A double-blind placebo-controlled trial of l-threonine in amyotrophic lateral sclerosis. J Neurol 1992;239:79–81.

43. Louwerse ES, Weverling GJ, Bossuyt PM, Meyjes FE, de Jong JMBV. Randomized, double-blind, controlled trial of acetylcysteine in amyotrophic lateral sclerosis. Arch Neurol 1995;52:559–564.

44. Appel SH, Stewart SS, Appel V, Harati Y, Mietlowski W, Weiss W, et al. A double-blind study of the effectiveness of cyclosporine in amyotrophic lateral sclerosis. Arch Neurol 1988;45:381–386.

45. Drachman DB, Chaudhry V, Cornblath D, Kuncl RW, Pestronk A, Clawson L, et al. Trial of immunosuppression in amyotrophic lateral sclerosis using total lymphoid irradiation. Ann Neurol 1994;35:142–150.

46. Tan E, Lynn DJ, Amato AA, Kissel JT, Rammohan KW, Sahenk Z, et al. Immunosuppressive treatment of motor neuron syndromes. Attempts to distinguish a treatable disorder. Arch Neurol 1994;51:194–200.

47. Smith SA, Miller RG, Murphy JR, Ringel SP. Treatment of ALS with high dose pulse cyclophosphamide. J Neurol Sci 1994;124(Suppl):84–87.

48. Gouriedevi M, Nalini A, Subbakrishna DK. Temporary amelioration of symptoms with intravenous cyclophosphamide in amyotrophic lateral sclerosis. J Neurol Sci 1997;159:167–172.

49. Caroscio JT, Mulvihill MN, Sterling R, Abrams B. Amyotrophic lateral sclerosis: its natural history. Neurol Clin North Am 1987;5:1–8.

50. Cedarbaum JM, Wittes J, Brittain E, Brooks BR, Sanjak M, Neville H, et al. Correlation between rates of change in functional rating scales and muscle strength measures in amyotrophic lateral sclerosis (ALS) patients. Neurology 1994;44:A256–A257.

51. Cedarbaum JM, Stambler N. Performance of the Amyotrophic Lateral Sclerosis Functional Rating Scale (ALSFRS) in multicenter clinical trials. J Neurol Sci 1997;152:S1–S9.

52. Ringel SP, Murphy JR, Alderson MK, Bryan W, England JD, Miller RG. The natural history of amyotrophic lateral sclerosis. Neurology 1993;43:1316–1322.

53. Stambler N, Charatan M, Cedarbaum JM, ALS CNTF Treatment Study Group. Prognostic indicators of survival in ALS. Neurology 1998;50:66–72.

54. Dawson JD. Comparing treatment groups on the basis of slopes, areas-under-the-curves, and other summary measures. Drug Inform J 1994;28:723–732.

55. Meininger V, Bensimon G, Lacomblez L, Salachas F. Natural history of amyotrophic lateral sclerosis: discussion. In: Serratrice G, Munsat T, editors. Pathogenesis and therapy of amyotrophic lateral sclerosis. Adv Neurol 1995;68:199–207.

56. Louwerse ES, de Jong JMBV, Kuether G. Critique of assessment methodology in amyotrophic lateral sclerosis. In: Rose FC, editor. Amyotrophic lateral sclerosis-progress in clinical neurologic trials. New York: Demos, 1990:151–179.

57. Sanjak M, Belden D, Cook T, Brooks B. Muscle strength measurement. In: Lane R, editor. Handbook of muscle disease. New York: Marcel Dekker, 1996:19–31.

58. Hoagland RJ, Mendoza M, Armon C, Barohn RJ, Bryan WW, Goodpasture JC, et al. Reliability of maximal voluntary isometric contraction testing in a multicenter study of patients with amyotrophic lateral sclerosis. Syntex/Synergen Neuroscience Joint Venture rhCNTF ALS Study Group. Muscle Nerve 1997;20:691–695.

59. Subcommittee on Motor Neuron Diseases of the World Federation of Neurology Research Group on Neuromuscular Diseases, Airlie House "Therapeutic Trials in ALS" Workshop Contributors. Airlie House Guidelines:-therapeutic trials in amyotrophic lateral sclerosis. J Neurol Sci 1995;129:1–10.

60. Stoller JK, Buist AS, Burrows B, Crystal RG, Fallat RJ, McCarthy K, et al. Quality control of spirometery testing in the registry for patients with severe alpha(1)-antitrypsin deficiency. Chest 1997;111:899–909.

61. Bach JR. Amyotrophic lateral sclerosis: predictors for prolongation of life by noninvasive respiratory aids. Arch Phys Med Rehabil 1995;76:828–832.

62. Brooks BR, Sanjak M, Singel S, England J, Brinkmann J, Pestronk A, et al. The Amyotrophic Lateral Sclerosis Functional Rating Scale: assessment of activities of daily living in patients with amyotrophic lateral sclerosis. Arch Neurol 1996;53:141–147.

63. Hillel AD, Miller R. Bulbar amyotrophic lateal sclerosis: patterns of progression and clinical management. Head Neck 1989;11:51–59.

64. Hillel AD, Miller RM, Yorkston K, McDonald E, Norris FH, Konikow N. Amytrophic lateral sclerosis severity scale. Neuroepidemiology 1989;8:142–150.

65. Hillel AD, Yorkston K, Miller RM. Using phonation time to estimate vital capacity in amyotrophic lateral sclerosis. Arch Phys Med Rehabil 1989;70:618–620.

66. Schiffman PL, Belsh JM. Pulmonary function at diagnosis of amyotrophic lateral sclerosis: rate of deterioration. Chest 1993;103:508–513.

67. Martifaregas J, Sanchis J, Casan P, Miralda R, Garciapachon E, Illa I. Forced vital capacity deterioration in amyotrophic lateral sclerosis has an inflexion point. Eur J Neurol 1996;3:40–43.

68. Munsat TL, Andres PL, Finison L, Conlon T, Thibodeau L. The natural history of motoneuron loss in amyotrophic lateral sclerosis. Neurology 1988;38:409–413.

69. Munsat TL. Development of measurement techniques. Neurology 1996;47:S83–S85.

70. Munsat TL, Andres PL, Skerry LM. The use of quantitative techniques to define amyotrophic lateral sclerosis. In: Munsat TL, editor. Quantification of neurologic deficit. Boston: Butterworth, 1989:129–142.

71. Schrank B, Wurffel W, Naghibi-Saber SA, Giess R, Ochs G, Toyka KV, et al. Amyotrophic lateral sclerosis: patterns of disease dynamics are invariant [abstract P02.113]. Neurology 1997;48(Suppl):A127–A128.

72. Brooke MH, Fenichel GM, Griggs RC, et al. Clinical investigation in Duchenne dystrophy. 2. Determination of the "power" of therapeutic trials based on the natural history. Muscle Nerve 1983;6:91–103.

73. Brooke MH, Griggs RC, Mendell JR, et al. Clinical trial in Duchenne dystrophy. 1. The design of the protocol. Muscle Nerve 1981;4:186–197.

74. Brooke MH, Florence JM, Heller SL, Kaiser KK, Phillips D, Gruber A, et al. Controlled trial of thyrotropin releasing hormone in amyotrophic lateral sclerosis. Neurology 1986;36:146–151.

75. Florence JM, Pandya S, King WM, et al. Intra-rater reliability of manual muscle test (Medical Research Council scale)

grades in Duchenne's muscular dystrophy. Phys Ther 1992; 72:115–126.

76. Tawil R, Griggs RC, McDermott MP, Cos L, Personius KE, Langsam A, et al. A prospective quantitative study of the natural history of facioscapulohumeral muscular dystrophy (FSHD): implications for therapeutic trials. Neurology 1997; 48:38–46.

77. Mendell JR, Moxley RT, Griggs RC, et al. Randomized, double-blind six-month trial of prednisone in Duchenne's muscular dystrophy. N Engl J Med 1989;320:1592–1597.

78. Tawil R, McDermott MP, Mendell JR, et al. Facioscapulo-humeral muscular dystrophy (FSHD): design of natural history study and results of baseline testing. Neurology 1994;44:442–446.

79. Personius KE, Pandya S, King WM, Tawil R, McDermott MP, The FSH DY Group. Facioscapulohumeral dystrophy natural history study: Standardization of testing procedures and reliability of measurements. Phys Ther 1994;74:253–263.

80. Kilmer DD, Abresch RT, McCrory MA, et al. Profiles of neuromuscular diseases: facioscapulohumeral dystrophy. Am J Phys Med Rehabil1995;74:131–139.

81. Medical Research Council. Aids to the investigation of peripheral nerve injury. War memorandum, 2nd ed. London: HMSO, 1943:11–46.

82. National Isometric Muscle Strength (NIMS) Database Consortium. Muscular weakness assessment: use of normal isometric strength data. Arch Phys Med Rehabil 1996;77: 1251–1255.

83. Brinkmann JR, Andres P, Mendoza M, Sanjak M. Guidelines for the use and performance of quantitative outcome measures in ALS clinical trials. J Neurol Sci 1997;147:97–111.

84. Kuther G, Struppler A, Lipinski HG. Therapeutic trials in ALS: the design of a protocol. In: Cosi V, Kato AC, Parlette W, Pinelli P, Poloni M, editors. Amyotrophic lateral sclerosis – therapeutic, psychological, and research aspects. Adv Exp Med Biol 1987;209:265–276.

85. Agre JC, Magness JL, Hull SZ, Wrigth KC, Baxter TL, Patterson R, et al. Strength testing with a portable dynamometer: Reliability for upper and lower extremities. Arch Phys Med Rehabil 1987;68:454–458.

86. Barker L, Smith C, Perkins B, BurhansK, Newman R, Zimmerman L, et al. Clinical trials in spinal muscular atrophy: protocol development and reliability of quantitative strength assessment method. J Neurol Rehabil 1992;6:175–183.

87. Appel V, Stewart SS, Smith G, Appel SH. A rating scale for amyotrophic lateral sclerosis: Description and preliminary experience. Ann Neurol 1987;22:328–333.

88. Brooks BR. The Norris ALS score: Insight into the natural history of ALS provided by Forbes Norris. In: Rose FC, editor. ALS: from Charcot to the present and into the future". London: Smith-Gordon, 1994.

89. Mitsumoto H, Chad DA, Pioro EP. Treatment trials. In: Mitsumoto H, Chad DA, Pioro EP, editors. Amyotrophic lateral sclerosis. Philadelphia: FA Davis, 1998:329–359.

90. Nobler MS, Sackeim HA, Moeller JR, Petkova E, Waternaux C. Quantifying the speed of symptomatic improvement with electoconvulsive therapy: comparison of alternative statistical methods. Convuls Ther 1997;13:208–221.

91. Feinstein AR. P-values and confidence intervals: two-sides of the same unsatisfactory coin. J Clin Epidemiol 1998;51:355–360.

92. Feuer EJ, Hankey BF, Gaynor JJ, Wesley MN, Baker SG, Meyer JS. Graphical representation of survival curves associated with a binary non-reversible time dependent covariate. Stat Med 1992;11:455–474.

93. Gehan EA, Lemak NA. Statistics in medical research: developments in clinical trials. New York: Plenum, 1994:1–214.

94. Horwitz RI, Singer BH, Makuch RW, Viscoli CM. Clinical versus statistical considerations in the design and analysis of clinical research. J Clin Epidemiol 1998;51:305–307.

95. Kazdin AE. Methodological issues and strategies in clinical research, 2nd ed. Washington, DC: American Psychological Association, 1998:1–780.

96. Laupacis A, Sackett DL, Roberts RS. An assessment of clinically useful measures of the consequences of treatment. N Engl J Med 1988;318:1728–1733.

97. Ludbrook J. Comparing methods of measurement. Clin Exp Pharmacol Physiol 1997;24:193–203.

98. Miller TQ. Statistical methods for describing temporal order in longitudinal research. J Clin Epidemiol 1997;50:1135–1168.

99. Dawson JD. Comparing treatment groups on the basis of slopes, areas-under-the-curves, and other summary measures. Drug Inform J 1994;28:723–732.

100. Peto R, Pike MC, Armitage P, Breslow NE, Cox DR, Howard SV, et al. Design and analysis of randomized clinical trials requiring prolonged observation of each patient. II. Analysis and examples. Br J Cancer 1977;35:1–39.

101. Bland JM, Altman DG. Statistics notes: transformations, means, and confidence intervals. Br Med J 1996;312:1079.

102. McGuire D, Garrison L, Armon C, Barohn R, Bryan W, Miller R, et al. Relationship of the Tufts Quantitative Neuromuscular Exam (TQNE) and the Sickness Impact Profile in measuring progression of ALS. Neurology 1996;46:1442–1444.

103. McGuire D, Garrison L, Armon C, Barohn RJ, Bryann WW, Miller RG, et al. A brief quality-of-life measure for ALS clinical trials based on a subset of items from the Sickness Impact Profile. J Neurol Sci 1997;152(Suppl 1):518–522.

104. Shields RK, Ruhland JL, Ross MS, Saehler MM, Smith KB, Heffner ML. Analysis of health-related quality of life and muscle impairment in individuals with amyotrophic lateral sclerosis using the Medical Outcome Survey and the Tufts quantitative neuromuscular exam. Arch Phys Med Rehabil 1998;79:855–862.

105. Bayliss MS, Woolley JM, Keller SD, Brooks BR, Munsat TL, Neville H, et al. Measuring health-related quality of life in patients with amyotrophic lateral sclerosis. Submitted.

106. Lee JR-J, Annegers JF, Appel SH. Prognosis of amyotrophic lateral sclerosis and the effect of referral selection. J Neurol Sci 1995;132:207–215.

107. McGuire V, Longstreth WT, Koepsell TD, van Belle G. Incidence of amyotrophic lateral slcerosis in three counties in western Washington state. Neurology 1996;47:571–573.

108. Mazzini L, Corra T, Zaccala M, Mora G, Del Piano M, Galante M. Percutanoeus endoscopic gastrostomy and enteral nutrition in amyotrophic lateral sclerosis. J Neurol 1995;242:695–698.

109. Marthus-Vliegen LMH, Louwerse LS, Merkus MP, Tytgat GNJ, Vianney de Jong JMB. Percutaneous endoscopic gastrostomy in patients with amyotrophic lateral sclerosis and impaired pulmonary function. Gastrointest Endosc 1994;40: 463–469.

110. Anderson JJ, Delson DT, Meenan RF, Williams HJ. Which traditional measures should be used in rheumatoid arthritis clincal trials? Arthritis Rheum 1989;32:1093–1099.

111. Anonymous. International classification of impairments, disabilities, handicaps. Geneva: World Health Organization, 1980.

112. Bromberg MB, Brooks BR. Issues in clinical trial design. II. Selection of end point measures. Neurology 1996;47: S100–S102.

113. Cummings SR, Strull W, Nevitt MC, Hulley SB. Planning the measurements: precision and accuracy. In: Hulley SB, Cummings SR, editors. Designing clinical research. Baltimore: Williams & Wilkins, 1988:31–41.

114. Felson DT, Anderson JJ, Boers M, Bombardier C, Chernoff M, Fried B, et al. American College of Rheumatology Core Preliminary core set of disease activity measures for rheumatoid arthritis clincal trials. Arthritis Rheum 1993;36:729–740.

115. Deyo RA, Patrick DL. The significance of treatment effects: the clinical perspective. Med Care 1995;33:AS286–AS291.

116. Kasarskis EJ, Berryman S, English T, Nyland J, Vanderleest JG, Schneider A, et al. The use of upper extremity anthropometrics in the clinical assessment of patients with amyotrophic lateral sclerosis. Muscle Nerve 1997;20:330–335.

117. Katz JN, Larson MG, Phillips CB, Fossel AH, Liang MH. Comparative measurement sensitivity of short and longer health status instruments. Med Care 1992;30:917–925.

118. van Gestel AM, Prevoo MLL, van't Hof MA, van Rijswijk MH, van de Putte LBA, van Riel PLCM. Development and validation of the European League Against Rheumatism response criteria for rheumatoid arthritis. Arthritis Rheum 1996; 39:34–40.

119. Zwerling C, Daltroy LJ, Fine LJ, Johnston JJ, Melius J, Silverstein BA. Design and conduct of occupational injury intervention studies: a review of evaluation strategies. Am J Ind Med 1997;32:164–179.

120. Bulpitt CJ. Randomized controlled clinical trials. The Hague: Martinus Nijhoff, 1983.

121. Deyo RA. Measuring functional outcomes in therapeutic trials for chronic disease. Control Clin Trials 1984;5:223–240.

122. Deyo RA, Centor RM. Assessing the responsiveness of functional scales to clinical change: an analogy to diagnostic test performance. J Chron Dis 1989;39:897–906.

123. Deyo RA, Diehr P, Patrick DL. Reproducibility and responsiveness of health status measures. Control Clin Trials 1991;12:142s–158s.

124. Deyo RA, Inui TS. Toward clinical applications of health status measures: Sensitivity of scale to clinically important changes. Health Serv Res 1984;19:275–289.

125. Fisher WP. Measurement-related problems in functional assessment. Am J Occup Ther 1993;47:331–338.

126. Friedman LM, Furberg CD, DeMets DL. Fundamentals of clinical trials, 3rd ed. Berlin Heidelberg New York: Springer, 1998.

127. Meinert CL. Clinical trials: design, conduct and analysis. New York: Oxford University Press, 1986.

128. Meinert CL. Clinical trials dictionary: termination and usage recommendations. Baltimore: Johns Hopkins Center for Clinical Trials, 1996.

129. Murray DM, Hannan PJ, Wolfinger RD, Baker WL, Dwyer JH. Analysis of data from group-randomized trials with repeat observations on the same groups. Stat Med 1998;17:1781–1600.

130. Aquilonius SM, Askmark H, Eckernas SA, Gillberg PG, Hilton-Brown P, Rydin E, et al. Cholinesterase inhibitors lack therapeutic effect in amyotrophic lateral sclerosis. A controlled study of physostigmine versus neostigmine. Acta Neurol Scand 1986;73:628–632.

131. Askmark H, Aquilonius SM, Gillberg PG, Hartvig P, Hilton-Brown P, Lindstrom B, et al. Functional and pharmacokinetic studies of tetrahydroaminoacridine in patients with amyotrophic lateral sclerosis. Acta Neurol Scand 1990;82:253–258.

132. Askmark H, Aquilonius SM, Gillberg PG, Liedholm LJ, Stalberg E, Wuopio R. A pilot trial of dextromethorphan in amyotrophic lateral sclerosis. J Neurol Neurosurg Psychiatry 1993;56:197–200.

133. Ernst E, Resch KL. The optional crossover design for randomized controlled trials. Fundam Clin Pharmacol 1995;9:508–511.

134. Norris FH, Tan Y, Fallat RJ, Elias L. Trial of oral physostigmine in amyotrophic lateral sclerosis. Clin Pharmacol Ther 1993;54:680–682.

135. Redelmeier DA, Tibshirani RJ. Interpretation and bias in case-crossover studies. J Clin Epidemiol 1997;50:1281–1287.

136. Guyatt GH, Keller JL, Jaeschke R, Rosenbloom D, Adachi JD, Newhouse MT. The n-of-1 randomized controlled trial: clinical usefulness. Our three-year experience. Ann Intern Med 1990;112:293–299.

137. Larson EB, Ellsworth AJ, Oas J. Randomized clinical trials in single patients during a 2-year period. JAMA 1993;270:2708–2712.

138. Johannessen T. Controlled trials in single subjects. 1. Value in clinical medicine. Br Med J 1991;303:173–174.

139. Mahon J, Laupacis A, Donner A, Wood T. Randomized study of n of 1 trials versus standard practice. Br Med J 1996; 312:1069–1074.

140. Rodney WM, Balestra DJ, Larson EB, Ellsworth AJ. Randomized clinical trials in single patients. JAMA 1994;271:1159–1160.

141. Larson EB. N-of-1 clinical trials: a technique for improving medical therapeutics. West J Med 1990;152:52–56.

142. Guyatt GH, Jaeschke R. N-of-1 randomized trials; where do we stand? West J Med 1990;152:67–68.

143. Irwig L, Glasziou P, March L. Ethics of n-of-1 trials. Lancet 1995;345:469.

144. Zucker DR, Schmid CH, McIntosh MW, D'Agostino RB, Selker HP, Lau J. Combining single patient (N-of-1) trials to estimate population treatment effects and to evaluate individual patient responses to treatment. J Clin Epidemiol 1997;50:401–410.

145. Byar DP. The use of databases and historical controls in treatment comparisons. In: Scheurlen H, Kay R, Baum M, editors. Cancer clinical trials: a clinical appraisal. Berlin Heidelberg New York: Springer, 1988:95–98.

146. Cantor AB. Power calculation for the log rank test using historical data. Control Clin Trials 1996;17:111–116.

147. Farewell VT, D'Angio GJ. A simulated study of historical controls using real data. Biometrics 1981;37:169–176.

148. Pocock SJ. The combination of randomized and historical controls in clinical trials. J Chron Dis 1976;29:175–188.

149. Sacks H, Chalmers TC, Smith H Jr. Randomized versus historical controls in clinical trials. Am J Med 1982;72:233–240.

150. Sacristan JA, Soto J, Glaende I, Hyland TR. A review of methodologies for assessing drug effectiveness an a new proposal: randomized database studies. Clin Ther 1997;19:1510–1517.

151. Byar DP. Why databases should not replace randomized trial. Biometrics 1980;180:337–342.

152. Byar DP. Problems with using observational data bases to compare treatments. Stat Med 1991;10:663–666.

153. Haverkamp LJ, Appel V, Appel SH. Natural history of amyotrophic lateral sclerosis in a database population. Brain 1995;118:707–719.

154. Miller RG, Anderson F, Bradley W, Brooks BR, Mitsumoto H, Munsat T, Ringel SP, ALS CARE Study Group. The ALS Patient Care Database. I. Goals, structure, and early results, Neurology, in press.

155. Schmoor C, Olschewski M, Schumacher M. Randomized and nonrandomized patients in clinical trials: experiences with comprehensive cohort studies. Stat Med 1996;15:263–271.

156. Schulz KF, Chalmers I, Hayes RJ, Altman DG. Empirical evidence of bias. Dimensions of methodological quality associated with estimates of treatment effects in controlled trials. JAMA 1996;273:408–412.

157. Ottenbacher K. Impact of random assignment on study outcome: an empirical examination. Control Clin Trials 1992;13:50–61.

158. Ottenbacher KJ. Evaluating clinical change: strategies for occupational and physical therapists. Baltimore: Williams & Wilkins, 1986.

159. Norman GR, Stratford O, Regehr G. Methodological problems in the retrospective computation of responsiveness to change: the lesson of Cronbach. J Clin Epidemiol 1997;50: 869–879.

160. O'Brien PC, Geller NL. Interpreting tests for efficacy in clinical trials with multiple endpoints. Control Clin Trials 1997;18:222–227.

161. O'Brien PC, Shampo MA. Statistical consideration for performing multiple tests in a single experiment. 1. Introduction. Mayo Clin Proc 1988;63:813–815.

162. O'Brien PC, Shampo MA. Statistical consideration for performing multiple tests in a single experiment. 2. Comparisons among several therapies. Mayo Clin Proc 1988;63: 816–820.

163. O'Brien PC, Shampo MA. Statistical consideration for performing multiple tests in a single experiment. 3. Repeated measures over time. Mayo Clin Proc 1988;63:918–920.

164. O'Brien PC, Shampo MA. Statistical consideration for performing multiple tests in a single experiment. 4. Performing multiple statistical tests on the same data. Mayo Clin Proc 1988;63:1043–1045.

165. O'Brien PC, Shampo MA. Statistical consideration for performing multiple tests in a single experiment. 5. Comparing two therapies with respect to several endpoints. Mayo Clin Proc 1988;63:1140–1143.

166. O'Brien PC, Shampo MA. Statistical consideration for performing multiple tests in a single experiment. 6. Testing accumulating data repeatedly over time. Mayo Clin Proc 1988;63:1245–1250.

167. O'Brien PC, Shampo MA, Dyck PJ. Statistical analysis in clinical laboratory medicine: fundamentals and common uses. Crit Rev Clin Lab Sci 1989;27:319–340.

168. Munoz A, Hoover DR. Use of cohort studies for evaluating AIDS therapies. In: Finkelstein DM, Schoenfeld DA, editors. AIDS clinical trials. New York: Wiley-Liss, 1995:423–446.

169. Gail MH. Use of observational data for evaluating AIDS therapies. In: Finkelstein DM, Schoenfeld DA, editors. AIDS clinical trials. New York: Wiley-Liss, 1995:403–422.

170. Milliken GA, Johnson DE. Analysis of messy data: nonreplicated experiments. London: Chapman & Hall, 1989.

171. Copas JB, Li HG. Inference for nonrandom samples, J R Stat Soc Ser B 1997;59:55–77.

172. Milliken GA, Johnson DE. Analysis of messy data: designed experiments. London: Chapman & Hall, 1992.

173. Dorman JD. Treatment of amyotrophic lateral sclerosis. JAMA 1969;209:112.

174. Dorman JD, Engel WK, Fried DM. Therapeutic trial in amyotrophic lateral sclerosis. JAMA 1969;209:257–258.

175. Ioannidis JPA, Cappelleri JC, Sacks HS, Lau J. The relationship between study design, results, and reporting randomized clinical trials of HIV infection. Control Clin Trials 1997;18:431–444.

176. Fowler WM Jr, Abresch RT, Aitkens S, et al. Profiles of neuromuscular diseases: design of the protocol. Am J Phys Med Rehabil 1995;74:62–69.

177. Carter GT, Abresch RT, Fowler WM Jr, et al. Profiles of neuromuscular diseases: spinal muscular atrophy. Am J Phys Med Rehabil 1995;74:150–159.

178. Carter GT, Abresch RT, Fowler WM Jr, et al. Profiles of neuromuscular diseases: hereditary motor and sensory neuropathy, type I and II. Am J Phys Med Rehabil 1995;74:140–149.

179. Fowler WM, Abresch RT, Koch TR, Brewer ML, Bowden RK, Wanlass RL. Employment profiles in neuromuscular diseases. Am J Phys Med Rehabil 1997;76:26–37.

180. McDonald CM, Johnson ER, Abresch RT, et al. Profiles of neuromuscular diseases: limb girdle syndrome. Am J Phys Med Rehabil 1995;74:117–130.

181. McDonald ER, Hillel A, Wiedenfeld SA. Evaluation of the psychological status of ventilatory-supported patients with ALS/MND. Palliat Med 1996;10:35–41.

182. Munsat TL. Issues in clinical trial design. I. Use of natural history controls: a protagonist's view, Neurology 1996;47: S96–S97.

183. Munsat TL, Hollander D, Andres P, Finison L. Clinical trials in ALS: measurement and natural history. In: Rowland LP, editor. Amyotrophic lateral sclerosis and other motor neuron diseases. Adv Neurol 1991;56:515–519.

184. Sufit RL. Issues in clinical trial design. I. Use of natural history controls: an antagonist's view. Neurology 1996;47: S98–S99.

185. Kazdin AE. Single case research designs. Oxford: Oxford University Press, 1982:1–380.

186. Moses LE. Measuring effects without randomized trials? Options, problems, challenges. Med Care 1995;33:AS8–AS14.

187. D'Agostino RB, Kwan H. Measuring effectiveness: what to expect without a randomized control group. Med Care 1995;33:AS95–AS105.

188. Kunz R, Oxman AD. The unpredictability paradox: review of empirical comparisons of randomised and nonrandomised clinical trials. Br Med J 1998;317:1185–1190.

189. Reboussin DM, Morgan TM. Statistical considerations in the use and analysis of single subject designs. Med Sci Sports Exerc 1996;28:639–644.

190. Roberts I. An amnesty for unpublished trials. Br Med J 1998;317:763–764.

191. Aboussouan LS, Khan SU, Meeker DP, Stelmach K, Mitsumoto H. Effect of non-invasive positive-pressure ventilation on survival in amyotrophic lateral sclerosis. Ann Intern Med 1997;127:450–453.

192. Pinto AC, Evangelist T, Carvalho M, Alves MA, Sales Luis ML. Respiratory assistance with a non-invasive ventilator [BiPAP] in MND/ALS patients: survival rates in a controlled trial. J Neurol Sci 1995;129:19–26.

193. Trochim WMK. The knowledge base: an online research methods textbook, 1996:1–188. *http://trochim.human.cornell .edu/kb/contentl.htm*

194. Ahn C. An evaluation of phase I cancer clinical trial designs. Stat Med 1998;17:1537–1549.

195. Kelly F, Bratty JR. Measurement of CNS effects. In: O'Grady J, Joubert PH, editors. Handbook of phase I/II clinical drug trials. Boca Raton: CRC Press, 1997:295–303.

196. Lumpkin M, Woodcock J, Zoon K. Content and format of investigational new drug applications (INDs) for phase I studies of drugs, including well-characterized, therapeutic, biotechnology-derived products, 1995:1–17.

197. O'Grady J, Joubert PH. Handbook of phase I/II clinical drug trials. Boca Raton: CRC Press, 1997:1–562.

198. Reele SB. Decision points in human drug development. In: O'Grady J, Joubert PH, editors. Handbook of phase I/II clinical drug trials. Boca Raton: CRC Press, 1997:67–80.

199. Rosenzweig P, Brohier S, Zipfel A. The placebo effect in health volunteers: influence of experimental conditions on physiological parameters during phase I studies. Br J Clin Pharmacol 1995;39:657–664.

200. Simon RM, Freidlin B, Rubinstein LV, Arbuck S, Collins J, Christian M. Accelerated titration designs for phase. I. Clinical trials in oncology, J Nat Cancer Inst 1997;89:1138–1147.

201. Thomas M. Study design and assessment of wanted and unwanted drug effects in phase I/II trials. In: O'Grady J, Joubert PH, editors. Handbook of phase I/II clinical drug trials. Boca Raton: CRC Press, 1997:157–167.

202. Von Hoff DD, Kuhn J, Clark GM. Design and conduct of phase I trials. In: Buyse ME, Staquet MJ, Sylvester RJ, editors. Cancer clinical trials: methods and practice. Oxford: Oxford University Press, 1984:210–219.

203. Wade DT. Measurement in neurological rehabilitation. Oxford: Oxford University Press, 1992:1–388.

204. Yao Q, Wei LJ. Play the winner for phase II/III clinical trials. Stat Med 1996;15:2413–2423.

205. Zhang J, Quan H, Ng J, Stepanavage ME. Some statistical methods for multiple endpoints in clinical trials. Control Clin Trials 1997;18:204–221.

206. Gibbons RD, Hedeker D, Elkin I, Waternaux C, Kraemer HC, Greenhuse JB, et al. Some conceptual and statistical issues in analysis of longitudinal psychiatric data: application to the NIMH treatment of Depression Collaborative Research Program dataset. Arch Gen Psychiatry 1993;50:739–750.

207. World Federation of Neurology, Research Group on Neuromuscular Diseases, Subcommittee on Motor Neuron Disease. Clinical trial electronic data entry resource book, 1996:1–72.

208. World Federation of Neurology, Research Group on Neuromuscular Diseases, Subcommittee on Motor Neuron Disease. Airlie House "Workshop on Therapeutic Trials in ALS" resource book, 1994:1–272.

209. World Federation of Neurology, Research Group on Neuromuscular Diseases, Subcommittee on Motor Neuron Disease. Airlie House II "Current Issues in ALS Therapeutic Trials" resource book, 1994:1–200.

210. Edwards SJL, Lilford RJ, Hewison J. The ethics of randomised controlled trials from the perspectives of patients, the public, and healthcare professionals. Br Med J 1998;317:1209–1212.

211. Featherstone K, Donovan JL. Random allocation or allocation at random? Patients' perspectives of participation in a randomised controlled trial. Br Med J 1998;317:1177–1180.

212. Feinstein AR, Concato J. The quest for "power": contradictory hypotheses and inflated sample sizes. J Clin Epidemiol 1998;51:537–545.

213. Finison LJ, Munsat TL, George P, Hollander D, Thornell B, Greenyer J. A model for reducing sample size in amyotrophic lateral sclerosis therapeutic trials [abstract P87]. Ann Neurol 1993;34:268.

214. Hauck WW, Anderson S, Marcus SM. Should we adjust for covariates in nonlinear regression analyses of randomized trials? Control Clin Trials 1998;19:249–256.

215. Hsieh FY, Block DA, Larsen MD. A simple method of sample size calculation for linear and logistic regression. Stat Med 1998;17:1623–1634.

216. Hulley SB, Siegel D, Cummings SR. Implementing the study: pretesting, quality control and protocol revisions. In: Hulley SB, Cummings SR, editors. Designing clinical research. Baltimore: Williams & Wilkins, 1988:171–183.

217. Browner WS, Black D, Newman TB, Hulley SB. Estimating sample size and power. In: Hulley SB, Cummings SR, editors. Designing clinical research. Baltimore: Williams & Wilkins, 1988:139–150.

218. Julious SA, Campbell MJ. Sample size calculations for paired or matched ordinal data. Stat Med 1998;17:1635–1642.

219. Juniper EF, Guyatt GH, Steiner DL, King DR. Clinical impact versus factor analysis for quality of life questionnaire construction. J Clin Epidemiol 1997;50:233–238.

220. Kalbfleisch JD, Prentice RL. The statistical analysis of failure time data. New York: Wiley, 1980.

221. Kaplan EL, Meier P. Non-parametric estimation from incomplete observations. Am Stat Assoc J 1958;53:457–481.

222. Koch GG, Tangen CM, Jung JW, Amara IA. Issues for covariance analysis of dichotomous and ordered categorical data from randomized clinical trials and non-parametric strategies for addressing them. Stat Med 1998;17:1863–1892.

223. Lachin JM, Foulkes MA. Evaluation of sample size and power for analyses of survival with allowance for nonuniform patient entry, losses to follow-up, noncompliance, and stratification. Biometrics 1986;42:507–519.

224. Laird NM, Ware JH. Random-effects models for longitudinal data. Biometrics 1982;38:963–974.

225. Lakatos E. Sample sizes based on the log-rank statistic in complex clinical trials. Biometrics 1988;44:229–241.

226. Lakatos E. Sample sizes for clinical trials with time-dependent rates of losses and noncompliance. Control Clin Trials 1986;7:189–199.

227. Lakatos E, Lan KKG. A comparison of sample size methods for the long rank statistics. Stat Med 1992;11:179–191.

228. Lang TA, Secic M. How to report statistics in medicine: annotated guidelines for authors, editors and reviewers. Philadelphia: American College of Physicians, 1997.

229. Law MG, Kaldor JM. Survival analysis of randomized clinical trials adjusted for patients who switch treatments. Stat Med 1997;15:2069–2076.

230. Law MG, Kaldor JM. Survival analysis of randomized clinical trials adjusted for patients who switch treatments [reply]. Stat Med 1997;16:2620–2621.

231. Leber PD, Davis CS. Threats to the validity of clinical trials employing enrichment strategies for sample selection. Control Clin Trials 1998;19:178–187.

232. Makuch RW, Simon RM. Sample size requirements for comparing time-to-failure among k treatment groups. J Chron Dis 1982;38:801–809.

233. Oxman AD, Guyatt GH. A consumer's guide to subgroup analysis. Ann Intern Med 1988;108:263–273.

234. Peduzzi P, Concato J, Kemper E, Holford TR, Feinstein AR. A simulation study of the number of events per variable in logistic regression analysis. J Clin Epidemiol 1996;49:1373–1379.

235. Shih JH. Sample size calculation for complex clinical trials with survival endpoints. Control Clin Trials 1995;16:395–407.

236. Waubant EL, Goodkin DE. Assessing efficacy in clinical trials of treatments for multiple sclerosis: issues and controversy. CNS Drugs 1996;6:462–273.

237. Williams PL. Sample size calculations for failure time data. In: Finkelstein DM, Schoenfeld DA. AIDS clinical trials. New York: Wiley-Liss, 1995:143–154.

238. Williams WN, Seagle MB, Nackashi AJ, Marks R, Boggs SR, Kemker J, et al. A methodology report of a randomized prospective clinical trail to assess velopharyngeal function for speech following palatal surgery. Control Clin Trials 1998;19:297–312.

239. Wright JC, Weinstein MC. Gains in life expectancy from medical interventions: standardizing data on outcomes. N Engl J Med 1998;339:380–386.

240. Wright JG, Young NL. A comparison of different indices of responsiveness. J Clin Epidemiol 1997;50:239–246.

241. Wu M, Fisher M, DeMets D. Sample sizes for long term medical trials with time-dependent noncompliance and event rates. Control Clin Trials 1980;1:109–121.

242. Subcommittee on Motor Neuron Diseases of the World Federation of Neurology Research Group on Neuromuscular Diseases. Consensus guidelines for the design and implementation of clinical trials in ALS. Second Airlie House Workshop 1998. *http://www.wfnals.org/Articles/Airlie1998.htm*

243. Iwane M, Palensky J, Plante K. A user's review of commercial sample size software for design of biomedical studies using survival data. Control Clin Trials 1997;18:65–83.

244. Braitman LE. Confidence intervals assess both clinical significance and statistical significance. Ann Intern Med 1991;114:525–527.

245. Brown BW. PHASE1. Planning and conduction of phase I trials designed to find the maximum tolerated doses: a rational successor to the three-plus-three rule, version 3.0, 1996:8–9. *http://odin.mdacc.tmx.edu/anonftp.page_2.html*

246. Brown BW. STPLAN. Study planning, version 4.0, 1996:11–12. *http://odin.mdacc.tmx.edu/anonftp.page_2.html*

247. Brown BW. SURVAN. Survival analysis, version 1.0, 1996:12. *http://odin.mdacc.tmx.edu/anonftp.page_2.html*

248. Brown BW. Department of Biomathematics Statistical Software Archives. How to get it, 1997:1–2. *http://odin.mdacc .tmx.edu/anonftp.page_4.html*

249. Efron B, Tibshirani R. Bootstrap methods for standard errors, confidence intervals, and other measures of statistical accuracy. Stat Sci 1986;1:54–77.

250. Elashoff J. nQuery Advisor. Software for planning research studies, release 2.0, 1997. *http://www.statsol.ie/nquery.html*

251. Frison LJ, Pocock SJ. Linearly divergent treatment efects in clinical trials with repeated measures: efficient analysis using summary statistics. Stat Med 1997;16:2855–2872.

252. Frison LJ, Pocock SJ. Repeated measures in clinical trials: analysis using mean summary statistics and its implications for design. Stat Med 1992;11:1685–1704.

253. Gardner MJ, Altman DG. Statistics with confidence: confidence intervals and statistical guidelines. London, 1989.

254. Gardner MJ, Machin D, Campbell MJ. Use of check lists in assessing the statistical content of medical studies. Br Med J 1986;292:810–812.

255. Hughes MD, Pocock SJ. Interim monitoring of clincal trials. In: Finkelstein DM, Schoenfeld DA, editors. AIDS clinical trials. New York: Wiley-Liss, 1995:177–198.

256. Luo XL, Turnbull BW, Clark LC. Likelihood ratio tests for a changepoint with survival data. Biometrika 1997;84:555–565.

257. Moher D, Dulberg CS, Wells GA. Statistical power, sample size, and their reporting in randomized controlled trials. Statistics and Peer Review, 13 July 1994. International Congress on Biomedical Peer Review and Global Communications. *http://www.arms-assn.org/public/ppeer/7_13_94/pv3037x .htm*

258. NCSS Statistical Software. PASS 6.0. Power analysis and sample size, 1997. *http://www.ncss.com/html/paas/html*

259. Neely E. EXPSURV. Exploratory survival, version 1.0, 1995:2. *http://odin.mdacc.tmx.edu/anonftp.page_2.html*

260. Niklaon IA, Reimitz PE, Sennef C. Factors that influence the outcome of placebo-controlled antidepressant clinical trials. Psychopharmacol Bull 1997;33:41–51.

261. Pocock SJ. Clinical trials with multiple outcomes: a statistical perspective on their design, analysis, and interpretation. Control Clin Trials 1997;18:530–545.

262. Roe DJ, Korn EL. Time-period effects in longitudinal studies measuring average rates of change. Stat Med 1993;12:893–900.

263. Thall PF. MULTC. Multiple outcomes in clinical trials, version 1.2, 1996:7. *http://odin.mdacc.tmx.edu/anonftp.page_2.html*

264. Thall PF, Simon R, Estey EH. Bayesian sequential monitoring designs for single-arm clinical trials with multiple outcomes. Stat Med 1995;14:357–379.

265. Turnbull BW, Jiang WX, Clark LC. Regression models for recurrent event data: parametric random effects models with measurement error. Stat Med 1997;16:853–864.

266. Pezzullo JC. Web pages that perform statistical calculations, 1998:1–9. *http://members.aol.com/johnp71/javastat.html*

267. Pezzullo JC. Interactive statistical pages, part 2, 1998:1–10. *http://members.aol.com/johnp71/javasta2.html*

268. Hung HMJ. Two-stage tests for studying monotherapy and combination therapy in two-by-two factorial trials. Stat Med 1993;12:645–660.

269. Paulus HE. Clinical trial design for evaluating combination therapies. Br J Rheumatol 1995;34:92–95.

270. Paulus HE. History of combination therapy of rheumatoid arthritis. J Rhematol 1996;23:38–42.

271. Schoenfeld DA. Issues in the testing of drug combinations. In: Finkelstein DM, Schoenfeld DA, editors. AIDS clinical trials. New York: Wiley-Liss, 1995:257–266.

272. Sim I, Rennels G. Standardized reporting of clinical trials into electronic trial banks: in support of computer-assisted evidence-based medicine SMI-96-0630. *http://smi-web .stanford.edu/pubs/SMI_Abstracts/SMI-96-0630.html*

273. Smith GD, Egger M. Incommunicable knowledge? Interpreting and applying the results of clinical trials and meta-analyses. J Clin Epidemiol 1998;51:289–295.

274. Schulz KF. The quest for unbiased research: randomized clinical trials and the CONSORT reporting guidelines. Ann Neurol 1997;41:569–573.

35. Motor Neurone Disease: Experience with Large Multicentre Trials

T.J. Steiner

Introduction

All multicentre trials are challenging, whatever the disease under study. Motor neurone disease (MND; USA: amyotrophic lateral sclerosis, ALS) brings to the challenge a particular set of difficulties. Here is a condition that exists in different forms and presents extremely variably. It has its onset in a wide age range with, accordingly, a range of concomitant illnesses, progresses inexorably but somewhat unpredictably and again very variably, and offers no *obvious* manner of measurement. In pathophysiological terms, reversal of the condition is unattainable, arrest is the Holy Grail and slowed rate of progression the most realistic outcome to hope for. In other words, patients at the conclusion of a trial will be *worse off* than at entry.

Compared with other major neurological degenerations such as cerebrovascular disease, MND is uncommon. Whereas large multinational collaborative stroke trials are now almost commonplace, experience of this sort in MND is still limited. Yet, because MND is uncommon, adequate trials require costly multinational collaborations whilst at the same time commercial interest is relatively lacking, favouring more common illnesses. Without commercial support it is extraordinarily difficult not only to set up and do large trials but also to apply to them the sort of quality control rightly demanded by drug regulatory authorities.

Nonetheless, and at what may have been high commercial risk, there have been such trials. One of these was academically controlled, an initiative arising from patient-led demand rather than commercial interest although, eventually, it was not without the latter. These trials have resulted in, if no more, the gathering of experience.

Some Foreseeable Problems

There are important general issues of science, ethics and judgements of cost/benefit, some of which predictably produce particular problems in MND trials.

Some Problems of Science

Scientific requirements in MND trials are entirely the usual ones: adequate experimental design combined with valid assessments in appropriately selected patients. In MND, adequate design and valid assessment obtain special significance because the nature of the illness makes both difficult to achieve. Patients, too, bring special problems in selection, although they are not generally in short supply nor unwilling to participate.

There is an important distinction in assessment of a treatment between *efficacy* and *safety* on the one hand – absolute qualities – and *utility*, a context-dependent quality deriving in part from the former. Treatments that are inefficacious or unsafe are not expected to have utility. Since trials that measure efficacy and safety require fewer patients (albeit more highly selected), logically, and perhaps ethically, these are the first requirement. There is a widely expressed belief that clinical trials invariably should replicate clinical practice, as that is the context in which treatments will be used; in this argument, assessments in other contexts are not only unhelpful but misleading. This is the pragmatic approach defined by Schwartz and Lellouch [1], and it lies behind intention-to-treat protocols in which compliance failures, inconsistencies and extraneous determinants of outcome are accepted as reflecting the "real world" of routine management of the disease.

Patients who do not, for any reason, take the treatment are assessed as though they have done – a problem (if not a nonsense) if drop-out rates are high.

Pragmatism may be appropriate if a new treatment, having efficacy, requires assessment in comparison with others that are already in use and determining a standard clinical practice which is unlikely to be fundamentally affected by the arrival of another treatment option. What meaning does this have when, as in MND, there is no current or universally accepted treatment? The one thing that is certain in that situation is that, when a treatment is found, "routine" management will change. This, in my opinion, raises significant questions about the validity of the pragmatic approach.

Pragmatic trials may be methodologically tolerant but they need no less adequate controls. Control is foreseeably difficult in MND: the problems brought by the variabilities of the disease are compounded by ethical pitfalls. Not least amongst these are issues arising from the use of placebo (see below). In other life-threatening conditions, a standard treatment as active comparator might ethically be greatly preferred to placebo control, and this would be true of MND if a generally accepted standard existed. Many might agree that the scientific methodology of MND trials has been considerably complicated by the emergence of an active treatment because the actual benefits it offers are uncertain and come at a cost in terms of adverse events [2,3].

In my view, trials that begin tomorrow must measure efficacy and safety in an explanatory (per-protocol) trial [1]. Utility comes later when efficacy is proven and its limits understood. The implications of per-protocol design and analysis fall mainly on admissibility of patients, with more rigid entry criteria defining what is being treated, on compliance control and assurance to define the treatment being assessed, and on rigorous follow-up to establish exactly its effect on the disease and its consequences rather than on health more generally. Several of these issues are discussed below.

Whereas clinical trials are usually discussed in the context of drug treatments, potential treatments for MND include remedial (physical) therapy. This is a discipline in which objective research is anyway problematic because of the nature of the intervention, depending as it does upon patient–therapist interaction. The double-blind conditions of drug trials cannot be reproduced. Nor can physical therapy be dispensed in fixed doses within a standard regimen. The difficulties special to trials of physiotherapy have been described previously in some detail [4].

Some Problems Related to Ethics

Ethical pitfalls are everywhere in the study of terminally ill patients, many of whom in desperation will try, even demand, any treatment available. Consent is too easily obtained. To the physician investigator, freed from many constraints normally imposed by what patients will not allow to be done to them, high risk for limited promise of gain is acceptable as a way forward. The same factor creates tensions over allocation of patients to untreated or placebo-treated comparative groups, even though it is in the nature of clinical trials that the treatment may be found to be ineffective or even harmful. For the patient, all hope is invested in the new treatment and why, in any circumstances, would he accept a placebo [5]?

Robinson's arguments [5] on this and related issues are worth reading, although few answers are found to the problems he presents. One issue he addressed is that of too small trials. Cure of MND is not a realistic goal, nor total arrest of progression a likely outcome of any treatment. Why are trials done with statistical power to show only such an outcome [6]? On the other hand, trials, especially placebo-controlled ones, ought not to be too large: one patient more than is needed on the less beneficial treatment serves no ethical purpose.

If several hundred patients must be recruited, several tens of centres, necessarily from several countries, need to participate over many months. Availability of resources is in question, in terms of interested investigators and adequately equipped centres (actual numbers of patients are a less limiting factor than the ability to locate them). The ethical implication is that a single major trial substantially ties up most of the resources in an area as large as Western Europe or North America. If this is so, the trial that is done must be the one that most needs doing, and "need" is the need of patients. It is not clear that any force exists to bring this about, and more likely that commercial interests will determine the issue [7]. Amongst the considerable harms that this may directly lead to is a financially motivated abandonment of a half-completed trial, wasting the commitment of patients to it, in order to start another.

Problems of Cost/Benefit

The need to put a price on benefit is a consequence of limited resources in health care provision. For clinical trialists one ethical issue is that resources may not be available for the treatment to continue even if found successful. Physical therapy, for example, is very expensive, and so are some drugs, especially those emerging from biotechnology programmes. Brooke and Steiner [4] referred to "the almost unanswerable question of what cost society should bear to postpone death of an individual, or to improve quality of life until a foreseeable death, assuming either of those benefits is attainable. What cost should society bear for merely a reasonable prospect of such benefits?" The equations are not easy: what weight is to be given to the unfortunate but recognisable truth that extending the life of an MND patient generally increases costs? If cost of a treatment per patient is high, but the disease is rare, does that increase the obligation on society (lower cost), or make it lower priority (benefit to fewer)?

Society, not trialists, makes these decisions. But, if these questions are raised because of a trial outcome [2], it is the trialists' ethical responsibility to generate the knowledge society needs to give informed answers. Furthermore, the extent to which outcomes in *groups* participating in clinical trials can be extrapolated to *individuals* who did not – but whose needs are as great – and, in particular, to individuals who would not have met the entry criteria for the trial in question is often indeterminable. Where treatment carries a cost (which might be financial, or a cost in adverse reactions), it is insufficient if the objectives of trials are limited to learning whether patients *as a group* can expect to gain from the treatment: they must ask also which patients have the greatest expectation, and how much of the therapy (e.g., for how long a period) gives the best cost/benefit ratio. Single clinical trials are not a good instrument for answering all such questions, and may need to be very large indeed to do so: multiple secondary and subgroup analyses on ever-declining numbers increase the risk of both type I and type II statistical errors. For this reason, drug development programmes would normally consist of several pivotal trials, each with a different principal objective. This has not so far been seen in MND.

Some Sources of Experience

The SPECIALS Trial of Branched-Chain Amino Acids (BCAA)

This study [8] came about almost wholly as a result of patient pressure, following publication in *The Lancet* of a very small study claiming benefit from BCAA [9]. These amino acids are purchasable from health-food shops in many countries but, in the

doses suggested, at significant annual cost. Efficacy had not been proven, in the long term was unknown, and safety was yet to be established. Patients, on the other hand, were seeking advice on whether, and how, to use them.

There had been no earlier multinational trial conducted to Good Clinical Practice (GCP) standards in MND, and the methodology had to be worked out. The study was conducted by the academic collaboration, the Scientific Pan-European Collaboration in Amyotrophic Lateral Sclerosis (SPECIALS). Financial sponsorship to cover costs only was raised from Ajinomoto Inc., Tokyo. The trial was a double-blind, placebo-controlled, parallel groups comparison. Recruitment began in November 1990 in 23 centres in six countries and ended in June 1993. The diagnostic criteria (as an issue for later discussion) are set out in Table 35.1, and other recruitment criteria in Table 35.2.

Patients were stratified according to whether the disease was bulbar or non-bulbar, and randomly allocated to BCAA (L-leucine, L-isoleucine and L-valine in the proportions 3:2:1.6 to a total of 6.6 g per dose) or matching placebo, taken orally four times daily. Treatment and follow-up were for 1 year. Assessments were made at entry and every 3 months for 1 year of muscle strength (using MRC score) in 22 groups, Norris score, 6.5 m timed walk and Barthel score (in some centres only). Forced vital capacity (FVC) measurements were made every 6 months. Conduct and quality assurance were to European (CPMP) standards of GCP.

In all, 450 patients were recruited from Denmark ($n = 3$), France ($n = 49$), Portugal ($n = 27$), Spain ($n = 88$), Turkey ($n = 52$) and the United Kingdom ($n = 231$). Of these, 18 (4.0%) were protocol violations. The Danish patients were withdrawn (see below) before completion, so the potentially evaluable population was $n = 429$ (male 287, female 142; bul-bar onset 232, non-bulbar 197; mean age 57.4 years, range 25–78 years; mean duration of illness 13.3 months, range 3–24 months; mean FVC as % of predicted 79.3, range 50–152; mean 6.5 m walk-time at entry 12.1 s, range 3–180 s).

Of the 429 patients, deaths occurred in 112 (26.1%). A further 136 (31.7%) provided incomplete datasets due to withdrawal or other failure to complete follow-up, and 181 patients (42.2%) had all data available for material events. In the principal per-protocol analysis excluding French patients (for reasons set out below), 72.0% survived to trial end in each treatment group. Factors adversely affecting survival (Cox regression analysis) were as follows and did not include either treatment: older age ($p < 0.001$), lower FVC ($p < 0.0001$), lower score for

Table 35.1.   Diagnostic criteria employed by the SPECIALS collaboration in the branched-chain amino acids trial

---

1. *Clinical diagnosis of primary ALS*
   (The diagnosis of primary ALS requires involvement of upper *and* lower motor neurones and involvement of more than one limb or the tongue, and is to be confirmed by clinical examination by a fully trained neurologist)
   This definition excludes:
   (a) progressive muscular atrophy (PMA) with *only* lower motor neurone signs, but includes all cases with unequivocal upper motor neurone involvement even if this is minimal and lower motor neurone signs strongly predominate
   (b) pure bulbar palsy (PBP) with *only* bulbar signs, but includes predominantly bulbar cases with even minimal limb involvement *provided that* both upper and lower motor neurone signs (bulbar or spinal) can be demonstrated
   (This implies that a patient with only lower motor neurone involvement when first seen may not be entered at that time, but could later become eligible if other signs appear within the first 24 months
   Similarly, a patient with only bulbar involvement when first seen may not be entered at that time, but could later become eligible if spinal signs appear within the first 24 months)
2. *Second opinion*
   The confirmatory second opinion may be given by another fully trained neurologist, or by a senior trainee in a post recognised for neurological training
3. *EMG support*
   An EMG requires the following features to support a clinical diagnosis of ALS:
   The EMG must in the opinion of the investigator
   (a) support the diagnosis *and*
   (b) show evidence of chronic partial denervation in more than one site *and* exclude peripheral neuropathy

---

EMG, electromyogram.

swallowing on the Norris scale ($p < 0.0001$), bulbar involvement at entry ($p = 0.0004$) (whereas bulbar involvement at onset or during the first 3 months of the course of the illness were not: $p = 0.3$), weaker upper limbs ($p = 0.0008$), slower 6.5 m walk-time ($p = 0.002$), lower Norris score for self-feeding ($p = 0.03$), lower Norris score for walking, and weaker lower limbs ($p = 0.03$), and male sex ($p = 0.07$). Disease duration had no clear effect ($p = 0.2$).

All patients entered to this trial (except for the protocol violators) were independent in swallowing, self-feeding and walking, as indices of bulbar, upper limb and lower limb function respectively. Rates of loss of independence by 12 months (the principal efficacy end-point) are shown in Table 35.3 for bulbar and non-bulbar groups, and were unaltered by treatment.

What Has Been Learnt from This Trial?

The trial was successful in that it led to a definitive conclusion that BCAA are not effective generally in the treatment of MND, having no effect discernible from that of placebo on survival alive and independent. As a treatment, BCAA have since effectively disappeared, which may have been a service to patients in view of what they might have spent on them, and they were not pleasant to consume. But the trial could not draw conclusions about subgroups who might respond differently. There were other lessons concerning international collaborations, and rates of reaching various important milestones were defined.

Some Unforeseeable Problems

The protocol ran in parallel and was harmonised with a similar trial conducted in Italy, which began about a year earlier using BCAA from a different source and with a slightly differing recipe. This trial was halted on the advice of a local data monitoring committee who were not a part of the SPECIALS collaboration. Their finding was that, in Italy, deaths were running at a higher rate in the active treatment arm. Although this was not statistically significant, a conclusion was drawn that the trial, in Italy, could not show benefit and should be terminated on safety grounds. The Italians investigators sought to publish their study and, after delaying, did so [10]. On receipt of the news of the trial-stop in Italy, the Danish investigators unilaterally halted the trial in Denmark and withdrew their three patients. The SPECIALS coordinators were forced to suspend recruitment but, after urgent discussions with the investigators, did not stop the trial in other centres.

The SPECIALS own data monitoring committee was convened, including a representative of the Italian committee. The potential harms here were, on the one hand, of continuing a relatively or actually harmful treatment in one group of patients and, on the other, of throwing away the trial and the resources it had already consumed, including patient commitment, and then finding the original important question unanswered [11]. Evidence from all published and other BCAA trials was adduced and cumulated with the data so far gathered from the SPECIALS trial itself, and all of it analysed with code-

Table 35.2. Entry criteria employed by the SPECIALS collaboration in the branched-chain amino acids trial

Inclusion criteria
(a) Clinical diagnosis of primary ALS with confirmatory second opinion and EMG support (see Table 35.1)
(b) Less than 2 years from onset
(c) History of progression over at least 3 months
(d) Forced vital capacity > 50% predicted
(e) Independence, defined as
   feeding by mouth (i.e., not nasogastic tube or gastrostomy *and* swallowing score of 3 or 2 on the Norris scale [32])

   and

   self-feeding (score of 3 or 2 on the Norris scale [32])

   and

   ambulatory (walking 6.5 m unassisted, with aids if needed [assistance may be given to stand up])
(f) Other medication optimised (especially anti-spasticity drugs)
(g) Aged 25–80 years
(h) Informed consent given

Exclusion criteria
Familial ALS
Known antecedent polio infection
CSF protein > 100 mg/dl (if known)
Other neurological degenerative illness (including dementia)
Other severe physical disability
Other illness:
   metabolic disorders (e.g., dysthyroid state) not controlled by treatment
   diabetes mellitus
   hepatic or renal disease with impaired function
   autoimmune disease
   known malignancy (affecting general health or life expectancy)
   disabling cardiac disease (angina or heart failure)
Need for neuroleptics or steroid medication
Therapeutic administration of BCAA in the past

EMG, electromyogram.

Table 35.3. Loss of independence rates at 12 months (% of *n* at entry) (*n* = 429, including French patients)

	Non-bulbar	Bulbar	*p* (bulbar vs non-bulbar)
Swallowing	54.8	72.0	0.0003
Feeding	68.5	72.8	0.27
Walking	73.1	75.0	0.74
All	77.2	85.8	0.03

The recruitment target had been 600 including the Italian cases. In the event, with the Italian and Danish cases excluded from the principal analysis, there were 447 but 18 were protocol violators at entry. However, in France the trial had been punctuated by various problems, and several centres had meanwhile begun recruiting to the newly started and fully commercially sponsored riluzole trial [14]. Of their 49 cases entered, only eleven were evaluable from a total of nine centres, and these were excluded as non-viable. (There were a variety of reasons but, in 38 cases, the protocol was violated; of the many patients withdrawn, some were subsequently recruited to the riluzole trial, which would have caused an interesting difficulty for intention-to-treat analysis.) The final per-protocol analysis was conducted in 380 patients, or 84.4% of those recruited.

Dose-Ranging Study of Riluzole in ALS

This study [14] was commercially supported by Rhône-Poulenc Rorer and followed a smaller trial of a fixed dose (100 mg) of riluzole [15] which "seemed to retard disease progression". Riluzole is believed to be neuroprotective, perhaps through presynaptic inhibition of glutamate release, but, in the earlier trial, an effect on survival greater in patients with bulbar onset and apparent at 12 months diminished during subsequent treatment.

The second study was a double-blind, placebo-controlled, parallel groups comparison of riluzole in three doses: 50 mg, 100 mg or 200 mg daily. Recruitment began in December 1992, midway through the SPECIALS trial, which suffered in France as a consequence. Patients with clinically probable or definite MND [16] were eligible within 5 years of onset, aged 18–75 years and with vital capacity >60% of predicted. Stratification was according to site of *onset*: bulbar or limbs (the SPECIALS trial had found this not prognostic, whereas both this study ($p = 0.03$) and SPECIALS ($p = 0.0004$) found bulbar involvement at entry predictive of poor outcome). Conduct and quality assurance were to European (CPMP)

breaks but in secrecy from the investigators, monitors and coordinators. In the light of this analysis, it was agreed that there was no serious safety issue and the study should proceed. Recruitment recommenced after a break of several weeks.

This was the best demonstration I have encountered of the need in every large multicentre trial for an independent *and authoritative* monitoring committee (the SPECIALS committee included recognised specialists in MND and in multinational trials, a clinical pharmacologist, a statistician and a lawyer). Over this I disagree with Barnett and Sackett [12]. This trial was seriously endangered. The threat came partly from within the collaboration responsible for the trial; for other trials it could arise from the release of results of quite independent studies [13].

standards of GCP. The principal efficacy measure was survival without tracheostomy, but patients continued treatment even after tracheostomy. Secondary measures were of strength assessed in seated patients by MRC scores summed in 22 muscle groups, limb and bulbar function separately assessed on the respective (modified) Norris scales, and vital capacity. An independent advisory board monitored accumulating data for safety or "overwhelming evidence of efficacy" on interim analysis. Final analysis was by intention-to-treat with follow-up at least to establish survival in those otherwise defaulting.

In 12 months, 959 patients were enrolled, 295 with bulbar onset and 664 with limb onset. A year later, with a median follow-up of 18 months, 55% were alive without tracheostomy and <1% had been lost to follow-up. Cox modelling was used to assess the power of a variety of prognostic factors and, on the basis of a general formula produced by this method, a prognostic score was derived for each patient and applied as an adjustment. Only after this process was it deduced that active treatment had significantly reduced the risk of tracheostomy or death within 12 and 18 months in a dose-related manner (adjusted risks: 0.76 on 50 mg, $p = 0.04$; 0.65 on 100 mg, $p = 0.002$; 0.61 on 200 mg, $p = 0.0004$). Per-protocol analysis of this end-point produced similar findings. Site of disease onset did not influence treatment effect, contrary to the findings of the earlier trial. None of the secondary measures detected a treatment effect.

Effect on quality of life, if any and whether positive or negative, could not be determined. Adverse experiences were reported by 90% of patients and 21% had treatment withdrawn, even amongst those on placebo. Asthenia and nausea were particularly more frequent amongst active treatment groups, the former being a principal reason for withdrawal. Some 6–8% of patients had evidence of dose-related liver toxicity with transaminase levels above 3× normal, reversing months after treatment withdrawal.

What Has Been Learnt from This Trial?

The meaning of these results to a patient considering whether or not to take riluzole might be expressed as a one-third reduction of risk of tracheostomy or death in 18 months, which could translate into survival extended by a few months, without apparent functional benefit and at the risk of some adverse reactions including hepatotoxicity. It is not known whether all patients might benefit to a similar extent, or whether some might be worse off [2].

Study of Recombinant Human Insulin-Like Growth Factor-I (IGF-I) on ALS Progression

This North American study [17] was supported by Cephalon. Outpatients over 20 years of age diagnosed by the El Escorial criteria [16], with mild or moderate disease only, were entered within 36 months of symptom onset. Measurable progression of the disease was required over a 2–3 month pre-randomisation period, with FVC remaining above 50% of predicted. Patients with progressive bulbar palsy were excluded. Thus, there was an intention to include patients who would significantly deteriorate but not die during a relatively short 9 month follow-up. There was no stratification. The study was multi-centre and 266 patients were randomised between January 1993 and April 1995 to three parallel groups. Their mean age was 57 years, mean time from onset was 16 months and from diagnosis 7 months. Low (0.05 mg/kg per day) or high (0.1 mg/kg per day) doses of IGF-I or placebo were injected subcutaneously twice daily. Conduct and quality control were presumably according to FDA GCP.

Assessments monthly used the Appel ALS (AALS) rating scale [18] which sums, to give a single number, subjectively and objectively quantified estimates of bulbar function, respiratory function, muscle strength and function in upper and lower limbs (normal = 30, maximum = 164; at 135, patients are likely to be bedridden and requiring total care). End-points were survival to 9 months, an earlier AALS score ≥ 115 (equivalent to severe physical disability) or an FVC < 39% of predicted. The primary outcome measure was the slope, on treatment, of the AALS score. The Sickness Impact Profile (SIP) [19] was also used as a health-related quality of life measure.

Only 53% of patients completed the 9 month follow-up, and 11% failed to achieve a minimum of three post-randomisation measurements in order to plot a slope. Protocol-defined early end-points were reached by 25% and deaths occurred in 10%. A dose-related reduction in slope of deterioration in AALS score was noted in the groups on IGF-I, and the difference between high-dose and placebo was that deterioration was 26% slower ($p = 0.01$) on the former. In terms of the actual changes in scores from baseline, statistically significant differences between placebo and high dose were recorded for bulbar function, muscle strength and upper limb function. Survival analysis of time to either AALS score ≥ 115 or FVC < 39% as indices of treatment failure showed a relative risk of encountering one or other within the follow-up period of 0.56 for the high-dose group compared with the placebo group ($p = 0.04$). There was no difference between low-dose and placebo groups. The SIP scores, too, showed statistically significant differences between high-dose and placebo groups, overall ($p = 0.01$) and in the psychosocial dimension ($p = 0.02$). What this means, if anything, in terms of quality of life for these patients is uncertain.

The results of this study were distingushed by the authors from those of the riluzole study in that they showed evidence of retarded disease symptom progression. This IGF-I study was not designed to show an effect on mortality, so it is not known if one exists. Significantly more frequent adverse events on IGF-I were injection site inflammation, hair changes, knee pain or joint swelling, and face oedema.

What Has Been Learnt from This Trial?

The meaning of these results to a patient considering whether or not to take IGF-I is that *signs* and, less clearly, *symptoms* of the disease might show slower progression on IGF-I. The risk of reaching either a state of severe physical disability (by one partly subjective criterion) or substantial respiratory disability is reduced by 44% over 9 months. Cost in terms of adverse reactions appears low and quality of life measures suggest some benefit of treatment, but how much is unclear. Whether benefits are maintained is crucial. Although the trial design built in extended observation of willing patients for a further 9 months after they completed the trial, treatment with IGF-I was open and follow-up uncontrolled and incomplete.

Further, a European trial with IGF-I failed to demonstrate beneficial effects and regulatory approval for the drug is not any longer pursued [47].

Some Observations

Problems of Diagnosis, Variability and Prognosis

Mitsumoto et al. [20] noted that diagnosis of MND was made with "surprising uniformity by physicians," whilst Li et al. [21] found striking differences in diagnostic behaviour between three countries. How to make the diagnosis is not the subject of this chapter but diagnostic uncertainty and variability are. Criteria are often more strict in clinical trials than in conventional therapy to reduce uncertainty [22]. One consequence is that results apply even less well to the larger group more "loosely" diagnosed. Another may be acceptance into a trial only of patients with unequivocal diagnoses, preferentially selecting those with advanced disease [22]. Apart

from being unrepresentative, intuitively it seems that these are the least likely to gain from treatment. The El Escorial criteria for diagnosis [16,23] at least standardise the diagnostic process. The regulated compromise between specificity and sensitivity has been widely accepted. The SPECIALS approach to diagnosis (Table 35.1) is perhaps better for including all patients who, in the ordinary way, would be treated for MND. Whilst setting basic diagnostic rules, this approach accepts as MND whatever two independent neurologists agree in an individual case is MND.

Wide disparities in presentation coupled with equally large variations in the clinical course determined by differing rates and patterns of disease progression create substantial difficulties for controlled studies of effects of intervention. Rates of progression in certain pathological terms may be linear: Munsat et al. [24] found deterioration rates indicative of motor neurone loss to be remarkably linear and Andres et al. [25], using their Tufts quantitative neuromuscular examination (TQNE), found an average deterioration of 4.5% per month. Nevertheless, at critical times, small decrements in muscle power cause major *functional* declines. In the three trials described, diagnostic criteria were supplemented by additional requirements to limit variability and thereby make prognosis more nearly uniform. Additionally or alternatively, stratification can to some extent minimise the confounding effects of known prognostic factors. The SPECIALS trial confirmed that bulbar involvement at the time of entry carries a poor prognosis, but so does lower FVC. In fact, most markers of disease advancement were associated with a poor prognosis, whereas disease duration was not (see below).

Problems of Recruitment

The SPECIALS trial also showed, which had not been known, that patients were conditionally willing to enter long-term placebo-controlled trials, and dropout rates were acceptable. Nonetheless, with some 30% not completing the prescribed treatment course for a variety of reasons, they would give intention-to-treat analysis a hard time. In the trial of IGF-I, only 53% completed the follow-up needed for the principal efficacy analysis. The riluzole trial, with loss to follow-up in <1%, shows a practical benefit of choosing death as the principal end-point in an intention-to-treat analysis.

The references in Table 35.1 to 24 months relate to the inclusion criteria in the SPECIALS trial (Table 35.2). This upper limit on time since disease onset was the *single factor most responsible for exclusion of potential recruits to the trial*. Restrictive entry criteria underlie Lasagna's law of clinical trials [26], which states that as soon as a clinical trial begins the supply of patients becomes one-tenth of what it was thought to be beforehand. Glasberg [27] described a typical MND trial exemplifying Lasagna's law perfectly. Because Lasagna is almost invariably right, there should be no exclusion criterion that is not based on sound argument.

Does duration of illness prior to entry to a treatment trial matter? The answer is affirmative if there is an effect upon prognosis, but the SPECIALS trial found none. Of course, entered patients had durations in a restricted range of 3 to 24 months (Table 35.2). The Committee on Health Care Issues of the American Neurological Association [28] noted a possible therapeutic window that might be missed: "beneficial effects may not be seen . . . if the patient was examined too soon or too late". As Robinson observed [5], "there are grounds for believing that not all points in a trajectory of neurological deterioration are equally amenable to therapeutic attention". Again the implications are that subgroup selection within the overall diagnosis of MND on the one hand is a prerequisite for seeing a treatment effect at all and on the other presents a genuine danger in extrapolating from trial populations to others, different in perhaps a fundamental way, coming for routine management.

If time from onset is very short, a greater degree of diagnostic uncertainty is likely: a recognisable pattern of progression over time is an important contributor to diagnostic probability, and was built into the entry criteria for the SPECIALS trial and, for a different reason, the IGF-I trial. There is a problem also with very long times from onset, which led to the limitation in the SPECIALS trial. A patient who has had the illness already for 5 years demonstrates quite a slow progression and, if still independent, does not fit the ideal of a "typical" patient. More importantly, if the slope of deterioration is maintained, the follow-up period will need to be long indeed to observe a change at all, let alone an effect of treatment on it.

Respiratory Function

The importance of poor respiratory function to trial recruitment lies in the adverse prognosis attaching to it. Notwithstanding that its measurement can be technically difficult, particularly in those in whom it is impaired, respiratory function is commonly measured as forced vital capacity (FVC) and values below 60% of predicted are rarely compatible with long survival. Stratification for low FVC, perhaps above and below 60%, is in most cases strongly advisable, but should patients with low FVC be excluded? Robinson [5] referred to the need to ensure that severely affected patients are expected to survive to the end of the trial, perhaps on the basis of pulmonary function at entry. It is clear what he meant, but he further observed that atypical cases of MND might be preferentially selected if follow-up is intended to be long term relative to the ordinary course of MND. All depends on the end-point and anticipated treatment effect. The SPECIALS and IGF-I trials excluded patients with FVC < 50% and the riluzole trial <60% of predicted. The higher limit in the riluzole trial, principally measuring survival without tracheostomy, is surprising. If a treatment may postpone death, it needs to be tested in those in whom death is expected but might be postponed, if not averted. Otherwise the usual view – though not necessarily correct – is that patients "predestined" to die are beyond help. Inclusion of numbers of patients in whom a treatment effect cannot be demonstrated merely reduces statistical power, and increases the numbers of other patients who must enter the analysis.

Primary Exclusions, and Numbers

The experience of SPECIALS was that the 2 year limit on disease duration was responsible for many exclusions of patients otherwise eligible. In retrospect it was a mistake. Lasagna's law [26] warns against *unnecessary* exclusions, which can imperil recruitment even when patients queue up to be entered. Requirements for group size are usually held to be statistically determined, and depend on what is expected of the treatment upon what outcome measure in the face of what natural history. Numbers needed to show a statistically significant treatment effect might be low where a treatment postpones death in a group selected for high expectation of death. More modest expectations call for higher numbers.

These factors lie behind power calculations, but they are not the only factors to be considered. The wider the net is cast amongst variable patients the larger the numbers necessary to ensure group matching. In other words, a smaller sample less adequately represents the population from which it is drawn. In acute stroke, for an altogether different reason, trials of tens of thousands of patients are contemplated: stroke clinicians, desensitised to trials, are impressed only by those with grossly large numbers, and only such trials change practice. MND patients who, untreated, get worse are more in control, and maintain the drive to introduce new treatments (too) speedily. Regulators obey, with expedited approval in what has been an "orphan" illness. But it is reasonable to ask whether the numbers included in the riluzole trials were really sufficient to inform prescribers and patients about *who* should have the drug and for *how long*.

Problems of Measurement

MND affects the integrity of nerve cells (*impairment*), but manifests principally as reducing muscle strength (*disability*) and the patient complains of loss of a range of functional abilities important to him or her (*handicap*). What, then, to measure and how to measure? End-point frequencies and times to failure were established for future trials in the SPECIALS trial. However, Borasio [29] points out that measures of disability and handicap are surrogates for motoneuronal degeneration which cannot itself be quantified directly. Maybe so, but patients would probably ask trialists to measure outcome in terms that mattered to them rather than to the pathologist in the final examination. The principal lesson in the riluzole trial may be that, where end-points of greatest concern to patients are not the object of principal analysis, the trial can fail to inform.

Mortality

Death is an outcome unquestionably meaningful to the patient. It is measurable in absolute terms or in terms of time until it happens, but is a less unequivocal outcome than might be expected [29]. Although the great majority of MND sufferers die of the disease, death can be "artificially" postponed by artificial ventilation. Need for ventilation is sometimes, for the purpose of outcome measurement, equated with death as the final ending of independent life, but the patient presumably would not be of this view or would decline to be ventilated (some, of course, do [30]). The problems are that artificial ventilation is not everywhere available, not always offered where it is or accepted when it is. In other words, as an outcome it is only partially illness-determined.

Apart from these problems, mortality is insensitive unless the impact of treatment is great and the stage of disease such that, without the treatment, a substantial proportion of entered patients will die shortly. Otherwise, follow-up must be very prolonged. Arguably, since treatment as part of normal care is likely to continue until death is at least near, follow-up should anyway be prolonged. Death is always an end-point in MND trials, but how are the needs of patients in a miserable existence met by a treatment that does no more than delay death?

Independence, and Its Loss

By no means all patients with MND may ever be described thus, but many are destined to reach that stage. A more appropriate end-point might be loss of independence (Table 35.2). However this is defined, it is a consequence of MND in every case and one, when it occurs, that is of great significance for the sufferer. Its delay, unlikely postponing death, should always be desirable and without adverse financial consequence in the way that delaying death has. If loss of independence is the end-point of interest, all patients entered must be independent. It is true that benefits of a treatment effective in *this* subgroup of patients may not accrue as well to those in routine management who are already dependent, but the objective once such a treatment is available will be to use it early. Further discussion is below.

Muscle Strength

Isometric contractions produce muscle cramps in many MND patients and isokinetic measures are unhelpful in severe weakness. The Medical Research Council [31] clinical grading system for muscle strength, scoring 0–5, was not developed for such purposes as this and is limited by insensitivity and subjectivity. Greatly unequal intervals between grades [25] mean that summation, often practised, is misleading. In my experience MRC scoring nonetheless works well *if* it is applied expertly (not by the most junior assistant) and with care over standardising the patient's position in the assessment.

The same requirements apply to dynamometry before it will yield any more accurate or reproducible results. Measures of muscle strength are altered where there is significant or, worse, variable spasticity. Muscle testing in MND patients is further hampered by muscle contractures and painful joints, general fatigue, dyspnoea, communication difficulty and emotional lability. Muscle strength in MND is also subject to fluctuations during the day, and from day to day. It may be unaltered yet functioning greatly changed through modification of muscle tone, body position and posture, and emotional state. Medication taken to reduce spasticity may have paradoxical consequences for function when, for example, loss of lower limb tone causes loss of posture, or support in gait.

Functional Measures

Gait at least is an activity whose measurement is relevant to the illness, but it is soon lost in many patients whilst remaining hardly impaired in a few. Gait is objectively quantifiable in many ways, not all good. *Timed* measures of gait ignore and may destroy quality of gait, are dangerous where gait is impaired, and wisely avoided.

Scores of *"overall" function* [e.g., 18,25,32–34] tend to produce figures whose meaning is difficult to conceptualise. The Norris scale [32–34] and modifications thereof gained popularity in a vacuum of alternatives whilst being non-linear and difficult to repeat accurately at home where function, according to common sense, is most appropriately measured. Many factors affecting functional assessment are subjective, and Robinson [5,35] debated whether or not these assessments are valid contributors to group outcome measurement. The SPECIALS protocol included a modification of the Barthel score [36], devised by a physiotherapist for patients undergoing rehabilitation. The intention was more to assess its validity in MND [37] than actually to make use of it. But such a simplistic approach to functional measurement, with categorical assessments of "can" or "cannot", is beset with difficulties if what is really to be measured is *handicap*. For example, can a patient comfortably able to walk 6.5 m unaided benefit from this "independence" if he cannot first get out of his chair? What is the real-life meaning of "independence in feeding" if the food initially has to be brought to the patient? In the real world, a patient may one day lose the ability independently to clean his teeth because the last user of the toothpaste tube replaced the top too tightly!

Quality of Life, and Independence Again

Quality of life and independence are not disease-specific and therefore not necessarily disease-determined, notwithstanding that they particularly matter to patients. "Fundamentally," wrote Robinson [5], "the issue is to what extent trials should be concerned with the precise measurement of motor neurone loss and possible regeneration, or be concerned with functional changes which may or may not be correlated with such loss or regeneration." Robinson saw this issue reflecting the debate on whether trials should be concerned with therapeutic efficacy alone, or had a role also in exploring pathogenesis. But, more relevant to the present discussion, Robinson questioned the whole status of objective measurements, whether fundamental or functional in emphasis, in relation to subjective indicators of improvement. Wynne [38] expressed a similar message: the ultimate response might be to abandon all indices of illness in favour of a single, necessarily subjective measure of quality of life.

The problem for the trialist is that quality of life, whilst of undeniable importance, is not wholly disease-determined. Borasio [29] observes, also, that current measures are unreliable because different patients attach different priorities to various elements that might contribute to quality of life. This brings the discussion back to *loss of independence*, the principal end-point in the SPECIALS trial. Although it avoided some of the problems outlined above, it faced two major difficulties. First was that of defining independence when some patients who could be independent were not because of indulgent carers and some who really were not managed nevertheless to exist without day-to-day support through dogged insistence or, more often, through lack of provision of carer support so that they simply had to. The way around this, to "measure" what reasonably could be done rather than what usually was done, is the opposite approach to that of the Barthel system [36]. The second difficulty was that dependence might come about in several quite different ways, reflecting bulbar, upper limb, lower limb or respiratory involvement, yet adoption of such an end-point made these equivalent. At least they might be equivalent in a cost/benefit sense, and they might be in their impact upon the patient.

Where to Assess?

The central feature of MND is progressively increasing disability which eventually becomes severe in all cases. Greatly disabled patients cannot travel distances for assessment and those merely disabled do it at considerable cost to themselves. Rarely can they do so repeatedly. If hospital admission for this purpose is the response, the upset to the patient's routine during a stay of any length can be detrimental in its own way. Altered diet and enforced inactivity affect health and mobility. Aids to mobility, however thoughtfully provided, never replicate home, where a clutter of strategically placed pieces of furniture can be the key to a patient's movement about his house, and his independence. What this means to a trial is that *patients whose disability is increasing will not return again and again to the hospital for serial assessments* even if they were able to initially.

The consequence is a loss of patients to the trial in whom worsening continues apace. This is a source of serious bias. If it is to be avoided, and to be fair to patients who enter MND trials with prolonged follow-up, they must be offered the option of reassessment at home. This is quite obviously so notwithstanding the logistic problems for the investigator (in any case, if there is to be difficulty either way, should it be placed on the patient rather than the investigator?) and the fact that testing then does not take place under ideally standardised conditions (assessments made in difficult circumstances are better than none at all). Equally importantly, because it affects validity, home assessment offers the opportunity for direct observation of carer input, and of what is provided in aids and services.

Problems of Treatment

One obvious point is the need to be aware of other treatments the patient may be receiving. Drug trial protocols as a matter of course draw up lists of excluded concomitant medication, partly because of possible interaction but also because of their potential effect on what is being measured [17]. Intention-to-treat trials, required to analyse outcome in all patients randomised, are particularly problematic: they expect patients who for some reason are not continuing the treatment to remain under review for the originally envisaged follow-up period, which may be acceptable, but *without entering other trials*, which is not. They would be "locked in without further hope". Intention-to-treat trials are not mandatory (see above) and, in consequence of this issue alone, perhaps should be avoided.

Do trials, ever, consider the impact of a newly started course of hydrotherapy, for example, or the functional improvement suddenly achieved by provision of a much-needed aid? These matters are highly patient-specific: what can bring about profound change for one may have no impact whatsoever on another. Trial protocols cannot legislate for all possibilities even if there were ethical freedom to do so. Perhaps these should be added to Munsat's "external" factors referred to below [24].

Controls

It is immensely difficult to recruit MND patients without offering them the therapy. The ethical concept of equipoise makes no difference: patients envisage but a single chance for themselves. For those with a life-expectancy of a few months, that period on placebo treatment is a sacrifice of everything, and the possibility that the treatment may be on trial for safety as well as efficacy has little meaning. At least one patient in the SPECIALS trial is known to have had his treatment analysed: it was BCAA, and he stayed in.

Is there a mandate for controlled trials at all in MND? According to Munsat et al. [24], longevity in MND is as dependent on "external" health factors such as emphysema, smoking history, general medical care and respiratory support as on actual motor neurone loss. In this argument, controls "matched" for disease variables but not the external factors are poor controls. Furthermore, there are other important "external" factors such as qualities of the carer, and of the home, availability of other treatments, mobility aids, provision of services, and a variety of personality factors that determine ability to cope. Against the background of chronic progressive incurable disease, Munsat pleads, cannot patients act as their own controls, and in such a context does placebo effect really have such lasting power that it needs to be isolated and corrected for?

Compliance

Cooperation with treatment programmes in MND trials rarely seems to be a problem initially. Many patients, eager to help themselves, will have queued to participate in a project that is a collaborative venture against the disease and, sometimes, the only prospect of getting *any* treatment. They are suspicious of placebo, of course, and hope not to receive it, as the patient in the SPECIALS trial who analysed his treatment demonstrated. Sooner or later, compliance with treatment is adversely influenced by this and three other factors.

Firstly, it may be affected by treatment side-effects. These of course are generally treatment-specific, and can be an important factor in breaching blinding, as was discovered in many of the TRH trials [39–41]. Secondly, the start of a treatment programme for an incurable disease risks hopes being inappropriately raised with the proposition that therapy can help. Whilst Wynne [38] showed that multiple sclerosis patients were not necessarily driven to unreasoning optimism, unrealistically high expectations have led in terminal cancer patients to later anger, frustration and disillusionment [42]. All of these promote the growth of non-compliance. The opposite side of this coin is sometimes seen in patients who argue that "more of a good thing must be better", and increase the dose of self-administered therapy. Thirdly, simple treatment failure, real or apparent, with disease progression, can dull the motivation of anyone. It also raises suspicions, right or wrong, that the treatment *is* placebo.

These several circumstances establish the importance of compliance monitoring, both to promote compliance (a concept foreign to intention-to-treat trial design) and to be aware of compliance failures. There is a danger not only of non-random drop-out but also of non-random non-compliance. Non-randomness leads to bias, and reduction of risk of bias is seen as a compelling argument for intention-to-treat analyses, but this does not solve this problem. It may reduce, for example, the risk of *overestimating* efficacy but, in this disease, to miss identifying real benefit by diluting it with the non-response of non-compliers is ethically at least as bad. Errors in the other direction are also possible.

Duration of Treatment and Follow-up

The dilemma regarding duration of treatment and follow-up results from a multiple conflict. To obtain the trial result in as short a time as possible is a wish for the benefit of all future patients as well as those involved in it presently. Consideration for those involved in it brings awareness that longer follow-up makes greater demands and possibly consigns them to a useless therapy for the remainder of their lifetimes. The concern for the trial is that longer follow-up results in more drop-outs and falling compliance. The duration of therapy might be chosen so that it is statistically most likely to reveal benefit but there is awareness too that, as it is life-long treatment that may subsequently be offered, that is what should be tested.

A short follow-up time is likely to identify only a fairly remarkable change from the natural history. Even if such occurred, it would still be of major importance to know whether the effect was maintained over longer follow-up. This was true, for example, of the IGF-I trial with a 9-month follow-up. Periods of a year or longer may be a minimum but, of course, MND patients tend to vote with their feet. If doubts about continuing arise, they look at once for another trial because they are very short of time.

Conclusions

Most issues in MND trials stem from the problem of outcome measurement, and disagreements over how to do it [29]. Once these are settled, inclusion criteria, numbers and duration of follow-up are largely determined by following certain rules. Yet, even in stroke trials, of which there have been a far larger number over a much longer period, there is no consensus over what, other than death, should be measured [43]. Stroke patients differ fundamentally from MND patients in that, generally, they are recovering rather than declining, but regaining *independence* is a significant milestone in recovery just as its loss is in decline.

There is, since recently, with the three trials described here and a few others [e.g., 44–47], a corpus of experience to guide the design and conduct of future MND trials. These trials were developed in rather quick succession, with little opportunity to learn from the errors of those going before. This was a pity but, on the other hand, the consequence of each doing things somewhat differently is an enriched cumulative experience to which an eclectic approach can best inform future trials. There should not be further wheels to invent.

References

1. Schwartz D, Lellouch J. Explanatory and pragmatic attitudes in therapeutic trials. J Chron Dis 1967;20:637–648.
2. Guiloff RJ, Goonetilleke A, Emami J. Riluzole and amyotrophic lateral sclerosis. Lancet 1996;348:336–337.
3. Anon. Riluzole for amyotrophic lateral sclerosis [editorial]. Drugs Ther Bull 1997;35:11–12.
4. Brooke AS, Steiner TJ. Special problems of physiotherapy trials in motor neuron disease. In: Clifford Rose F, editor. Amyotrophic lateral sclerosis. New York: Demos, 1990:181–193.
5. Robinson I. Ethical issues and methodological problems in the conduct of clinical trials in amyotrophic lateral sclerosis. In: Clifford Rose F, editor. Amyotrophic lateral sclerosis. New York: Demos, 1990:195–213.
6. Munsat TL, Brooks BR. Don't throw the baby out with the bathwater [letter]. Neurology 1987;37:544–545.
7. Chaturvedi S. Clinical trials and financial reimbursement [letter]. Stroke 1998;29:1256.
8. Steiner TJ. Branched-chain amino-acids in ALS: the European trial. In: Clifford Rose F, editor. New Evidence in MND/ALS Research. London: Smith-Gordon, 1991:315–316.
9. Plaitakis A, Smith J, Mandeli J, Yahr MD. Pilot trial of branched-chain aminoacids in amyotrophic lateral sclerosis. Lancet 1988;I:1015–1018.
10. The Italian ALS Study Group. Branched-chain amino acids and amyotrophic lateral sclerosis: a treatment failure. Neurology 1993;43:2466–2470.
11. Breteler MMB. Selegiline, or the problem of early termination of clinical trials [editorial]. BMJ 1998;316:1182–1183.
12. Barnett HJM, Sackett DL. Monitoring clinical trials [editorial]. Neurology 1993;43:2437–2438.
13. Josefson D. Breast cancer trial stopped early [news item, with commentary: British researchers say that American trial was stopped prematurely]. BMJ 1998;316:1187.
14. Lacomblez L, Bensimon G, Leigh PN, Guillet P, Meininger V. For the Amyotrophic Lateral Sclerosis/Riluzole Study Group II. Dose-ranging study of riluzole in amyotrophic lateral sclerosis. Lancet 1996;347:1425–1431.
15. Bensimon G, Lacomblez L, Meininger V. ALS/Riluzole Study Group. A controlled trial of riluzole in amyotrophic lateral sclerosis. N Engl J Med 1994;330:585–591.
16. Brooks BR. El Escorial World Federation of Neurology criteria for the diagnosis of amyotrophic lateral sclerosis. J Neurol Sci 1994;124(Suppl):96–107.
17. Lai EC, Felice KJ, Festoff BW, Gawel MJ, Gelinas DF, Kratz R, et al. and the North American ALS/IGF-I Study Group. Effect of recombinant human insulin-like growth factor-I on progression of ALS. a placebo-controlled study. Neurology 1997; 49:1621–1630.
18. Appel V, Stewart SS, Smith G, Appel SH. A rating scale for amyotrophic lateral sclerosis. description and preliminary experience. Ann Neurol ••;22:328–333.
19. Bergner M, Bobbit RA, Carter WB, Gilson BS. The Sickness Impact Profile: development and final revision of a health status measure. Med Care 1981;19:787–805.
20. Mitsumoto H, Hanson MR, Chad DA. Amyotrophic lateral sclerosis: recent advances in pathogenesis and clinical trials. Arch Neurol 1988;45:189–202.
21. Li TM, Swash M, Alberman E, Day SJ. Diagnosis of motor neuron disease in three countries. J Neurol Neurosurg Psychiatry 1991;54:980–983.
22. Kuether G, Struppler A, Lipinski HG. Therapeutic trials in ALS: the design of a protocol. In: Cosi V, Kato AC, Parlette W, Pinelli P, Poloni M, editors. Amyotrophic Lateral Sclerosis. New York: Plenum Press, 1986:265–276.
23. Swash M, Leigh N. Criteria for diagnosis of familial amyotrophic lateral sclerosis [Workshop report]. Neuromusc Disord 1992;2:7–9.
24. Munsat TL, Andres P, Taft J. The nature of clinical change in amyotrophic lateral sclerosis. In: Tsubaki T, Yase Y, editors. Amyotrophic lateral sclerosis: recent advances in research and treatment. Amsterdam: Excerpta Medica, 1988:203–206.

25. Andres PL, Hedlund W, Finison L, Conlon T, Felmus M, Munsat TL. Quantitative motor assessment in amyotrophic lateral sclerosis. Neurology 1986;36:937–941.

26. Gorringe JAL. Initial preparation for clinical trials. In: Harris EL, Fitzgerald JD, editors. The principles and practice of clinical trials. Edinburgh: Livingstone, 1970:41–46.

27. Glasberg MR. Selection of patients in therapeutic trials. In: Clifford Rose F, editor. Amyotrophic Lateral Sclerosis. New York: Demos, 1990:33–38.

28. Committee on Health Care Issues of the American Neurological Association. Current status of thyrotropin-releasing hormone therapy in amyotrophic lateral sclerosis. Ann Neurol 1987;22:541–543.

29. Borasio GD. Amyotrophic lateral sclerosis: lessons in trial design from recent trials. J Neurol Sci 1997;152(Suppl 1):S23–S28.

30. Albert SM, Murphy P, Del Bene M, Rowland LP. Patient preferences for treatment in amyotrophic lateral sclerosis (ALS): relationship to outcomes one-year post-diagnosis. Proc Am Acad Neurol 25 April–2 May, no.28. 1998.

31. Medical Research Council. Aids to the examination of the peripheral nervous system. Memorandum 45. London: HMSO, 1976:1–2.

32. Norris FH, Calanchini PR, Fallat RJ, Panchari S, Jewett B. The administration of guanidine in amyotrophic lateral sclerosis. Neurology 1974;24:721–728.

33. Hillel AD, Miller RM, McDonald E, Konikow N, Norris FH. Amyotrophic lateral sclerosis severity scale. In: Tsubaki T, Yase Y, editors. Amyotrophic lateral sclerosis: recent advances in research and treatment. Amsterdam: Excerpta Medica 1988:247–252.

34. Hillel AD, Miller RM, Yorkston K, McDonald E, Norris FH, Konikow N. Amyotrophic lateral sclerosis severity scale. In: Clifford Rose F, editor. Amyotrophic lateral sclerosis. New York: Demos, 1990:93–97.

35. Robinson I. Analysing the structure of 23 clinical trials in multiple sclerosis. Neuroepidemiology 1987;6:46–76.

36. Mahoney FI, Barthel DW. Functional evaluation: the Barthel index. Maryland State Med J 1965;14:61–65.

37. Louwerse ES, de Jong JMBV, Kuether G. Critique of assessment methodology in amyotrophic lateral sclerosis. In: Clifford Rose F, editor. Amyotrophic lateral sclerosis. New York: Demos, 1990:151–179.

38. Wynne A. Is it any good? The evaluation of therapy by participants in a clinical trial. Soc Sci Med 1989;29:1289–1297.

39. Caroscio JT, Cohen JA, Zawodniak J, et al. A double-blind, placebo-controlled trial of TRH in amyotrophic lateral sclerosis. Neurology 1986;36:141–145.

40. Brooke MH, Florence JM, Heller SL, et al. Controlled trial of thyrotropin releasing hormone in amyotrophic lateral sclerosis. Neurology 1986;36:146–151.

41. Mitsumoto H, Salgado ED, Negroski D, et al. Amyotrophic lateral sclerosis: effects of acute intravenous and chronic subcutaneous administration of thyrotropin-releasing hormone in controlled trials. Neurology 1986;36:152–159.

42. Chatterton P. Physiotherapy for the terminally ill. Physiotherapy 1988;74:42–46.

43. Roberts L, Counsell C. Assessment of clinical outcomes in acute stroke trials. Stroke 1998;29:986–991.

44. Lotz B, Brooks B, Sanjak M, et al. A double-blind placebo-controlled clinical trial of subcutaneous recombinant human ciliary neurotrophic factor (rHCNTF) in amyotrophic lateral sclerosis. Neurology 1996;46:1244–1249.

45. Miller RG, Petajan JH, Bryan WW, et al. A placebo-controlled clinical trial of recombinant human ciliary neurotrophic (rhCNTF) factor in amyotrophic lateral sclerosis. Ann Neurol 1996;39:256–260.

46. Miller RG, Moore D, Young LA, et al. Placebo-controlled trial of gabapentin in patients with amyotrophic lateral sclerosis. Neurology 1996;47:1383–1388.

47. Borassio GD, Robberecht W, Leigh PN, Emile J, Guiloff RJ, Jerusalem F et al. Effect of recombinant human insulin – like growth factor I in amyotrophic lateral sclerosis. Neurology 1998;51:583–586.

36. Peripheral Neuropathies: Controlled Clinical Trials

P.J. Dyck and P. O'Brien

Definition and Characteristics

The term "controlled clinical trials" at a minimum implies testing whether a prospectively administered intervention (a drug, diet, activity or other therapy) prevents, stabilizes or ameliorates clinical polyneuropathy to a clinically beneficial degree when compared with a sham intervention, similar in all respects to the intervention with the exception that the intervention is not included. It is also understood that neither the investigators or patients can identify the intervention from the sham intervention except perhaps by the response. The term "controlled clinical trial" also implies rigorous pre-planning, written design, choice of carefully selected outcomes, estimation of statistical power, written permission agreed to, and supervised by, an institutional review board, periodic evaluation for safety, meticulous record keeping, quality assurance and detailed statistical analysis. Often controlled clinical trials are multicenter studies and funded by a pharmaceutical house, disease advocacy agency or governmental research agency. Typically, the study is registered, modified and monitored by an agency such as the Federal Drug Administration (FDA; in the USA).

Often controlled clinical trials are a final step in testing the efficacy of an intervention. Usually there is earlier evidence, in a hierarchy of evidence, suggesting efficacy. This evidence may come from several sources: animal studies, anecdotal reports, study of previous open or controlled trials on individual or small groups of patients, or rigorous phase II or phase III trials.

In definitive phase III studies, one seeks unequivocal evidence that the intervention induces a favorable effect which is better than for the sham intervention group. In the USA, the FDA usually requires evidence from two multicenter studies to accept a drug as being efficacious. For an intervention to be accepted as efficacious, it must be shown to produce a statistically significant better outcome than the placebo and additionally this beneficial effect must be of sufficient magnitude to be considered clinically useful or meaningful.

When Are Controlled Clinical Trials Needed?

The degree to which controlled clinical trials are used varies among studies and medical specialties. Although open trials of small series of patients may provide a preliminary indication of whether an intervention may be efficacious, it generally takes one, or perhaps two, controlled clinical trials to prove efficacy. Controlled trials have generally not been used before introducing new surgical procedures, but perhaps this was not wise. It seems self-evident to us that evidence for the health value of a surgical procedure should be as rigorous as for any medical therapy. Quite complex and expensive interventions, such as plasma exchange or immune globulin infusion in acute or chronic inflammatory demyelinating polyneuropathy (CIDP) [1], or in dysproteinemic polyneuropathy (MGUS neuropathy) [2], can be tested using sham-controlled trials.

Controlled clinical trials should be performed:

1. prior to the introduction of any new therapeutic intervention irrespective of the medical or surgical specialty;
2. when there is preliminary experimental or anecdotal evidence that an intervention may have a useful effect on symptoms, course or outcome for a variety of neuropathies or nerve conditions, and more definitive evidence is needed to confirm this beneficial and clinically meaningful effect;
3. when there is preliminary or anecdotal evidence that an intervention may be more effective, safer, cheaper, freer of complications, or a better route of administration than was previously available.

Unethical Studies and Bias

It is not always a simple matter to judge whether a planned therapeutic trial is ethical or unethical, mainly because the extent and magnitude of potential risks and benefits are usually not known with certainty ahead of time.

Unethical studies are ones in which:

1. The potential benefits are unlikely to outweigh risks. The rule that potential benefits should outweigh risks is self-evident but actually hard to judge. It is usually held that for severe diseases with potential for death, such as Guillian– Barré syndrome, CIDP or amyloidosis, a greater degree of potential risks for the intervention can be accepted than for a disease with mild involvement and a known good outcome. The same rule may also apply to the expense of treatments – more expensive treatments may be justified in serious death-threatening disease.
2. The potential benefits are not expected to equal an already known available efficacious treatment which is inexpensive, readily available and given in an acceptable form.
3. No biologic effect, only a placebo effect, is anticipated.
4. No or insufficient preceding evidence or scientific rationale provides a basis for the study.
5. The study is to be performed on persons who by nature of their age (e.g. children), status (e.g. prisoners or mental hospital patients) or other condition may not be able to give free and informed consent.
6. Only marketing, but no medical or scientific questions are pursued.
7. Outright falsification of conduct of the study or analysis of results is planned.
8. Design or conduct of the trial is unable to answer the question.

Here are several examples to make the point that the risk, discomfort and inconvenience of a trial may vary depending on the severity of the disease. In recent controlled clinical trials of CIDP and acute inflammatory demyelinating polyneuropathy (AIDP), which are paralytic diseases that can cause death, trials of plasma exchange and intravenous gamma globulin were justifiable despite the high frequency of mild side effects of the putative treatments (light-headedness, postural hypotension, headache) and infrequent severe complications (e.g. anaphylaxis, hepatotoxicity, and even death). In mild diabetic polyneuropathy, a disorder which is much less severe, one would perhaps not be justified in trying these risky treatments, at least not for mild cases.

For study of therapy in diabetic polyneuropathy the issue of potential benefits versus risks has been discussed for one evaluative procedure, the sural nerve biopsy. An earlier committee of the FDA had permitted use of pathologic endpoints of nerve biopsy for the study of aldose reductase inhibitors (ARI). In the minds of proponents of this point of view, the advantage of these markers to the resolution of efficacy of ARI outweighed the known paresthesia, pain and sensation loss which would ensue from nerve biopsy of both sides of the body and in treated and sham-treated patients. At a later time a committee from the Peripheral Neuropathy Association favored other approaches to nerve biopsy for these studies.

The following strategies help in minimizing unethical practices:

1. The preliminary animal data and clinical data along with all adverse event data should be available to all participating investigators, institutional review boards and governmental health regulatory agencies.
2. The planned design of the trial, efficacy measures, degree of improvement sought and calculated power estimates should be available for inspection.
3. Quality assurance centers should be used to independently assess the quality and accuracy of neurologic endpoints.
4. An external scientific review committee with access to all data and adverse events might be appointed to conduct an interim analysis and decide whether the study needs to be stopped (because of adverse outcomes, unequivocal lack of efficacy or unequivocal benefit) or should be continued. This committee might also approve the final statistical analysis.
5. Oversight by a governmental committee (e.g., the FDA in the USA) is needed.

For most large-scale studies, the concern is more about subtle factors which may introduce bias at evaluation of patients or analysis of results. Many of the problems of bias in the conduct of the study can be minimized by a good double-blind design in which both patients and observers are blinded as to which intervention is used. Unfortunately, it may be difficult to provide a totally satisfactory sham intervention in some studies, so the patient or the observer may not be truly blinded. In our studies of prednisone in CIDP, we were unable to find a suitable sham-intervention drug, similar in all respects to prednisone except for its putative beneficial effect on neuromuscular symptomatology. We simply gave the sham group no treatment. In a study of plasma exchange and immune globulin infusion, we were able to prevent patients or observers from knowing what treatment was being given by using the strategy of instructing all personnel not to discuss treatment with patients or evaluating physicians, providing a physical screen between patient and treating instruments and giving sham plasma exchange (with actual separation of cellular elements from plasma, recombining them and giving this recombined blood to the sham group) and bandaging injection sites identically for treatment and sham group during the neurologic examination. After completion of the study, patients were asked which treatment they had been on. Their responses indicated that they had remained blinded as to treatment.

A further source of bias may occur with the handling of drop-outs and of data. Conceptually non-responders in the intervention and sham-intervention groups might drop out, biasing results. Although, they cannot be prevented from dropping out (it is their right) perhaps they could be encouraged to have periodic, or end of study, evaluations so that intent-to-treat analysis would be optimized.

Controlled Clinical Trials Should Be Tailor-Made for the Type of Neuropathy Being Studied

In the differential diagnosis of peripheral neuropathy, there are perhaps 19 different anatomico-pathologic patterns of peripheral neuropathy [3]. The outcome variables for a study, therefore, should be chosen with the clinical pattern, the natural history and putative action of the drug in mind. To illustrate, diabetic neuropathy is made up of quite dissimilar entities, i.e., distal sensorimotor polyneuropathy, lumbosacral radiculoplexus neuropathy, thoracolumbar radiculoneuropathy, upper limb mononeuropathies (median neuropathy at the wrist and ulnar neuropathy at the elbow), autonomic, abnormality, hypoglycemic neuropathy and oculomotor neuropathy. It would not be appropriate to treat these disorders using the same protocol – pathogenetic mechanisms are different and outcome variables need to be different. The endpoints will need to be different for a disease which primarily affects motor neurons, from one which affects sensory neurons and from one that affects autonomic neurons. In some diseases, death may be an appropriate outcome (motor neuron disease, diseases due to severe inborn errors of metabolism), whereas in other diseases, death is a quite an inappropriate outcome. In some diseases, it may be necessary to show prevention of neurologic impairment (e.g., many genetic diseases).

In others, one is trying to prevent, stabilize or ameliorate symptoms, impairments or functional derangements. In still others, one may look for recovery or near recovery (e.g., Guillain–Barré syndrome).

Neuropathic Markers, Overall Estimates of Severity or Outcomes

To conduct a controlled clinical trial in a given type of neuropathy, is it sufficient to assess one marker of neuropathy or is it necessary to measure several or many symptoms, impairments or test abnormalities? If one marker is to be used, it is necessary to show that the marker is a sufficiently reliable identifier of the presence and severity of neuropathy. Unfortunately, for most varieties of neuropathy, such a favorable marker does not exist [4]. In diabetic polyneuropathy (DPN), various individual markers have been employed, such as reduced or absent ankle reflexes, decreased vibration sensation or abnormalities of nerve conduction. None of these markers, however, is as reliable a marker of DPN as desirable. More important, the information derived is dichotomous. It provides information only about whether the patient has or does not have polyneuropathy. It provides no information about characteristics or overall severity. It may, therefore, be preferable to develop an overall impairment score which takes into account sensory loss, autonomic dysfunction, muscle weakness and test abnormalities. It is then possible using the same composite score to define abnormality at a given percentile, e.g., 95th, 97.5th, or 99th, depending on the study for which it will be used.

In Table 36.1 we show how we derive Neuropathy Impairment Score (Lower Limbs) + 7 tests [NIS(LL) + 7] for diabetic polyneuropathy. In this example, note that the basis is a transformation of a percentile to a point abnormality. In longitudinal follow-up of a population-based diabetic cohort, the NIS(LL) + 7 was found to show a monotonic worsening with magnitude [4].

Another approach which might be considered is to stage overall severity taking into account symptoms, impairments, and perhaps outcome. In our staging approach for DPN polyneuropathy we have identified levels of abnormality based on overall neuropathic severity, symptoms and outcomes [5]. The staging approach we developed for DPN used disease gradations – insights coming from our study of the Rochester Diabetic Neuropathy Study (RDNS) cohort and using a representative healthy subject cohort for comparison. The following criteria were used to stage DPN: presence or absence of minimal criteria for DPN, decreased or absent ankle reflexes,

Table 36.1. Calculating the Neuropathy Impairment Score of Lower Limbs +7 tests (NIS(LL) +7 Tests) score[a]

- Sum individual scores of the NIS for the lower limbs, NIS (LL)
- In NIS(LL), substitute transformed points for percentile abnormality[b] of VDT for each great toe (obtained with CASE IV) for the clinical vibration sensation point score of great toes
- Add transformed points for percentile abnormality[a] of HB DB (1× only)
- Summate transformed points for percentile abnormality[b] of the five attributes of NC of lower limb [peroneal nerve (CMAP, MNCV and MNDL), tibial nerve (MNDL) and sural nerve (S SNAP)], divide by the number of attributes with obtainable values,[c] multiply by 5 (the number of attributes), and add this number to the global score

CMAP, compound muscle action potential; HB DB, heart beat variation with deep breathing; MNCV, motor nerve conduction velocity; MNDL, motor nerve distal latency; NC nerve conduction; S SNAP, sural sensory nerve action potential; VDT, vibration detection threshold.

[a] Items 17–24, 28, 29 and 34–37 of NIS.
[b] <95th = 0, ≥95th–99th = 1, ≥99th–99.9th = 2, and ≥99.9th = 3 (or ≥5th = 0 to ≤0.1th = 3, whichever end of the distribution is abnormal).
[c] MNCV and MNDL cannot be estimated when CMAP is 0.

inability to walk on the heels or comparable degrees of ankle dorsiflexor muscle weakness, neuropathic symptoms, and sufficiently severe sensory, autonomic or motor abnormality to be disabling.

Another approach is to measure such outcomes as death, inability to perform certain tasks, or development of such complications as Charcot joints. In Guillain–Barré syndrome, death, ability to walk, feed oneself, perform independent acts of daily living, may be excellent outcome measures. In DPN, such outcomes as Charcot joints, plantar ulcers and ability to work might be considered. There are several reasons why these measures of outcome may be problematic: (1) multiple factors other than the disease studied may relate to the poor outcome, and therefore the outcome may not be a very accurate measure of severity of neuropathy, (2) scoring may not be independent of motivational factors, and (3) the score may not be continuous. Take the case of plantar ulcers. Although this is an important outcome in DPN, multiple factors other than sensory loss are implicated, such as previous injury, use of or failure to use shoes, inadequate treatment of injury, overweight and attitude. The size of the ulcer and whether the foot and leg ultimately have to be amputated (perhaps a measure of graded severity) may relate to various factors other than simply severity of neuropathy. Take another example: the ability to work and to perform acts of independent living. This is greatly dependent on motivation, ingenuity, previous training and education, and other factors such as support from family and community.

Neuropathy Symptoms as Outcome Measures

Because symptoms are what patients complain of they need to be measured in treatment trials of neuropathy, but they are quite variable, hard to measure and do not relate closely to severity of impairments. To test for the efficacy of an analgesic, the pain experience itself must be measured. In other cases, the severity of a variety of pain may need to be measured, i.e., lancinating, deep aching, restless legs, or other. One may also want to measure other positive neuropathy experiences directly, such as prickling, hypersensitivity, or other. Symptoms of this kind may be measured by having the patient compare their symptom with an externally applied stimulus or, more usually, with a visual analog or numerical scale from 1 (least) to 10 (most). Subjective symptoms can also be judged by a combination of intensity, frequency and duration. When and how often should the pain experience be assessed? Various approaches have been used: (1) it is evaluated by medical personnel at the time of the medical evaluation – the patient recalls the frequency, duration and severity of symptoms for a preceding period of time, (2) it is evaluated at periodic intervals by medical personnel by office interview, telephone, telefax or electronic mail, or (3) is evaluated by the patient him- or herself, recording the information in a diary or transmitting it by electronic mail.

We have introduced three standard approaches to survey both positive and negative motor, sensory and autonomic symptoms encountered in neuropathy. The Neuropathy Symptom Score (NSS) is a standard tally of 18 symptoms abstracted from a neurologist's notes and assumes that the questions have been inquired after [6]. Any score greater than 0 is abnormal. The Neuropathy Symptom Profile (NSP) is a patient-completed questionnaire about 32 symptoms encountered in neuropathy. The answers to the questions are grouped into scales, i.e., neuropathy, weakness, sensory, autonomic and others (see below) [7]. The Neuropathy Symptoms and Change (NSC) is a 38 question instrument, shown in abbreviated form (Table 36.2) and is completed by the interviewing physician who makes the final judgment as to whether symptoms are or are not present. Each question takes the general form "Do you experience this symptom?", which is then answered yes or no. If the answer is "yes," its severity is graded mild (1), moderate (2) or severe (3). Finally, the symptom is compared with a previous time, e.g., 3 months ago, and is graded as the same, better [slightly (+1), moderately (+2) or much (+3)] or worse [slightly (−1), moderately (−2) or much (−3)]. For certain questions, the

Table 36.2. Neuropathy Symptoms And Change (NSC)[a]

Instructions to neurologist

1. All 38 questions must be answered yes or no, except for questions 35 and 36 in women. Use a #2 pencil
2. A given symptom is marked as present if, in the judgment of the examining neurologist, it occurs more frequently or more severely than in healthy persons of the same age and gender and is due to diabetic neuropathy. If the neurologist is in doubt as to whether a symptom is present or whether it is due to diabetic neuropathy, it should be scored "no." To illustrate, impotence in a man who is ≥60 years old is scored "no"
3. If a symptom is present, its severity should be graded as + (slight), ++ (moderate) or +++ (severe)
4. The change in symptoms are to be compared with the week just preceding the screening visit #1
5. Determine whether the symptom is the same, better or worse; this must be answered for every question whether or not the symptom is present. Indicate the degree of change (slight [+/−], moderate [++/−−], or much [+++/−−−]). The change in symptoms for each visit (screening visit #1 and subsequent visits) are to be compared with symptoms in the week preceding the screening visit #1
6. A good strategy is to ask patients to provide two answers for each question: the first answer is for "at this time" (for the week of the visit), and the second for "the week preceding the week of the screening visit #1." If the patient answers "yes" and "yes", the examiner knows that the symptom is present now and was present in the week preceding the screening visit #1. Assuming that the examiner judges that the positively answered symptom is due to diabetic neuropathy, he or she must then determine whether the severity is slight (+), moderate (++) or severe (+++) and degree of change is the same, better [slight (+)], moderate (++) or much (+++)] or worse [slight (−), moderate (−−) or much (−−−)]. If the answer is "yes" and "no", one infers that the symptom has developed since the week preceding the week of screening #1; in this case severity and degree of change are recorded. If the answer is "no" and "yes", one infers that the symptom has improved since the week preceding the week of screening #1; in this case only degree of change is recorded
7. If the question (20–29) is answered "yes", complete only one of the regions of the body affected, i.e., in legs only, in arms only . . . other than any of the above

Symptoms of weakness

			If "yes" Severity			Are the symptoms the same, better, or worse than the week preceding screening #1?						
	Yes	No				Same	Better			Worse		
			(+)	(++)	(+++)		(+)	(++)	(+++)	(−)	(−−)	(−−−)
16. Weakness of the legs so that you slap your feet in walking or cannot carry your weight on your heels	☐	☐	☐	☐	☐	☐	☐	☐	☐	☐	☐	☐
17. Weakness of the legs so that you cannot walk on your toes or forefoot	☐	☐	☐	☐	☐	☐	☐	☐	☐	☐	☐	☐

Sensory symptoms

Do you experience these symptoms in one region or over the surface of your body to an abnormal degree? Do not include the brief symptoms of "prickling" or "asleep numbness" and discomfort which come from lying too long on an arm, or sitting or lying too long in one position on a leg

			If "yes" Severity			Are the symptoms the same, better, or worse than the week preceding screening #1?						
	Yes	No				Same	Better			Worse		
			(+)	(++)	(+++)		(+)	(++)	(+++)	(−)	(−−)	(−−−)
20. Decrease (or inability) to feel the surface features, size, shape, or texture of what your touch	☐	☐	☐	☐	☐	☐	☐	☐	☐	☐	☐	☐
If "yes", choose only one:												
in legs only (feet are included)	☐											
in arms only (hands are included)	☐											
in legs and arms only	☐											
in mouth, face, or head only	☐											
other than any of the above	☐											
22. Decrease (or inability) to feel pain, cuts, bruises, or injuries	☐	☐	☐	☐	☐	☐	☐	☐	☐	☐	☐	☐
If "yes", choose only one:												
in legs only (feet are included)	☐											
in arms only (hands are included)	☐											
in legs and arms only	☐											
in mouth, face, or head only	☐											
other than any of the above	☐											

Table 36.2.   (Continued)

Autonomic symptoms													
Do you experience these symptoms to an abnormal degree?						Are the symptoms the same, better, or worse than the week preceding tscreening #1?							
	Yes	No	If "yes" Severity			Same	Better			Worse			
			(+)	(++)	(+++)		(+)	(++)	(+++)	(−)	(−−)	(−−−)	
30. Feel faint or actually faint, which only comes upon sitting or in standing, and which cannot be explained by use of blood pressure medication or psychologic stress (e.g., sight of blood)	☐	☐	☐	☐	☐	☐	☐	☐	☐	☐	☐	☐	

a Incomplete; only examples of test questions are included.

anatomic location has to be designated. The NSC tallies number of symptoms, severity of symptoms (at this time) and change of symptoms (as compared with a preceding time).

The NSP questionnaire was completed by more than 300 healthy persons and percentile responses were estimated for the various scales and as corrected for age, sex and other physical variables. Since the questionnaire was completed by the patients themselves, no bias of medical [3] personnel was involved. We have studied its use in a DPN cohort (RDNS). The questionnaire did not perform as well as a physician-completed questionnaire. Over time, patients in the RDNS worsened slowly by the criteria of the overall neuropathic impairment as measured by Neuropathy Impairment Score (NIS) and also by the number of neuropathy symptoms as measured by NSS. By contrast, NSP scores tended to improve. Perhaps patients on the study learned with time which symptoms were related to neuropathy and which were not. Physicians made more consistent judgments of symptoms related to neuropathy. The results suggest that a trained physician may need to be involved in determining which symptoms are due to DPN and which are not due to DPN.

What is the least degree of change which a symptoms score such as the NSC questionnaire can recognize over time? It is quite clear that the number of symptoms, their severity, and their duration and magnitude of change tracks with the direction of change as measured by NIS, summated compound muscle action potentials, summated sensory nerve action potentials and quantitated sensory test results in such diseases as CIDP, if the change over time is large. In this case, the scores will clearly mirror improvement or worsening. The least degree of change which will be recognized is not known

and may depend on the quality of patients and the expertise of physicians.

The Neurologic Examination as Outcome Measure

In the USA, for the purposes of setting social security disability, it is necessary to get objective evidence from a physician's examination of abnormality. To be disabled, a person must be found to have more than claims or symptoms of disease – he or she must be found to have objective evidence of disease (impairment). Thus, abnormality from the neurologic examination is a major indicator of neuropathic impairment and, therefore, is useful in efficacy trials.

We have developed the Neuropathy Impairment Score (NIS) and NIS (lower limb) [NIS] (LL) to provide a disease scale for polyneuropathy [6]. A standard representative group of muscles are assessed for weakness. First a judgment is made whether the muscle is weak (considering age, gender, physical characteristics and physical fitness) and whether this is due to neuropathy. If it is not due to neuropathy, the weakness is not graded. Weakness is graded by the following criteria: 1 = 25%, 2 = 50%, 3 = 75%, 3.25 = movement against gravity just possible; 3.5 = movement with gravity eliminated is just possible; and 3.75 = only a flicker of muscle activity is possible. The scoring is based with modification on the system of neurologic grading used at Mayo Clinic and with further modification on the Medical Research Council approach for war nerve injuries. Reflexes are graded as normal (0), decreased (1) or absent (2). Touch-pressure, vibration, joint position and pin prick are evaluated on index finger and great toe and are scored as decreased (−1) and absent (−2). If scores greater than 0 are entered, it indicates unequivocal abnormality. By comparison with percentile abnormality, a score of 1 point is to represent a percentile value of ≥95th–99th (or ≤5th–1st, whichever applies) and 2 points a percentile value of ≥99th (or ≤1st, whichever applies). In Table 36.3 we show selective items of the NIS and provide further instructions for scoring.

The NIS scale was the primary endpoint in several prospective controlled trials showing efficacy of prednisone, plasma exchange, and intravenous gamma globulin infusion in CIDP and in neuropathy associated with monoclonal protein. It is the primary endpoint in diabetic trials using recombinant human (rhNGF) and the anti-oxidant alpha-lipoic acid.

Nerve Conduction Abnormality as an Efficacy Measure

Abnormality of attributes of nerve conduction are useful measures of impairment, particularly as they are quantitative, sensitive (recognizing an effect given that it is present), reproducible and objective (results cannot be willed or influenced by the bias of the patient). On the other hand, attributes of nerve conduction are weak measures of severity and of clinical meaningfulness. Attributes of nerve conduction which may be used include amplitude (AP), conduction velocity (CV) and latency (NL) of motor fibers (CMAP, MNCV and MNDL) and sensory nerve fibers (SNAP, SNCV and SNDL).

The value of testing for nerve conduction abnormality is also limited because the tests are cumbersome, time-consuming, expensive and uncomfortable. Because not all the abnormalities of nerve conduction are directly related to weakness, sensory loss or autonomic impairment, one must take into account many disparate measurements. Also an estimate of conduction velocity or distal latency is not possible when a response is absent.

Because of its high sensitivity, abnormality of attributes of nerve conduction is an excellent minimal criterion for polyneuropathy, e.g., DPN. Because abnormality of nerve conduction is not a good measure of severity or of clinical meaningfulness, it is usually not a good primary outcome measurement for use in controlled clinical trials for neuropathies such as DPN. As a secondary endpoint or as a component of a composite score, it is a very useful measurement. It is particularly useful if the results can be calculated as a normal deviate or as a specific percentile value considering the tested nerve, attribute, age, sex, height, weight, surface area and

body mass index of the patient [8,9]. For use in DPN, we have introduced an approach which takes into account the number of nerves with nerve conduction abnormality, severity of abnormality and missing values, and combined nerve conduction abnormalities with clinical and other abnormalities [4].

Quantitative Sensory Tests as Outcome Measures

Quantitative sensory tests (QST) are important outcome measures of neuropathy if sensory loss is a feature of the neuropathy studied [4]. The QST which are available are vibration (VDT) and cool (CDT) detection threshold and heat pain: 0.5 (detection) and 5 (HP:5) levels. The tests are performed on parts of limbs known to be affected. In DPN, the suitable anatomic location is the foot.

The tests used should be standard and validated [8,9]. The stimulus waveform used should be appropriate for the test, be reproducible, and provide only one stimulus modality. Stimuli should be available over a broad range of intensities so that sensitive and insensitive regions and young and old can be studied. Testing at defined levels of intensity (e.g., in steps from small to large) is preferable over continuously increasing the intensity of the stimulus to perception. Use of defined small exponential steps permits the subject to take whatever time is needed to decide whether the stimulus was felt (or not felt) at a given stimulus intensity. Continuously increasing the stimulus magnitudes results in an overestimate of threshold because of delay due to reaction time. Longer reaction times may result in higher thresholds in deliberative persons. A variety of algorithms have been developed to estimate threshold. It is important to use ones that have been validated so that results are not due to build-in problems. Two algorithms that we have extensively tested are our forced-choice and our 4, 2 and 1 stepping algorithm.

The details of methodology and different systems available for testing are beyond the scope of this chapter.

For use in multicenter tests, it is mandatory that all aspects of the test be the same at all centers. This implies that microprocessor-controlled systems be used, that all aspects of testing and finding threshold be standard and that calibration be performed using the same standards for all participating medical centers. For VDT all aspects of testing should be the same: (1) the site of test (e.g., at the base of the nail, terminal phalanx of great toe), (2) the static load, (3) the mass of the stimulating head, (4) the area and shape of the waveform, (5) the precise steps of

Table 36.3.   Lower Limb Function Test (LLF) and Neuropathy Impairment Score[a]

Lower Limb Function Test (LLF)
This is a preliminary functional test carried out before doing the NIS.

Persons up to 75 years old are usually able to carry their weight in walking on toes or heels unless they are markedly overweight. Patients over 60 years of age may not be able to rise from a kneeling position when they are overweight, physically unfit or have knee disease. Do not score as abnormal if the disability is due to age, physical unfitness or knee disease

	Right				Left			
1. Walk on toes	Normal	☐	Abnormal	☐	Normal	☐	Abnormal	☐
2. Walk on heels	Normal	☐	Abnormal	☐	Normal	☐	Abnormal	☐
3. Rise from kneeling position	Normal	☐	Abnormal	☐	Normal	☐	Abnormal	☐

Neuropathy Impairment Score (NIS)
Objective: To provide a single score of neuropathic deficits and subset scores: cranial nerve, muscle weakness, reflexes and sensation. Abnormalities are abstracted from a neurologic examination in which all the assessments are made

Scoring: The examiner scores deficits by what he or she considers to be normal considering the test, anatomic site, age, gender, height, weight and physical fitness

MUSCLE WEAKNESS
Score

0 = Normal	3.25 = move against gravity
1 = 25% weak	3.5 = movement, gravity eliminated
2 = 50% weak	3.75 = muscle flicker, no movement
3 = 75% weak	4 = paralysis

	Right								Left							
	0	1	2	3	3.25	3.5	3.75	4	0	1	2	3	3.25	3.5	3.75	4
21. Ankle dorsiflexors	☐	☐	☐	☐	☐	☐	☐	☐	☐	☐	☐	☐	☐	☐	☐	☐
22. Ankle plantar flexors	☐	☐	☐	☐	☐	☐	☐	☐	☐	☐	☐	☐	☐	☐	☐	☐
23. Toe extensors	☐	☐	☐	☐	☐	☐	☐	☐	☐	☐	☐	☐	☐	☐	☐	☐

REFLEXES
For patients 50–69 years old, ankle reflexes which are decreased are graded 0 and when absent are graded 1. For patients ≥70 years, absent ankle reflexes are graded 0

Score
0 = normal   1 = decreased   2 = absent

	Right			Left		
	0	1	2	0	1	2
28. Quadriceps femoris	☐	☐	☐	☐	☐	☐
29. Triceps surae	☐	☐	☐	☐	☐	☐

SENSATION
Touch-pressure, pin prick and vibration sensation are tested on the dorsal surface, at the base of the nail, of the terminal phalanx of the index finger and great toe. Touch-pressure is assessed with long-fiber cotton wool. Pin prick is assessed with straight pins. Vibration sensation is tested with a 165 Hz tuning fork (V. Mueller, Chicago, length 25 cm, made from $\frac{1}{2} \times 1\frac{1}{4}$ inch stock; 165 Hz with counterweights). Joint motion is tested by moving the terminal phalanx of the index finger and great toe

Score
0 = normal   1 = decreased   2 = absent

Great toe	Right			Left		
	0	1	2	0	1	2
34. Touch pressure	☐	☐	☐	☐	☐	☐
35. Pin prick	☐	☐	☐	☐	☐	☐
36. Vibration	☐	☐	☐	☐	☐	☐
37. Joint position	☐	☐	☐	☐	☐	☐

[a] Incomplete; only selected items are included.

stimulus magnitude, (6) the algorithm to find threshold and (7) the basis of abnormality. For CDT and HP:5 it is critically important that in addition to having exactly the same testing systems and tests at each medical center, careful calibration, especially of temperature be conducted of each system at various times throughout the study. In studies we are involved with, we use a highly reproducible platinum resistor (Goodrich-Rosemount Engineering, Minneapolis, MN) to calibrate the temperature of the thermode at 20 °C and 40 °C. It is further important that for cooling detection threshold, the initial skin temperature be accommodated to 30 °C and for heat-pain to 34 °C so that constant steps of stimulus magnitude be used. There is a further important consideration that excessive heat stimuli that will be damaging to tissue should be avoided.

Quantitative Autonomic Test Abnormality

Many autonomic functions can be tested. Among those that have been most extensively studied and are involved in certain neuropathies are heart beat response to deep breathing (HB DB) or the same response to the Valsalva maneuver (HB Val) [10]. These two can readily be used in controlled clinical trials and can be incorporated into a composite score of neuropathy. Other tests, such as of sudomotor dysfunction, could also be studied, but the test is quite complex, time-consuming, associated with some discomfort and expensive. Sudomotor tests are not currently recommended for multicenter trials because of their complexity.

Sural Nerve Morphometric and Teased Fiber Studies

Evaluation of the number and size distribution of myelinated fibers of semithin transverse epoxy sections of glutaraldehyde and osmium tetroxide fixed sural nerves stained with paraphenylenediamine may be used as the endpoint for controlled clinical trials. There are some confounding variables that need to be taken into account when using morphometric results [11]. It may not always be possible to recognize a myelinated fiber from a non-intact myelin ovoid. In addition, one is not certain that the fiber which is counted is innervating target tissue. Concern has also been expressed that the procedure is too invasive (the sural nerve is taken from one side before the study is begun, and from the other side

after it has ended) for many contemplated studies. The potential benefits of the future therapy may not outweigh the discomfort and risk of the procedure.

Skin Biopsy

Evaluating the number of dermal nerve fibers in a 3 or 4 mm punch biopsy taken from a region of the body affected by neuropathy has been advocated as a primary outcome measure in controlled clinical trials for certain neuropathies such as the sensorimotor neuropathy of diabetes mellitus and of acute immune deficiency disease. The concern that tallied fibers may not be functional is perhaps not as great in the skin biopsy as it is for the sural nerve biopsy because fibers are near or at termination. The main concerns about using this measure are perhaps four: (1) it is not useful for neuropathies with motor involvement, (2) adequacy of recognition of all nerve fibers, (3) adequacy of controls and (4) adequacy as a meaningful clinical measure. The degree to which all neurites are identified may still need further assessment. Also needed is a thorough evaluation of the density of fibers considering site, age, gender and physical variables. Large numbers of punch biopsies from healthy subjects without neuropathy or diseases predisposing to neuropathy randomly selected from the community are needed to ensure that normal values (percentiles) can be estimated. It may be that the variability in later decades of life is simply too great to allow this technique to be a useful primary endpoint for controlled clinical trials, especially of old people. A further major concern is that the endpoint will not be seen by the general medical community as a clinically meaningful endpoint of the neuropathy to be studied. It may be difficult to extrapolate from a change in density of fibers of a skin biopsy to overall severity of polyneuropathy.

Functional Scales of Activities of Daily Living

The activities of daily living which a person can or cannot perform may be a useful measure of the severity of neuromuscular disease in a given patient. Generally, the scales define broad categories especially of severe motor dysfunction, and therefore tend to be more useful for paralytic than for sensory and autonomic disorders. Because defined categories or stages of dysfunction tend to represent large differences in neuromuscular dysfunction, a recognized statistically significant change between groups should be clinically useful or meaningful. The approach, therefore, may be a good measure in such conditions as AIDP, CIDP and MGUS neuropathy. Because dysfunction is influenced by motivation and secondary gain, functional scales may not be as objective as desired. The work and lifestyle implications of neurologic impairment are quite variable, depending on psychologic outlook, education, kind of work, and many other variables.

Here we will not comprehensively review the many scales of function which have been published. To illustrate the approaches, two such scales will be given. In the modified Rankin scale, five grades of severity are used: 1 = no symptoms; 2 = slight disability, unable to carry out all previous activities, but able to look after their own affairs without assistance; 3 = moderate disability, requiring some help, but able to walk without assistance; 4 = moderately severe disability, unable to walk without assistance and unable to tend to own bodily needs without assistance; and 5 = severe disability, bedridden, incoherent, and requiring constant nursing care and attention.

The Rankin score might be considered for studies of AIDP, CIDP or MGUS neuropathy, but probably would not be useful for many neuropathies, e.g., DPN. Many of the disabilities would be dependent on motivation, physical characteristics (e.g., weight), age, sex, and activities which need to be performed. It is conceivable that a patient may have little impairment (as evaluated by a physician) and have a high score on the Rankin score and vice versa.

Hughes [13] developed a functional scale for assessment of therapy in AIDP (see Chapter 37, Table 37.1). This scale categorized patients by their ability to walk with or without support and for a given distance, need for assisted ventilation, and death. The scale tends to be useful only for disorders with generalized paralysis such as AIDP. It has some of the limitations of the Rankin scale.

Composite Scores of Overall Neuropathy Impairment

There are several reasons why an overall assessment of severity of neuropathy is better than a simple determination of whether neuropathy is present or not based on one or a few markers. The assessment that is needed is not unlike an appraisal of a house after a fire or an automobile after a collision. One needs a tally of the components which need to be repaired and the cost of replacement of the faulty components. The ill-health of a person, e.g., neuropathy, might similarly be comprehensively surveyed by a list of the motor, sensory and autonomic symptoms and impairments (the kind and severity)

which have become dysfunctional from a given disease. Increasingly physicians have had to list the extent and severity of such diseases as cancer, retinopathy and neuropathy.

For peripheral neuropathy, approaches have been introduced to quantitate all the symptoms into an overall score of symptoms. In an earlier section of this chapter we described how this may be done using a tally of symptoms (the NSS) or number of symptoms, severity of symptoms and change in symptoms (the NSC). Likewise, in the NIS, we summate all neurologic abnormalities in one overall score based on a standard examination encompassing the neurologic examination. This technique provides a useful way of having one number represent overall impairment. One can combine symptoms and overall impairment in a staging approach. We have developed a staging approach for DPN: N0 = no neuropathy, N1 = asymptomatic DPN, N1a = abnormality of NC or HB DB without neurologic abnormality, N1b = abnormality of NC or HB DB with neurologic abnormality, N2 = symptomatic DPN, N2a = able to walk on heels, N2b = unable to walk on heels, and N3 = disabling neuropathy.

Abnormal Limits of Tests and Composite Evaluations Using Percentiles

There are measurable advantages to providing defined abnormal limits (≥95th percentile, ≥99th percentile, or other) for test results specific for test, site, age, gender and applicable physical variables. Expressing a patient's test abnormality as a percentile response, considering these variables, one can more accurately express the change attributable to the disease studied and how it is influenced by treatment. One can, therefore, directly compare the influence of a therapeutic agent free from the influence of age, gender, weight or other variables. To develop such normal percentile values, it is important to evaluate a representative and sufficiently large (e.g., 300 to 1000 persons) cohort of healthy subjects drawn from the same population as the study population. Further, one would like to exclude patients with neurologic disease or neuropathy or diseases known to predispose to neuropathy. Obviously the tests should be performed exactly as they are in the study population.

Quality Assurance

The subject of quality assurance is a broad one. To begin with, tests should be obtained under optimal conditions, by standard and the best approaches, results should be accurately and fully recorded and transmitted to a data center. Quality assurance comprises all the procedures and surveillance necessary to ensure that data are accurately obtained, stored, transmitted and analyzed. For the study of peripheral neuropathy, it may be necessary to have a reading and quality assurance center to validate that certain neurologic tests are adequately performed and interpreted. Neuropathic symptoms, neurologic examination abnormalities, nerve conduction abnormalities, quantitative sensory test abnormalities and quantitative autonomic test abnormalities are test items that may need such quality assurance. In the first place one wants to grade only those abnormalities related to the variety of neuropahy studied. Neurologic abnormalities related to concurrent physical abnormalities or neurologic disease simply add noise to the data. In the second place, one wants to measure only disease abnormality and with low inter- and intra-observer variability. The quality assurance center tries to ensure that these goals are met. These points may be illustrated by consideration of conduct of the nerve conduction examination. An expert electromyographer may be able to detect that the limb temperature was too low, that there was anatomic cross-over of a nerve, that the recorded action potential came from a nerve other than that which was to have been stimulated, and so on. Such quality control may be necessary to achieve an accurate and statistically significant result. It should be appreciated that even a good-quality assurance center cannot overcome poor-quality data from participating centers. There is a trade-off between use of many participating centers sending a mixture of good and mediocre data and fewer centers sending only good data.

To improve this variability, we advocate the following: (1) use of standard tests with all aspects of testing and estimating results following the same rules that are, if possible, pre-programmed, (2) the abnormal limit to be used should be the same and a rigorous one, e.g., 99th or 1st percentile for individual test, and 97.5th for a composite score, (3) for the neurologic examination, board-eligible or certified specialists should do the examinations – particularly to recognize other disease conditions causing neuropathy, (4) the same neurologists should do all the examinations in a given patient, (5) the neurologist should be blinded not only to treatment schedule but also to side effects which might allow him or her to surmise which treatment was involved, (6) at the end of the trial, the patient and investigator should state whether they thought treatment or placebo was being given, (7) the order of testing should emphasize performing the primary test before others (e.g., NIS before NSC), (8) primary clinical tests should be done in duplicate at the beginning and end of trials, and (9) there should be quality assurance of clinical records, QST and nerve conduction by experts to correct or repeat inadequately obtained endpoints.

Quality control for the clinical examination in multicenter trials is facilitated by having: (1) specially prepared instructional material – how-to-do manuals, (2) a demonstration video, (3) training sessions and (4) quality reading centers. For nerve conduction evaluation, certified electromyographers should be used and they should use standard electrodes, placements and stimulation and recording techniques. Abnormality should be expressed as a percentile (and normal deviate) specific for test, site, age, gender and other applicable physical variables. The quality assurance electromyographer should actually review the submitted tracings and values to detect the influence of low temperature, spurious or incorrect waveform, anatomic cross-over, disease conditions other than the ones studied and gross errors. If an error has occurred, the patient will probably have to be recalled. If inaccurate and consistent results cannot be achieved by a center, that center should be disqualified from participation.

For the clinical neurologic evaluation, the quality reading and assurance center may stress to participating investigators that specificity is to be emphasized over sensitivity. Neurologists should grade only neurologic abnormalities they judge to be due to the disease process studied. They should judge disease abnormality beyond what is attributed to be due to age, sex, height, weight, unfitness, and so on. The quality assurance center may wish to compare functional tests (e.g., walking on toes, on heels, or rising from a kneeling position) with manual testing of these functions. If excessive variability is uncovered, the evaluations are repeated. The quality assurance neurologist looks especially for unbelievable results: findings not appropriate for the diagnosis, excessive variability in repeat examinations, and so on.

As discussed below, measurements of endpoints are usually made at the beginning and end of a trial, and perhaps once or twice between (to recognize an early effect). Assuming the initial double evaluations to be satisfactory, one uses the mean of the assessments. If they are not, a third measurement is made and the median value is used.

Statistical Considerations

Interim Analyses

It is desirable to monitor the results of clinical trials as they progress with a view towards terminating early if the results become overwhelmingly apparent prior to the scheduled end of the study. There are several reasons for wanting to have the option to terminate early. Perhaps one of the most compelling is the ethical requirement to make a new treatment available as soon as possible. There are also obvious financial considerations, which include the costs of continuing a trial and the desirability of bringing a new drug to market as soon as possible. In addition, by terminating a trial early, patients may become available for alternate trials. Another factor which may become relevant is the availability of alternate treatments and the results of other studies which may become available during the course of a trial.

However, there are also important factors which militate against early termination. These may often be less apparent than the reasons for early termination, but they need to be considered in arriving at the ultimate decision. One concern is that, although adequate information may be available to conclude that the new treatment is efficacious, the available information may be insufficient to answer all the scientific questions of interest. These may relate to mechanisms of action and identifying subgroups of patients that may respond differently from the overall group.

Another concern results from the fact that early termination occurs when the effects of treatment are observed to be especially positive or negative, thus biasing estimates of the true magnitude of the effect. Although statistical techniques are available in some instances to adjust for this bias, they are often quite complicated and difficult to interpret.

Early termination may also increase the probability of coming to a wrong conclusion about efficacy. One concern is that, by assessing efficacy on multiple occasions, one may be overly impressed by an optimistic result, increasing the chances of incorrectly concluding that a treatment is efficacious. Again statistical techniques are available for dealing with this problem. However, one must be alert to the concern that some of these techniques may markedly increase the total number of subjects required to complete the trial if early termination does not occur. Alternatively, terminating early to conclude that the new treatment is not efficacious will increase the possibility that an efficacious treatment may go undetected. Again, statistical techniques are available to assess the magnitude of this effect.

In order to allow for the possibility of terminating a trial early to conclude efficacy, the criteria which will be used must be stated in the protocol prior to initiating the trial. Various statistical stopping rules are available. The most commonly used approach is called group sequential testing. An example of this method is the O'Brien–Fleming boundary. To illus-

trate, if one wished to plan for two interim analyses at equally spaced points during the trial as an alternative to performing a single two-sided test at the end, the p values which would need to be exceeded at each of these analyses or at the end in order to achieve statistical significance would be 0.001, 0.015 and 0.047.

Notice that, with these interim analyses built into the study design, it will no longer suffice to obtain a p value less than 0.05 at the end of the study. Thus, in order to maintain the original power (probability of detecting a treatment effect), it is necessary to increase the maximal sample size (the number of patients required if early termination does not occur). Since many factors need to be considered in arriving at the decision whether or not to terminate a trial early, of which crossing the statistical boundary is just one, that statistical stopping "rule" should be viewed as providing guidelines for early termination rather than a hard and fast rule requiring termination.

Group sequential methods are less helpful in determining whether a trial should be terminated early due to lack of efficacy. The reason is that convincing evidence is required to conclude that a new treatment is efficacious. However, if the effect is observed to go in the wrong direction, one would not want to require convincing evidence that the treatment is harmful to stop the trial, just a high level of confidence that, were the study to continue to the end, a conclusion of efficacy would not occur.

The statistical approach used to determine the chances of achieving statistical significance if the study is continued to the end, given the existing results, is called conditional power. Specifically, one might ask what the probability is of achieving significance if the treatment effect was of the magnitude originally hypothesized in the study design. Although of interest, this question becomes less relevant if the available data suggest that such an effect is quite implausible. In some instances, formal statistical algorithms are not especially helpful in judging the need to stop early for lack of an effect. Particularly important in these circumstances are the risks to the patients of participating in the trial, the costs of continuing, and whether the negative results observed in the primary endpoint is also observed uniformly in the secondary analyses.

Multiple Endpoints and Time to Event Endpoints

In order to control the type I error rate (falsely declaring a treatment to be efficacious) at the 0.05 level, it is necessary for the protocol to specify a single statistical test or composite measure which will be used in the determination of efficacy. This is referred to as the primary analysis, and it usually specifies a single endpoint which will be used. However, in some instances there are several equally important endpoints. In these situations, it may be undesirable to arbitrarily specify one as the primary endpoint, effectively disregarding the information available from the other endpoints in the primary analysis.

Ideally, one would combine the information from the various endpoints in a clinically meaningful way, thus arriving at a single "combined endpoint." Methods for combining endpoints in peripheral neuropathy have been discussed previously. Unfortunately, in some instances, it may not be feasible to obtain such a clinically meaningful overall assessment which will be acceptable to the medical community at large. When a clinically meaningful method for combining multiple endpoints is not available, an alternate statistical algorithm which weights the endpoints equally may be helpful [12].

The method is as follows. For each endpoint considered individually, rank the response from each subject in the study from best to worst. (The best response is assigned a rank of 1, the second best a rank of 2, and so forth. If ties are observed when assigning ranks, assign the mean rank.) Then, for each subject in the study, sum the ranks assigned to the various endpoints, obtaining a rank sum score for each subject. Using the rank sum scores as the combined endpoint, any of the usual two-sample statistical tests (such as the two-sample t-test) can be used.

Endpoints which pose special statistical issues are "time to event" endpoints. An example would be time to progression of disease (suitably defined), in which not all patients will experience progression. When time to progression is the only primary endpoint, suitable statistical techniques (life table methods, using Kaplan–Meier survival curves and log rank tests, for example) are available. When time to progression is one of multiple primary endpoints, a rank sum score can be obtained by ranking the log rank scores used in computing the log rank test.

An additional concern arises when using time to event endpoints: the experience of patients after experiencing the event will not be considered. For example, one might define progression to be worsening of NIS(LL) + 7 by 1 point. The possibility exists that a new treatment may delay progression so defined, and yet at the end of a 3 year study treated patients may have higher NIS(LL) + 7 scores than untreated patients.

This problem with time to event endpoints is of particular concern in interim testing. For example, the percent of patients experiencing the endpoint at

1 year might be markedly less for the treated patients, but by 2 years the percentages may be no different or even reversed.

Heterogeneous Treatment Effects

A central focus of the primary analysis assessing efficacy is whether or not the apparent treatment effect might occur by chance. The convention is that, if the observed superiority of the new treatment would occur in the absence of a true benefit (that is, by chance) less than 5% of the time, then the results are judged to be statistically significant. The standard statistical tests for making this comparison (the t and rank sum tests) assume that the beneficial effects of the new treatment are homogeneous: that they improve response by exactly the same amount in every patient. Of course, this is quite unrealistic. However, if the assumption is at least approximately true, the tests will perform well in identifying a treatment effect. On occasion, however, the nature of the heterogeneity is such that obvious treatment effects will be missed by the standard tests and judged to be not significant.

One way to investigate the possibility of heterogeneous effects is to develop a mathematical model which will include terms which identify and quantify the factors which account for the heterogeneity, then identify additional terms in the model which will accurately relate these factors to treatment effects. Unfortunately, these factors are often unknown or difficult to measure, and developing a model which accurately reflects their association with treatment effects may be tenuous.

An alternate approach is to test for the existence of heterogeneous effects. If significant evidence of heterogeneity is observed, then one must typically take a closer look at the data to identify the nature of the true treatment effect. Examples illustrating the use of this approach are provided in O'Brien and Dyck [9] and Dyck et al. [8].

References

1. Dyck PJ, Litchy WJ, Kratz KM, et al. A plasma exchange versus immune globulin infusion trial in chronic inflammatory demyelinating polyradiculoneuropathy. Ann Neurol 1994;36: 838.
2. Dyck PJ, Low PA, Windebank AJ, et al. Plasma exchange in polyneuropathy associated with monoclonal gammopathy of undetermined significance. N Engl J Med 1991;325: 1482.
3. Dyck PJ, Dyck PJB, Grant IA, Fealey RD. Ten steps in characterizing and diagnosing patients with peripheral neuropathy. Neurology 1996;47:10.
4. Dyck PJ, Davies JL, Litchy WJ, O'Brien PC. Longitudinal assessment of diabetic polyneuropathy using a composite score in

the Rochester Diabetic Neuropathy Study cohort. Neurology 1997;49:229.

5. Dyck PJ, Kratz KM, Karnes JL, et al. The prevalence by staged severity of various types of diabetic neuropathy, retinopathy, and nephropathy in a population-based cohort: the Rochester Diabetic Neuropathy Study. Neurology 1993;43:817.

6. Dyck PJ, Sherman WR, Hallcher LM, et al. Human diabetic endoneurial sorbitol, fructose, and myo-inositol related to sural nerve morphometry. Ann Neurol 1980;8:590.

7. Dyck PJ, Karnes J, O'Brien PC, Swanson CJ. Neuropathy symptom profile in health, motor neuron disease, diabetic neuropathy, and amyloidosis. Neurology 1986;36:1300.

8. Dyck PJ, Litchy WJ, Lehman KA, Hokanson JL, Low PA, O'Brien PC. Variables influencing neuropathic endpoints: the Rochester Diabetic Neuropathy Study of Healthy Subjects (RDNS-HS). Neurology 1995;45:1115.

9. O'Brien PC, Dyck PJ. Procedures for setting normal values. Neurology 1995;45:17.

10. Low PA. Clinical autonomic disorders: evaluation and management. Boston: Little, Brown, 1993.

11. Dyck PJ. Diabetic polyneuropathy in controlled clinical trials: consensus report of the Peripheral Nerve Society. Ann Neurol 1995;38:478.

12. O'Brien PC. Procedures for comparny samples with multiple endpoints. Biometrics 1984;40:1079–1088.

13. Guillain-Barré syndrome Steroid Trial Group. Double blind trial of intravenous methylprednisolone in Guillain-Barré Syndrome, Lancet 1993;341:586–590.

37. Peripheral Neuropathies: Experience with Large Multicentre Trials

V. Bril

Introduction

Peripheral neuropathies pose a peculiar challenge in assessing response to therapeutic interventions. Superficially, one would expect it to be a simple matter to assess the presence or lack of response to any intervention in peripheral neuropathies. After all, the peripheral nervous system is readily available to examination by both non-invasive and invasive tests. Experience has proved this to be a false expectation when dealing with chronic axonal neuropathies. For the most part, no therapy is available for these neuropathies. Generally, the elimination of cause (e.g. toxic drug) or minimisation of metabolic derangement (e.g. impaired glycaemic control) are the only therapies available for chronic neuropathies. As more therapeutic interventions are proposed (e.g. aldose reductase inhibitors in diabetic polyneuropathy, nerve growth factor for small-fibre neuropathies), accurate methods of assessing response are essential. In the case of autoimmune neuropathies – e.g. acute inflammatory demyelinating polyneuropathy (AIDP), chronic inflammatory demyelinating polyneuropathy (CIDP) – positive clinical and electrophysiological therapeutic responses are shown more readily, and successful therapies are available.

Demyelinating Versus Axonal Neuropathies

In the autoimmune demyelinating polyneuropathies, efficacy end-points are straightforward, and mainly clinical. For example, in AIDP, or Guillain–Barré Syndrome (GBS), therapeutic trials of corticosteroids, plasma exchange and intravenous immunoglobulin have used clinical grading scales successfully [1–4] (Table 37.1). The degree of clinical deficit in GBS typically is large and readily assessed by clinical examination alone, and significant clinical change between grades is easily agreed upon and measured. Therefore, efficacy can be followed clinically. Other measures such as electrophysiological changes are ancillary, and useful for prognosis more than for response to treatment since clinical testing alone is sufficient to show efficacy [5]. Even with large clinical changes in a relatively uniform disorder such as GBS, power analysis indicates a requirement for large numbers of patients in multicentre trials for adequate statistical evaluation of outcomes [2,3] due to the inherent variability in natural history. As a result, multicentre trials are essential in order to obtain sufficient numbers of patients to prove a therapy's efficacy. This requirement carries with it an inevitable increase in variability due to centre effect. With large clinical changes, easy grading system and statistical adjustments for study centre, variability across sites due to different investigators is not a major drawback, and trials in GBS have been successful in providing both positive [2,3] results for plasma exchange and intravenous immunoglobulin, and negative results [4,6] for high-dose corticosteroid therapy.

In CIDP, large clinical and electrophysiological changes can occur, and can be demonstrated in trials with smaller numbers of patients since the course is more uniform, and often unremitting without therapy [7,8]. The efficacy of various interventions is shown and assessed more readily in this demyelinating form of neuropathy [7,8].

In chronic axonal neuropathies, the challenges are far greater. Development of these neuropathies takes place over many years: approximately 10 years for diabetes mellitus (DM), and a similar duration for alcoholic and uraemic neuropathy. Although the diagnosis of non-insulin-dependent diabetes mellitus (NIDDM) may be made at the time of presentation of peripheral neuropathy, it is generally accepted that the patient has had preceding, undiagnosed DM for some time prior to the onset of the neuropathy.

Table 37.1. Hughes' clinical grades in Guillain–Barré syndrome [4]

Grade 0	Healthy, no signs or symptoms of Guillain–Barré syndrome
Grade 1	Minor symptoms or signs and able to run
Grade 2	Able to walk 5 m across an open space without assistance
Grade 3	Able to walk 5 m across an open space with the help of one person and waist-level walking-frame, stick or sticks
Grade 4	Chairbound/bedbound; unable to walk as in grade 3
Grade 5	Requiring assisted ventilation (for at least part of the day or night)
Grade 6	Dead

Chronic axonal neuropathies develop insidiously. An overt relationship between symptoms and pathology can be lacking [9]. The pathophysiology of neuropathic symptoms is unclear in many chronic axonal neuropathies [10]. The clinical presentations even in the same metabolic disorder (e.g. DM) are highly variable and inconsistent from patient to patient [11]. Increasing symptoms may indicate nerve regeneration with discharges from immature axons [10,11], while a reduction in painful symptoms may indicate total loss of nerve fibres with progression of neuropathy [9]. Therefore, following response on the basis of symptomatic improvement can be misleading and erroneous.

Successful therapy will depend on nerve regeneration in these chronic axonal processes. The regenerating axons will need to form functional connections with end-organs for successful recovery from neuropathy. Nerve sprouts develop at the distal axon terminals and recovery will occur along the length of the neurone. Whether reversal of chronic axonal pathological processes can occur is debatable. Slowing of progression and some clinical improvement have been observed [12,13], but total reversal may be an unrealistic goal. Interventions producing even limited clinical recovery are likely to require long treatment intervals if they are to be successful, e.g. a minimum of 3 years and probably 5 years or more [13]. Most pharmaceutical firms are unwilling to continue double-blind studies for this long due to the costs involved. Clinical improvements are unlikely to be observed earlier. Additionally, the improvement is most evident in those with less severe neuropathy when the intervention is started [12].

Given these considerations, surrogate end-points have been advocated. A primary surrogate marker in peripheral nerve disease is electrophysiological testing, or nerve conduction studies (NCS). Electrophysiological testing which measures peripheral nerve function has a major role in demyelinating peripheral neuropathies [14–18]. The utility of NCS in chronic axonal processes is more limited. When monitoring nerve function by NCS, the changes observed in 12 months are small as most chronic axonal neuropathies by their nature will not show major changes in nerve conduction velocity or amplitudes in this period of time [12,19]. Additionally, a single surrogate measure of improvement in peripheral neuropathies is inadequate to prove therapeutic efficacy for many governmental agencies (Federal Drug Administration Advisory Board Meeting, US Government). Additional surrogate measures are necessary. Sural nerve biopsy has been used successfully in some therapeutic trials ([12], D.A. Greene et al. [13]); this is an invasive method of assessing peripheral nerve activity. Other surrogate markers used include quantitative sensory testing (QST) and quantitative autonomic testing (QAT). These are useful in the definition of peripheral neuropathy as well as for efficacy testing, but all surrogate markers have drawbacks as discussed below.

In summary, efficacy has been easier to demonstrate in primary demyelinating polyneuropathies with major motor deficits than in chronic axonal neuropathies, on both clinical and electrophysiological grounds. These large-fibre neuropathies are easier to treat in the clinic. Chronic axonal neuropathies have failed to show major clinical improvements with therapy other than with prolonged treatment intervals of at least 5 years, such as in diabetic polyneuropathy in the Diabetes Control and Complications Trial (DCCT) [14]. Planned trials of any new intervention in peripheral nerve disease must consider these limitations.

Definition

In AIDP, definition is not difficult clinically. A certain profile of neurological symptoms and signs defines the disorder. Clinical criteria are available, and agreed upon [20]. Misdiagnoses can occur, but are infrequent. The staging of severity is not difficult [1].

In diabetic chronic peripheral polyneuropathy, criteria for diagnosis are available and accepted by consensus panels [21,22]. Abnormalities in at least two of five areas of peripheral nerve activity are required to define peripheral neuropathy (symptoms, signs, NCS, QST, QAT). Standardisation of measurement techniques has been advocated in all these areas to make testing comparable across multiple centres [23]. As a result of these deliberations, there is general agreement on how to make an appropriate diagnosis of peripheral polyneuropathy in diabetic patients in research trials. Most current trials use these criteria and standards. Similar criteria and standards should be advocated for any research trials in other forms of chronic axonal neuropathy.

Efficacy Parameters

In AIDP, outcome measures are clinical and widely accepted as relevant and meaningful [2,3].

Debate still persists with respect to how to measure therapeutic outcome in chronic axonal neuropathies. The optimal outcome is the complete resolution of both clinical symptoms and abnormal signs, keeping in mind the discrepancy which can be observed between symptoms and pathological alteration in peripheral nerves [9]. Most patients and physicians would consider an improvement towards normal on routine clinical assessments as the optimal outcome in research trials. This result cannot be achieved in brief, 6 to 18 month, trials in disorders which evolve over 5 or 10 or more years. "Resolution of symptoms" is meaningless in cases which are asymptomatic to begin with. Most authorities agree with the use of surrogate measures, although the degree of change needed in those measures is greatly debated. The surrogate measures include NCS, QST, QAT and nerve biopsy. Some agreement is being reached on how surrogate measures are used and interpreted [21].

Electrophysiological Studies

Nerve conduction studies provide the most reliable, sensitive and reproducible measure of peripheral nerve function [15–17,24]. These studies measure peripheral nerve function directly and objectively without contamination by central processes or psychological factors which may confound the results. NCS measure the function of large nerve fibres easily, accurately and reproducibly. In early neuropathy trials, nerve conduction studies were not standardised. Therefore, comparison across multiple centres became problematic. The tests were not monitored by sophisticated reviewers, and major errors entered databases. Specific NCS protocol requirements in a trial extending over 3 years (recruitment 1 year, double-blind therapy 18 months) with testing at the beginning and the end of the study are difficult to remember accurately. Triplicate assessments at the beginning and end might be required by protocol, but at the conclusion of the study the electrophysiologist may not recall the exact procedural requirements. In addition, the training and experience of the personnel performing NCS was not mandated, sometimes resulting in poorly trained and inexperienced individuals carrying out the procedures with inevitable reduction in the quality of the data.

Early trials had a minimum coefficient of variation of nerve conduction velocity of 10–15%, and of nerve potential amplitude of 30–50%. These numbers resulted in a reduction in power of these studies and complete inability to show small changes in amplitude. With insufficient numbers of patients, even small changes in conduction velocity would not be detected. Generally, a small change in conduction velocity of the order of 1 m/s was observed in multiple trials of improved glycaemic control and aldose reductase inhibitor therapy in diabetic polyneuropathy [12,14,19,25–31]. This magnitude of change was disputed to be insignificant, i.e. without any clinical meaning, in the evolution of the disorder.

Monitoring of quality was instituted in early trials and has been continued and refined to the present time with the development of expert "core laboratories". These core laboratories are staffed by expert reviewers who develop specific protocols in concordance with the consensus group views, review qualifications of all electrophysiological personnel in multicentre trials, train these individuals in the study-specific methodology and requirements, and then review acceptability of all curves, worksheets and case report forms for that trial. After corrections of obvious errors, and repeat NCS in cases of protocol violations, the core laboratory functions resulted in optimal NCS with the variability of repeat measures in single patients for conduction velocity of 3% and for amplitudes of 10% across 60 sites (Table 37.2); dramatic results achieving the same variability levels as repeat NCS in single, excellent laboratories [24]. This type of core laboratory increases the power of a study dramatically, and necessitates fewer patients to show significant changes in conduction velocity, and even in amplitude. This was not possible in previous studies.

The limitations of nerve conduction studies are: measurement of only large-fibre function, functional changes in conduction velocity which may not persist with time, inability to show changes in amplitude prior to recent core laboratory developments, inadequate numbers of patients, and inadequate duration of therapy to show amplitude changes.

In AIDP the NCS are useful as large changes in conduction velocity can be expected, and even changes in motor amplitudes are prognostic for outcome [5]. In CIDP, changes in nerve conduction studies can provide a useful measure of efficacy [7].

Quantitative Sensory Testing

QST is a psychophysical measure of peripheral nerve function. Quantifying peripheral sensory function is

Table 37.2. Variability of repeat electrophysiological testing (60 centres)

Parameter	Control subjects (n = 253)	Patients Baseline (n = 1345)	Completion (n = 1144)
Median motor DL	4	4	4
Median motor amplitude wrist	7	10	9
Median motor amplitude elbow	8	11	10
Median motor CV	3	3	3
Median sensory DL	4	4	4
Median sensory amplitude wrist	8	11	11
Median sensory Distal CV	3	4	4
Median sensory amplitude elbow	13	17	17
Median sensory Proximal CV	3	4	3
Peroneal motor DL	5	6	6
Peroneal motor amplitude ankle	9	13	12
Peroneal motor amplitude knee	10	15	13
Peroneal motor CV	3	3	3
Right sural DL	5	6	6
Right sural amplitude	10	16	15
Right sural CV	3	5	4
Left sural DL	4	6	5
Left sural amplitude	10	16	15
Left sural CV	3	5	4

Values are expressed as percentages.
DL, distal latency (ms); amplitude: motor (mV), sensory (μV); CV, conduction velocity (m/s).

an admirable goal. In general, large fibres (Aδ) are assessed by vibratory perception thresholds (VPT) and small fibres (unmyelinated C fibres and thinly myelinated fibres) by thermal perception thresholds (TPT). QST methods are non-invasive and non-painful.

There is controversy about the testing paradigm, the appropriate equipment, and the reproducibility of QST [23,32–34]). Clearly, VPT is more reproducible than TPT, but generally, the variability of repeat testing in the same patient is at least 15% in multicentre trials with the Vibratron (Physitemp Instruments, Clifton, NJ) and 10% with the Neurothesiometer (Scientific Laboratory Supplies, Nottingham, UK). Quantitative thermal thresholds show considerably higher variability (>50% in most trials) unless artificially limited.

In our experience with psychophysical measures, variability can be enormous due to psychological factors completely unrelated to current peripheral

nerve function. As a result, large numbers of patients are needed to show significant changes. No pivotal (phase III) study to date has shown significant QST change as an efficacy parameter; perhaps due to the variability and inadequate numbers of patients studied, or perhaps due to inadequate duration of therapy. QST is valuable as a screening tool, quick if using the method of limits testing (Neurothesiometer), and non-invasive. Utility in large-scale multicentre research trials remains to be proven, although several current trials employ QST as an efficacy parameter in the hope that significant improvement will be detected.

The CASE IV device (W.R. Medical, Minneapolis, MN) is expensive with the same variability found with other equipment, and a very lengthy testing paradigm. The Neurothesiometer examines only Aδ fibre function, not small-fibre activity. However, the testing is rapid and the results show low variability on repeat testing in single subjects [33]. The Vibratron tests the same fibres and is more variable than the Neurothesiometer with the two-forced choice testing paradigm. QST equipment is not readily available, or standardised, and is costly with unreliable results. Its utility in routine diagnosis is uncertain as the site of the lesion accountable for abnormal QST results is unknown and the testing is subjective and may not represent true pathological changes, creating doubts as to how the results are to be interpreted. However, QST can be a useful ancillary efficacy parameter in research trials.

QST has not been used to any great extent in AIDP or CIDP.

Quantitative Autonomic Testing

QAT investigates autonomic fibre function. The importance of this testing in a chronic axonal process such as diabetic peripheral polyneuropathy is well recognised [35,36]. However, QAT is more difficult than QST because of multiple methods, great variability in repeat testing in single subjects, difficulty in testing sympathetic function adequately, and much controversy over the appropriate methods and equipment to be used [37]. An abnormal test result does not predict the outcome reliably. The magnitude of positive change necessary to indicate an efficacious clinical result is uncertain, and no pivotal trials have shown significant change in autonomic function. Large numbers of patients and standardised techniques are required to assess autonomic function adequately [38]. Current tests easily assess cardiovascular reflexes. No routine investigations are widely accepted and used for sweating regulation, gastrointestinal, bladder or sexual function. Multiple difficulties persist with many false positive results which cannot be controlled in the assessments. The role of QAT remains strictly investigative currently. QAT must be standardised and quality-controlled with respect to testing procedures, and data resulting from the testing. The practical significance of QAT is still limited because of high variability (at least 15% in carefully controlled studies [38]), uncertainty about the meaning of the results, and uncertainty whether changes can be effected, particularly in a short treatment interval.

QAT has not been used widely in AIDP or CIDP.

Symptoms

The assessment of symptoms can be the most difficult with respect to their meaning, presence and implication in chronic axonal neuropathies. Their assessment should be done by a neurologist, well-trained internist, or physician with some insight into neurological disorders [11]. In spite of such precautions, symptoms are highly variable in the same patient on repeated assessments within a short period of time, and very variable over longer intervals of time. Symptoms are highly variable from patient to patient with the same severity of neuropathy. Symptoms can be absent in end-stage neuropathy. It is undisputed that the symptomatic state is important to the patient's sense of well-being, but symptoms cannot be used in isolation or even for secondary efficacy very easily or meaningfully in large-scale trials at this time.

Symptoms are more useful in AIDP as weakness can be profound. The pathophysiology of CIDP is also usually reflected more accurately by the symptomatic state.

Signs

Signs are easier to standardise than the symptoms in chronic axonal neuropathies. Typically, patients have a peripheral glove-and-stocking sensory loss and depression of ankle reflexes [11]. The meaning of some findings in patients over 60 years of age can be debatable (for example, absence of ankle reflexes may be considered a normal variant). Comparison of the findings with a reference population is optimal, but not always possible as reference populations may not be uniform in all geographic areas. The findings in chronic axonal neuropathies develop slowly over many years, and reversal or major improvement over 6–18 months of treatment is unlikely. The sensory levels detected on clinical examination are also a psychophysical measure with high variability. The typical experience in neurological clinics is that the findings can change within a few minutes as different examiners assess the same patient. The deficits are not fixed, but change from examination to examination for uncertain reasons. This observation indicates that sensory levels are not reliable, or reproducible. However, the deficits are very important to the patient.

In AIDP and CIDP, measurement of motor deficits is more reliable and reproducible. In AIDP, diffuse motor weakness, areflexia and minimal sensory loss are found. Using the British MRC scale of 0–5 for muscle strength, and a grading scale such as that proposed by Hughes [4], makes evaluation more straightforward.

Summary

Multicentre therapeutic trials in demyelinating polyneuropathies have been successful largely due to the ease with which these neuropathies can be assessed clinically. Therapeutic trials in chronic axonal neuropathy have been plagued by the limitations of clinical evaluation, uncertainty as to the clinical relevance of surrogate markers, controversy over efficacy parameters, and lack of knowledge on how surrogate markers should best be measured. The degree of positive, detectable change in surrogate markers in a short, 12 month trial is very small and leads to questions concerning the adequate duration of therapy necessary to prove efficacy of investigational drugs and/or other interventions. Much has been learned about how trials should be designed and run in the last 15 years, but these lessons are often overlooked in the design of new trials, with not unexpected negative outcomes.

References

1. Hughes R, Newsom-Davis J, Perkin G, Pierce J. Controlled trial of prednisolone in acute polyneuropathy. Lancet 1978;II: 750–753.
2. Guillain–Barré Syndrome Study Group. Plasmapheresis and acute Guillain–Barré syndrome. Neurology 1985;35:1096–1104.
3. Plasma Exchange/Sandoglobulin Guillain–Barré Syndrome Trial Group. Randomised trial of plasma exchange, intravenous immunoglobulin, and combined treatments in Guillain–Barré syndrome. Lancet 1997;349:225–229.
4. Guillain–Barré Syndrome Steroid Trial Group. Double-blind trial of intravenous methylprednisolone in Guillain–Barré syndrome. Lancet 1993;341:586–590.
5. Cornblath D, Mellitts E, Griffin J, McKhann GM, Albers JW, Miller RG, et al. Motor conduction studies in Guillain–Barré syndrome: description and prognostic value. Ann Neurol 1988;23:354–359.
6. Hughes R. Ineffectiveness of high-dose intravenous methylprednisolone in Guillain–Barré syndrome. Lancet 1991;338: 1142.

7. Hahn A, Bolton C, Pillay N, Chalk C, Benstead T, Bril V, et al. Plasma-exchange therapy in chronic inflammatory demyelinating polyneuropathy. Brain 1996;119:1055–1066.

8. Dyck P, Litchy W, Kratz K, Suarez G, Low P, Pineda A, et al. A plasma exchange versus immune globulin infusion trial in chronic inflammatory demyelinating polyradiculoneuropathy. Ann Neurol 1994;36:838–845.

9. Britland S, Young R, Sharma A, Clarke B. Association of painful and painless diabetic polyneuropathy with different patterns of nerve fiber degeneration and regeneration. Diabetes 1990; 39:898–908.

10. Ochoa J. Positive sensory symptoms in neuropathy: mechanisms and aspects of treatment. In: Asbury A, Thomas P, editors. Peripheral nerve disorders 2. Oxford: Butterworth-Heinemann, 1995:44–58.

11. Dyck P. Quantitating severity of neuropathy. In: Dyck P, Thomas P, Griffin J, Low P, Poduslo J, editors. Peripheral neuropathy. Philadelphia: Saunders, 1993:685–697.

12. Sima A, Bril V, Nathaniel V, McEwen T, Brown M, Lattimer S, et al. Regeneration and repair of myelinated fibers in sural nerve biopsies from patients with diabetic neuropathy treated with sorbinil, an investigational aldose reductase inhibitor. N Engl J Med 1988;319:548–555.

13. Green DA, Arezzo JC, Brown MD. The Zenarestat Study Group, Effect of aldose reductase inhibition on nerve conduction and morphometry in diabetic neuropathy. Neurology 1999;53: 580–591.

14. Diabetes Control and Complications Trial Research Group. The effect of intensive treatment of diabetes on the development and progression of long-term complications in insulin-dependent diabetes mellitus. N Engl J Med 1993;329:977–986.

15. Arezzo J. The use of electrophysiology for the assessment of diabetic neuropathy. Neurosci Res Commun 1997;21:13–23.

16. Bril V. Role of electrophysiological studies in diabetic neuropathy. Can J Neurol Sci 1994;21:S8–S12.

17. Daube J. Electrophysiologic Testing in diabetic neuropathy. In: Dyck P, Thomas P, Asbury A, Winegrad A, Porte DJ, editors. Diabetic Neuropathy. Philadelphia: Saunders, 1987;162–176.

18. Lamontagne A, Buchthal G. Electrophysiological studies in diabetic neuropathy. J Neurol Neurosurg Psychiatry 1970; 33:442–452.

19. Macleod A, Till S, Sonksen P. Discussion of the clinical trials of the aldose reductase inhibitor, tolrestat. Int Proc J 1991;4: 17–24.

20. Ad Hoc Subcommittee of the American Academy of Neurology AIDS Task Force. Research criteria for diagnosis of chronic inflammatory demyelinating polyneuropathy (CIDP). Neurology 1991;41:617–618.

21. Peripheral Nerve Society. Diabetic polyneuropathy in controlled clinical trials: consensus report of the peripheral nerve society. Ann Neurol 1995;38:478–482.

22. Consensus Statement of the American Diabetes Association and the American Academy of Neurology. Report and recommendations of the San Antonio conference on diabetic neuropathy. Diabetes 1988;37:1000–1004.

23. Consensus Statement. Proceedings of a consensus development conference on standardized measures in diabetic neuropathy. Neurology 1992;42:1823–1829.

24. Bril V, Ellison R, Ngo M, Bergstrom B, Raynard D, Gin H, Roche Neuropathy Study Group. Electrophysiological monitoring in clinical trials. Muscle Nerve 1998;21:1348–1393.

25. Judzewitsch R, Jaspan J, Polonsky K, Weinberg C, Halter J, Halar E, et al. Aldose reductase inhibition improves nerve conduction velocity in diabetic patients. N Engl J Med 1983; 308:119–125.

26. Macleod A, Boulton A, Owens D, Van Rooy P, Van Gerven JM, Macrury S, et al. A multicentre trial of the aldose-reductase inhibitor, tolrestat, in patients with symptomatic diabetic peripheral neuropathy. Diabete Metab 1992;18:14–20.

27. Malone JI, Lowitt S, Korthals JK, Salem A, Miranda C. The effect of hyperglycemia on nerve conduction and structure is age dependent. Diabetes 1996;45:209–215.

28. Reichard P, Nilsson B, Rosenqvist U. The effect of long-term intensified insulin treatment on the development of microvascular complications of diabetes mellitus. N Engl J Med 1993;329:304–309.

29. Service F, Rizza R, Daube J, O'Brien P, Dyck P. Near normoglycaemia improved nerve conduction and vibration sensation in diabetic neuropathy. Diabetologia 1985;28:722–727.

30. Troni W, Carta Q, Cantello R, Caselle MT, Rainero I. Peripheral nerve function and metabolic control in diabetes mellitus. Ann Neurol 1984;16:178–183.

31. Young R, Ewing D, Clarke B. A controlled trial of sorbinil, an aldose reductase inhibitor, in chronic painful diabetic neuropathy. Diabetes 1983;32:938–942.

32. Arezzo J, Schaumburg J, Petersen C. Rapid screening for peripheral neuropathy: a field study with the Optacon. Neurology 1983;33:626–629.

33. Bril V, Kojic J, Ngo M, Clark K. Comparison of a Neurothesiometer and Vibratron in measuring vibration perception thresholds and relationship to nerve conduction studies. Diabetes Care 1997;20:1360–1362.

34. Yarnitsky D. Quantitative sensory testing. Muscle Nerve 1997;20:198–204.

35. Ewing D, Campbell I, Clarke B. The natural history of diabetic autonomic neuropathy. Am J Med 1980;49:95–108.

36. Rathmann W, Ziegler D, Jahnke M, Haastert B, Gries F. Mortality in diabetic patients with cardiovascular autonomic neuropathy. Diabet Med 1993;10:820–824.

37. Low P. Pitfalls in autonomic testing. In: Low P, editor. Clinical autonomic disorders: evaluation and management. Boston: Little, Brown, 1993:355–365.

38. Low P, Pfeifer M. Standardization of clinical tests for practice and clinical trials. In: Low P, editor. Clinical autonomic disorders: evaluation and management. Boston: Little, Brown, 1993: 287–296.

38. Disorders of the Neuromuscular Junction: Outcome Measures and Clinical Scales

J.B.M. Kuks and H.J.G.H. Oosterhuis

Introduction

In this chapter disorders of the neuromuscular junction are described. The main symptom of these diseases is fluctuating weakness of voluntary muscles associated with fatigability. Myasthenia gravis (MG), the most well-known disorder in this group, is caused by a postsynaptic disturbance, while the Lambert–Eaton myasthenic syndrome is a prototype of a presynaptic defect. In addition a number of rare diseases of the neuromuscular junction are recognised: kinetic abnormalities of the acetylcholine receptor (the slow channel syndrome), or structural deficits such as end-plate acetylcholinesterase deficiency, paucity of synaptic vesicles, and others. Presynaptic and congenital disorders will not be considered here. The same rules as for MG will hold for trials in patients with these syndromes.

Clinical and Epidemiological Characteristics of Myasthenia Gravis

MG may affect any voluntary muscle but the involvement of one or more cranial muscles is almost obligatory. The diagnosis can be surmised from a history with fluctuating symptoms of weakness. Clinical examination with prolonged testing of muscle strength may render further evidence. The presence of autoantibodies to the acetylcholine receptor (see below), reaction to anticholinesterases, decrement at repetitive nerve stimulation [1] and increased jitter at single-fibre electromyography [2,3] provide further support for the diagnosis.

In most patients MG is a disease acquired during life. However, congenital MG exists and should be differentiated from the acquired type as clinical characteristics and therapeutic management vary for the two entities [4].

The prevalence of MG is reported to be around 50–100 per million, with an increased prevalence in more recent studies [5,6], reflecting both improved diagnosis and a better prognosis in the latter years. MG may become manifest at any age, with a peak age at onset in the twenties for women and some 10 years later for men. A second peak is reported between 51 and 60 years [7].

Because of the use of several dramatic therapies the natural course of MG has become uncertain. Before the introduction of immunomodulating therapies a disease-related mortality rate of 25–30% was found, with most patients dying in the first 5 years of MG; 40% of patients were reported to improve spontaneously after several years. In most patients the disease gradually develops to a maximum intensity in the initial 3–5 years. Spontaneous transitory remissions may occur in 20% in the first year. Patients who survive the first years usually improve subsequently or maintain a steady state; a spontaneous remission rate of 21% and an improvement rate of 37% were found in a cohort study of 62 patients with a mean follow-up of 21 years [5]. These percentages may be still higher because mild cases of MG might previously have remained undiagnosed.

Pathophysiology of MG

It is now clear that MG results from a deficiency of normally functioning acetylcholine receptors (AChR) on the postsynaptic muscle membrane. Circulating antibodies directed to the acetylcholine receptor (a-AChR) accelerate the degradation of AChRs by cross-linking the receptor molecules, others interfere with neurotransmitter binding, channel opening or with ionic fluxes, and finally a-AChR may lead to complement-mediated membrane lysis [8].

There is a poor correlation between a-AChR serum levels and the clinical state across individuals

[9], but within an individual patient serum levels fluctuate with the clinical course [10].

In spite of sensitive a-AChR assays a category of patients seronegative for a-AChR antibodies remains. It is not established whether these patients have another type of pathophysiology and whether seronegative patients can be compared clinically with seropositive ones.

Thymic abnormalities are found in more than 85% of MG patients seropositive for a-AChR. In about 15% a thymoma is found while follicular hyperplasia or a diffuse thymitis is common in the others.

Subgroups of MG Patients

The bimodal age-related incidence peak, the prevalence of thymic abnormalities and HLA phenotypes led to the separation of several patient groups (Table 38.1). The distinction between early onset and late onset is made around the age of 40 years in most studies, although it is suggested that the dividing line should be at the age of 50 years because of incidence rates [6].

Osserman [11] subdivided patients according to clinical characteristics. Although this system dates from 1958, before the era of immunomodulation, many authors classify their patients following Osserman using the modifications by Oosterhuis [12] or Perlo et al. [13]. A description of the Osserman classification with modifications is given in Table 38.2.

Clinical Symptoms

The degree of weakness of individual muscles in a given patient may vary considerably. Ocular symptoms are very common in MG some patients even have MG restricted to the extraocular muscles. In another category bulbar weakness may dominate, and some patients with severe bulbar symptoms

never experience ptosis or double vision. Most patients have ocular and extremity muscle weakness alone or in combination with bulbar weakness; both types are labelled "generalised MG". All skeletal muscles may be involved and in severe cases ventilatory insufficiency may occur leading to a so-called myasthenic crisis.

Clinical Fluctuations

The degree of weakness may vary within minutes depending on the degree of effort or the use of anticholinergic medication. These rapid variations can be explained by a decline in the efficiency of transmitter release that accompanies repeated neuromuscular stimulation under physiological conditions. In the normal situation there is an abundant number of normally functioning AChRs ready for binding transmitter. Thus the end-plate potential evoked by a single release is amply above the threshold for a muscle action potential, and even in the case of decreased efficiency a normal muscle fibre action potential will occur. In MG the end-plate potential is reduced and with that the safety factor of neuromuscular transmission. Thus a single release of acetylcholine may not always lead to a muscle fibre action potential and this failure becomes more striking after repetitive stimulation such as occurs in

Table 38.1. Classification of patients with acquired myasthenia gravis

A *Patients seropositive for a-AChR*
1. Ocular MG
2. Early-onset generalised MG, no thymoma
3. Late-onset generalised MG, no thymoma
4. MG with thymoma

B *Patients seronegative for a-AChR*
1. Ocular MG
2. Generalised MG

a-AChR, antibody to acetylcholine receptor.

Table 38.2. Osserman classification of myasthenia gravis [2]

I Ocular or otherwise localised MG, without progression, good prognosis
II Generalised MG with gradual onset, fluctuating course, fairly well controllable with anticholinesterase medication, good prognosis
III Generalised MG with insidious onset, severe bulbar symptoms, often leading to a crisis at the beginning of the disease, poor reaction to anticholinesterases, very poor prognosis
IV Generalised MG with a late (>2 years) progression to a severe state, gradually developing from type I, IIa, IIb
V Generalised MG with muscle atrophy, usually developing from type II

Modification by Perlo et al. [13]
IIa Mild generalised MG, including ocular involvement
IIb Moderately severe generalised MG including ocular involvement with usually mild bulbar involvement
V Omitted

Modification by Oosterhuis [12]
IIa Mild symptoms, not severely interfering with the patient's health and ability to work, and which tend to disappear in the course of time
IIb Moderate symptoms, usually more generalised, running a fluctuating course over many years, and which may handicap the patient to a variable extent
V Omitted

exertion. If the number of functional intact AChR exceeds 30–40% of the normal value the patient will be able to recuperate after a short rest because the amount of acetylcholine has physiologically increased.

On the other hand more gradual fluctuations in the clinical course over weeks to months may occur. This is a reflection of variations in the number of normally functioning AChRs available, related to the activity of the autoimmune process. Momentary rapid fluctuations related to exertion become increasingly prominent as the number of residual intact AChRs diminishes. A period of rest will then not relieve the weakness sufficiently and anticholinesterases become less and less effective. Such a situation eventually may lead to a myasthenic crisis if the number of residual intact AChRs falls below 20–30% of the normal value.

Therapies in MG

The mortality rate reported in early studies now belongs to the past given the availability of efficient therapies for MG. Patients who do not react sufficiently to anticholinesterase are nowadays treated with immunomodulating drugs to improve the quality of daily life, to stop a life-threatening myasthenic crisis or to prevent them from progressing to a severe myasthenic condition.

Anticholinesterases are first-line drugs in MG. Pyridostigmine is most commonly used up to a daily total of 720 mg in divided doses at 2–6 h intervals. Muscarinic side effects such as salivation, abdominal cramps and diarrhoea can be counteracted with parasympathicolytics. These drugs are fairly well tolerated but also moderately potent.

Steroids are highly effective for the treatment of MG but the notorious side effects are a limiting factor for their use. Usually a start is made with a daily dose of 60–100 mg to be tapered to an alternate-day dose just sufficient to suppress myasthenic symptoms. The final maintenance dosage varies between individuals and may come down to 10–60 mg per 2 days for a prolonged period of several years or longer. A difficult problem with steroids is the initial worsening of myasthenic symptoms which may occur within 1–2 weeks after starting this therapy. If the clinical condition of the patient is brittle there is a substantial hazard of a prednisone-induced myasthenic crisis.

To reduce the need of steroids *azathioprine* may be added to the medication in a dose of $2\frac{1}{2}$–3 mg/kg body weight. This drug is effective after 3–6 months and may eventually lead to a complete independence of steroids. Side effects are mild although severe bone marrow depression, liver disturbances and incidental lymphomas have been described.

Cyclosporine is a possible alternative to steroids at a starting dose of about 5 mg/kg body weight. There is less experience with this drug, which has been in use for some 10 years. Intensive monitoring for renal side effects is very important.

Cyclophosphamide and *other cytostatic drugs* are used but reports on such therapies are scarce. Side effects are considerable and therefore azathioprine is preferred to these drugs.

Plasmapheresis is known as an effective therapy to force an improvement of myasthenic symptoms and is thus used to stop a myasthenic crisis or to turn a chronic unsatisfactory myasthenic condition. Additional immunomodulating therapy is required as the effect lasts for some weeks at the most.

Intravenous administration of *immunoglobulins* may be equivalent to plasma-exchange therapy and studies comparing the two therapies are in progress.

Thymectomy is generally recognised as an effective therapy for MG; nevertheless there is no consensus about the indication for this operation in different situations. There is divergence of opinion about restrictions with respect to age of onset of MG, whether patients with ocular MG should be operated on or not, the operative technique (trans-sternal, cervical or a combined approach) and the question of whether the use of immunomodulatory drugs should be preferred over an operation. We advocate a trans-sternal thymectomy in all patients with a thymoma and all patients with generalised MG in whom the disease became manifest before the age of 50 years. Thymectomy is always an elective intervention and should never be performed in the case of an increased operative risk. It may take 6 months to about 3 years before the effect of the operation becomes manifest. In our experience about 25% of patients do not benefit from the operation while more than 40% enter a remission.

Clinical Examination

Clinical examination of a patient with MG should be performed both at rest and after exercise. Signs in rest may be inconspicuous but in most patients some weakness of the facial musculature is evident (e.g. a vertical laugh or snarl, asymmetric ptosis probably compensated by contraction of the frontalis muscles or head tilt). The lower jaw may be supported by one hand to prevent the mouth from falling open or the head from inclining. There may be horizontal and/or vertical squinting of the eyes. In some cases a footdrop may be noted on the way to the consulting room. The patient may not be able to close his eyes completely, to knit her forehead or to push a profile in the cheek with the tongue. Weakness of the jaw musculature may be found in the rest condition and weakness of the neck musculature is not uncommon.

There may be no weakness of the skeletal musculature at direct testing. However, after exercise, weakness may become prominent in the muscles affected. A number of provocation tests are summarised in Table 38.3. Some of these are semiquantitative (e.g. degree of ptosis, dysarthria after counting or reading) but results of others can be expressed as a number, being thus suitable for follow-up examination. It is most useful to compare muscle force before and after exercise in the case of apparently normal test results. The patient may, for example, be able to lift his arms straight forward for 3 min but afterwards there may be a notable weakness (MRC III–IV) in the deltoid muscle at direct testing which was not present before.

Devices such as a hand-held dynamometer [14], a peak flow meter or a vital capacity meter may be helpful at the bedside.

Table 38.3. Clinical investigation of myasthenia gravis

Ptosis
- Looking straight towards a bright light provokes ptosis
- Looking aside for 30 s provokes ptosis, especially of the lid on the side of abduction
  Note the degree of ptosis at several time points:
  0   No ptosis
  25%   Drooping of the eyelid until the pupil
  50%   Cover of half the pupil
  75%   Total cover of the pupil
  100% Complete ptosis

Diplopia
- After sustained lateral/vertical gaze (maximum 30 s)

Bulbar functions
- Peak expiratory flow with and without nose clips
- Eye closure becomes weak(er) after repeatedly closing the eyes tightly
- Nasal speech after counting 101–199. Note the number at which dysarthria or nasality occurs
- Chewing with click and subsequent test of masseter function 100×[a,b]
- Swallowing a glass of water is not possible without coughing or regurgitation through the nose

Neck musculature
- Keeping the head raised for 1 min when in a horizontal position ('look at your feet')[a]
- Raising the head repeatedly 20×[a,b]

Arm
- Arms stretched forward (90°) for 180 s[a,b]
  – note the beginning of trembling or shaking of the arm/hand
  – note drooping of individual fingers

Hand
- Inflation of sphygmomanometer to 300 mmHg
- Fist closing/opening with fingers joined together (no digital abduction allowed) 70×[b]

Leg
- Hip flexion (45°, supine) for 60 s
- Deep knee bends 20×[b]
- Raising from a normal chair without use of the hands 20×[b]

Ventilatory function
- Vital capacity or peak flow in resting condition
- Vital capacity or peak flow decreases after repeated testing (5–10×)

[a] Test muscle force directly before and after exercise.
[b] Upper limit.

Other Parameters for Following the Course of MG

Auto-antibody levels – especially a-AChR – may fluctuate with the clinical state of MG both in the case of therapeutic interventions [15–18] and in the natural course of the disease. However, discordances between antibody fluctuations and clinical course are not uncommon, partly because immunomodulating drugs may directly suppress immunoglobulin levels – and thus a-AChR-levels – without achieving a prominent clinical improvement. Therefore the course of auto-antibody levels by itself is not suitable for assessment of the efficacy of a therapy and may only be considered as an additional datum. If serial measurements of auto-antibodies are performed it is crucial to use the same batch of antigen or even better to test all sera from one patient in the same assay.

Neurophysiological tests may reasonably be used to quantify myasthenia in selected muscles but very few studies to validate electromyography (EMG) for follow-up of MG symptoms have been published and the results are equivocal [2,19,20]. Cholinesterase inhibitors may blind the findings of EMG and are thus required to be stopped at least 24 h before testing.

Clinical Scales

Several systems have been developed to define the clinical condition of the MG patient at any point in time. This may be useful for follow-up studies and to assess the effect of therapeutic interventions. Osserman's scale (Table 38.2) is still used for this purpose but, in fact, his system describes types of myasthenia instead of the clinical state at a point in time, and a shift from one category to another (except from I or II to IV) is, strictly speaking, impossible. Oosterhuis' modification [12] and the later modification by Perlo (from the Osserman group) [13] tried to meet this problem but did not provide a good solution. Both authors, however, realised that bulbar symptoms deserved special categorisation because of their greater impact on the clinical state of the patient.

In fact, it is difficult to lump scores from several systems (ocular, bulbar and limb muscle symptoms) together in one number reflecting the overall clinical state. Some patients are severely disabled by one category of symptoms (e.g. bulbar weakness) while other systems (e.g. limb muscles) are affected only mildly or not at all. This point may be met by introducing weighting factors: ventilatory disabilities are by far the most severe and thus deserve a greater weight than, for example, bulbar disturbances; the latter, in turn threaten vital functions far more than ocular symptoms do. These considerations are valuable for assessing the clinical state in a severe myasthenic condition such as an (impending) crisis. However, it should be realised that the handicap of an ambulant patient may differ from the overall clinical severity. Ocular symptoms may be of great importance in daily living and make the patient functionally blind without being life-threatening, while mild bulbar symptoms may be coped with. In these situations it might be more appropriate to score the different functional systems separately.

Disability may be expressed in numerical values as the amount of time the patient is able to sustain an effort (e.g. keeping the arms outstretched). This is quite an exact way of measuring disability and results may be compiled using parametric statistics. Using numerical expressions demands standard values and these remain a matter of debate. Table 38.3 comprises the standards we use in practice. Many functions (especially from the bulbar and ocular systems) can only be expressed in an ordinal scale eventually labelled with a number (e.g. Appendices A, B [21,22]). Some scaling systems try to supply an overall score by combining values assigned to functions from different systems by using weighting factors (e.g. Appendices C–E [23–25]). However, the introduction of weighting factors – which greatly affects the numerical results – remains arbitrary. Moreover such overall scores consist of a mixture of numerical values and ordinal rank-numbers which makes parametric statistics more hazardous.

On the other hand purely ordinal scales have been developed (e.g. Appendices F–J [26–30]), using information from both clinical history and examination. In this context it should be noted that patients' reports of oculobulbar symptoms are reliable but spinal muscle weakness may be unobserved by some patients and therefore underestimated in a purely history-based system (e.g. Appendix D). Some of these scales (Appendices F, G) closely resemble the generally used and well-defined Rankin scale. In such scales overall disability scores may composed of subscores from different systems. A prominent problem of these classifications may be that they do not imply a linear correlation between numerical class and the actual condition of an individual patient. This may easily be seen in the classifications depicted in Appendices H and I. Compare a patient who is severely disabled by bulbar symptoms and only mild limb girdle weakness (and thus prone to falling into a crisis) with a patient with moderate generalised weakness (who can be treated in an ambulant setting). The first patient is classified with a 3 while the latter gets a score of 4 in both systems. Qualitative descriptions such as "slight", "mild", "moderate" and "severe" are used, introducing interobserver variability. This may be further enhanced by a certain overlap between successive categories.

Szobor's score (Appendix J) is very detailed and may therefore be difficult to use in clinical practice. Furthermore the system of "other functions" seems less to the point.

Overall disability scales are obviously not suitable for patients with ocular myasthenia. Ocular disability is, for example, confined to the first two classes of Oosterhuis' scale (Appendix F) and hardly fits in the Arsura system (Appendix G) or the Besinger score (Appendix A). Schumm constructed a sophisticated system for ocular myasthenia using separate scores for degrees of ptosis and diplopia, combining these two in an overall ocular score (Appendix K [31]).

In the case of ordinal scales non-parametric statistics are required for analysis, and arithmethic manipulations (e.g. subtracting pre- and post-event scores) only are allowed with the greatest caution – conditions which are not always respected in literature. Differences between scores in several clinical conditions (e.g. before and after an intervention) cannot be expressed in simple subtractions of the numerical lables assigned to the ordinal categories but should be defined more precisely. For example, we defined an "unequivocal effect of thymectomy" as "complete remission or a shift of at least 2 points on the Oosterhuis disability scale" [32].

Clinical Trials in MG

As is the case in many other diseases much of our knowledge on treatment efficacies is obtained from open studies and controlled studies concerning the treatment of MG are scarce. In this perspective it is interesting to consider the history of the origin of thymectomy in the treatment of MG illustrating role of a correctly performed analysis:

> A role of the thymus in the pathogenesis of MG was already surmised in the beginning of this century after the autopsy findings that many patients with MG had thymic abnormalities. The American surgeon Blalock was in 1936 the first to perform a thymectomy for an attempt to treat MG. Afterward it might be doubted whether this really was a therapeutic intervention as it concerned a patient with a thymoma (see below) after a pre-operative course of radiotherapy. Anyway, the patient improved, and encouraged by this success he and others thymectomised several dozens of patients with MG in the next 10 years. However the enthusiasm waned in the second half of the forties when a retrospective analysis of the results showed only marginal advantages of the operation in comparison to medical treatment. In fact the operation was then abandoned in the USA. However, in the beginning of the 1950s the British surgeon Keynes had amassed a respectable series of thymectomies and after a retrospective analysis (with help of an outside investigator) it turned out that thymectomy really was beneficial to MG patients without a thymoma while patients with a thymic tumour often got worse. Reconsidering the US series it appeared that patients with a thymoma were overrepresented there and after a new analysis American results were also encouraging and thymectomy yet became an established therapy for MG. [33]

Further steps in the evolution of MG treatment were the introduction of prednisone and of azathioprine in the 1960s. Almost all reports on these drugs concerned uncontrolled open studies. To our knowledge only one double-blind study [34] has been performed comparing prednisone with placebo and results were inconclusive. Nevertheless clinical experience with steroids now is large and several non-controlled series have been studied since.

Azathioprine as single therapy is well established too after the publication of several open studies [22], but the period of 6–12 months needed for obtaining a final effect makes it less suitable for treating the severely affected MG patient.

The addition of azathioprine to steroids was not found to show benefit in either the duration of improvement or treatment tolerance compared with single therapy with steroids but a greater response was found with the combination of both treatments [35]. This combination treatment is used in many centres both in order to keep the dose of steroids as low as possible and to obtain a greater effect [36].

Cyclosporine has been introduced in an era in which clinical trials to assess the effect of a treatment are mandatory for acceptance of a new drug. Furthermore side-effects and financial costs counted against cyclosporine when compared with standard therapies. Therefore this imunomodulator has been brought to trial more extensively than the older drugs. First cyclosporine was found to be effective compared with placebo in a double-blind study with patients not taking other immunomodulatory drugs [37]. Subsequently, preliminary results of a study with cyclosporine compared with azathioprine were inconclusive [38]. However, in a more recent trial cyclosporine was more effective than placebo in patients on the lowest tolerable steroid dose and there were indications that addition of cyclosporine might reduce the need for steroids [39].

Recently a clinical trial comparing high-dose intravenous immunoglobulin and plasma-exchange for myasthenia gravis was published. Both therapies appeared similarly efficacy while immunoglobulins were tolerated better [40].

Prospects for Further Trials

Although steroids are cheap and quite efficacious in the treatment of MG, a proportion of patients still do not respond sufficiently or remain dependent on high daily doses. Furthermore long-term side-effects and the risk of initial worsening of MG remain problems to be solved. Therefore testing new strategies for treatment with prednisone – e.g. the use of pulse doses of steroids, whether or not to offer the patient plasma exchange at the start of steroids, how to induct steroids – remain of interest. It also remains worthwhile to look for additional drugs reducing the long-term need of steroids or for alternative drugs with fewer side-effects.

The places of cyclosporine, cyclophosphamide and possibly other immunomodulatory drugs is not well established and there is still hope for a more specific immunomodulating therapy. The use of plasma exchange (e.g. only in crises or also for long term treatment in the ambulant setting) and the efficacy of intravenous immunoglobulin remain points of debate.

Trials for MG therapies self-evidently should be performed following general rules. There are, however, some points of special interest:

1. It is nowadays almost unethical to test new therapeutic modalities against placebo instead of steroids (with or without azathioprine) in patients who are moderately to severely affected. Testing a new intervention against placebo remains possible in a patient poorly controlled with steroids remaining on the lowest tolerable steroid or azathioprine dose [39].

2. Before starting a new trial it should be ensured that the effect of the intervention to be tested will not be confounded with that of other therapies. This means that no thymectomy should have been

performed in the 4 years preceding a trial as patients improve gradually after thymic surgery [41, own experience]. Furthermore changes in steroid dose in the 4 weeks before and azathioprine in the 6 months before the start of a trial may interfere with the study.

3. A strategy for emergency situations and how to handle the data obtained in such cases should be established. It should, for example, be clear in what situations plasma exchange may be performed.

4. It is important to decide which type of patients should be included in the study (Table 38.2). Patients with a thymoma or with late-onset MG may react differently on interventions from others. Seronegative patients probably suffer from a subtype of MG with its own characteristics and mode of response to therapy. Patients with prominent bulbar symptoms (Osserman category IIb) are difficult to compare with other categories (e.g. Osserman IIa). Patients with MG restricted to the ocular muscles should always be considered separately.

5. The method of assessing the clinical state will be of importance. Several global scales have been developed (see above), all with their particular shortcomings and advantages. It is advisable to use a test scheme, for example as presented in Table 38.3, or a modification of this. In many situations it may be sufficient to use part of the outline to test only the most affected muscles. As MG may produce rapidly fluctuating symptoms it is crucial to standardise the conditions in which the patient is tested. It might be ideal to assess the clinical state in the evening hours after about 30 min of rest, followed or not by a standardised excercise. Interference from anticholinesterases should be minimised, by testing the patient 12 h after the last dosage. In addition, the patient may be asked to do simple self-assessments at home (e.g. lifting the arms for as long as possible) following instructions from the investigator.

6. The choice of an end-point or measure of efficacy depends on the question to be answered. Prevention of relapse of MG, possible reduction of steroids, clinical improvement after a defined period as established by clinimetry or a move on an appropriate scale may be used for this.

Appendix A. Besinger Score [21]

Test items	None 0	Mild 1	Moderate 2	Severe 3
A Muscles of limbs and trunk				
Arms outstretched (90°, standing)	>240 s	90–240 s	10–90 s	<10 s
Leg outstretched (45°, supine)	>100 s	30–100 s	0–30 s	0 s
Head lifted (45°, supine)	>120 s	30–120 s	0–30 s	0 s
Grip strength[a]	<15%	15–30%	30–75%	>75%
Vital capacity				
(Males)	3.5 l	2.5–3.5 l	1.5–2.5 l	<1.5 l
(Females)	2.5 l	1.8–2.5 l	1.2–1.8 l	<1.2 l
B Oropharyngeal muscles				
Facial muscles	Normal	Mild weakness on lid closure, snarl	Incomplete lid closure	No mimic expressions
Chewing	Normal	Fatigue on chewing solid foods	Only soft foods	Gastric tube
Swallowing	Normal	Fatigue on normal foods	Incomplete palatal closure, nasal speech	Gastric tube

[a] Vigorimeter, decrement after 10 maximal closures.

Appendix B. Assessment of muscular strength and performance in myasthenia gravis [22]

	General criteria	Ocular muscles	Faciopharyngeal muscles	Skeletal muscles
100%	Almost total and temporarily complete paralysis. Unable to do any work	Total ophthalmoplegia externa and complete ptosis	Complete paralysis of deglutition. Feeding possible only by tube and respiration through tracheostoma. Speech unintelligible. Amimia	Patient virtually unable to move, constantly confined to bed. Artificial respiration necessary. Inability to lift the head. Arms practically paralytic
80%	Severe paralysis, increased exhaustibility. Unable to do any work	Minimal oculogyration. Upper eyelid covers the pupils	Severe dysphagia. Feeding by tube necessary. Respiration often possible only through tracheostoma. Speech difficult to understand. The tongue is hardly moved. Lower jaw usually hanging down	A few steps possible on even ground, but only if supported. The head is held up with difficulty. The arms can only be raised slightly
60%	Moderately severe paralysis, considerable reduction in performance, Unable to do manual work	Oculogyration from the mean position not possible in any direction beyond 30°, or severe paresis of individual muscles. Impairment of vision due to ptosis	Patients frequently swallow "the wrong way". Slurred speech; tongue extended to the teeth; chin supported by hand. Flaccid face	Short walks possible. Rising from the lying, sitting and squatting positions only possible with assistance. Ability to climb a few steps if supported. Ability to raise arms up to the horizontal position
40%	Moderate muscular weakness with greatly restricted ability to work	Paresis of individual ocular muscles. Constant double vision. Serious impairment of vision due to ptosis is rare	Patients find swallowing of solid foods strenuous and chewing quickly fatigues them. "Lumpy" speech. Tongue extended to the middle of the lips. Unable to whistle	Knee-bending exercise and climbing on chairs possible with effort. Patients able to raise arms above the horizontal position and to comb their hair
20%	Slight muscular weakness. Slightly to moderately restricted ability to do manual work	Slight paresis of individual ocular muscles. Double vision only in terminal position. Eyelids raised incompletely	Increased exhaustibility on prolonged swallowing and speaking. Indication of myopathic facies	Increased general fatiguability, possibly with predilection for individual muscle groups. Ability to raise the arms above the head
0%	No paresis. Full working capacity			

Appendix C. Scoring System Following Gajdos et al. [23]

Maintain *upper limbs* horizontally outstretched
15   150 seconds
10   100 seconds
 5   50 seconds

Maintain *lower limbs* above bed plane, while lying on back
15   75 seconds
10   50 seconds
 5   25 seconds

Raise *head* above bed plane, while lying on back
10   Against resistance
 5   Without resistance
 0   Impossible

Trunk muscles
Sit up from lying position
10   Without help of hands
 5   With help of hands
 0   Impossible

Extrinsic *ocular musculature*
10   Normal
 5   Ptosis
 0   Double vision

Eyelid occlusion
10   Complete
 5   Incomplete
 0   Impossible

Chewing
10   Normal
 5   Weak
 0   Impossible

Swallowing
10   Normal
 5   Impaired without aspiration
 0   Impaired with aspiration

Speech
10   Normal
 5   Nasal
 0   Blurred

Appendix D. Disability Scale Following d'Alessandro et al. [24]

Eye muscles
Ptosis
0   Absent
1   Observed or reported sometimes in one or both eyes, but vision never impaired
2   Always present in one or both eyes but vision never impaired
3   Vision sometimes impossible in one or both eyes
4   Vision always impossible in one or both eyes

Diplopia
0   Absent
1   Sometimes present, but only in lateral gaze
2   Always present, but only in lateral gaze
3   Sometimes present in primary gaze position
4   Always present in primary gaze position

Bulbar muscles
Dysphagia
Dysphonia/dysarthria
Chewing difficulties
0   Absent
1   Sometimes present, but function still possible
2   Always present, but function still possible
3   Function sometimes impossible
4   Function always impossible

Spinal muscles
Scapular girdle weakness
Pelvic girdle weakness
Neck muscle weakness
0   No dysfunction
1   Weakness observed or reported sometimes, but functions still possible
2   Always weakness, but function still possible
3   Function sometimes impossible
4   Function always impossible

Appendix E. Assessment Following Peluchetti et al. [25]

Ocular level

0   Normal
1   Paretic nystagmus and/or blurred vision and/or provoked ptosis
2   Diplopia in one or two cardinal directions and/or monolateral ptosis
3   Diplopia in primary position and/or bilateral ptosis
4   Mono- or bilateral ophthalmoplegia

Generalised level

Facial muscles

0   Normal
10 Orbicularis oculi and/or oris are weak but can overcome external resistance, snarl smile
20 Orbicularis oculi and/or oris are weak and cannot overcome external resistance
30 Lagophthalmos and/or severe weakness of orbicularis oris

Anterior head and neck flexors muscles
Deltoid muscles

0   Normal
10 Weakness but ability to overcome external resistance
20 Weakness, inability to overcome external resistance, but possibility of acting against gravity
30 Weakness, impossibility of acting against gravity
40 Visible action but no effective contraction
50 No visible action

Abdominal muscles: ability to flex the vertebral column

0   Normal
10 With hands clasped behind the head
20 With forearms folded across the chest
30 With forearms extended forward
40 Ability to flex the cervical spine with forearms extended forward
50 Inability to curl the trunk

Lower extremity muscles

0   More than 15 squats
10 6–14 squats
20 1–5 squats
30 Squats with the aid of the hands
40 Rising from a normal chair
50 Inability to rise from a normal chair

Bulbar level

Chewing

0   Normal
1000   Chewing fatiguability
2000   Weakness of masseters against resistance
3000   Ptosis of the jaw

Tongue

0   Normal
1000   Inability to press the tip against the cheek
2000   Inability to curl the tongue and reach the upper lip frenulus
3000   Inability to protrude the tongue

Swallowing

0   Normal
1000   Fatigue with normal foods
2000   Dysphagia for solid foods, necessity of soft foods
20 000 Impossible, nasal tube feeding

Phonation

0   Normal
1000   Slight nasality
2000   Severe nasality but speech still intelligible
3000   Speech difficult to understand

Respiratory level

0   Normal
200 000 Vital capacity 15–25 ml/kg body weight
500 000 Impossible, artificial ventilation

Appendix F. Disability Score Following Oosterhuis [26]

Class 0
No complaints, no signs after exertion or at special testing

Class 1
No disability. Minor signs, minor complaints
The patient knows that he or she (still) has MG, but family members or outsiders do not perceive it. The experienced doctor may find minor signs at appropriate testing, e.g. diminished eye closure, some weakness of the foot extensors or triceps muscles, the arms cannot be held extended for 3 min. The patient may have complaints such as heavy eyelids or diplopia only when fatigued; inability to perform heavy work

Class 2
Slight disability, clear signs after exertion
The patient has some restrictions in daily life, e.g. he or she cannot lift heavy loads, cannot walk for more than half an hour, has intermittent diplopia. Bulbar signs are not pronounced. Family members are aware of the signs, but outsiders (inexperienced doctors included) are not. Weakness is obvious at appropriate testing

Class 3
Moderate disability, clear signs at rest
The patient is restricted in domestic activities, needs some help in dressing, meals have to be adapted. Bulbar signs are more pronounced. Signs of MG can be observed by any outsider

Class 4
Severe disability
The patient needs constant support in daily activities. Bulbar signs are pronounced. Respiratory function is decreased

Class 5
Repiratory support is needed

Comments
1. The clinical score is calculated independently of the medication. The qualification "remission" is to be restricted to class 0, when the patient is not using medication.
2. Patients with purely ocular signs are classified as class 1 or 2.
3. It is sometimes difficult to decide between classes 2 and 3. The attitude of the patient and the adaptation to the disease may play a role.
4. The development of respiratory difficulties obviously depends on external factors such as respiratory infections, inadequate drug regimen or other intercurrent diseases.
5. The function of individual muscle groups may be scored on a 4-point scale:
   0   normal function (i.e. the specific function tests can be carried out, the patient has no complaints)
   1   mild or intermittent signs
   2   moderate signs
   3   severe signs
   A reasonable use of this semi-quantification can be made by scoring O(cular), B(ulbar), U(pper extremities), L(ower extremities) and V(entilatory functions) together. For instance a patient with constant diplopia and ptosis, dysarthria after only 3 min of reading aloud, inability to extend the arms for 1 min, not able to walk a stairway and a vital capacity of 75% would be scored as O3 B1 U2 L2 V1.

Appendix G. Disability Scale Following Arsura et al. [27]

1   Asymptomatic (no signs or symptoms of disease, except for orbicularis oculi weakness)
2   Minor symptoms with repetitive exercising, but not interfering with daily living
3   Mildly disabled with symptoms apparent on examination, restriction of more demanding activities
4   Restricted in daily activities; symptomatic at rest, symptoms easily apparent in basal state
5   Completely dependent on skilled care for support

Appendix H. Virginia University Muscle Weakness Classification [28]

1   Ocular and facial weakness
2   Mild ocular, facial and limb-girdle weakness
3   Mild ocular, facial, limb-girdle and bulbar weakness
4   Moderate generalised weakness
5   Severe generalised weakness

Appendix I. Classification Following Mann et al. [29]

I   Only ocular symptoms
II   Predominantly ocular and mild limb-girdle symptoms
III   Predominantly faciopharyngeal plus mild limb-girdle and/or ocular symptoms
IV   Moderate generalised symptoms
V   Severe generalised symptoms

Appendix J. Assessment Following Szobor [30]

Assessment

I *Ocular functions*

0   No symptoms
1   Periodic (unilateral) ptosis, pupil is free
2   Moderate, unilateral permanent ptosis, (pupil is free); moderate, bilateral, fluctuating ptosis,[a] mild diplopia ("blurred vision") in the evening or upon severe exhaustion[b]
3   Permanent, hardly fluctuating bilateral ptosis;[b] severe, unilateral ptosis (with partially covered pupil); periodic diplopia;[a] bilateral lagophthalmos (facial weakness)[b]
4   Serious bilateral ptosis (pupil completely covered on one side);[a,b] permanent diplopia; severe ptosis + diplopia (despite optical correction); bilateral ptosis + lagophthalmos;[a,b]
5   Severe or total bilateral ptosis (both pupils are covered);[b] permanent diplopia + ptosis, or dissociated paresis of the ocular muscles

II *Facial and chewing functions*

0   No symptoms
1   Mild chewing difficulty upon exhaustion; difficulty in pursing the lips and in whistling
2   Chewing fatigue;[a] periodic fatiguability in all facial functions (smiling, showing the teeth, snarling, pursing the lips, sucking, whistling)
3   "Facies myasthenica"; permanent, though fluctuating disorder in the facial and chewing functions
4   "Facies myasthenica"; open mouth and hanging lip symptom; serious and permanent chewing and sucking disorder;[a] "supporting head symptom"
5   "Facies myasthenica"; inability of voluntary and emotional facial movements, amimia; permanent inability to chew and suck.

III *Bulbar functions*

0   No symptoms
1   Softer speech or nasal phonation upon exhaustion;[a] mild dysphagia in tiredness
2   Permanently softer speech, dysphonia; unmodulated toneless speech;[a] nasal phonation;[a] mild, permanent dysphagia (stagnation in the piriform recesses); hyporeflexia of the soft palate and the pharynx; temporary disorder of the movements of the tongue[a]
3   Permanently soft and nasal phonation;[b] pronounced dysphagia with periodic nasal regurgitation; hanging soft palatal arch, lack of pharyngeal reflex; definitely disturbed tongue movements
4   Serious dysarthria, dysphonia; severe dysphagia, permanent regurgitation; severe disturbance of tongue movements
5   Aphonia, anarthria; aphagia (nasal probe is necessary for feeding); minimal tongue movements

IV *Skeletal functions*

0   No symptoms
1   Positive "head drop symptom"; "supporting head symptom" on exhaustion, increased fatiguability during running or climbing stairs[a]
2   "Hair comb disability"; difficulty in washing oneself; difficulty in standing up from squatting; moderate exhaustion on walking[a]
3   Pronounced fatiguability on walking; inability to climb stairs; myopathy-like movements on sitting up or standing up; pronounced difficulty in stretching out the arms ("arm stretch symptom"); quick exhaustion of gripping and squeezing strength[a]
4   Severe and permanent disorder in walking;[b] inability to get up from the lying position; permanent "supporting head symptom"; inability to grip and squeeze;[b] weakness of the skeletal (supporting) muscles
5   Abasia, astasia; permanent, severe weakness of the arms and hands; inability to grasp and hold; inability to look after oneself ("inability state")

V *Respiratory functions*

0   No symptoms
1   Mild, periodic dyspnoea (only on exhaustion); respiratory deficit upon climbing stairs or cycling;[a]

Appendix J. (*Continued*)

2   Permanent, mild tachypnoea; dyspnoea during working;[a] mild difficulty in coughing and expectorating[b]

3   Permanent or prolonged respiratory deficit (hypoxia); definite dyspnoea even during light work; signs of increased functioning of the auxiliary respiratory muscles (intercostal muscle retraction, Harrison's groove, respiration through the wings of the nose, tension of the cervical muscles, increased activity of the abdominal muscles); severe disability in coughing and expectorating[b]

4   Severe and permanent dyspnoea, tachypnoea, cyanosis (permanent hypoxia); hypocrisis, precrisis; possibility of apnoea on any mild exertion; inability to cough and expectorate

5   Myasthenic, cholinergic (or oscillating) respiratory crisis, apnoea (assisted or controlled artificial respiration, IPPR is necessary

VI   *Other functions*

0   No symptoms

1   Periodic, pseudoneurasthenia-like exhaustion; disorder in concentration and tenacity of attention

2   Definite psychic fatiguability[a]; mild depression syndrome

3   Severe, permanent psychic fatiguability; disturbance of the pursuit of an intellectual occupation; temporary disorder of urination and defaecation[a] (fluctuating weakness of the abdominal press)

4   Severe psychic inactivity, disability of intellectual activity; sensitive-paranoid character symptoms; pathological personality reactions (asthenic, sthenic reactions, querulence, cenaesthesia, depression, hysteric symptom augmentation, affective reactions, "short ciruit"-like actions); pathological personality development (precise-meticulous, hypochondriac, psychasthenic personality)

5   Intellectual and emotional stupor; apathy; negativism; inability of bowel function

Disability status scale [30]

0   *Negative history and neurological status.* Muscle fatiguing tests are negative, 0 scale in every functional system

1   *The patient continues working in his or her original occupation.* Minimal symptoms (degree 1) in one or two functional systems, such as the ocular, facial, skeletal or other functions, but the bulbar and respiratory systems are completely healthy

2   *Minimal disability, the patient works in his or her original occupation.* Periodic symptoms (degree 2) in one or two functional systems, or permanent symptoms (degrees 1–2) in some functional systems with the exception of the respiratory system

3   *Moderate disability, the patient works part time only in his or her original occupation, or does light physical work full time.* Symptoms (degree 2) in some functional systems with degree 3 in one system with the exception of the respiratory system

4   *Definite disability, the patient can look after him- or herself and can do light work (housework) part time.* Degree 3 in the facial and/or bulbar functions + degree 2 in the skeletal system; degree 4 in the ocular system + degree 3 in one or two further functional systems; degrees 1–2 in the respiratory system + degree 3 in one additional functional system or degree 2 in several further systems

5   *Severe disability, the patient is able to look after him- or herself but is unable to work.* Degree 4 in two functional systems; degree 3 in the majority of the systems; degree 3 in the respiratory system; degree 2 in the respiratory system + degree 3 in the other functional systems

6   *Serious disability, the patient is able to move but requires assistance.* Degree 4 in two or three functional systems; degrees 3–4 in the majority of the systems with the exception of the respiratory system; degree 3 in the respiratory system + degrees 2–3 in the other systems

7   *Serious disability, the patient is bedridden or can sit up with assistance, and is able to move the limbs.* Degree 4 in the skeletal, facial and/or bulbar systems; degrees 3–4 in the majority of systems including the respiratory system

8   *Inability, the patient is bedridden with minimal hand movements.* Degree 5 in the skeletal system + degree 4 in the facial and bulbar systems; degree 5 in more than two systems, degree 4 in the respiratory system, degrees 4–5 in three or more systems

9   *Total inability, the patient is bedridden, incapable of any movement; patient receiving artificial respiration.* Degree 5 in the skeletal, facial and bulbar systems; degree 5 in the respiratory system; degrees 4–5 in every functional system

10   *Death due to myasthenia.* Due to crisis, syncope, pneumonia, convulsions or other causes

[a] Symptoms showing strong fluctuation.
[b] Drug resistance, hardly changing symptoms.

Appendix K. Schumm's Eye-score [31]

I *Symptoms of the external ocular muscles*

0   No paresis of the external ocular muscles. No double vision
1   Paresis observable in extreme position of the eyes. Double vision in up to two gaze directions (more than 20° excentricity)
2   Paresis observable in a gaze position more than 20° from the midline. Double vision in up to three gaze directions
3   Paresis of more than three external ocular muscles. No double vision in the midline position
4   Nearly continuous double vision
5   Continous double vision
6   Marked paresis of three external ocular muscles
7   Marked paresis of four external ocular muscles
8   Only very small eye movements
9   One eye cannot be moved
10 Both eyes cannot be moved

II *Ptosis*

0   No ptosis after continued upward gaze for more than 1 min (Simpson test)
1   Simpson test positive prior to 60 s (one or both sides)
2   Simpson test positive prior to 30 s (one or both sides)
3   Slight spontaneous ptosis on one side
4   Slight spontaneous ptosis on both sides
5   Marked ptosis with pupils visible
6   Eyelid covers pupil on one side
7   Eyelid covers pupil on both sides
8   Iris visible on both sides
9   Iris visible on one side
10 Both eyes closed

$$\text{Score} = \frac{I + II}{2}$$

References

1. Desmedt JE, Borestein S. Double-step nerve stimulation test for myasthenic block: sensitization of postactivation exhaustion by ischemia. Ann Neurol 1977;1:55–64.
2. Sanders DB, Howard JF. Single-fiber electromyography in myasthenia gravis. AAEE minimonograph 25. Muscle Nerve 1985;8:809–819.
3. Stålberg E. Clinical electrophysiology in myasthenia gravis. J Neurol Neurosurg Psychiatry 1980;43:622–633.
4. Engel AG. Congenital myasthenic syndromes. In: Lisak RP, editor. Handbook of myasthenia gravis and myasthenic syndromes. New York: Marcel Dekker, 1994:33–62.
5. Oosterhuis HJGH. The natural course of myasthenia gravis: a long term follow up study. J Neurol Neurosurg Psychiatry 1989;52:1121–1127.
6. Somnier FE, Keiding N, Paulson OB. Epidemiology of myasthenia gravis in Denmark. Arch Neurol 1991;48:733–739.
7. Grob D, Brunner NG, Namba T. The natural course of myasthenia gravis and effect of therapeutic measures. Ann NY Acad Sci 1981;377:652–669.
8. Drachman DB. Myasthenia gravis: immunobiology of a receptor disorder. Trends Neurosci 1983;6:446–451.
9. Limburg PC, The TH, Hummel-Tappel E, Oosterhuis HJGH. Anti-acetylcholine receptor antibodies in myasthenia gravis. 1. Relation to clinical parameters in 250 patients. J Neurol Sci 1983;58:357–370.
10. Oosterhuis HJGH, Limburg PC, Hummel-Tappel E, The TH. Anti-acetylcholine receptor antibodies in myasthenia gravis. 2. Clinical and serological follow-up of individual patients. J Neurol Sci 1983;58:371–385.
11. Osserman K. Myasthenia Gravis. New York: Grune & Stratton, 1958.
12. Oosterhuis HJGH. Studies in myasthenia gravis. 1. A clinical study of 180 patients. J Neurol Sci 1964;1:512–546.
13. Perlo VP, Poskanzer DC, Schwab RS, Viets HR, Osserman KE, Genkins G. Myasthenia gravis: evaluation of treatment in 1355 patients. Neurology 1966;16:431–439.
14. Van der Ploeg RJO, Oosterhuis HJGH, Reuvekamp J. Measuring muscle strength. J Neurol 1984;231:200–203.
15. Kuks JBM, Oosterhuis HJGH, Limburg PC, The TH. Anti-acetylcholine receptor antibodies decrease after thymectomy in patients with myasthenia gravis: clinical correlations. J Autoimmun 1991;4:197–211.
16. Oosterhuis HJGH, Limburg PC, Hummel-Tappel E, van den Burg W, The TH. Anti-acetylcholine receptor antibodies in myasthenia gravis. 3. The effect of thymectomy. J Neurol Sci 1985;69:335–343.
17. Kuks JBM, Limburg PC, Horst G, Oosterhuis HJGH. Antibodies to skeletal muscle in myasthenia gravis. 3. Relation with clinical course and therapy. J Neurol Sci 1993;120:168–173.
18. Kuks JBM, Djojoatmodjo S, Oosterhuis HJGH. Azathioprine in myasthenia gravis: observations in 41 patients and a review of literature. Neuromusc Disord 1991;1:423–431.
19. Campbell WW, Leshner RT, Swift TR. Plasma exchange in myasthenia gravis: electrophysiological studies. Ann Neurol 1980;8:584–589.
20. Konishi T, Nishitani H, Matsubara F, Ohta M. Myasthenia gravis: relation between jitter in single-fiber EMG and antibody to acetylcholine receptor. Neurology 1981;31:386–392.
21. Besinger UA, Toyka KV, Hoemberg M, Heininger K, Hohlfeld R, Fateh-Moghadam A. Myasthenia gravis: long-term correlation of binding and bungarotoxin blocking antibodies against acetylcholine receptors with changes in disease severity. Neurology 1983;33:1316–1321.
22. Mertens HG, Balzereit F, Leipert M. The treatment of severe myasthenia gravis with immunosuppressive agents. Eur Neurol 1969;2:321–339.

23. Gajdos Ph, Simon N, Rohan-Chabot P de, Raphael J-C, Goulon M. Effets à long terme des écharges plasmatiques au cours de la myasthénie: résultats d'une étude randomisée. Presse Med 1983;12:939–942.

24. D'Alessandro R, Casmiro M, Benassi G, Rinaldi R, Gamberini G. Reliable disability scale for myasthenia gravis sensitive to clinical changes. Acta Neurol Scand 1995;92:77–82.

25. Peluchetti D, Cornelio F, Shirlanzoni A, Corrarlile C. The course of MG in patients treated with different immunosuppresive measures. Presented at the Congress on Neuromuscular Diseases, Milan, 1986.

26. Oosterhuis HJGH. Clinical aspects. In: Oosterhuis HJGH. Myasthenia gravis. Edinburgh: Churchill Livingstone, 1984: 21–50.

27. Arsura E, Brunner NG, Namba T, Grob D. High-dose intravenous methylprednisolone in myasthenia gravis. Arch Neurol 1985;42:1149–1153.

28. Pascuzzi RM, Coslett HB, Johns TR. Myasthenia gravis treatment with long-term corticosteroids: a report of 116 cases. Semin Neurol 1983;3:250–264.

29. Mann JD, Johns TR, Campa JF, Muller WH. Long-term prednisone followed by thymectomy in myasthenia gravis. Ann NY Acad Sci 1976;274:608–622.

30. Szobor A. Myasthenia gravis: a quantitative evaluation system. Disability Status Scale applied for myasthenia gravis. Eur Neurol 1976;18:439–446.

31. Schumm F, Wiethölter H, Fateh-Moghadam A, Dichgans J. Thymectomy in myasthenia with pure ocular symptoms. J Neurol Neurosurg Psychiatry 1985;48:332–337.

32. Kuks JBM, Lems SPM, Oosterhuis HJGH. HLA type is not indicative for the effect of thymectomy in myasthenia gravis. J Neuroimmunol 1992;37:217–224.

33. Viets HR. Historical introduction. In: Viets HR, Schwab RS, editors. Thymectomy for myasthenia gravis. Springfield, IL: Thomas, 1960:3–18.

34. Howard FM, Duane DD, Lambert EH, Daube JR. Alternate-day prednisone: preliminary report of a double-blind controlled study. Ann NY Acad Sci 1976;274:596–607.

35. Palace J, Newsom-Davis J, Lecky B. A randomized double-blind trial of prednisolone alone or with azathioprine in myasthenia gravis. Myasthenia Gravis Study Group. Neurology 1998;50:1778–1783.

36. Matell G, Wedlund JE, Osterman PO, Pirskanen R. Effects of long-term azathioprine alone and combined with steroids in the course of myasthenia gravis. In: Satoyoshi E, editor. Myasthenia gravis: pathogenesis and treatment. Tokyo: Tokyo University Press, 1981:373–382.

37. Tindall RSA, Rollins JA, Phillips JT, Greenlee RG, Wells L, Belendiuk G. Preliminary results of a double-blind, randomized, placebo-controlled trial of cyclosporine in myasthenia gravis. N Engl J Med 316:1987;719–724.

38. Schalke B, Kappos L, Dommasch D, Rohrbach E, Mertens HG. Cyclosporin A treatment of myasthenia gravis: initial results of a double-blind trial of cyclosporin A versus azathioprine. Ann NY Acad Sci 1987;505:872–875.

39. Tindall RSA, Phillips T, Rollins JA, Wells L, Hall K. A clinical therapeutic trial of cyclosporine in myasthenia gravis. Ann NY Acad Sci 1993;681:539–551.

40. Gajdos P, Chevret S, Clair B, Tranchant C, Chastang C. Clinical trial of plasma exchange and high-dose intravenous immunoglobulin in myasthenia gravis. Myasthenia Gravis Clinical Study Group. Ann Neurol 1997;41:789–796.

41. Papatestas AE, Genkins G, Kornfeld P, Eisenkraft JB, Fagerstrom RP, Pozner J, Aufses AH. Effects of thymectomy in myasthenia gravis. Ann Surg 1987;206:79–88.

42. Wolfe GI, Herbelin L, Nations SP, et al. Myasthenia Gravis activities of daily living profile. Neurology 1999;52:1487–1489.

43. Weijnen FG. Quantitative and qualitative evaluation of bulbar symptoms in patients with myasthenia gravis. Thesis, Utrecht, The Netherlands 2000. Several publications in press.

After finishing this chapter an "activities daily living profile" for myasthenia gravis was published by Wolf et al. [42] that can serve as a secondary efficacy measurement in clinical trials. Furthermore, Weijnen et al. developed a unique laboratory setup to quantify bulbar muscle function in Myasthenia Gravis [43].

39. Myasthenia Gravis: Basic Designs, Sample Sizes and Pitfalls

J. Palace

Myasthenia gravis (MG) is a well-characterised antibody-mediated autoimmune disorder. The target of attack is the acetylcholine receptor (AChR) situated at the neuromuscular junction, and the resultant loss of AChRs leads to fatiguable weakness which is variable in distribution between patients. Patients with MG often respond dramatically to anticholinesterases, which increase the amount of acetylcholine (ACh) available to bind to the reduced number of AChRs. However this action is short-lived (hours) and has no effect on the underlying disease process. Immune manipulation with immunosuppressive drugs, plasma exchange (PE) and intra venous immunoglobins (IVIG) is more effective and, in the former case, long-term treatment for many patients. Clinical trials in MG aim to find the optimum of the present available treatments and the effectiveness of new, usually immune-modulating treatments.

Basic Designs

There have been few fully randomised double-blind controlled trials in MG. This may be because the established treatments such as anticholinesterases, corticosteroids, thymectomy and PE have been used since the 1970s before properly conducted trials were required by ethics committees.

Ethics

All trials now set up should be randomised, controlled and double-blind whenever possible. New long-term treatments should be tested against or in addition to older established ones rather than placebo for ethical reasons. This means that the old established treatments are unlikely to be tested for efficacy now against placebo.

Diagnosis

The diagnosis of MG should take into account three factors: the clinical picture, the electromyographic findings and the anti-AChR antibody status.

The clinical findings are of muscle weakness, often affecting extraocular muscles and often worse as the day goes on.

The electromyogram should show evidence of fatiguability with >10% decrement when the fifth shock of a train at 3 Hz is compared with the first (or at 2 min after exercise), or evidence of increased jitter and/or blocking on the single-fibre EMG.

Ninety per cent of patients with generalised MG have detectable anti-AChR antibodies. It is simpler to include only anti-AChR antibody positive patients unless a clinical trial of seronegative MG is specifically being undertaken. This is because the clinical picture and the presence of jitter and blocking on EMG are not specific for MG. Additionally, it can occasionally be difficult to differentiate between seronegative MG and congenital myasthenia, two conditions with similar EMG findings and absent anti-AChR antibodies. However, their disease mechanisms differ, the former being immune-mediated and responsive to immune modulation whereas the latter is genetic and non-responsive to such treatments.

Inclusions and Exclusions

All patients must have MG as defined under "Diagnosis". It may be necessary to exclude patients with ocular MG or Ossermann category I and include only the more severe cases of MG in treatment trials of immunosuppressive agents. The inclusion criteria may be set to ensure sufficient numbers of patients can be recruited to obtain a high level of statistical power. For example, when comparing two long-term immunosuppressive therapies, including patients already taking such treatment rather than only patients about to start such treatment, would increase the number of eligible patients.

Exclusion criteria will include the following:

1. any diseases in which the treatments are contraindicated;
2. other general medical conditions which might affect the outcome measures (e.g. myopathies or neuropathies which also cause muscle weakness);
3. serious medical conditions which are likely to shorten the follow-up period, such as malignancy;
4. pregnancy, unless the risks are equivalent in the treatment arms and no greater than established treatments;
5. age, usually >16–18 years.

Whether to set an upper age limit is open to debate. The management of elderly patients with MG is an important clinical consideration but including them inevitably causes an increase in the number of withdrawals and deaths due to unrelated medical problems. This was seen in one study [1] which did not set an upper age limit and had a large number of elderly deaths and withdrawals compared with another [2] which set an upper age limit of <75 years.

Stratification

Because MG affects different patients in different ways, and because some patients may have had previous treatments that can modify the disease process, it is desirable to stratify the treatment groups at randomisation. The clinical heterogeneity may affect how responsive a patient is to a specific treatment and thus the randomisation should ensure equal numbers of patients within each category entered into each treatment arm. For example, patients can be classified according to their clinical picture in association with the thymic pathology, age of onset and anti-AChR antibody titre [3] (Table 39.1).

Alternatively stratification according to disease severity, such as a modified Osserman classification (Table 39.2) or other measures of muscle strength, can be used to ensure that patients are equally distributed on entry to the trial. Additionally, a previous thymectomy may influence long-term outcome and should be included in any stratification.

Therapeutic Schedules

Corticosteroid schedules vary widely between centres and countries. Prednisone and prednisolone are the most commonly prescribed. Starting regimes

Table 39.1. Classification of MG patients according to age of onset, clinical features, thymus pathology and anti-AChR titre

Age of onset	Clinical features	Thymus pathology	Anti-AChR titre
<40 years	Generalised	Hyperplasia	+++
>40 years	Generalised	Involution	+
Any	Generalised	Thymoma	++
Any	Ocular	Thymoma excluded	+, ±, 0
Any	Generalised	Thymoma excluded	0

Table 39.2. Modified Osserman classification of MG

I	Ocular
IIA	Mild generalised
IIB	Moderate generalised
III	Acute severe
IV	Chronic severe

vary between slowly incrementing the dose to using the full dose immediately [4]. Variations include an initial high dose of between 1 and 1.5 mg/kg and alternate-day versus daily therapy. Once remission has been achieved the rate of corticosteroid reduction and the eventual maintenance dose also varies. Table 39.3 demonstrates the different corticosteroid schedules used in two similar treatment trials performed recently.

Other treatments vary in their schedules although probably less so than corticosteroids. It is important when setting up the trial to use treatment protocols acceptable to the treating neurologists. This may be particularly problematic at an international level because treatment schedules often differ between countries. For example, efficacy and side effects of daily prednisolone may differ from those observed in an alternate-day regime.

Where possible the outcome variable should be measured at a time when variations in regimes are unlikely to differ in their effect. In the case of immunosuppressive treatments, most variations only make a substantial difference early on. This allows some comparison to be made between trials which use different treatment schedules.

It is important to decide when setting up the study what additional treatments will be allowed during the course of the trial. This decision will take into consideration ethical issues such as whether the patient would be worse off if the additional treatment (e.g. PE) were withheld or whether the trial has sufficient flexibility to increase the study treatment to offset this disadvantage. One study, for example,

Table 39.3. Corticosteroid schedules used in two recent treatment trials for MG

	Palace et al. [1]	MG Clinical Study Group [2]
Corticosteroid:	Prednisolone	Prednisone
Induction:	Increments of 10 mg/ad (slower as an out-patient)	Start full dose
Alternate vs daily:	Alternate days	Daily
Top dose:	1.5 mg/kg (100 mg if lower)	1 mg/kg
Reduction instituted:	At clinical remission	After 1 month
Rate of reduction:	5–10 mg/kg monthly	1 mg/kg monthly for 5 months, then half this rate

allowed the prednisolone dose to be tailored to the patient's needs and then used the prednisolone dose as a measure of outcome [1]. Additional short-acting treatments such as PE and intravenous gamma-globulin (IVIG) should not affect long-term outcome if the outcome measurements are taken at times outside such treatment effects, and the requirement of such additional treatment could be a measure of "treatment failure". Two trials comparing corticosteroids and azathioprine treatments differed; one allowed PE [1], and the other allowed only it during the first 2 weeks of the trial, stratifying for such prior to randomisation [2].

Trial Personnel

All trials will need a blinded assessor in each participating centre, who will document the outcome measures. If the trial is assessing any treatment that requires long-term follow-up or has possible side effects it will also require a non-blind assessor to monitor blood tests and other side effects. It is also desirable to have a clinical manager if the trial requires the treatment to be modified in the light of the clinical state of the patient. This person would in theory be blinded to the treatment the patient was receiving so as not to be influenced in his or her decision. However, the clinical manager may correctly identify the treatment from the clinical clues.

Withdrawal Criteria

A non-blind doctor should monitor side effects, and withdraw or reduce the treatment according to the protocol. To minimise the likelihood of the blinded assessors/managers guessing which treatment group the patient is in, it may be necessary to withdraw or reduce the placebo treatment from a similarly stratified patient in the opposite arm.

Follow-up Visits and the Timing of Outcome Measurements

Myasthenic weakness fluctuates on an hourly and daily basis. This is partly due to the fatiguability which causes the motor function to deteriorate as the day progresses and also to the treatments commonly prescribed. Anticholinesterases are short-acting drugs which, when taken orally, work within an hour and last for several hours only. PE or IVIG are quick-acting but the effects are short-lived, whereas immunosuppressive treatment with, for example, corticosteroids or azathioprine, is slow in its initial action but effective in its long-term action. Additionally corticosteroid therapy may be given on alternate days in order to minimise the side effect profile. The timing of the outcome measures is therefore critical to reduce such variability. It is important that the measurements are taken (a) at the same time of day, (b) at a constant interval after anticholinesterase dosage and (c) consistently on an "on" (or "off") corticosteroid day. In addition, the delayed onset of action (e.g. 1 year) of long-acting immunosuppressive agents such as azathioprine needs to be recognised. Follow-up visits of between 2 and 6 months are usually sufficient. It may also be necessary to see patients at additional times to the scheduled follow-up periods, when relapses or side effects occur.

Sample Sizes

The number of patients needed for a study should be calculated by conventional methods [5]. Although most MG therapies have a large treatment effect they cannot ethically be tested against placebo. This means that the estimated difference in treatment effects between the two arms will be small and the sample size will need to be larger. In two recent studies comparing prednisolone and azathioprine it was estimated that 100 and 105 patients respectively were needed [1,2]. However, the slow accession rate resulted in both groups having to extend the time of entry to the trial, and led to termination of the trial with only 36 and 41 patients entered respectively, demonstrating the difficulty in finding sufficient MG patients for such randomised controlled trials. It is interesting nevertheless that both trials still showed statistically significant advantages from using azathioprine, suggesting that the difference in treatment effect was larger than originally estimated. Only if very short-acting treatments are studied (similar to the short action seen with anticholinesterases) can a placebo arm ethically be included. This may make it possible for a single-centre study to be performed, because the numbers of patients needed are likely to be lower. One study reported in 1987 did use a placebo arm when looking at the effectiveness of long-term immunosuppression with cyclosporine, and showed a significant effect during the 12 month trial using only 20 patients [6].

In addition, because of the clinical heterogeneity of MG, sufficient numbers of patients need to be recruited to ensure that patients can be stratified equally into the treatment arms.

Pitfalls

Timing of Outcome Measures

As discussed previously, the timing of outcome measures has to fulfil tight criteria which make the organisation of clinical trials in MG very demanding. Additionally the delayed onset of action of immunosuppressive agents means that it takes up to 1 year to reach remission. To allow for a subsequent reduction to a maintenance dose, the outcome measures have to be analysed from 1 year onwards. This means that such clinical trials need to follow each patient for 2–3 years. Because of the additional difficulty in recruitment, trials of immunosuppression in MG are prolonged; the two trials comparing azathioprine and corticosteroids lasted 7 [1] and 9 [2] years from randomising the first patient to final follow-up of the last.

Double-Blinding

In MG, some treatments are difficult to blind because of the procedure itself (e.g. PE) or because the patients may recognise the side effects of the active treatment (e.g. in the majority of patients, paraesthesia develops shortly after taking 3,4-diaminopyridine). In others such blinding would be ethically unacceptable (e.g. sham thymectomy). One solution is to set up a single-blind trial with the outcome assessor having no knowledge of the treatment received and, where possible, to back up clinical outcome measures with anti-AChR antibody levels and EMG measurements. However, the dramatic improvement seen immediately after thymectomy in some patients might be a direct effect of the trauma of the thoracotomy itself, similar to the way burn injuries result in upregulation of AChRs [7]. Single-blind would not differentiate between improvement due to thymectomy and improvement due to thoracotomy.

Clinical Heterogeneity

Although, as already mentioned, stratification at randomisation can distribute patients with different clinical classifications equally into each treatment arm, there is a wide variation in the pattern of weakness between patients even within these groups. The mean overall strength measurement for each patient would not distinguish between severe weakness of only a few muscle groups causing major disability and minimal weakness in all muscle groups. This problem has been approached by measuring the worst three of nine outcomes in one trial [1] and a five-scale functional scale in another [2].

References

1. Palace J, Newson-Davis J, Lecky B. A randomized double-blind trial of prednisolone alone or with azathioprine in myasthenia gravis. Myasthenia Gravis Study Group. Neurology 1998;50:1778–1783.
2. Myasthenia Gravis Clinical Study Group. A randomised clinical trial comparing prednisone and azathioprine in myasthenia gravis: results of the second interim analysis. J Neurol Neurosurg Psychiatry 1993;56:1157–1163.
3. Newsom-Davis J. Myasthenia gravis and myasthenic syndromes. In: Appel SH, editor. Current neurology. Chicago: Year Book Medical, 1986:47–72.
4. Sebold ME, Drachman DB. Gradually increasing doses of prednisolone in myasthenia gravis: reducing the hazards of treatment. N Engl J Med 1974;290:81–84.
5. George SL, Desu MM. Planning the size and duration of a clinical trial studying the time to some critical event. J Chron Dis 1974;87:15–24.
6. Tindall RSA, Rollins JA, et al. A double-blind randomised placebo-controlled trial to assess the safety and efficacy of cyclosporin a in the treatment of myasthenia gravis. Ann NY Acad Sci 1988;505:854–856.
7. Ward JM, Martin JA. Burn injury-induced nicotinic acetylcholine receptor changes on muscle membrane. Muscle Nerve 1993;16:348–354.

40. Myopathies: Ethics, Outcome Variables and Clinical Scales

R.W. Orrell and R.J. Guiloff

Introduction

Large-scale trials of therapy in muscle disease have been relatively rare. This may be related to the rarity of many individual muscle diseases, the lack of understanding of the pathogenesis of these diseases, and the limited number of rational therapies available. The chronic nature of some of the muscle diseases makes short-duration clinical trials of limited value.

The issues of ethics, outcome variables and clinical scales will be considered in the context of some of the muscle diseases in which they have been utilised. These muscle diseases illustrate the different issues involved. For example:

1. Duchenne muscular dystrophy: a childhood progressive, disabling and fatal disease.
2. Facioscapulohumeral dystrophy: a later onset, slowly progressive and non-fatal disease.
3. Mitochondrial myopathies: a heterogeneous group of biochemically definable diseases.
4. Myotonic dystrophy: a complex disease, both in its effects on muscle function and in its variable severity.
5. Inflammatory myopathies: a range of acquired, and often treatable, muscle diseases including polymyositis, dermatomyositis and inclusion body myositis.

Duchenne Muscular Dystrophy

Duchenne muscular dystrophy (DMD) is an X-linked muscle wasting disease, affecting males only, with typical features including a progressive proximal muscle weakness developing by age 5 years, loss of independent walking by age 12 years, and death due to respiratory failure before around 20–30 years. The biochemical abnormality is a deficiency of the cytoskeletal protein dystrophin in muscle fibres, due to mutations of the large dystrophin gene on chromosome Xp21.2. Lesser abnormalities of dystrophin may cause less severe forms of disease, explainable on the basis of the form of mutation (the more severe DMD being an out-of-frame mutation). The range of disease may better be called dystrophinopathies, and includes the milder presentation of Becker muscular dystrophy (BMD), and presentations with quadriceps myopathy, cardiomyopathy, myalgia and cramps, and sometimes no symptoms [1].

Steroids

Trials of prednisolone were performed in the 1970s [2], and earlier, and have been repeatedly performed and reported over the years. Initial scepticism [3] has matured into a general acceptance of the efficacy of this form of treatment in DMD [4,5]. Steroids appear to be effective in slowing the course of DMD, but do not halt or reverse the progressive muscle disease. With prednisone, the progress of the disease appears to be slowed by at least 3 years [6]. The clinical trials have recently been summarised [5]. The methodology includes double-blind, randomised control, crossover, and open studies. Measurements have been of muscle force, and functional assessments in relation to timed activities [4]. By selecting patients to study who are ambulant and within a narrow age range, the study may be more sensitive to detecting changes in shorter periods of time. Some studies have included patients with too early or late a stage of disease to detect, for example, a loss of ambulation. Muscle strength has been measured using the MRC scale in 26 muscle groups, and an electronic dynamometer in 24 muscle groups. Timed functions include walking 10 m and climbing stairs [4].

The design of satisfactory clinical trials has required a documentation and understanding of the natural history of the disease. Clinical trials in the dystrophinopathies are most usefully performed in the patients with the more severe and fatal DMD, but the results may then be transferable to milder forms. All patients may now be categorised at a molecular and histological level, which may improve the homogeneity of the population studied. Patients may discontinue treatment for reasons including lack of improvement or unacceptable side effects. With steroids the latter include excess weight gain, mood changes and skin changes [4].

Therapeutic trials using natural history controls have been proposed as an alternative to randomised placebo-controlled trials, as they require fewer patients and may be less expensive to perform, allowing screening of new agents [7]. Measurements used include muscle strength (average muscle score); joint contractures (average contracture score); timed functional tests (standing from a lying position on the floor, climbing four standard stairs, traversing 9 m as fast as possible); pulmonary function (forced vital capacity, maximum voluntary ventilation and maximum expiratory pressure); and amount of functional grade in legs and arms. Mendell et al. [7] pointed out that the ideal measurement is a single clinically relevant interval measure, with a linear change with age throughout the course of the disease. The closest match to this was the average muscle strength of 34 muscles. More difficult is the "roller-coaster" measurement, for example the time to walk 9 m, which is relatively stable until a rapid decline occurs, and then the test may no longer be performed. One possibility is to use a form of age standardisation. The disadvantages of natural history controlled trials are not addressed here.

A benefit for prednisone versus placebo in DMD was demonstrated in a randomised, double-blind, controlled trial in 103 boys, using two doses of prednisone and placebo [8]. Improvement was seen in scores of muscle strength and function; in time to rise from supine to standing, to walk 9 m, to climb four stairs, to lift a weight; and forced vital capacity. Urinary creatinine excretion was also increased, suggesting an increase in muscle mass. The initial study was 6 months of treatment, and a long-term study of 3 years confirmed a sustained benefit, using natural history controls [9]. Arguably a placebo group would be inappropriate in further studies given the demonstrated benefit. Another study demonstrated that daily therapy was superior to alternate-day therapy [6].

It is difficult to blind the assessor to the effect of a medication such as prednisone, and tests of muscle strength and function should ideally be performed by an assessor who has not enquired into the side effects. A study in 99 boys with DMD investigated a lower dose of prednisone (0.3 mg/kg versus 0.75 mg/kg, versus placebo) using the natural history control methodology. This demonstrated a beneficial effect of the higher dose [10]. It was pointed out that by performing early measurements, an improvement in strength was noted at 10 days, which is before the side effects of prednisone manifest, excluding the possibility of unblinding.

The mechanism of action of prednisone and prednisolone is uncertain, but is probably due to a membrane stabilising effect. Steroids have an immunosuppressant effect, and other agents have been tested in small pilot studies. These have again been natural history controlled, allowing smaller numbers of patients, and minimising financial costs. A comparison of placebo, prednisone, and prednisone and azathioprine (demonstrating no beneficial effect of azathioprine) used manual muscle testing of 34 muscle groups graded according to the MRC 10 point scale, and a score for average muscle strength was defined [11]. Muscle strength was also measured on the right side for shoulder abduction, elbow flexion and extension, and hip abduction, using a myometer. The myometry values were standardised by measures made at the initial two visits, and a composite value calculated, the composite score reflecting a change from baseline. Pulmonary function tests, timed functional tests, and the maximum hand-held weight which could be lifted were also assessed. Biochemical markers included creatine kinase (which did not change), and creatinine excretion (which increased with prednisone treatment indicating an increase in muscle mass).

A pilot study, the results suggesting a double-blind placebo controlled trial, was carried out in 10 DMD patients with an anabolic steroid, oxandrolone [12]. This was given for 3 months, and showed significant improvement in average muscle score, using natural history controls.

These studies demonstrate varying degrees of efficacy of steroids in DMD, but do not give a clear indication of the long-term effects on the disease. These studies are more difficult to perform. A study of 16 prednisone-treated and 38 untreated patients investigated age at loss of ambulation as an endpoint, using a survival curve analysis [13]. The study was initially an open trial, without simultaneous randomised controls, but the inability to stand or ambulate independently appears to be a well-defined and simple measure which is clinically relevant. The duration of prednisone treatment varied from 1 to 11 years, and ambulation was prolonged by around 2 years in treated patients.

Other Immunosuppressants

Another immunosuppressive drug, cyclosporine, has been investigated in a small non-randomised, unblind 2 month trial [14]. This was based on a preceding 4 month natural history study and 4 month post-treatment washout study. Measurements were performed specifically on tibialis anterior muscle isometric force, including twitch tension, maximum voluntary isometric contraction, tetanic force and compound muscle action potential amplitude. Tetanic force and maximum voluntary contraction increased during treatment, and further longer-term controlled studies were suggested. Studies of toxicity and tolerability of medication were also an important part of this pilot study.

Other Interventions

Other interventions in DMD include physiotherapy and orthopaedic treatment, including correction of contractures and scoliosis, and application of orthoses. Studies in this field are less strongly controlled, and may have a significant descriptive component. Outcome measures include medium- and long-term functional recovery, and the short- and long-term morbidity of surgical procedures [15–17].

Gene Therapy

The genetic abnormality which causes DMD (mutations of the dystrophin gene) is well characterised. The application of potential gene therapy to DMD patients reflects some of the issues relating to gene therapy in general [18,19]. The ideal treatment would correct the defect at all sites in the body, with physiological and anatomical reversal of the lesions [1]. Gene therapy may be considered as somatic cell gene therapy and genetic therapy [1]. In somatic cell gene therapy, normally functioning genes are inserted into the affected cells. In genetic therapy the abnormal gene expression is modified by genetic manipulation. For example it has been suggested that utrophin upregulation in DMD may correct the functional dystrophin deficit [20].

One method of gene therapy has been tested in patients with DMD. This is myoblast transfer, which is a form of somatic cell gene therapy. This involves injecting normal myoblasts into abnormal DMD muscle, in the hope that the myoblasts will fuse with the DMD fibres, introducing normal dystrophin to these fibres. Studies in *mdx* mice suggested that this was possible, and a study of 8 boys with DMD was performed, injecting a total of 55 million myoblasts at 55 sites in one biceps, giving placebo injections into the other biceps used as a control [21]. Cyclophosphamide immunosuppression was necessary. There were no serious complications, but there was a lack of improvement in maximum voluntary force generation, dystrophin content of the muscle and magnetic resonance imaging of the muscle, and

a lack of donor-derived DNA and dystrophin messenger RNA in the injected muscle. Other studies have also been performed in small numbers of patients. In one study expression of normal dystrophin was demonstrated in DMD, but no clinically relevant measurements were reported [22]. The limitations of these methods of myoblast transfer include the multiple injections required, the inaccessibility of many muscles, and apparent lack of efficacy.

Further clinical trials are awaiting improvements in the design of appropriate genes, gene delivery and gene expression systems [16]. Functional measures in clinical trials will be similar to those in more conventional pharmacological interventions, but with careful design for the unique ethical and long-term complications which may be associated with gene therapy. Extensive studies must be performed in animal models of the disease, if possible, before progressing to clinical studies. These may include studies of efficacy and adverse effects.

Current lines of research include the development of adenovirus vectors to introduce the gene into the muscle, and in DMD the *mdx* mouse has been used as a model of disease. Problems in adenovirus-mediated dystrophin minigene transfer include the immune response triggered by the viral proteins, a reduced muscle contraction due to direct vector toxicity, difficulty in infecting mature muscle fibres and an appropriate method of vector administration [19]. Potential problems in the patient include the unregulated expression of the gene in target, and non-target, cells. Transgene expression in germ cells may produce unpredictable effects and, more importantly, genetic manipulation of future generations.

The progressive, severe and fatal nature of DMD may make some of these risks potentially acceptable. Ethical considerations in gene therapy in DMD include [19] the expense of the treatment for society and the individual patient, and the fact that promoting longevity may increase the possibility of affected individuals having children, leading to an increase in the defective gene pool. Issues relating to therapy in DMD in general include the delivery of an experimental treatment to children who are unable to give consent, especially when it appears the treatment should ideally be given as early as possible in the disease. Kakulas [1] discusses the implications of gene therapy, or indeed any therapy, in DMD having a modest effect, and whilst not halting the disease, slowing the disease to give a milder Becker-like phenotype. Benefits include retained ability to walk, prevention of complications, arrest of progression and extension of lifespan. But limitations include a continuing dependency, no improvement in intelligence quotient, obligate carrier female offspring, and a change from an early death due to respiratory failure to a later death due to cardiac disease (the cardiac muscle dystrophin is also affected).

Facioscapulohumeral Dystrophy

Facioscapulohumeral dystrophy (FSHD) is the third most common form of muscular dystrophy. The distribution of muscle weakness is characteristic, affecting facial, scapular and humeral muscles predominantly, although other groups are also affected. The weakness is generally slowly progressive and, although it may cause significant disability in some patients (around 20% eventually requiring a wheelchair), it does not generally affect life expectancy [23]. FSHD is now a genetically defined disease, although the pathogenesis remains unknown. Most patients with FSHD have a reduced number of 3.3 kb repeats in the telomeric region of chromosome 4q. The inheritance is autosomal dominant, although around 30% may be de novo spontaneous mutations [23]. Although generally not causing death, the progressive weakness is disabling, and studies of therapeutic agents have been carried out. Following the observation that prednisone improved strength in DMD, and also the finding of inflammatory infiltrates in muscle biopsies of some patients with FSHD suggesting an inflammatory component to the myopathy, prednisone was tried in individual patients with FSHD, some with initial improvement in strength.

A pilot study was performed in 8 patients with FSHD [24], prednisone being given for 12 weeks. Methods of assessment used included manual muscle testing (MMT) and maximum voluntary isometric contraction (MVIC) in nine pairs of muscle groups; muscle mass estimation by measurement of lean body mass using dual-energy X-ray absorptiometry (DXA) [25]; and urinary creatinine excretion. No change was demonstrated over the 12 week period. DXA utilises the differential attenuation by tissues of transmitted photons to assess body composition. It takes around 30 min to perform. The primary outcome measure was change from baseline to 12 weeks in an arbitrary average MMT score (using an average of MMT grades; 5 = 5, 5− = 4.67, 4+ = 4.33, etc.). A secondary measure was the change from baseline to 12 weeks in average standardised MVIC score found after converting MVIC scores from individual muscles to the number of standard deviations from average normal strength (using a normal group rather than a patient group), and accounting for age, gender and height [23]. This was based on a previous study of the natural history of

81 FSHD patients over a period 3 years [26]. The progress in muscle weakness is slow in FSHD, but a decline in muscle strength was detectable. This study also allowed a calculation of sample size; for example, a two-armed clinical trial involving 160 patients per group and 1 year follow-up would provide 80% power to detect complete arrest of progression of disease. The inclusion of age, gender and height gives allowance for the wide variety of the patient population with FSHD, and the possible decline in muscle strength with age and sex in the normal population. The standardisation in children is more complex, as effects of underlying growth may complicate the interpretation of results. Also, in a disease such as FSHD, testing of involved muscles such as serratus anterior, peroneal, upper abdominal and facial muscles is difficult. The results of MVIC and MMT were compared, and whilst MVIC may be more sensitive, more cost and time is involved (MVIC of 18 muscle groups took nearly 1 h), and it was concluded that both MVIC and MMT have a place in clinical trials in FSHD [26].

Subsequently a pilot trial of albuterol has been conducted in FSHD, using similar methods [27]. Albuterol (or salbutamol) is a β2 adrenoceptor agonist, (commonly used in the treatment of asthma). This has previously been studied in a short duration (14 and 21 day) trial in healthy men [28]. In this study MVIC of quadriceps and hamstrings of both legs was measured using a transducer. Grip strength was measured using a dynamometer. Stimulated contraction–relaxation of adductor pollicis muscle of both hands was also measured. A significant increase in strength in quadriceps and hamstring muscles was demonstrated. Another β adrenoceptor agonist, clenbuterol, which has been abused by athletes to increase performance, was investigated in a double-blind, randomised, placebo-controlled study in 20 healthy men, studying operated (medial meniscectomy) and unoperated legs. Measurements included muscle strength by MVIC of knee extensor muscles, and CT images of muscle cross-sectional area in mid-thigh [29]. In the pilot trial of albuterol in FSHD [27], 15 FSHD patients were given albuterol for 3 months. Primary outcome measure was a change from baseline to 12 weeks in lean body mass using DXA. Secondary measures included the 3 week change in muscle mass (DXA), and 3 and 12 week changes in composite MVIC score. Albuterol significantly increased DXA lean body mass, and strength with composite MVIC scores increased by 12%. Strength was measured using MVIC and MMT as previously described [24,26]. A standardisation of the testing procedures and reliability has been demonstrated in FSHD patients and normal volunteer controls [30].

These effects are now being studied in a prospective, randomised, double-blind, placebo-controlled trial of 90 patients, involving three groups of 30 patients receiving placebo, low-dose albuterol or high-dose albuterol. Assessments are being done at baseline and at months 3, 6 and 12, using DXA, MVIC and MMT together with functional assessments and a subjective patient quality of life rating scale.

One of the ethical issues, or complications in trial design, relating to a readily available medication such as salbutamol/albuterol, which is readily prescribable and safe, and used in the treatment of asthma, is that patients may confuse the placebo arm by taking medication surreptitiously if they believe in the results of a pilot study.

Mitochondrial Myopathies

The mitochondrial diseases are a result of abnormalities of mitochondrial function, which may be due to a primary genetic abnormality in either the mitochondrial or nuclear genome. The result is a deficiency in oxidative phosphorylation and aerobic ATP production. In muscle this may lead to impaired exercise and tolerance, lactic acidosis and myopathy. The deficiency in other tissues may lead to other phenotypes [31]. The specific biochemical defects in the electron transport chain may be identified, and specific strategies to correct the deficit, or bypass it, have been tried [32]. Gene therapy strategies are being investigated, including approaches to selectively inhibit the replication of the mutant DNA (the cells being heteroplasmic, with both mutant and normal forms of the gene) [33]. The mitochondrial myopathies are rare, and may be a heterogeneous group with different biochemical defects. Many of the studies are in individual patients, or small groups, where the outcome measure may be biochemical.

For example, in an open study of a patient with cytochrome oxidase deficiency, a combination of oral dichloroacetate (DCA) and aerobic training resulted in improvement in biochemical indices of lactate response to exercise, phosphorus magnetic resonance spectroscopy, submaximal treadmill exercise test and the Medical Outcome Study Short Form Health Survey Questionnaire (SF-36) [34].

In a patient with a complex III defect of the electron transport chain, nuclear magnetic resonance determination of the ratio of phosphocreatine to inorganic phosphate was used, and improved following treatment with vitamins K_3 and C (these vitamins being supposed to allow electrons to bypass cytochrome b). A very subjective measure of distance walked or climbed and feeling of well-being also improved [35].

In an open study of 16 patients with a heterogeneous group of mitochondrial disorders, not all including myopathy, coenzyme Q_{10} (which has been found to be deficient in some patients with mitochondrial disease) together with other vitamins was tested [36]. Measures included lactate production and exercise response, phosphorus magnetic resonance spectroscopy studies at rest and during metabolic recovery from exercise, and change in deltoid or iliopsoas power. No significant changes were observed in these measures.

In a patient with MELAS syndrome (myoclonic encephalomyopathy, lactic acidosis, and stroke-like episodes), due to a mutation of mitochondrial $tRNA^{Leu(UUR)}$ [37], there was only mild proximal limb weakness (other features, including encephalopathy, seizures and sensorineural deafness, being more prominent). Treatment was with riboflavine and nicotinamide for 18 months, in an "N of one" crossover trial. Sural sensory action potential amplitude and magnetic resonance spectroscopy of the muscle bellies of finger flexor muscles, at rest, during exercise and during recovery, were measured. The two clinical endpoints were peripheral nerve dysfunction and encephalopathic stupor. Encephalopathic stupor occurred suddenly, suggesting a threshold phenomenon. The magnetic resonance spectroscopy phosphocreatine/adenosine triphosphate recovery rate fell in parallel with sural nerve sensory amplitude, and a fall in a measure of muscle bioenergetic efficiency coincided with development of encephalopathy. The symptoms and measures improved with treatment and deteriorated on withdrawal of medication. The full crossover was not completed as the initial withdrawal of vitamins (the patient already having taken them for 18 months) led to deterioration of symptoms, and blinding was felt to be superfluous.

Myotonic Dystrophy

Myotonic dystrophy is the most common adult form of muscular dystrophy. It is a multisystem disease, with muscle pathology including both a muscle wasting due to dystrophy and a stiffness due to myotonia or increased muscle excitability. Other features include cataracts, cardiac conduction defects, insulin resistance and testicular atrophy [38]. The underlying genetic defect is an unstable trinucleotide CTG repeat in the region of the DM gene on chromosome 19q13.3. Inheritance is autosomal dominant, with the clinical phenomenon of anticipation, i.e. the disease manifests in a more severe form in successive generations due to increased expansion of the repeat. Myotonia is also present in other rarer disorders such as sodium channelopathies (e.g. paramyotonia congenita) and chloride channelopathies (myotonia congenita).

For clinical trials, problems include the multisystem nature of the disease and the wide variation in clinical severity. There is also a perception that patients with myotonic dystrophy are sometimes reluctant to participate in clinical studies, as they may be unaware of their symptoms. The measurement of myotonia is different from that of weakness. A study of disopyramide and procainamide in the relief of myotonia in myotonic dystrophy [39] included 10 patients in a crossover trial. Both grip strength and timed hand opening were measured. Improvement with both drugs was variable between patients. Assessments were performed at 14 days. It should be possible to assess the response to myotonia in a short period of time as myotonia is thought to be improved through a membrane stabilising effect of the treatment.

In a study of nifedipine (used for its presumed effect on calcium transport in membrane stabilisation) in 10 patients with myotonic dystrophy [40], severity of myotonia was assessed by measuring finger extension time after maximum voluntary finger flexion, using a goniometer which included a potentiometer and chart recorder. A subjective measure of change in myotonia – no change, worse or improved – was also made. A significant improvement in myotonia was detected.

Testosterone was demonstrated to increase muscle mass and creatinine excretion and lean body mass (estimated by total body potassium measurement) in patients with myotonic dystrophy [41]. A 12 month, randomised, double-blind therapeutic trial of testosterone in 40 patients with myotonic dystrophy [41] evaluated strength by MMT, hand-held myometry and hand-grip dynamometry. Timed function testing, pulmonary function and forearm volume (water displacement) were also measured. Muscle mass was assessed by 24h urinary creatinine excretion, and lean body mass by whole-body potassium estimations. Myometry values were transformed into Z-scores based on a mean and standard deviation calculated for each muscle in all subjects at baseline evaluation. An average myometry strength score was calculated by averaging the Z-scores across all muscles for each patient evaluated, i.e. a "megascore". It was pointed out that the statistical design would require an improvement in strength to detect a benefit due to the slow progression and period of stabilisation in patients with myotonic dystrophy, unlike the more predictable course of progression

in DMD. In this study no improvement in strength was noted but an increase in muscle mass was detected.

In a placebo-controlled study in 27 patients with myotonic dystrophy, using selenium and vitamin E [42], main outcome measures used were muscle strength (knee extension, knee flexion, hand grip) using a dynamometer, maximal walking speed for 30 m, a functional status questionnaire, and two tests of cognitive functioning. No clear effect of treatment was observed, but the authors concluded that simple tests such as measurements of hand grip strength and walking speed demonstrated a deterioration over 2 years, which an effective therapy might be expected to change.

A study of recombinant human insulin-like growth factor I (rhIGF-I) (used on the basis of overcoming insulin resistance) investigated 7 patients with myotonic dystrophy on treatment and 9 on placebo [43]. Glucose metabolism was assessed by stable lactate IV glucose tolerance test; amino acid metabolism by stable labelled leucine turnover, oxidation and incorporation; body composition by DXA and nitrogen excretion; muscle response by graded MMT; and muscle function by patient perception of neuromuscular function. The patient's perception neuromuscular function scale was devised to test predominantly the fine motor function of the peripheral muscle, with 28 function activities (e.g. opening bottles, opening jars, putting on socks). The ability to perform the task was graded from 0 to 5. In this study, in addition to an increase in the metabolic indices and lean body mass, there was an increase in manual muscle strength and neuromuscular function in the 4 patients receiving the higher dose of rhIGF-I, over a period of 4 months.

Inflammatory Myopathies

The inflammatory myopathies include the syndromes of polymyositis and dermatomyositis, and inclusion body myositis, all of which have distinctive pathological features and are different diseases. Within these there are further distinctive subgroups, e.g. childhood dermatomyositis and adult dermatomyositis [44]. Clinical trials require a precise diagnosis and classification of the inflammatory muscle diseases, including full clinical assessment, muscle biopsy and electromyography. Corticosteroids are very effective in the acute management of many, but not all, inflammatory myopathies – so much so that is it difficult to perform a study with a placebo only. However, the long-term management with steroids is associated with significant side effects, and optimum therapeutic regimes and alternative agents, especially in subtypes of disease, may be tested in a clinical trial.

The severity and course of disease varies markedly between individuals, causing difficulty in the design of clinical trials. A controlled, prospective, double-blind therapeutic trial of azathioprine was performed in 16 patients receiving 60 mg of prednisone daily, plus either azathioprine or placebo for 3 months [45]. Disease activity was measured by time to normalisation of CPK level. MMT was performed on 18 muscle pairs, graded from 0 to −4, with scores totalled. A muscle biopsy was performed at baseline and at 3 months from the contralateral muscle, and the separate histological features (inflammation, degeneration, regeneration, necrosis, oxidative enzyme change, perifascicular atrophy, increased connective tissue, selective type II fiber atrophy, and other structural changes) were scored. There appeared to be no benefit of azathioprine, although this was a short-duration study of only 3 months and the immunosuppressant effect of azathioprine may take at least 3 months to become effective. It was possible to use the data to correlate serum CPK level with other levels of disease activity, and whilst in most cases a fall correlated with improvement in muscle strength and histopathological abnormalities, in 10 of 16 patients inflammatory cells persisted in muscle where CPK was normal.

In dermatomyositis, another variable – the rash – is available for study. In a double-blind, placebo-controlled study of 15 patients with biopsy-proven, treatment-resistant dermatomyositis [46], patients continued prednisone and randomly received either immunoglobulin infusion or placebo infusion. Clinical response was assessed by a neuromuscular symptom score (based on 20 activities that test function of a specific muscle group: e.g. raising arm above head, turning keys, graded from 0 to 3 and summed), an activities of daily living (ADL) score based on the Barthel index (used only for patients with severe muscle weakness, where this has been validated) and MMT of 18 proximal muscle groups rated on the MRC scale (with modification and summed [47]). Photographs of the rash were compared before and after treatment. Repeat muscle biopsies were performed in 5 patients with major improvement – quantified measures included muscle fibre diameter, and mean number of capillaries and their diameter. There was a significant improvement in muscle strength scores and neuromuscular symptoms in the patients treated with immunoglobulin. There was an increase in muscle fibre diameter, an increase in number and decrease in diameter of the capillaries, resolution of complement deposits on the capillaries,

and a reduction in expression of intercellular adhesion molecule 1 and major histocompatibility complex (MHC) class I antigen.

Unlike the other inflammatory myopathies, inclusion body myositis is considered poorly responsive to corticosteroid treatment. A retrospective review of 25 patients suggested a modest benefit in 40% [48]. A concomitant open randomised crossover prospective trial of combined oral azathioprine and methotrexate, and of biweekly intravenous methotrexate with leucovorin rescue, was performed in 11 patients [48]. For inclusion, all patients had to have at least two muscle groups graded 3 or less on an MMT scale of 0 to 5, and a reduction of at least 1 functional level below normal in at least 1 group on assessment of activities of daily living for functional capabilities. MMT of strength in 16 muscle groups was grade on a scale of 0 to 5 and scored. Ability to perform activities of daily living was assessed using an adaptation of the Convery Assessment Scale [49], i.e. feeding, grooming, wheelchair use and perineal care were deleted, and a question about reaching above eye level was added. Muscle biopsies were scored, and magnetic resonance imaging of the proximal leg performed with a fat-suppression technique to maximise the signal from inflammation. Other laboratory markers were measured. Outcome decisions were based on an improvement, stabilisation or worsening of MMT and ADL, defined as a change of at least 1 grade in two muscle groups and a net change in score of at least 2 on MMT and a net change of least 1 functional level in at least 1 category in the ADL score. There was clinical improvement in 3 trials, stabilisation in 11 and worsening in 5.

Conclusion

These examples of clinical trials in specific muscle diseases illustrate the variety of methods of clinical assessment and trial design which may be applied. Individual muscle diseases have specific variables and endpoints which may be uniquely appropriate. In some diseases it may be possible to quantify biochemical, molecular or histological changes, which whilst giving an early indication of an effect of the intervention do not necessarily indicate long-term clinical benefit.

The measurement of muscle strength, by manual grading or myometry, has been used repeatedly in these trials, and successful clinical trial centres and groups have devised consistent and validated methods. Some of these methods are similar to those discussed in the chapters on motor neurone disease

(Chapters 33–35). Natural history studies have been performed in some of these diseases, and when carefully performed these provide an important understanding of the relevance of outcome variables, a validation of the testing methods specific to that disease, and the possibility of anticipating the number of patients required in potentially expensive and time-consuming fully powered trials.

Unlike some of the other diseases discussed in this book, the muscle diseases, especially the muscular dystrophies, cause significant disability and death in very young children, raising specific ethical issues. The muscular dystrophies were the first neurological diseases to be understood by molecular genetics, and there is much research effort devoted to developing genetic therapies. There has not been any successful gene-based therapy for patients, but the development, testing and administration of any genetic therapy, especially to children, requires very careful consideration of ethical elements and well-designed, adequately powered studies with complete preparation.

References

1. Kakulas BA. Problems and potential for gene therapy in Duchenne muscular dystrophy. Neuromusc Disord 1997;7: 319–324.
2. Drachman DB, Toyka KV, Myer E. Prednisone in Duchenne muscular dystrophy. Lancet 1974;II:1409–1412.
3. Munsat TL, Walton JN. Prednisone in Duchenne muscular dystrophy. Lancet 1975;I:276–277.
4. Dubowitz V. 47th ENMC International Workshop: treatment of muscular dystrophy. Neuromusc Disord 1997;7:261–267.
5. Dubrovsky AL, Angelini C, Bonifati DM, Pegoraro E, Mesa L. Steroids in muscular dystrophy: where do we stand? Neuromusc Disord 1998;8:380–384.
6. Fenichel GM, Mendell JR, Moxley III RT, et al. A comparison of daily and alternate-day prednisone therapy in the treatment of Duchenne muscular dystrophy. Arch Neurol 1991;48:575–579.
7. Mendell JR, Province MA, Moxley III RT, et al. Clinical investigation of Duchenne muscular dystrophy: a methodology for therapeutic trials based on natural history controls. Arch Neurol 1987;44:808–811.
8. Mendell JR, Moxley RT, Griggs RC, et al. Randomized, double-blind six-month trial of prednisone in Duchenne's muscular dystrophy. N Engl J Med 1989;320:1592–1597.
9. Fenichel GM, Florence JM, Pestronk A, et al. Long-term benefit from prednisone therapy in Duchenne muscular dystrophy. Neurology 1991;41:1874–1877.
10. Griggs RC, Moxley III RT, Mendell JR, et al. Prednisone in Duchenne dystrophy. Arch Neurol 1991;48:383–388.
11. Griggs RC, Moxley III RT, Mendell JR, et al. Duchenne dystrophy: randomized, controlled trial of prednisone (18 months) and azathioprine (12 months). Neurology 1993; 43:520–527.
12. Fenichel G, Pestronk A, Florene J, Robison V, Hemelt V. A beneficial effect of oxandrolone in the treatment of Duchenne muscular dystrophy: a pilot study. Neurology 1997;48:1225–1226.
13. DeSilva S, Drachman DB, Mellitis D, Kuncl RW. Prednisone treatment in Duchenne muscular dystrophy: long term benefit. Arch Neurol 1987;44:818–822.
14. Sharma KR, Mynhier MA, Miller RG. Cyclosporine increases muscular force generation in Duchenne muscular dystrophy. Neurology 1993;43:527–532.
15. Granata C, Merlini L, Cervellati S, et al. Long-term results of spine surgery in Duchenne muscular dystrophy. Neuromusc Disord 1996;6:61–68.
16. Scheuerbrandt G. DMD meeting. Treatment of Duchenne muscular dystrophy. Neuromusc Disord 1998;8:213–219.
17. Vignos PJ, Wagner MB, Karlinchak B, Katirji B. Evaluation of a program for long-term treatment of Duchenne muscular dystrophy. J Bone Joint Surg AM 1996;78:1844–1852.
18. Karpati G, Gilbert R, Petrof BJ, Nalbantoglu J. Gene therapy research for Duchenne and Becker muscular dystrophies. Curr Opin Neuro 1997;10:430–435.
19. Karpati G, Lochmuller H. The scope of gene therapy in humans: scientific, safety and ethical considerations. Neuromusc Disord 1997;7:273–276.
20. Dennis CL, Tinsley JM, Deconinck AE, Davies KE. Molecular and functional analysis of the utrophin promoter source. Nucleic Acids Res 1996;24:1646–1652.
21. Karpati G, Ajdukovic D, Arnold D, et al. Myoblast transfer in Duchenne muscular dystrophy. Ann Neurol 1993;34:8–17.
22. Gussoni E, Paviath GK, Lanctot AM, et al. Normal dystrophin transcripts detected in Duchenne muscular dystrophy patients after myoblast transplantation. Nature 1992;356:435–438.
23. Tawil R, Figlewicz DA, Griggs RC, Weiffenbach B. Facioscapulohumeral dystrophy: a distinct regional myopathy with a novel molecular pathogenesis. FSH Consortium. Ann Neurol 1998;43:279–282.
24. Tawil R, McDermott MP, Panya S, et al. A pilot trial of prednisone in facioscapulohumeral muscular dystrophy. Neurology 1997;48:46–49.
25. Tawil R, Herr BE, Moxley RT, et al. Dual-energy x-ray absorptiometry: quantifying muscle mass in therapeutic trials [abstract]. Ann Neurol 1994;36:320.
26. FSH-DY Group. A prospective, quantitative study of the natural history of facioscapulohumeral muscular dystrophy (FSHD): implications for therapeutic trials. Neurology 1997; 48:38–46.
27. Kissel JT, McDermott MP, Natarajan R, et al. Pilot trial of albuterol in facioscapulohumeral muscular dystrophy. Neurology 1998;50:1402–1406.
28. Martineau L, Horan MA, Rothwell NJ, Little RA. Salbutamol, a β2-adrenoceptor agonist, increases skeletal muscle strength in young men. Clin Sci 1992;83:615–621.
29. Maltin CA, Delday MI, Watson JS, et al. Clenbuterol, a β-adrenoceptor agonist, increases relative muscle strength in orthopaedic patients. Clin Sci 1993;84:651–654.
30. Personius KE, Pandya S, King W, Tawil R, McDermott MP, FSH DY Group. Facioscapulohumeral dystrophy natural history study: standardization of testing procedures and reliability of measurements. Phys Ther 1994;74:253–263.
31. Hirano M, DiMauro S. Clinical features of mitochondrial myopathies and encephalomyopathies. In: Lane RJM, editor. Handbook of muscle disease. New York: Marcel Dekker, 1996:479–504.
32. Cooper JM, Schapira AHV. Clinical features of mitochondrial myopathies and encephalomyopathies. In: Lane RJM, editor. Handbook of muscle disease. New York: Marcel Dekker, 1996:519–531.
33. Taylor RW, Chinnery PE, Turnbull DM, Lightowler RN. Selective inhibition of mutant human mitochondrial DNA replication in vitro by peptide nucleic acids. Nature Genet 1997; 15:212–215.

34. Taivassalo T, Matthews PM, De Stefano N, et al. Combined aerobic training and dichloroacetate improve exercise capacity and indices of aerobic metabolism in muscle cytochrome oxidase deficiency. Neurology 1996;47:529–534.

35. Eleff S, Kennaway NG, Buist NRM, et al. ^{31}P NMP study of improvement in oxidative phosphorylation by vitamins K_3 and C in a patient with a defect in electron transport at complex III in skeletal muscle. Proc Natl Acad Sci USA 1984; 81:3529–3533.

36. Matthews PM, Ford B, Danduran RJ, et al. Coenzyme Q_{10} with multiple vitamins is generally ineffective in treatment of mitochondrial diseases. Neurology 1993;43:884–890.

37. Penn AMW, Lee JWK, Thuillier P, et al. MELAS syndrome with mitochondrial tRNA$^{Leu(UUR)}$ mutation: correlation of clinical state, nerve conduction, and muscle ^{31}P magnetic resonance spectroscopy during treatment with nicotinamide and riboflavin. Neurology 1992;42:2147–2152.

38. Lane RJM, Shelbourne P, Johnson KJ. Myotonic dystrophy. In: Lane RJM, editor. Handbook of muscle disease. New York: Marcel Dekker, 1996:311–328.

39. Finlay M. A comparative study of disopyramide and procainamide in the treatment of myotonia in myotonic dystrophy. J Neurol Neurosurg Psychiatry 1982;45:461–463.

40. Grant R, Sutton DL, Behan PO, Ballantyne JP. Nifedipine in the treatment of myotonia in myotonic dystrophy. J Neurol Neurosurg Psychiatry 1987;50:199–206.

41. Griggs RC, Pandya S, Florence JM, et al. Randomized controlled trial of testosterone in myotonic dystrophy. Neurology 1989;39:219–222.

42. Orndahl G, Grimby G, Grimby A, Johansson G, Wilhelmsen L. Functional deterioration and selenium–vitamin E treatment in myotonic dystrophy: a placebo-controlled study. J Intern Med 1994;235:205–210.

43. Vlachopapadopoulou E, Zachwieja JJ, Gertner JM, et al. Metabolic and clinical response to recombinant human insulin-like growth factor I in myotonic dystrophy: a clinical research center study. J Clin Endocrinol Metab 1995;80: 3715–3723.

44. Lane RJM, Hudgson P. Idiopathic inflammatory myopathies. In: Lane RJM, editor. Handbook of muscle disease. New York: Marcel Dekker, 1996:539–573.

45. Bunch TW, Worthington JW, Combs JJ, Ilstrup DM, Engel AG. Azathioprine with prednisone for polymyositis. Ann Intern Med 1980;92:365–369.

46. Dalakas MC, Illa I, Dambrosia JM, et al. A controlled trial of high-dose intravenous immune globulin infusions as treatment for dermatomyositis. New England Journal of Medicine 1993;329:1993–2000.

47. Soueidan SA, Dalakas MC. Treatment of inclusion-body myositis with high-dose intravenous immunoglobulin. Neurology 1993;43:876–879.

48. Leff RL, Miller FW, Hicks J, Fraser DD, Plotz PH. The treatment of inclusion body myositis: a retrospective review and a randomized, prospective trial of immunosuppressive therapy. Medicine 1993;72:225–235.

49. Convery FR, Minteer MA, Amiel D, Connett KL. Polyarticular disability: a functional assessment. Arch Phys Med Rehabil 1997;58:494–499.

41. Myopathies: Basic Designs, Sample Sizes and Pitfalls

M.H. Brooke

Introduction

Clinical researchers in neuromuscular diseases and, indeed, in neurologic diseases in general have been slow to adopt the methodology of clinical trials that were commonplace in some of our sister disciplines. At a time when the cardiologists were mining gold from large-scale epidemiologic trials, neurologists persisted in the belief that if a drug really worked it would not take more than a few patients to recognize it. Unconsciously, perhaps, it reflected the experience with penicillin, a drug which may have been as devastating to the idea of the controlled clinical trial as to the pneumococcus.

There have been relatively few clinical trials in myopathies, although Duchenne muscular dystrophy has come in for its share of the limelight [1–21]. On the other hand, we have learned a lot during the last decade about the methodology of trials in the myopathies. What once seemed a simple business of collecting a few patients and starting them on a medication has turned into a far more sophisticated system of enrolment, measurement and analysis. The following sections will reflect some of that experience and may provide a frame of reference for those wishing to determine the effect of therapeutic intervention on the myopathic patient.

The Right Question

This may seem absurd but the question answered by a clinical trial is often different from that originally intended. The CIDD group some years ago tested a number of agents in Duchenne muscular dystrophy (DMD) [2,3,10,11,14–18]. The trials were designed before there was any information on dystrophin deficiency as the cause of DMD. Muscle strength was (and is) the commonest variable that is measured in the clinic to follow such patients.

One of the trials undertook to determine whether prednisone was beneficial in DMD. The well-known Medical Research Council (MRC) manual muscle testing scale was adapted as the primary outcome measure of the study. This scale proved extremely reliable and was validated by inter- and intraobserver correlation [22]. It was shown to decline in a predictable linear fashion over the course of the disease in a number of different studies [10,11,14–18]. When the prednisone study was completed, there was an unequivocal effect of prednisone on strength. For the patients in the placebo group strength declined 0.2 ± 0.3 units. The treated group increased their strength by 0.2 ± 0.35 units. Statistical analysis using the familiar comparison of least square means showed a p value of <0.0001. This indicated that prednisone administration was associated with a difference in strength at the end of 6 months. A problem with the study was that it did not answer the question of whether this was useful to the patients or whether the increase in strength might have been due to a change in volition associated with a prednisone-induced euphoria, nor did it answer the question of whether prednisone had caused any change in the pathologic basis of the illness, all of which were important to physicians managing patients with DMD. The investigators had one other piece of information which was not tested scientifically but which was very convincing to those of us involved. In an earlier unblind pilot study of prednisone [23], the intent was to treat the patients for 6 months with prednisone, follow the strength change and subsequently to withdraw the patients from prednisone for 6 months. Appropriate measurements were planned to detect any change in the progression of the disease between the two phases. The design failed because at the end of the 6 months on active drug the families were so impressed by the effect of the drug on their children that they refused to discontinue the prednisone in spite of the urging of the investigators. We were told by several families that if we attempted to withdraw prednisone, they would go to their own physician to obtain it.

This aspect of clinical trials, the opinion of the subjects themselves, has been ignored until relatively recently and yet it is the crux. If the patient does not believe the drug to be efficacious, it is unlikely that it has a clinically significant effect. This has led to the development of global measures which are now considered an essential part of any trial. The question is usually put to the patients in a form which asks them whether they believe that they have had marked improvement, moderate improvement, no change, moderate worsening or marked worsening. This is not to recommend that measurements of strength be abandoned, but rather that they should be supplemented by functional measures and global measures of well-being.

You Must Be Mistaken

The perfect study is a hypothetical ideal that one cannot attain. Some errors can be avoided but others are inherent in the real world in which trials are conducted. By acknowledging that they exist, one can avoid drawing false conclusions.

Many of the patients in clinical trials are atypical. The population which is available to the investigator for testing is a subset of the patients attending the clinic, which is itself a subset of the patients in the region and world. All of us extrapolate the results obtained in our study subset and apply them to the entire population of patients, but this is not always justified. Certainly, some by the very act of volunteering for a clinical trial will set themselves apart from their more timid counterparts.

Consider recent trials in amyotrophic lateral sclerosis (ALS; UK: motor neurone disease, MND). When news of trials of experimental treatment reached the ALS community, clinics were understandably swamped with calls from patients desperate to enrol. Such patients represented a subset of all patients with the illness. They were highly motivated with access to information sources which even their family physician might not have had. They believed that the drug might work. They had the physical and financial resources which allowed them to travel. These characteristics set them apart from the general population of patients with ALS. These same characteristics also may have been the reason why some of these patients enrolled in two clinical trials simultaneously, without informing the investigators.

There are then two types of inference made in a clinical trial. The first is that the findings derived from the study represent some fundamental truth of the study. For example, the increase in the average MRC score in the trial of DMD implied that prednisone was beneficial to patients *in the study*. This being so, the study has internal validity. External validity implies that this finding can be extrapolated to the general population of DMD patients in all situations and depends on how well the selected population represents the larger population. An unlimited supply of patients is not available in most clinics. Further there are practical limits on how many patients can be accommodated in a particular trial. We will always have to select patients. It is wise to remember that truth, as discovered within a study population, only indicates truth in the general population if the characteristics of the two are identical for all important variables, and there may be some variables of which the investigator is unaware.

Selection Criteria

Inclusion Criteria

Investigators will correctly point out that the selection of inclusion and exclusion criteria is the single most important part of the trial design. Often the inclusion criteria are synonymous with diagnostic criteria and their purpose is to make certain that the population is homogeneous with regard to the disease entity. In the past, these criteria were often based on clinical findings. The selection of boys who were between 5 and 15 years old with the onset of the disease at 2 years of age or earlier, with a creatine kinase (CK) level of 10 times normal and with gastrocnemius hypertrophy would identify boys with DMD. As the basic mechanisms of the disease become apparent it may simplify the selection criteria. For example, boys younger than 15 years old with weakness and dystrophin deficiency would probably identify the same subset nowadays. One of the reasons that DMD, facioscapulohumeral dystrophy and myotonic dystrophy have been commoner subjects for clinical trials in the past [24–27] is that these diseases are clinically more stereotypic. It should not be long before trials in "limb girdle" dystrophy based on the genetic characterization of the populations become a reality. Inclusion criteria are also directly related to the research question which is being asked – an aspect which is often forgotten. If we turn back to the familiar example of prednisone in DMD, an investigator might be interested in one of the following three research questions: (1) Does prednisone have an effect in restoring dystrophin levels in the muscle toward normal? (2) Does prednisone have an effect in reducing secondary mechanisms of cell death? (3) How long does the effect of prednisone in DMD persist? Inclusion criteria for the first would need only to select patients who were dystrophin deficient, regardless of their phenotype. Similarly, the second question would require inclusion criteria that would set up some measure of cell damage not necessarily restricted to DMD. The third question would require the more familiar inclusion criteria to define the DMD patient and the patients would have to be young though to permit prolonged follow-up.

Exclusion Criteria

Exclusion criteria eliminate patients with diagnoses that may mimic the one intended. Thus, in studying facioscapulohumeral dystrophy, one might want to exclude patients with denervation changes on electromyography or biopsy, avoiding contamination of the group by unusual proximal spinal muscular atrophies. Criteria are also used to exclude patients who should not be recruited to the study for reasons unrelated to the diagnosis. Women who might be pregnant may be excluded because of the fear of unknown consequences to the fetus of an experimental drug. Patients with drug abuse or alcoholism, with significant general medical disease, or patients who are unlikely to be able to make the repeated visits for the evaluations are often excluded. The third use of exclusion criteria is to control confounding variables (see below). Inclusion criteria should be as simple as possible. A long and complicated set of inclusion criteria implies difficulty in characterizing the illness. Exclusion criteria, on the other hand, may be quite numerous as they exclude patients in specific situations.

Pitfalls

The wording of exclusion and inclusion criteria should be examined critically. It is very easy to provide accidental loopholes which will permit patients other than those intended to enter the study. This is not so detrimental if the study is limited to one or two investigators who have a clear idea of the intent of the criteria, but when a multicenter study is undertaken the dangers of misinterpretation increase. The following two examples illustrate the type of problem.

The OR Loophole

The OR loophole allows patients to slide in on the whim of the examiner. Let us say that a trial in myotonic dystrophy requires patients to have an objective measure of hand weakness. The criteria are "Grip strength <20 lb *or* cannot grasp a pen with thumb and forefinger *or* interosseous muscle strength ≤MRC 4". A grade of MRC 4 depends on a

judgment on the part of the examiner and is very difficult to apply to the small muscles of the hand. The criteria translate to the statement "The patient is weak because I say he is weak" rather than an objective measure. In designing diagnostic criteria, the investigator should avoid linking any subjective interpretation to objective measurements with an "or" statement.

The Nested AND

Sometimes, diagnostic criteria become unnecessarily complicated. This does not harm the protocol but does result in longer forms with investigator and patient fatigue as the clinical evaluation stretches out. A naive illustration would be a criterion which defines upper motor neurone damage by requiring "increased reflexes and ankle clonus". It is impossible to have ankle clonus without having increased reflexes. Since the set of patients defined by "ankle clonus" will always have "increased reflexes", one does not need to test for the latter.

The Tag Team Phenomenon

The tag team phenomenon is related to the nested "and" and occurs when one aspect of the disease is given undue emphasis in the inclusion criteria. In times before the discovery of dystrophin deficiency, clinical and laboratory findings were used to make the diagnosis of DMD. One way to define the disease might be to require five of the following eight criteria in boys under 10 years of age: progressive course, proximal muscle weakness, gastrocnemius hypertrophy, waddling gait, heel cord contractures, difficulty with stair climbing, myopathic electromyogram, elevated CK level. Because proximal muscle (hip) weakness is responsible for a waddling gait and difficulty in stair climbing, these are not independent criteria. Thus hip weakness accounts for three "points" whereas it should only account for one. Since one would only have to add a myopathic biopsy and a progressive course for a patient to be included in the study, a boy with any progressive myopathy would be eligible.

Confounding Variables

One of the most difficult tasks for the clinical investigator is the identification of confounding variables. A confounding variable is any factor which may itself have an effect on the outcome measures. To illustrate this, consider a study investigating the effects of percutaneous tenotomy on braced ambulation in DMD [28]. Twenty-nine patients who had subcutaneous tenotomy continued walking until almost 13 years of age whereas a group of 25 patients who refused surgery ceased walking soon after their tenth birthday – a clear difference. There are several possible confounding variables in this study. The success or failure of braced ambulation has much to do with the motivation of the patient and his family. In a natural history study, when the time to traverse 30 feet (9 m) was recorded on successive visits, some patients would slow down and then abruptly be unable to do the task. Others would keep performing the task even though they took 5 or 10 min to complete it. The latter group of boys placed great importance on ambulation and were strongly motivated. It is possible that patients who have strong motivation to continue ambulation will accept the recommendation for surgery. Those who do not care about walking will not. This postulates that motivation is a compounding variable, as the authors themselves pointed out. It is a very difficult one to control, but supposing that both groups were matched as far as motivation was concerned, would that indicate a valid study? There are other potential difficulties. Patients with DMD have variable intelligence. In general, it is believed that the population has a shift in the IQ curve of some 20 points to the side of lower intelligence. This means that although there are many bright children with the illness, others are of borderline or low normal intelligence. In addition many patients have an attention deficit disorder. Both could influence the ability to use braces and present as possible confounding variables. Finally, knee-foot orthoses were used in all children who underwent surgery but not in those who refused. This could be another confounding variable and may be the reason why these children walked for a longer period. Is it likely that percutaneous tenotomy prolongs the stage of braced ambulation? Yes it is. Are the conclusions drawn by the study justified? Only if the groups were balanced with regard to the confounding variables.

Types of Confounding Variables

Cause-Effect

The examples given above are all cause-effect variables, that is the variable itself has a direct effect on the outcome measure being studied.

Effect-Cause

Some confounding variables work in reverse fashion, the cart in front of the horse. Such errors are not likely to arise in cohort studies (the traditional placebo-controlled double-blind type) but may be seen in cross-sectional studies where the characteristics of a disease are being studied in a large population. Consider the situation in myasthenia in which

the patients who do best are those who are on immunosuppressive drugs but are taking no pyridostigmine. Does one conclude that pyridostigmine has a long-term deleterious effect on myasthenia or is the proper interpretation that this is an effect-cause and that patients who have an inherently milder disease can get by with no pyridostigmine?

Effect-Effect

Effect-effect confounding variables are probably the most difficult to control. Some other unknown factor controls both the variable in question and the outcome predictor. A hypothetical study might compare a group of patients who had scoliosis surgery with those who did not and conclude that the patients who had such surgery lived longer. In fact, socio-economic status may play a major role in determining both. Families who cannot afford the surgery might also have limited access to the medical system for the expensive treatment of the late complications of the disease and the boys may die earlier.

Dealing with Confounding Variables

There are three ways of dealing with such confounding variables. The first is to exclude them. This is the easiest to deal with statistically, but since there are often many variables and relatively few patients with muscle disease this reduces the power of the study to detect an effect. One can also balance the groups at baseline with regard to the variable. This essentially matches the groups and removes the influence of the variable. It is this principle which results in the traditional age-matched control, since age is simply one of the commonest confounding variables. Matching the patients in this way has a disadvantage since if the variable is of interest in its own right, one can not study it any further in the trial. Stratification of the patients is another way of dealing with confounding variables. This is the same as matching the groups at baseline except that the process is done during the statistical analysis at the end of the study rather than at the start. The disadvantage of baseline matching and stratification is again that there may be a large number of "strata" with few patients in each group and this will reduce the power to detect change. Finally multivariate analysis can be used to determine the effect of a number of variables on the outcome measures.

Dropouts and Survivor Bias

Very few studies will finish with all the patients having attended the clinic for all the visits, and in most studies some patients are completely lost to follow-up before the end of the study in spite of the investigators' best efforts. The causes vary from death to disenchantment and may be commoner in neuromuscular diseases with the attendant debilitation than in other illnesses. Statisticians have developed various ways of dealing with the problem which are beyond the scope of this chapter (see Chapter 13). However, the concept of survivor bias is an important one and implies that the characteristics of volunteers who successfully complete a study is different from those who drop out. It is probably best illustrated by considering a hypothetical study of DMD which is designed using historical controls. Since there is no concurrent placebo group, all are placed on the treatment being investigated. Patients with DMD progress at various rates, including one group who may progress extremely slowly and have been termed "outliers" [29]. Halfway through the study, which is now becoming tedious to the families, Mrs. Smith notices that her boy is progressing more rapidly than Mrs. Jones' son as they swap notes in the waiting room. She is depressed and discouraged by this and wonders whether the drug is worth the frequent arduous trips. The informed consent says that she can drop out at any time – so she does. Conversely, Mrs. Jones notices that her boy is doing surprisingly well and decides that, whatever the inconvenience, she had better continue. This will lead to a disproportionate number of the "good" DMD patients finishing the study and the conclusion that patients who were maintained on the drug for the whole course of the study did better than those who discontinued the drug earlier. The effect based on natural history may be mistaken for a therapeutic effect. This makes it imperative to study the group of patients who drop out in order to identify, as far as possible, any survivor bias.

Make the Right Measurements

Incorrect Data

Underlying all clinical trials is the assumption that the data are accurate. When comparing the statistics within a study, it is assumed that the measurements that went into deriving these parameters are correct. Good clinical evaluators and clinical investigators are not genetically determined but need training and constant practice. It is advisable in any new clinical trial to have a 2 to 3 month period during which data is collected, measurements standardized and which is, in general, the "shakedown" period. It is better to discover unacceptable and often unexpected variations in the measurement techniques at this stage than when one breaks the code and analyzes the final

data. Another aspect of data collection which is often overlooked is that the evaluator who makes the measurements should not have access to any of the previous measurements when the subject is being evaluated. If the strength of the biceps has been steadily declining over the last few months, the evaluator will "expect" the strength to be slightly lower and may not grade the muscle as objectively.

Missing Data

Before discussing the measurements themselves there are some important general principles to consider. Only measurements that are made at baseline and at the end of the protocol can be used to gain information. One cannot extrapolate the data points beyond their limit any more in a clinical trial than one can in the laboratory (see also Chapters 10 and 13). This does not simply mean that the patient must complete the study. For example, if timed ambulation is declared as the primary outcome measure, there must be some expectation that patients who are ambulatory at the beginning of the study will still be walking at the end of the study. Similarly, if the primary outcome measure is cessation of ambulation, patients should be selected who are likely to lose ambulation during the study.

Floor and Ceiling Effects

Related to the above, is the concept of floor and ceiling effects. Any measurement scale has a maximum and minimum point. If the patient reaches either of these points during the study, no more change can be measured. It was for this reason that DMD patients over the age of 15 years were excluded from several studies. They are often so weak that little increase in their weakness would be expected, making comparison between the treatment group and the placebo very difficult.

Measurements

There are many different types of measurements that can be made in patients with myopathies. Most are indirect measures of the illness and measure some aspect of either strength or function. Manual muscle testing, isometric and isokinetic myometry, pulmonary function testing, functional rating scales and timed functional tests have been described and validated.

Types of Data

There is often confusion about the way in which data points can be handled statistically and, to repeat the familiar review, data may be continuous or categorical. Continuous data implies that one end of the scale represents a quantity that is more than the other end and that the steps in between are related to each other. The ideal continuous scale has an infinite number of steps, hence the name continuous data. A discrete variable is one in which the steps are regularly ordered but not infinite. Thus, the number of cups of coffee drunk per day would be a discrete variable whereas the volume of coffee drunk is a continuous variable. In practice, most measurements are discrete variables. Take the example of the blood pressure as usually recorded. Although this is in theory a continuous variable, the markings on the average sphygmomanometer do not permit measurement more precise than about 2 mmHg.

One gets into more difficulty with data which are not continuous but are categorical. Categorical data implies that the measurement falls into a category, which may or may not be related in quantity. Nominal data, such as whether a patient is left- or right-handed or the patient's blood type, imply no quantitative relationship between the categories. Ordinal data, in which the categories bear some relationship – such as mild, moderate and severe – may be analyzed differently. Ordinal data with large numbers of categories may provide a considerable amount of useful information which can be analyzed with methods similar to continuous data. Manual muscle testing falls into this category in special situations.

There are two other characteristics of measurements which are often used synonymously although they imply quite different aspects of the data: accuracy and precision. The precision of a measurement reflects the degree to which it can be reproduced by more than one examiner or by the same examiner at different times. Accuracy implies the relationship of the test to the property which it is desired to measure. In a study attempting to alter the course of ALS, nerve conduction velocity would have high precision but very low accuracy.

Manual Muscle Test

Manual muscle testing is based on the MRC's recommendations. The well-known scale ranges from 0 to 5 but it has been modified to give a 10 point scale.

0   No movement.
1   Flicker of movement.
2   Moves the joint when the effect of gravity is eliminated.
3   Moves the joint through the full range against gravity but not against resistance.
3+ Moves the joint against gravity and a little resistance, but there is not enough additional strength

to sustain this and the limb collapses after a second or so of applied resistance. *Note*: this is quite different from the "sudden give" of the hysterical muscle. In this case the muscle exerts quite good strength (MRC 4) before abruptly collapsing.

4− Definitely weak, moves the joint against gravity and sustained resistance but the examiner has to exert little effort to overcome the strength.
4   Definitely weak and the examiner has to exert resistance but not to the point of strong effort.
4+ Definitely weak but still exerts enough resistance to make the examiner work at overcoming the resistance.
5− The examiner truly cannot identify the muscle as abnormal but has a suspicion that it might not be normal. It is not used for muscles that are slightly weak.
5   Full strength.

Manual muscle testing requires training of the evaluator. The commonest error in applying these grades is to underestimate the normal level of strength. Anyone who has tried to take a toy away from an unwilling child has a better appreciation of normal strength than many neurologists. The knee extensor, for example, even when tested with the knee semi-flexed, cannot be overcome by the examiner until it has lost considerable strength. After a period of training the test becomes extremely reliable [30]. Like many measurement scales, there are significant advantages and disadvantages.

The manual muscle test provides ordinal data and the various grades are not separated by a predictable interval. One of the reasons why the original MRC scale was expanded is that grade 4 in its original form covered a wide range of strength. Manual muscle testing is of little use if one or two muscles are being evaluated. Its comes into its own when a composite is used. The Average Muscle Score is an average of the values of 34 muscle groups (neck flexors and extensors, shoulder abductors and external rotators, elbow flexors and extensors, wrist flexors and extensors, finger and thumb abductors, hip flexors and extensors, knee flexors and extensors and ankle dorsiflexors, evertors and plantar flexors). The power of this measurement is that it markedly increases the sensitivity of the scale and provides ordinal data which behave as interval data and can be analyzed with similar methods. The Average Muscle Score is sensitive to change limited to one region of the body in a way which is undetected by a more limited survey of the muscles as is the case with fixed myometry. This makes it valuable in illnesses in which not all muscles are changing at the same rate or in which the weakness is regional or asymmetric. It is also very useful in children. As children grow, their strength increases. This means that if a child is weak and that weakness remains the same for 2 years, the muscle will be "stronger" at the end of the period when measured by fixed myometry, a technique without any internal reference. In manual muscle testing the evaluator judges the strength against what would be normal for a child of that particular age and build. This is at once one of the strengths and weaknesses of the scale. It requires subjective interpretation on the part of the examiner. In practical use in clinical trials it has proven very effective. In DMD it provided a measure of strength which declined linearly, was reproducible in several different trials and which was sensitive enough to detect a treatment effect of prednisone within 2 weeks. It also provided a reliable measure of strength in ALS [31].

Hand-Held Myometry

The hand-held myometer [32] is an attempt to improve the quantitation of manual muscle testing. These devices are basically portable strain gauges, often electronic, which provide a measurement of force in newtons. The myometer is placed by the examiner over a selected spot in the limb to be tested. For example, when the biceps is tested, the myometer is placed at the level of the wrist. The patient flexes the elbow and the examiner resists this movement. The force generated by the patient in a maximal effort is recorded. It is important that succeeding examinations are carried out with the limb in an identical position and with the myometer placed in the identical spot to avoid changing the length of the lever arm, which would obviously make a major difference in the force recorded. The advantage to hand-held myometry is that it gives a quantitative measure of strength. It is portable and not very expensive. It is therefore within reach of the average neurologist's office. There are some problems associated with this device. As mentioned, the consistency of the measurements is critically dependent on the exact placement of the myometer each time. Also the examiner's strength is a limiting factor. If the patient is stronger than the examiner then the maximum strength that will be recorded is the examiner's strength and not the patient's. This may be a practical problem if the patient is a burly 100 kg ex-football player and the examiner is not.

Fixed Myometry

The fixed myometer is a strain gauge which is attached to a rigid frame. Incorporated into this frame is a positioning device such as an adjustable examining table which allows the patient to be placed in a predetermined position for testing. The force is exerted through a strap or cable that is placed in a set position each time. The data are usually recorded electronically and may be expressed in a number of ways: graphs, curves of force, etc. Maximum voluntary isometric contraction (MVIC) has been validated in a number of studies, particularly in ALS [33]. It provides a linear measure of decline of strength in this illness. It is the only method to quantitate the force generated and is often regarded as the gold standard of strength measurement. If a study is limited to the measurement of strength in only one or two muscles, it is the only method that can be used since effective manual muscle testing requires measurements from many different muscles.

Fixed myometry provides useful measures of change in individual muscles. It has been more difficult to apply myometry across groups of patients. The force generated by the biceps of a frail 60-year-old is not the same as that from a 22-year-old weightlifter and yet both are normal. In order to provide some measure which could be used to standardize the data, comparisons with control groups defined by age, sex and body habitus may be used. Similarly the raw data may be expressed in relation to the values for the entire group of subjects and transformed into Z-scores [34].

The problems involved in fixed myometry are, again, practical ones. The test is time-consuming. Only large muscle groups can be tested, although adaptive devices can be designed which allow some of the smaller muscle groups to be evaluated. Common muscles to test include the hip flexors, extensors, the knee and elbow flexors and extensors and the shoulder abductors. Since these represent the major significant muscles in the body this may not be much of a disadvantage. Fixed myometry is affected much more by volition than some other tests since the myometer, unlike the evaluator, has no way of sensing whether the patient is trying his or her hardest. This may be a particular problem when myometry is included as the last test on a crowded morning. Perhaps the biggest disadvantage is that the myometer is a bulky and expensive piece of equipment and not likely to be found in the average neurologist's office.

Isokinetic Dynamometry

The isokinetic dynamometer is a popular measure of muscle function in exercise physiology laboratories and physiotherapy departments. Fixed myometry measures the force of the muscle exerted against an immovable strain gauge. The isokinetic dynamometer measures the patient's strength in a fashion which seems more physiologic. The force is exerted against a lever arm which moves at a constant angular velocity which can be varied from slow to fast speeds. This tests the muscle performance in a more realistic setting, moving the limb at a number of different speeds. This advantage may be somewhat theoretical and there are no studies which have shown that patients with neuromuscular diseases are more easily followed on this machine than with fixed myometry. Until such time as a clear advantage is noted, the additional cost of the equipment remains a strong deterrent.

Functional Rating Scales

Functional rating scales and the related timed functional tests are very useful in the setting of treatment protocols which are designed to detect a change in the course of the disease. It is sometimes hard to appreciate, but the patient is only interested in an improvement in strength insofar as it relates to a change in function. An increase in the MVIC of the quadriceps muscle of 15 newtons is not by itself as important as regaining the ability to use a zipper. For this reason functional scales are becoming increasingly important.

The Observational Functional Measurement (Functional Scale). Functional scales have been used for decades. One of the earliest in muscular dystrophies was that proposed by Vignos et al. [35] and later modified by the CIDD group (Table 41.1). In addition to its use in clinical trails this rating scale often provides information which is lacking from the routine

medical record. Many investigators have had the experience, in attempting to do a retrospective chart review, of not being able to find out whether the patient was ambulatory or not, quite apart from the niceties of how strong the muscles were. Because the clinical characteristics of diseases differ there has been a tendency for functional scales to be disease-specific. Thus a commonly used rating scale in ALS [36] is quite different from that used in DMD. There is nothing wrong with this and investigators may wish to design their own version of a rating scale to suit a particular illness. Some caveats should be heeded. Firstly a rating scale has to be validated by use in the clinical situation. It must be shown the scale changes consistently and progressively in the target disease.

Of interest in the functional rating scale that was used by the CIDD group was that during the course of several years of studies most patients dropped from leg functional grade 3 (walks and climbs stairs) to 5 (walks but cannot arise from a chair or climb stairs) without ever entering grade 4 (walks and arises from chair but cannot climb stairs). The reason for this is obvious in retrospect. In designing the scale the investigators believed that the DMD patient would cease to climb stairs before they ceased to arise from a chair. In fact, these two thresholds were crossed at the same time. Thus leg functional grade 4 should be abandoned and the scale telescoped to a 9 point scale. This scale is not linear in patients with DMD. Most of the change occurs in the years between 6 and 10 years of age. The scale does represent impor-

Table 41.1. Functional scale for muscular dystrophies

Functional grade: Legs
 1 Climbs stairs without assistance
 2 Climbs stairs with the aid of a railing.
 3 Climbs stairs slowly (over 12 seconds for four standard stairs)
 4 Walks unassisted and rises from chair but cannot climb stairs – see text
 5 Walks unassisted but cannot rise from chair or climb stairs
 6 Walks only with assistance or walks independently with long leg braces
 7 Walks with long leg braces but requires assistance for balance
 8 Stands in long leg braces but unable to walk even with assistance
 9 Confined to wheelchair
10 Confined to bed

Functional grade: Arms
 1 Starting with the arms by the sides, the patient can abduct the arms in a full circle until they touch above the head
 2 Can raise arms above the head by flexing the elbow (shortening the circumference of the movement)
   If grade 1 or grade 2, how many kilograms can be placed on a shelf above eye level, using one hand?
 3 Cannot raise hands above head but can raise and 8 ounce glass of water to mouth (using both hands if necessary)
 4 Can raise hand to mouth but cannot raise 8 ounce glass of water to mouth
 5 Cannot raise hands to mouth but can use hands to pick up coins from a table
 6 Cannot raise hands to mouth and has no useful function of hands

From Vignos et al. [36] as modified by the CIDD group.

tant stages in the life of the individual and for this reason it provides a clinically significant classification of the illness.

Pitfalls. There are some traps for the unwary in the design of rating scales. A common problem in designing functional scales is linking two or more clinical features with "and" statements when they are not related. To illustrate this consider a functional rating scale taken from the older literature [37] in which the investigator graded the severity of the patient's functional impairment as follows:

Grade 9:   Frequent collapse due to knees giving way, prefers being carried to walking.
Grade 10: Walks slowly with rolling gait and very marked lordosis, unable to arise from chair unaided.

The fact that "frequent" and "slowly" requires some standard of comparison will be overlooked. A bigger problem is that the set of patients designated by "Frequent collapse due to knees giving way" may be the same set as those defined by "walks slowly with rolling gait and very marked lordosis". There is no predictable progression from one state to the other. The grades could be redefined as follows to try to present an ordered progression:

Grade 9:   Walks slowly with a waddling gait, prefers to be carried.
Grade 10: Walks slowly with a waddling gait, falls daily, cannot arise from a chair.

Now there is a worse problem which involves the last part of the criteria. We are linking states by "and" that should not be linked. The investigator has assumed that the natural history of the disease goes from preferring to be carried to not being able to arise from a chair. These things have nothing to do with each other, however, One – "prefers being carried" – is an emotional preference; the other – "cannot arise from a chair" – a measure of physical strength. If there are boys who prefer to be carried even when they are not falling daily, or others who cannot arise from a chair but hate the "indignity" of being carried, then the criteria will be useless. Interestingly the conclusion of the investigator in this study was that the drug used caused marked benefit in the disease. It was followed by other better controlled trials which showed no effect [38]. This is an extreme example but other more subtle instances may be found. Consider the following two criteria for evaluating facial weakness:

Strong: Normal eye closure (buries eyelashes fully), purses lips fully.
Weak: Poor eye closure (buries eyelashes incompletely), cannot purse lips fully.

There will be patients who can be graded as neither normal nor weak (those who can purse their lips but not bury their eyelashes, for example). In this instance for the grading to be valid it would have to read:

1. Normal.
2. Weakness of either eye closure or lip pursing.
3. Weakness of both eye closure and lip pursing.

The rule in designing and evaluating accurate functional grades is to look at each grade. Do all characteristics in the grade which are linked by the Boolean "and" always coexist? If they do, you only need one of them! If they do not, then the characteristics must be ranked according to the progression of the disease and grades must be set up which will allow a progression through the sequence. If you wish to base a grading system on weekly falling, loss of stair climbing and loss of ambulation, which you believe always occur in a progressive sequence in the target illness, the necessary grades would be.

1. Ambulatory, falls less then weekly, can climb stairs.
2. Ambulatory, falls at least weekly, can climb stairs.
3. Ambulatory, cannot climb stairs.
4. Non-ambulatory.

Notice that you drop the need for rating "falling" and "stair climbing" from the later grades because of the rule in the preceding paragraph.

Quantitated Functional Measurement (Timed Functional Testing, Pulmonary Function). Among the most useful of the functional tests is the timed functional test. The common tasks are arising from the floor, climbing four standard stairs and walking 10 m or 30 feet. The advantage to these tests is that they provide the advantages of a functional test with the quantitation which can be used in more powerful statistical analysis. The major problem with timed tests is that are very susceptible to floor and ceiling effects during the course of the illness. The average life span of the child with DMD is around two decades. Until the age of 3 or 4 years, such children can arise from the floor within a couple of seconds or so, a time indistinguishable from normal, even though their illness is worsening. By the time they are 5 years old they can do the test reliably and it is usually abnormal. Assume, as is often true, that the boy will lose the ability to arise from the floor at all by 8 or 9 years old. This means that outside of these ages the test will either be performed so quickly that timing it is difficult (ceiling) or the test cannot be done at all (floor). If one were to embark on a 4 year study of DMD using this test as a primary outcome measure, patients (from 5 to 9 years old) who could provide a reliable measure at baseline would not be able to complete the test at the end of the study. Their data would therefore be useless as far as analysis of the timed aspect is concerned. It might be suggested that one could use the data from the first 1 or 2 years to provide useful information. This is correct, but then one has a 1 or 2 year study not a 4 year study. The recommendation is to match the functional tests to the knowledge of the natural history of the disease.

Pulmonary function testing is a special form of quantitated functional testing which has two major advantages. Firstly it represents a function that is of primary importance to the individual. Secondly, it does not exhibit a "floor" effect in the usual sense since, without assistance, the cessation of breathing is not compatible with life. Simple measures of pulmonary function such as forced vital capacity and maximum voluntary ventilation over 1 min are as useful as any of the more complicated tasks and, additionally, can be done in the office of the average neurologist.

Questionnaires

There is an increasing use of the questionnaire in present clinical trials. This is a form which is filled out by the subject or by the care giver. It measures the impact of the treatment on the patient and on the home environment in a way which is impossible with any of the measurements made in the clinic setting by the study evaluator. As such, these questionnaires are invaluable and are particularly useful in studies in which a small statistically significant effect may be mistaken for a clinically significant effect. There are a number of these tools. One well-standardized questionnaire is the Sickness Impact Profile [39] and its shorter version the SIP68.

It is of interest that in the recent ALS trials, the primary outcome measures were functional ones and not measures of muscle strength. In industry-driven clinical trials it is perhaps understandable that the sponsors are interested in whether the potential customer perceives the drug to have changed their quality of life. From the academic clinician's point of view, however, it is important that clinical trials should provide as much information as is practical about the pathology of the disease. This often provides the basis for future trials of other and better drugs. It would be regrettable if we forfeit this type of finding by a complete reliance on quality of life scales.

Pitfalls. There is a major pitfall which has to be avoided with the questionnaire. Investigators will usually ask the patient to fill the form out in the waiting room or similar environment. Often patients who are physically disabled need the help of the care giver to write in the answers. The form is then handed to the clinical investigator. This might seem perfectly acceptable but it will lead to erroneous data. Many of the questions may relate to how the patient feels about the home environment, about the patient's mood and about how the patient perceives their situation at home. The patient might be quite reluctant to provide an honest answer when the most significant person in their life is looking over their shoulder. The patient's relationship to the physician may also jeopardize the answers. The mere fact that the patient is enrolled in the study implies that the physician and the patient have established rapport. Patients often feel that it is insulting to the doctor to reply to a questionnaire in anything but positive terms. Patients always believe that if a form is handed to the doctor in charge, he or she will read it. The only way to avoid these errors is to have the patient fill out the form by themselves or with the aid of a completely neutral individual and for the form to be transmitted directly to the data coordinating center and not handed to the physician in charge.

Types of Clinical Trials

The gold standard for clinical trials remains the randomized double-blind controlled trial. Such a trial will rule out the effects of baseline confounding variables and will remove any investigator or patient bias. It will also rule out the effect of any change in the "background" therapy such as an improvement in pulmonary care or some other intervention. The practical problem in trials in myopathies is that the diseases are rare enough that in one clinic or even one region the number of available patients may constrain the trial. A randomized controlled clinical trial demands more patients when compared with other types of trials. For this reason other trial designs are often considered. The use of historical controls is controversial. In DMD a randomized controlled trial would require over 90 patients to be able to detect the same effect that could be detected by a total of 25 patients in a historically controlled trial [40]. The principle behind the controlled trial is that the natural history of the disease is so well known that it can be used as the standard to compare the effects of treatment without recourse to the concomitant control group. There are many requirements in the design of a historical control trial that must be met. In essence they demand that there has been no change in the patient population, in the medical management nor in the clinical measurement tools between the time and place when the natural history data were collected and the time and place of the clinical trial. Since many of us as clinic directors are unaware of the changes which can occur in our clinics with the change in personnel or in differences in treatment from one region to the other, it is quite difficult to be certain that the control group is in fact valid. One may argue the pros and cons of historical trials ad infinitum, but the observed fact is that a higher proportion of historical trials give a positive result (successful intervention) than do randomized controlled trials. The place of the historical controlled trial is probably as an initial study which, if positive, will lead to a larger, more definitive trial.

In the "crossover" trial, the population of patients is divided two groups, one being initially placed on placebo and the other on the active drug. Then, after some time period, the groups are switched to the opposite treatment arm. This trial has one major advantage: all patients will get the active medication at some stage and this makes patient recruitment easier. One problem with the crossover trial is that it may be relatively inefficient. Let us say that a crossover trial compares treatment X against treatment Y and that the groups are switched at the end of 6 months and continued on the opposite treatment (Y vs X) for another 6 months. Suppose that at the end of the first 6 months the treatment effect has almost reached significance but is not yet valid. When the groups are reversed, the difference will disappear after another 6 months whereas in a plain randomized controlled trial lasting the same (1 year) time period there might have been an unequivocal result. There are, in fact, statistical methods to handle this type of trial but they lack the clarity of the randomized controlled trial.

Sample Size and Power

One of the basic rules of trials is that the trial must have enough power to answer the question which is posed. There are several trials in myopathies over the years which failed this test. In a study testing the null hypothesis, the power of the study is the likelihood that it will detect the desired therapeutic effect if it is present. The concept of the β error is now familiar. "Beta" refers to the chance that patients who, in fact, demonstrate a therapeutic effect will be mistakenly identified as not different from the placebo group and the null hypothesis will not be rejected. The power of a study is the degree of certainty that this

will *not* happen. To calculate the power of a study requires knowing something of the natural history of the disease as well as of the measurements being used in this population.

We will again consider the trials in DMD. This is the only one of the myopathies that has been characterized repeatedly with enough accuracy to allow precise calculations of power and sample size. The decline in the average muscle score, derived from the average manual muscle score of 34 muscles, for a large population of boys with DMD, is 0.40 units per year. Obviously not all patients decline at this rate. The population is normally distributed around this mean value with a standard deviation of 0.39 units. This decline is as true for the ambulatory patients as for the wheelchair-bound. Postulate the use of a drug which will slow the disease. Now assume that one wishes to design a study which will reliable detect whether or not a drug slows the progress of the disease to 25% of its original progression. Ideally the patients would be randomized to a treatment group and a placebo group. The placebo group will continue to decline at the rate of 0.40 units in 1 year. The treatment group will decline at a quarter of this rate, 0.1 units. Thus, after 1 year there will be a difference of approximately 0.3 units between the groups. If this value is found in the actual trial, its significance will depend on the number of patients and, most importantly, on the variability of the measurement. We cannot measure this variability before the trial starts, but we can predict it by assuming that it will be the same as the known variability of the measurement in the natural history study, namely 0.39. We may now convert the observed difference between the two groups into a "standardized difference" by dividing the observed value by the standard deviation, in this case $0.3/0.39 = 0.75$. The simplest way to calculate power and sample size from this is to turn to a power table and use the value to relate power to the duration of the study and the necessary number of patients. An acceptable value for power is 0.80 which means that there is an 80% chance of detecting an effect if it is in fact present.

In a situation where the limiting factor is the number of available patients and little is known about the natural history of the disease, one can start with the number of available patient and the likely time period for the trial and then find what standardized difference should be sought to provide a power of 0.80. This will allow the investigator to determine the type of measurement that might be needed to provide a meaningful result. Another way of thinking about the problem is to relate the available sample size to the correlation coefficient. An effect which has perfect correlation with the intervention will have $r = 1.0$. If one has 30 patients available for a study, one would expect to detect (one-tailed $\alpha = 0.05$, $\beta = 0.10$) an effect having a correlation coefficient of 0.50.

Data Analysis: Alice in Wonderland and the Null Hypothesis

Traditionally, trials in neuromuscular disease, like their counterparts in general medicine, have relied on testing of the null hypothesis. Current trends are away from this type of analysis toward the analysis of confidence intervals, which give more meaningful data. The investigator using the null hypothesis sets out to prove that something is true by showing that it is not untrue. This is a little reminiscent of the conversation at the Mad Hatter's tea party. At the end of the study the investigator can draw the conclusion that two (or more) groups are extremely unlikely to belong to the same population. The leap is then made that, if the likelihood is very small indeed, the effect must be clinically useful to the patient. This is just not true. First, no two human populations could ever be completely identical in their behavior, so it is just a matter of choosing a huge sample size and then you are guaranteed a positive result, one way or another. This leads to the common phenomenon of an effect which is statistically significant but has no meaning for the patient. More meaningful information is conveyed by the use of confidence intervals [40].

In expressing the results as confidence intervals the same consideration is given to determining the difference in outcome between two groups but the results are presented indicating not only the mean difference but also the upper and lower boundaries of such a difference expressed with a degree of confidence which may be 95%, 90% or even 80%. Reworded, the upper limit of a 95% confidence interval implies that, if the trial were to be repeated, there is a 95% likelihood that the difference would again be recorded below the upper limit. Confidence limits are much less open to misinterpretation. Consider Fig. 41.1, which presents the manual muscle testing data for a DMD study. The upper box is the presentation of the original data. It illustrates that the effect over 6 months was to improve muscle strength and the 0 point is excluded, indicating significance. The "true" effect was unlikely (95% confidence) to have been a change in average muscle strength of less than +0.33 units and may have been as much as +0.57 units in comparison with the placebo group. Consider the hypothetical study A below this. The mean is similar but, since the lower confidence limits include 0, this study does not show any significance. However, notice that the upper confidence limit means that the treatment might have caused an increase in strength of one full unit which would be a striking improvement in strength. Finally, the third example (B) illustrates a hypothetical study which is statistically significant since it excludes the null point. It would be a precise study but the maximum change in strength to be expected would be very small and probably not of clinical significance.

In summary, expressing clinical data as confidence intervals provides more information than the familiar p value: (1) it indicates whether the study is statistically significant; (2) it provides information about the possible extent of the effect; (3) it indicates the precision of the measurements.

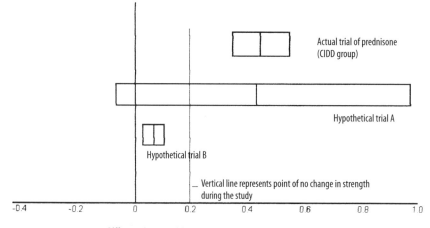

Actual trial of prednisone (CIDD group)

Hypothetical trial A

Hypothetical trial B

— Vertical line represents point of no change in strength during the study

-0.4   -0.2   0   0.2   0.4   0.6   0.8   1.0

Difference in strength between active treatment and placebo

Fig. 41.1. Manual muscle testing data (mean and 95% confidence intervals) for actual and hypothetical treatment trials in DMD. See text for details.

Postscript

One final word of caution. Clinical trials are back-breaking. One spends 2 or 3 years of one's life trying to persuade patients to persist in the study, making sure that the measurements are accurate and taking care of an inordinate amount of paperwork. One reaches the end of the study and finds that there is no benefit from the drug. This is hard to accept when it has consumed your waking hours for this length of time. The temptation is to go back and examine the patients' data to see if there isn't perhaps one group that responded or one measurement that hasn't been looked at in quite the right fashion. Don't. Retrospective dredging of the data is not productive. Declare your primary outcome measures at the beginning of the trial and stay with them. You could miss a potential small effect, perhaps, but at least you will avoid the fate of the rest of us who finish our papers with the doleful phrase "the results, although not significant, suggest that further studies are warranted."

References

1. Pernice W, Beckmann R, Ketelsen UP, Frey M, Schmidt-Redemann B, Haap KP, et al. A double-blind placebo controlled trial of diltiazem in Duchenne dystrophy. Klin Wochenschr 1988;66:565–570.
2. Fenichel GM, Brooke MH, Griggs RC, Mendell JR, Miller JP, Moxley RT III, et al. Clinical investigation in Duchenne muscular dystrophy: penicillamine and vitamin E. Muscle Nerve 1988;11:1164–1168.
3. Moxley RT III, Brooke MH, Fenichel GM, Mendell JR, Griggs RC, Miller JP, et al. Clinical investigation in Duchenne dystrophy. VI. Double-blind controlled trial of nifedipine. Muscle Nerve 1987;10:22–33.
4. Heckmatt JZ, Hyde SA, Gabain A, Dubowitz V. Therapeutic trial of isaxonine in Duchenne muscular dystrophy. Muscle Nerve 1988;11:836–847.
5. Gamstorp I, Gustavson KH, Hellstrom O, Nordgren B. A trial of selenium and vitamin E in boys with muscular dystrophy. J Child Neurol 1986;1:211–214.
6. Madsen KS, Miller JP, Province MA. The use of an extended baseline period in the evaluation of treatment in a longitudinal Duchenne muscular dystrophy trial. Stat Med 1986;5:231–241.
7. Zatz M, Betti RT, Frota-Pessoa O. Treatment of Duchenne muscular dystrophy with growth hormone inhibitors. Am J Med Genet 1986;24:549–566.
8. Dick DJ, Gardner-Medwin D, Gates PG, Gibson M, Simpson JM, Walls TJ. A trial of flunarizine in the treatment of Duchenne muscular dystrophy. Muscle Nerve 1986;9:349–354.
9. Jackson MJ, Coakley J, Stokes M, Edwards RH, Oster O. Selenium metabolism and supplementation in patients with muscular dystrophy. Neurology 1989;39:655–659.
10. Mendell JR, Moxley RT, Griggs RC, Brooke MH, Fenichel GM, Miller JP, et al. Randomized, double-blind six-month trial of prednisone in Duchenne's muscular dystrophy. N Engl J Med 1989;320:1592–1597.
11. Mendell JR, Province MA, Moxley RT III, Griggs RC, Brooke MH, Fenichel GM, et al. Clinical investigation of Duchenne muscular dystrophy: a methodology for therapeutic trials based on natural history controls. Arch Neurol 1987;44:808–811.
12. Bertorini TE, Palmieri GM, Griffin JW, Igarashi M, McGee J, Brown R, et al. Effect of chronic treatment with the calcium antagonist diltiazem in Duchenne muscular dystrophy. Neurology 1988;38:609–613.
13. Sharma KR, Mynhier MA, Miller RG. Cyclosporine increases muscular force generation in Duchenne muscular dystrophy. Neurology 1993;43:527–532.
14. Griggs RC, Moxley RT III, Mendell JR, Fenichel GM, Brooke MH, Pestronk A, et al. Duchenne dystrophy: randomized, controlled trial of prednisone (18 months) and azathioprine (12 months). Neurology 1993;43:520–527.
15. Fenichel GM, Mendell JR, Moxley RT III, Griggs RC, Brooke MH, et al. A comparison of daily and alternate-day prednisone therapy in the treatment of Duchenne muscular dystrophy. Arch Neurol 1991;48:575–579.
16. Fenichel GM, Florence JM, Pestronk A, Mendell JR, Brooke MH, et al. Long term benefit from prednisone therapy in Duchenne muscular dystrophy. Neurology 1991;41:1874–1877.
17. Griggs RC, Moxley RT, Mendell JR, Fenichel GN, Brooke MH, et al. Randomized, double-blind trial of mazindol in Duchenne dystrophy. Muscle Nerve 1990;13:1169–1173.
18. Griggs RC, Moxley RT, Mendell JR, Fenichel, Brooke MH, et al. Prednisone in Duchenne dystrophy: a randomized, controlled trial defining the time course and dose response. Arch Neurol 1991;48:383–388.
19. Reitter B. Deflazacort vs prednisone in Duchenne muscular dystrophy: trends of an ongoing study. Brain Dev 1995;17:39–43.
20. Angelini C, Pegoraro E, Turella E, Intino MT, Pini A, Costa C. Deflazacort in Duchenne dystrophy: study of long-term effect. Muscle Nerve 1994;17:386–391.
21. Mesa LE, Dubrovsky AL, Corderi J, Marco P, Flores D. Steroids in Duchenne muscular dystrophy: deflazacort trial. Neuromusc Disord 1991;1:261–266.
22. Florence JM, Pandya S, King WM, Robison JD, Baty J, Miller JP, et al. Intrarater reliability of manual muscle test (Medical Research Council scale) grades in Duchenne's muscular dystrophy. Phys Ther 1992;72:115–122.
23. Brooke MH, Fenichel GM, Griggs RC, Mendell JR, Moxley R, Miller JP, et al. Clinical Investigation of Duchenne dystrophy; interesting results in a trial of prednisone. Arch Neurol 1987;44:812–817.
24. Personius KE, Pandya S, King WM, Tawil R, McDermott MP. Facioscapulohumeral dystrophy natural history study: standardization of testing procedures and reliability of measurements. The FSH DY Group. Phys Ther 1994;74:253–263.
25. Tawil R, McDermott MP, Mendell JR, Kissel J, Griggs RC. Facioscapulohumeral muscular dystrophy (FSHD): design of natural history study and results of baseline testing. FSH-DY Group. Neurology. 1994;44:442–446.
26. Griggs RC, Pandya S, Florence JM, et al. Randomized controlled trial of testosterone in myotonic dystrophy. Neurology 1989;39:219–222.
27. Vlachopapadopoulou E, Zachwieja JJ, Gertner JM, Manzione D, Bier DM, Matthews DE, et al. Metabolic and clinical response to recombinant human insulin-like growth factor I in myotonic dystrophy: a clinical research center study. J Clin Endocrinol Metab 1975;80:3715–3723.
28. Smith SE, Green NE, Cole RJ, Robison JD, Fenichel GM. Prolongation of ambulation in children with Duchenne muscular dystrophy by subcutaneous lower limb tenotomy. J Pediatr Orthop 1993;13:336–340.

29. Brooke MH, Fenichel GM, Griggs RC, Mendell JR, Moxley R, Miller JP, et al. Clinical investigation in Duchenne dystrophy. 2. Determination of the "power" of therapeutic trials based on the natural history. Muscle Nerve 1983;6:91–102.

30. Brooke MH, Griggs RC, Mendell JR, Fenichel GM, Shumate JB, Pellegrino RJ. Clinical trial in Duchenne dystrophy. 1. Design of the protocol. Muscle Nerve 1981;4:186–197.

31. Brooke MH, Florence JM, Heller SL, Kaiser KK, Gruber A, Babcock D, et al. Controlled trial of thyrotropin releasing hormone in amyotrophic lateral sclerosis. Neurology 1986;36: 146–151.

32. Goonetilleke A, Modarres-Sadeghi H, Guiloff RJ. Accuracy, reproducibility, and variability of hand-held dynamometry in motor neuron disease. J Neurol Neurosurg Psychiatry 1994;57:326–332.

33. Andres PL, Thibodeau LM, Finison LJ, Munsat TL. Quantitative assessment of neuromuscular deficit in ALS. Neurol Clin 1987;5:125–141.

34. Munsat TL, Andres PL, Skerry LM. The use of quantitative techniques to define amyotrophic lateral sclerosis. In: Munsat TL, ed. 1989. Quantification of neurological deficit. Boston: Butterworth, 1989:129–142.

35. Vignos PJ, Spencer GE, Archibald KC. Management of progressive muscular dystrophy in childhood. JAMA 1963;184: 89–96.

36. ALS CNTF Treatment Study (ACTS) Phase I–II Study Group. The ALS functional rating scale: assessment of activities of daily living in patients with amyotrophic lateral sclerosis. Arch Neurol 1996;53:141–147.

37. Thomson WH, Smith I. X-linked recessive (Duchenne) muscular dystrophy (DMD) and purine metabolism: effects of oral allopurinol and adenylate. Metabolism 1978;27:151–163.

38. Mendell JR, Wiechers DO. Lack of benefit of allopurinol in Duchenne dystrophy. Muscle Nerve 1979;2:53–56.

39. Bergner M, Bobbitt RA, Carter WB, Gilson BS. The Sickness Impact Profile: development and final revision of a health status measure. Med Care 1981;19:787–805.

40. Borenstein M. The case for confidence intervals in controlled clinical trials. Controlled Clin Trials 1994;15:411–428.

Index